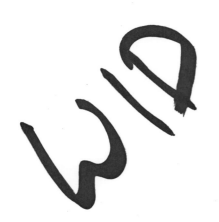

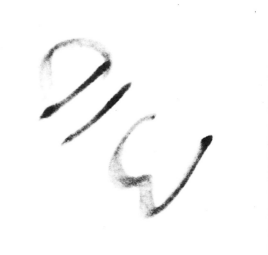

The GALE ENCYCLOPEDIA of FITNESS

FIRST EDITION

The GALE ENCYCLOPEDIA of FITNESS

FIRST EDITION

VOLUME

2

M–Z
GLOSSARY
GENERAL INDEX

JACQUELINE L. LONGE, EDITOR

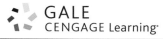

GALE
CENGAGE Learning·

Detroit • New York • San Francisco • New Haven, Conn • Waterville, Maine • London

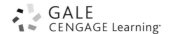

Gale Encyclopedia of Fitness

Project Editor: Jacqueline L. Longe

Editorial: Laurie Fundukian, Kristin Key, Brigham Narins, Joseph Palmisano, Alejandro Valtierra, Jeffrey Wilson

Product Manager: Anne Marie Sumner

Editorial Support Services: Andrea Lopeman

Indexing Services: Cathy Goddard, Laurie Dorricott, Dorricott Information Services

Rights Acquisition and Management: Margaret Chamberlain-Gaston

Composition: Evi Abou-El-Seoud

Manufacturing: Wendy Blurton

Imaging: John Watkins

Product Design: Kristine Julien

For product information and technology assistance, contact us at
Gale Customer Support, 1-800-877-4253.
For permission to use material from this text or product,
submit all requests online at **www.cengage.com/permissions.**
Further permissions questions can be emailed to
permissionrequest@cengage.com

While every effort has been made to ensure the reliability of the information presented in this publication, Gale, a part of Cengage Learning, does not guarantee the accuracy of the data contained herein. Gale accepts no payment for listing; and inclusion in the publication of any organization, agency, institution, publication, service, or individual does not imply endorsement of the editors or publisher. Errors brought to the attention of the publisher and verified to the satisfaction of the publisher will be corrected in future editions.

Library of Congress Cataloging-in-Publication Data

The Gale encyclopedia of fitness / Jacqueline L. Longe, editor. -- 1st ed.
    p. cm.
Summary: "Alphabetically arranged encyclopedia (about 250 entries) that covers a wide variety of fitness topics"-- Provided by publisher.
    Includes bibliographical references and index.
    ISBN 978-1-4144-9016-8 (hardback) -- ISBN 978-1-4144-9017-5 (vol. 1)
    -- ISBN 978-1-4144-9018-2 (vol. 2)
    1. Aerobic exercises. 2. Physical fitness. 3. Health. I. Longe, Jacqueline L. II. Title: Encyclopedia of fitness.
RA781.15.G35 2012
613.7'1--dc23   2012001472

Gale
27500 Drake Rd.
Farmington Hills, MI 48331-3535

ISBN-13: 978-1-4144-9016-8 (set)   ISBN-10: 1-4144-9016-X (set)
ISBN-13: 978-1-4144-9017-5 (vol. 1)   ISBN-10: 1-4144-9017-8 (vol. 1)
ISBN-13: 978-1-4144-9018-2 (vol. 2)   ISBN-10: 1-4144-9018-6 (vol. 2)

This title is also available as an e-book.
ISBN-13: 978-1-4144-9019-9 ISBN-10: 1-4144-9019-4
Contact your Gale, a part of Cengage Learning sales representative for ordering information.

Printed in China
1 2 3 4 5 6 7 16 15 14 13 12

CONTENTS

LIST OF ENTRIES

PLEASE READ—IMPORTANT INFORMATION

The first edition of *The Gale Encyclopedia of Fitness* is a health reference product designed to inform and educate readers about fitness, exercise and participating in sports. Gale, Cengage Learning believes the product to be comprehensive, but not necessarily definitive. It is intended to supplement, not replace, consultation with a physician or other healthcare practitioners. While Gale, Cengage Learning has made substantial efforts to provide information that is accurate, comprehensive, and up-to-date, Gale, Cengage Learning makes no representations or warranties of any kind, including without limitation, warranties of merchantability or fitness for a particular purpose, nor does it guarantee the accuracy, comprehensiveness, or timeliness of the information contained in this product. Readers should be aware that the universe of medical knowledge is constantly growing and changing, and that differences of opinion exist among authorities. Readers are also advised to seek professional diagnosis and treatment for any medical condition, and to discuss information obtained from this book with their healthcare provider.

INTRODUCTION

The *Gale Encyclopedia of Fitness* is a valuable source of information for anyone who wants to learn more about fitness, exercise, sports, and nutrition. This collection of approximately 250 entries provides in-depth coverage of sports; fitness exercises and types of training; body systems; fitness tests, therapies, and equipment; nutrition and nutritional needs of various fitness levels; and diseases and conditions. In addition, key government fitness initiatives from various countries have been included to facilitate understanding of how governments are promoting healthy lifestyle choices to combat the global spread of obesity.

This encyclopedia minimizes medical jargon and uses language that laypersons can understand, while still providing thorough coverage that will benefit health science students as well.

SCOPE

Entries follow a standardized format that provides information at a glance. Rubrics include, but are not limited to:

SPORTS

- Definition
- Purpose
- Demographics
- History
- Description
- Preparation
- Risks
- Results
- Key Terms
- Questions to Ask Your Doctor
- Resources

FITNESS EXERCISES, TESTS, TRAINING, THERAPY

- Definition
- Purpose
- Demographics
- Description
- Recommended dosage
- Precautions
- Side effects
- Interactions
- Key Terms
- Questions To Ask Your Doctor
- Resources

FITNESS EQUIPMENT

- Definition
- Purpose
- History
- Description
- Benefits
- Risks
- Key Terms
- Questions To Ask Your Doctor
- Resources

BODY SYSTEMS

- Definition
- Description
- Function
- Role in human health
- Common diseases and conditions

- Key Terms
- Questions To Ask Your Doctor
- Resources

DISEASES AND CONDITIONS

- Definition
- Description
- Demographics
- Causes and symptoms
- Diagnosis
- Treatment
- Prognosis
- Prevention
- Key Terms
- Questions To Ask Your Doctor
- Resources

INCLUSION CRITERIA

A preliminary list of sports and fitness topics was compiled from a wide variety of sources, including professional guides and textbooks, as well as consumer guides and encyclopedias. The advisory board, made up of professionals from a variety of fields including kinesiology, medicine, nutrition, sports medicine, and physical education, evaluated the topics and made suggestions for inclusion. Final selection of topics to include was made by the advisory board in conjunction with the Gale editor.

ABOUT THE CONTRIBUTORS

The essays were compiled by experienced medical writers. The advisors reviewed the completed essays to ensure that they are appropriate, up-to-date, and accurate.

HOW TO USE THIS BOOK

The *Gale Encyclopedia of Fitness* has been designed with ready reference in mind.

- Straight **alphabetical arrangement** of topics allows users to locate information quickly.

- **Bold-faced terms** within entries direct the reader to related articles.

- **Cross-references** placed throughout the encyclopedia direct readers from alternate names, brand names, and related topics to entries.

- A list of **key terms** is provided where appropriate to define unfamiliar terms or concepts. A **glossary** of key terms is also included at the back of Volume II.

- The **Resources** sections direct readers to additional sources of information on a topic.

- A comprehensive **general index** guides readers to all topics mentioned in the text.

GRAPHICS

The *Gale Encyclopedia of Fitness* contains over 200 illustrations, photos, and tables.

ADVISORY BOARD

Several experts have provided invaluable assistance in the formulation of this encyclopedia from defining the scope of coverage to reviewing individual entries for accuracy and accessibility. I would, therefore, like to express sincere thanks and appreciation for all of their contributions.

CONTRIBUTORS

Margaret Alic, PhD
Science Writer
Eastsound, Washington

William Atkins, BB, BS, MBA
Medical Writer
Pekin, Illinois

Julie Jordan Avritt
Medical Writer
Decatur, Georgia

Erin Braun
Freelance Writer
South Lyon, Michigan

Tom Brody, PhD
Science Writer
Berkeley, California

Laura Jean Cataldo, RN, EdD
Medical Writer
Myersville, Maryland

Stacey Chamberlin
Copyeditor
Fairfax, Virginia

Daniel M Cohen, PhD
Research Associate
University of Pennsylvania
Philadelphia, Pennsylania

Lance Dalleck, PhD
Senior Lecturer
Department of Sport & Exercise
   Science
University of Auckland
Auckland New Zealand

Emily Darr, MD
*Medical doctor, professional
volleyball player*
Spartanburg, South Carolina

Tish Davidson, AM
Medical Writer
Fremont, California

Stéphanie Islane Dionne Sherk
Medical Writer
Ann Arbor, Michigan

Doug Dupler, MA
Science Writer
Boulder, Colorado

Karen Ericson, RN
Medical Writer
Estes Park, Colorado

Karl Finley
Medical Writer
Fremont, California

Janie F. Franz
Writer
Grand Forks, North Dakota

Rebecca J. Frey, PhD
*Research and Administrative
Associate*
East Rock Institute
New Haven, Connecticut

Laith F. Gulli, MD
*Consultant Psychotherapist in
Private Practice*
Lathrup Village, Michigan

Crystal Heather Kaczkowski, M.Sc.
Medical writer
Dorval, Quebec, Canada

Monique Laberge, PhD
Visiting Scientist
Concordia University

Department of Biology
Montreal, Quebec, Canada

John T. Lohr, PhD
*Assistant Director, Biotechnology
Center*
Utah State University
Logan, Utah

Sally C. McFarlane-Parrott
Medical Writer
Ann Arbor, Michigan

Susan M. Mockus, PhD
Seattle, Washington

David E. Newton, AB, MA, EdD
Medical Writer
Ashland, Oregon

Melinda Granger Oberleitner, RN, DNS
*Acting Department Head and
Associate Professor*
Department of Nursing
University of Louisiana at
   Lafayette
Lafayette, Louisiana

Teresa G. Odle
Medical Writer
Albuquerque, New Mexico

J. Ricker Polsdorfer, MD
Medical Writer
Phoenix, Arizona

Richard Robinson
Medical Writer
Tucson, Arizona

Jennifer E. Sisk, MA
Medical Writer
Havertown, Pennsylvania

Contributors

Elizabeth Swain
Medical Writer
San Diego, California

Carol A. Turkington
Medical Writer
Lancaster, Pennsylvania

Ken R. Wells
Freelance Writer
Laguna Hills, California

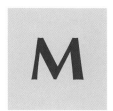

M

Male reproductive system *see* **Reproductive system, male**

Marathon and half marathon

Definition

A marathon is a foot race over a course that is 26 mi. 385 yd. (42.195 km) in length. Other long-distance races associated with the marathon is a half-marathon, a race that covers exactly half the distance of a full marathon and an ultra marathon, which extends over a distance of 31 mi. (50 km), 62.5 mi. (100 km), 50 mi. (80 km), or 100 mi. (160 km).

Purpose

The purpose of marathons, half-marathons, and ultra-marathons is for a runner to finish ahead of all other competitors in the race.

Demographics

The best available statistics on marathon participants are provided by the website MarathonGuide.com that publishes demographic data on marathon runners each year. The most recent data show that about 468,000 individuals completed at least one marathon race in 2009. Of this number, 59.6 % were males and 40.4% females. The average age for all runners was 38.7 years, averaged between 40.2 years for males and 36.5 years for females. The marathon runners ranged in age from teenagers to senior citizens over the age of 70. The lowest age group, consisting of those under the age of 19, accounted for 1.14 % of all male runners and 0.69 % of all female runners. The largest age groups among males were the 35–39 and 40–44 age groups, each of which accounted for 9.42% of all runners (and 15.8% of all male runners), while the largest

group of female runners came from the 25–29 age group, with 7.75 % of all runners (and 19.2% of all female runners). Virtually all marathon races now include a wheelchair division. One of the first major races to include a wheelchair division was the Boston Marathon, in which one wheelchair participant competed in 1975. Since that time, more than 1,000 wheelchair marathoners have competed in that race. The Boston Marathon (and other similar races) also include categories for the visually impaired/blind and the mobility handicapped.

History

Marathon has a famous history. The sport is named after a city in ancient Greece, where an important battle was fought in 490 BCE between the Persians and Athenians. At the conclusion of the battle, won by the Athenians, a messenger named Pheidippides was sent to Athens with news of the victory. Tradition has it that Pheidippides ran non-stop from Marathon to Athens, where he carried the news "We have won!" before collapsing and dying. Scholarly disputes about the accuracy of this story have not diminished its place in the heart of modern marathon runners and fans of the sport.

The tale of Pheidippides and his run from Marathon to Athens remained a part of Greek history and folklore until the late nineteenth century when plans for the first modern **Olympics** game were being formulated. In an effort to emphasize the role of Greek history in the games, a suggestion was made to include a marathon race in the first modern games, planned for 1896. The winner of that race was a Greek water-carrier, Spiridon "Spiros" Louis, after whom the major Greek Olympics stadium is now named. Louis completed the course in 2 hours, 58 minutes and 50 seconds. The marathon has been a part of the Olympics game every year in which it was held since 1896. The first woman to run a marathon is thought to be French runner Marie-Louise Ledru, who completed the Tour de Paris marathon in 1918 in a time of 5 hours and 40 minutes. It was

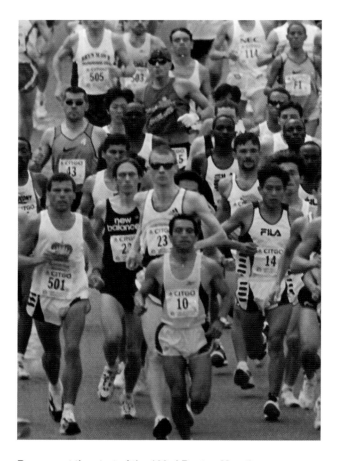

Runners at the start of the 103rd Boston Marathon, Hopkinton, Massachusetts on April 19, 1999. *(© AP Images/ Winslow Townson)*

a half century, however, before race organizers officially recognized women contestants, the first of whom was Kathrine Switzer, who actually finished second in the 1975 Boston marathon behind an unregistered, "illegal" runner, Bobbi Gibb. The top ten fastest marathon races ever run have all been won by participants from Ethiopia (one) or Kenya (nine), with the fastest time being that of Haile Gebrselassie, at 2:03:59 in Berlin in 2008. The fastest women's time is that posted in 2003 by Paula Radcliffe, of Great Britain, with a 2:15:25 in London.

Description

In contrast to many sports, marathon and its longer and shorter cousins have relatively few rules, most relating to the layout of the course and the proper registration and behavior of runners. According to the International Association of Athletics Federations, for example, a marathon can be run only on a hard surface, such as a road, and not on soft or grassy land. The course must also be clearly marked so that runners

are always aware of their progress. Runners must remain on the course at all times unless they find it necessary to leave the course for some reason, in which case they must be accompanied by a judge. Runners may also take refreshments only at stands specifically provided for that purpose, and at no other locations. A number of requirements also deal with the registration process to ensure that all runners are legitimately qualified to take part in a competition.

Preparation

Preparing for a marathon, half-marathon, or ultra-marathon requires, more than anything else, a range of **running** exercises, supplemented by various types of cross-training exercises, the proper mental attitude about the challenge, and a nutritional program that best prepares a person for the run.

Equipment

Marathon runners wear jerseys, shorts, and shoes especially designed for running. No additional equipment is needed.

Training and conditioning

By far the most important element in training for a marathon, half-marathon, or ultra-marathon is a program of running. Various coaches have somewhat different approaches to the proper running schedule, but a common theme is that runners should try to reach a maximum of about 20 mi. (32 km) in a single run two or three times a week in the weeks leading up to a marathon, with a maximum of about 100 mi. (160 km) total in a week for the best runners. Practice runs do not necessarily require full-out competition speeds, and slower runs, punctuated by periods of **walking**, may prove to be the best training regimen. Many coaches also recommend cross training in sports such as cycling, **swimming**, and walking that increase one's aerobic capacity.

Nutrition is a critical element in training for long runs. When a person first starts running, his or her body produces **energy** by means of aerobic respiration, a process in which energy is released by the breakdown of glycogen stored in the liver and muscles. Most people use up their supply of glycogen after a distance of about 20 mi. (32 km) of running, at which point their body switches over to anaerobic respiratory processes. These processes involve the breakdown of fat in the body to obtain needed energy. Anaerobic processes are slower and less efficient than aerobic processes that account for the common experience reported by runners of "hitting the wall" at distances of about 20 mi. (32 km). One way of compensating for this problem is to increase the amount of carbohydrate in a person's body at the start of the race. These excess **carbohydrates** are converted by the body to glycogen, increasing the supply of that substance in the body over its normal levels. This principle underlies the common practice among distance runners of "carbo-loading" in the 24 hours preceding a race.

Risks

The most common injuries and health problems associated with marathon running are those that result from repetitive activities related to running, problems such as **blisters**, calluses, discolored toenails, muscle cramps, and chafing. Other common problems that develop during a race include **sunburn** and windburn, diarrhea and nausea, **dehydration** and **hyponatremia** (salt deficiency). One of the most common marathon-related problems is exhaustion at a distance of up to 20 mi. (32 km), the so-called "hitting the wall" phenomenon. Sprains, strains, and fractures of the ankle and lower legs are also common, especially as one's body becomes more tired and less able to maintain proper balance.

A number of studies have been conducted to determine the most common injuries incurred by distance runners and the frequency of such injuries. A survey of the general findings of 17 such studies was reported in 2007. The survey focused on injuries to the lower extremities, by far the most common injuries for runners. Researchers found that the incidence of lower extremity injuries ranged from a low of 19.4–79.3% in the studies reviewed. Previous surveys of this kind had reported a similar range of injuries among distance runners, from a low of 26.0 % to a high of 92.4 %. An outside reviewer of the survey suggested that the wide range in reported injuries in these two overall surveys might reflect the differing subject populations and methodologies used in the individual studies reviewed.

A wide range in the incidence of injuries to specific parts of the body was also reported in the 2007 survey. The most common site of injury was the knee, with anywhere from 7.2–50.0% of runners reporting damage in this area. The next most common areas of injury were the lower leg (calf, shin, Achilles tendon, and heel), foot and toes, and upper leg (hamstring, thigh, and quadriceps) with incidences of 9.0–32.2%, 5.7–39.3%, and 3.4–38.1%, respectively. The lowest rate of injuries was reported for the ankle and the hip, pelvis, and groin, ranging from 3.9–16.6% and 3.3–11.5%, respectively. Researchers also reviewed a number of possible concomitants for these injuries, including conditioning and training, lifestyle factors, systemic factors (such as age and gender), and health factors. Among all the factors studied, only two appeared to have a strong correlation with rate of injuries: a history of previous injuries and a tendency among male runners to engage in longer-than-normal training sessions prior to a race.

Results

Existing evidence appears to suggest that well-designed programs of training and conditioning can contribute to the general fitness of men and women who engage in long distance running, although there may be some questions as to the possibility that overdoing the training (in terms of distance covered) may increase one's risk for lower extremity injuries.

Resources

BOOKS

Donovan, Joe. *Marathon Method: Essential Guide to Training for Your First Marathon: Selecting, Training, and Finishing Your First Marathon the Easy Way Title.* Milwaukee, WI: Donovan Group Holdings, LLC, 2008.

Fink, Don. *Mastering the Marathon: Time-Efficient Training Secrets for the 40-plus Athlete.* Guilford, CT: Lyons Press, 2010.

Galloway, Jeff. *Marathon: You Can Do It!* Bolinas, CA: Shelter Publications, 2010.

Higdon, Hal. *Marathon: The Ultimate Training Guide.* Emmaus, PA: Rodale, 2005.

Pfitzinger, Pete, and Scott Douglas. *Advanced Marathoning*, 2nd ed. Champaign, IL: Human Kinetics, 2009.

WEBSITES

How to Run Your First Marathon. active.com. http://www.active.com/running/Articles/How_to_Run_Your_First_Marathon.htm (accessed August 13, 2011).

How to Train for a Marathon or Half Marathon. Marathon Rookie.com. http://www.marathonrookie.com/index.html (accessed August 13, 2011).

What's New. halhigdon.com. http://www.halhigdon.com/ (accessed August 13, 2011).

ORGANIZATIONS

Association of International Marathons and Distance Races, borao@correcaminos.org, http://aimsworldrunning.org.

USA Track & Field, Inc., 132 East Washington St., Suite 800, Indianapolis, IN, 46204, (317) 261-0500, Fax: (317) 261-0481, http://www.usatf.org/about/directory/index.asp, http://www.usatf.org.

David E. Newton, AB, MA, EdD

Martial arts

Definition

Martial arts are various methods of armed and unarmed combat that originated centuries ago in Asia, primarily China, Japan, Korea, and the Philippines. The most popular styles include karate, kung fu, jujutsu, judo, aikido, tai chi, **tae kwon do**, sumo wrestling, and kendo.

Purpose

Martial arts usually have the dual purpose of physical fitness and self-defense. Some martial arts emphasize one purpose over the other, however, the very name of "martial" arts implies defense or combat.

Demographics

Almost anyone can learn and practice martial arts, from fitness beginners to those already fit. It has become equally popular among males and females and all **age** groups in Europe and North America. Most gyms, fitness centers, and community recreation facilities offer at least one martial arts class or program. There are several hundred styles and variations and each offers a unique regimen from gentle movements to violent kicks and hand chops. Most have mental or consciousness aspects attached, including meditation and a feeling of general well-being. These usually are not emphasized as much in North America as in Asia. The most violent martial arts, designed specifically for combat, are taught in many of the world's militaries.

History

Martial arts have traditionally represented a large number of offensive and defensive fighting techniques derived from Asia. Historically, the techniques were developed in India and then taken to China by Bodhidharma, the legendary founder of the famous Shaolin School. During the Sui and T'ang Dynasties these skills were spread to Korea, Japan, Indonesia, the Philippines, and Brazil. Throughout most of these early years the martial arts were secretly developed and transferred by word of mouth due, in large part, to repressive feudalism. Since World War II, members of various militaries carried the arts worldwide. Information technologies, such as the Internet and social media, have exposed a much broader world audience to the martial arts.

In China, exercises involving martial arts, such as tai chi, qi gong, and kung fu, developed at least 2,000 years ago. They are linked to Taoism, which uses the yin and yang symbol to show how strength should be balanced with compassion and gentleness. Japanese martial arts stretch back more than 600 years. Kendo is one of the most ancient. The four original styles of karate (shotokan, wado ryu, shito ryu and goju ryu) originated on the Japanese island of Okinawa and spread to the Japanese mainland in the early 1900s. Japanese martial arts were introduced into Korea around 1900. Since then, Korean martial artists developed their own styles, including tang soo do, hapkido and tae kwon do. Tae kwon do was introduced as an Olympic sport at the 2000 Olympic games in Sydney, Australia. Philippine martial arts, including eskrima, kali, and arnis (stick fighting), were developed hundreds of years ago. Filipino martial artists later incorporated blades and swords into their routines. In Brazil, a spinoff of Japanese jujutsu became Brazilian jiu jitsu in the early 1900s and has grown in popularity,

BRUCE LEE (1940–1973)

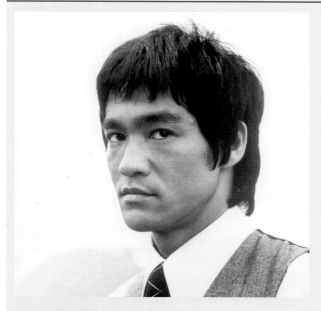

(© Michael Ochs Archives/Getty Images.)

On November 27, 1940, in the Chinese year of the Dragon, another son was born to the Lee family. The infant Lee made his film debut at age three months when he appeared as a stand–in for a baby in the American film, Golden Gate Girl. Shortly afterward, the Lee family returned to Hong Kong. With his father in the entertainment industry, Lee often visited movie sets. At four years old, he had his first walk–on, then two years later, he had his first real part. As the young Lee grew out of childhood, he became more and more involved with street gangs.

A strong, hot–tempered youth, Lee was constantly getting into trouble. On the streets, he became known as the Little Dragon. In order to develop himself into an invincible fighter, Lee decided to study the traditional martial art of kung fu. Lee began studying at the Wing Chun School, which offered a sophisticated Chinese martial arts system that stressed economy of movement and springing energy. Under the tutelage of wing chun master, Yip Man, it became clear that Lee was especially adept in martial arts. After quickly learning the techniques, Lee began to add his own adaptations and variations to the traditional moves. Frowned upon by the established wing chun community, Lee was asked to leave the school.

Not yet out of high school, Lee was offered a film contract with Run Run Shaw, a powerful producer in Hong Kong at the time. Lee announced to his mother that he would quit school and accept the offer. Although his mother was certain that Lee would someday be successful, she was also concerned that he at least earn his high school diploma. When Lee was picked up by the police for street fighting, his mother forbade him to accept Shaw's offer, and sent him to the United States to live with family friends and to finish high school. To support his education, Lee worked at Ruby Chow's, a popular Seattle restaurant, living in the restaurant attic and working at night as a busboy and waiter. After a few months of restaurant life, Lee quit and began teaching kung fu to his fellow students. One of those students was Linda Emery, whom Lee married in 1964.

Shortly after, the couple moved to California where Lee devoted all his time to teaching his new technique called Jeet kune do. Eventually, Lee operated three schools for jeet kune do, in Seattle, Oakland, and Los Angeles' Chinatown. He called these establishments the Jun Fan Kung Fu Institute, bearing his Chinese name. As Lee became more and more successful as a martial arts pioneer, he finally had his first big break in 1966 with "The Green Hornet" television series. When Lee felt he would not attain success in Hollywood, he returned to Hong Kong with his wife and two young children. It was in Hong Kong that Lee experienced the stardom he yearned for in the United States and his legacy consequently spread far beyond his death in 1973.

especially in North America and Latin America, over the last 100 years. In Thailand, martial arts started nearly 2,000 years ago with the development of muay thai, an extremely aggressive style. American kickboxing began in the 1970s and has quickly increased in popularity, especially in the United States.

Description

While the words "martial arts" may conjure up images of Bruce Lee films, they are in reality a group of usually graceful **exercise** movements that keep the body and mind strong and healthy. They can be performed by young and old, and range from simple **stretching** and meditative exercises to more complicated and demanding physical activities requiring mental concentration. The training is usually done without weights or special equipment and can be practiced alone or in a group. Most large gyms and fitness centers offer classes in at least one type of martial art. Some martial arts styles, such as karate and tae kwon do, are more challenging and emphasize general physical conditioning. Others, including tai ching and chi kung, are less physically challenging. Their benefits include more **energy**, balance, flexibility, and a general sense of well-being.

There are dozens of martial arts styles, including kung fu, a general term to describe Chinese martial arts. Among the most popular martial arts styles globally are:

- Karate: A Japanese martial art in which no weapons are used. The word, in Japanese, means "empty hand" and is thought to have originated in the 1300s. Karate uses primarily the hands, legs, and feet to disarm or disable an opponent.

- Tae kwon do: This martial art originated in Korea and combines physical skills with mental strength. It uses the hands and feet and is often demonstrated by a practitioner using a hand or foot to break a board or concrete brick. The Olympic sport teaches strength, stamina, speed, balance, and flexibility. It has an estimated 30 million followers in more than 100 nations, making it the most popular martial art.

- Judo: Another Olympic sport, judo was developed in Japan in the late 1800s by borrowing basic skills from other martial arts popular at the time. It is best known for its throwing techniques but also involves pins, control holds, and arm locks. Benefits include self-discipline, concentration, coordination, and flexibility.

- Jujutsu: Another of the many martial arts from Japan, jujutsu was practiced by samurai warriors hundreds of years ago, usually in situations where they were without their swords. It focuses primarily on self-defense techniques, including grappling, throwing, rolling, and locking.

- Tai chi: A Chinese martial art, also called tai chi chuan, that emphasizes slow movements and concentrates on breathing and balance. It is practiced worldwide and offers general health benefits, including improved concentration and stress reduction. It is not a combat or self-defense martial art. For this reason, it is an ideal martial art for beginners and seniors. Probably the most popular martial art among alternative health devotees, tai chi comes from the Chinese philosophy of Taoism and is based on the concept of yin and yang. Tai chi has a self-defense aspect based on counteracting an opponent's attack and then counterattacking, all in the same movement. As an exercise to maintain health, tai chi strengthens muscles and joints. It employs deep breathing techniques that increase blood circulation, benefiting the heart, lungs, and other organs.

- Chi kung (qigong) is another martial art from China that is done with slow and smooth movements, much like aikido. It is not a combat martial art. It focuses on balancing and increasing the body's energy, and improving general physical and mental health, strength, and well-being. It is usually practiced to reduce stress, develop flexibility, stamina, and coordination. It

KEY TERMS

Chi—In traditional Chinese culture, the life force or energy flow of all living things.

Feudalism—A system of legal, economic, and social repression in medieval Europe and Asia from the ninth century to the fifteenth century.

Social media—Internet technology and Web sites where people share information and interact socially, such as Facebook, Twitter, and You Tube.

Taoism—An ancient Chinese philosophy that advocates simple living and accepting the natural course of life.

Yin and yang—The Chinese philosophy that there are two opposing but complimentary forces in the universe.

is often recommended by alternative health practitioners to help relieve chronic back and joint pain. Chi kung is based on the idea of chi (life energy) and getting rid of the negative life energy. In China, there are hospitals that use chi kung to treat serious illnesses, particularly cancer.

- Kendo (way of the sword) is the Japanese martial art and sport of fighting with bamboo swords, with the fighters wearing protective armor and face masks. It is associated with the samurai (the warrior class of feudal or ancient Japan) of the ninth through fifteenth centuries and developed into its present form in the 1920s. It is popular in Japan and North America and primarily uses upper body muscles. Kendo is designed to build character and discipline. It is practiced by an estimated four million people in about 60 countries.

Other popular martial arts include: aikido, Brazilian jiu-jitsu, capoeira, arnis, escrima, kali, aikido, kung fu, sumo wrestling, jeet kune do, muay thai, krav maga, and American kickboxing.

Preparation

Most martial arts involve a **warm-up** to prevent injuries in training and promote joint, muscle, and tendon flexibility. A cool-down follows most regimens and serves to reduce the accumulation of blood and fluids in the muscles and reduce the breathing rate.

Risks

There are some risks in martial arts but generally they are not as great as in other sports. This is because in most martial arts, the body sets its own limits, making it difficult for sprains and other injuries to occur. Martial arts that use weapons carry a small but inherent risk of injury.

Results

Martial arts training usually does not greatly increase muscle mass; rather it replaces fat tissue with lean tissue and increases maximum endurance, flexibility, and mental well-being. In martial arts, the focus is on twisting the trunk, executing kicks, and counter-balancing hand movements. The high leg kick in many martial arts, such as judo and kickboxing, helps develop the muscles of the trunk and inner thighs. For women in particular, martial arts helps tone and strengthen the lower abdominal, hip, and thigh muscles.

Martial arts also offer other benefits, including improved concentration, vision clarity, body development, aerobic conditioning of the heart and lungs, and training in body control that is valuable in any other sport or physical activity, according to the United States Ju-Jitsu Federation.

Resources

BOOKS

Ashley, Scott. *Kickboxing: A Champion's Guide To Training*. Tamarac, FL: Llumina Press, 2011.

Austin, Andrew. *Tai Chi for Beginners*. New York: Rosen Publishing Group, 2011.

Goodman, Fay, et al. *The Complete Step-by-Step Guide To Martial Arts, Tai Chi, and Aikido*. London: Anness, 2011.

Link, Norman, and Lily Chou. *The Anatomy of Martial Arts: An Illustrated Guide to the Muscles Used for Each Strike, Kick, and Throw*. Berkeley, CA: Ulysses Press, 2011.

Scandiffio, Laura. *The Martial Arts Book*. Toronto: Annick Press, 2010.

PERIODICALS

Gwin, Peter. "Battle for the Soul of Kung Fu." *National Geographic* (March 2011): 100.

Rooney, Martin. "Build a Bruce Lee Body (and Defend It): 3 Time-Tested Martial Arts Training Moves That Will Transform Your Body and Your Life." *Men's Fitness* (May 2010): 26.

Rubin, Courtney. "Take Up the Ancient Chinese Exercise Tai Chi." *U.S. News & World Report* (November 26, 2010): 24.

Soo, Kim. "Taekwondo for Health: Train Smart Now or Pay the Price Later." *Black Belt* (September 2011): 72.

Young, Robert W. "Crash Course: 4 Judo Techniques Every Mixed Martial Artist and Self-Defense Practitioner Needs To Know." *Black Belt* (April 2011): 52.

WEBSITES

"Martial Arts: Jujutsu". Martial-arts-info.com. http://www.martial-arts-info.com (accessed October 30, 2011).

United States Martial Arts Association. http://www.mararts.org (accessed October 30, 2011).

ORGANIZATIONS

Karate Canada, 4400 Sherbrooke East, Montreal, Canada, QC, H1V 3S8, (514) 252-3209, Fax: (514) 252-3211, olivier@karatecanada.org, http://www.karatecanada.org.

National Association of Professional Martial Artists, 2578 Enterprise Rd., Suite 344, Orange City, FL, 32763, (727) 540-0500, Fax: (727) 693-9581, info@napma.com, http://www.napma.com.

United States Judo Federation, P.O. Box 338, Ontario, OR, 97914, (541) 889-8753, Fax: (541) 889-5836, http://www.usjf.com.

United States Martial Arts Federation, 1850 Columbia Pike, Suite 619, Arlington, VA, 22204, (703) 920-1590, natlhq@usmaf.org, http://www.usmaf.org.

Ken R. Wells

Maximum oxygen uptake

Definition

The cardiorespiratory fitness level of an individual can be defined as the highest rate at which oxygen is taken up and consumed by the body during intense **exercise**. The gold standard measurement for cardiorespiratory fitness is the maximal oxygen uptake (VO_2max). This measurement can be directly obtained from gas exchange measurement during maximal exercise testing or estimated from the results of submaximal or maximal exercise tests. The Fick equation can be used to properly define VO_2max: $VO_2max = Q(CaO_2 - CvO_2max)$; where Q refers to cardiac output, CaO_2

refers to the content of oxygen in arterial blood, and CvO_2max refers to the content of oxygen in venous blood.

Other terms frequently used when referring to cardiorespiratory fitness include cardiovascular fitness, fitness, aerobic power, aerobic fitness, and peak metabolic equivalents (METs). The units for reporting cardiorespiratory fitness levels are commonly either in absolute (L/min) or relative (mL/kg/min) terms.

Purpose

Traditionally, cardiorespiratory fitness has been viewed as a measure of overall health with studies consistently revealing an inverse relationship between VO_2max values and risk of death from all causes. Cardiorespiratory fitness can be used to accurately prescribe exercise intensity. Typically, intensity of exercise is prescribed as a range with a desirable lower and upper limit target workload established. These lower and upper limits can be defined in terms of a percentage of VO_2max or peak metabolic equivalents (METs). Compendiums of physical activity or metabolic calculations are then used to identify specific activities/exercises that fall within the target workload. Additionally, cardiorespiratory fitness has long been considered an attribute required for success in endurance-related events. A classic study conducted at Ball State University in the 1960s confirmed the importance of VO_2max to endurance performance. The results of the study demonstrated a strong correlation between VO_2max values and 10-mi. (16-km) run times. However, in a group of individuals with comparable levels of VO_2max, factors such as lactate threshold and economy become better predictors of performance.

Description

Maximal oxygen uptake may be determined using numerous exercise modes that activate large groups of muscle mass, provided the intensity of effort and protocol duration are sufficient to maximize aerobic **energy** transfer. **Treadmill** exercise and cycle ergometry are the most common modes utilized for VO_2 max testing. Other types of exercise modes, including bench stepping, free, tethered, and flume **swimming**, swim-bench ergometry, in-line skating, cross-country skiing, roller-skating, simulated arm-leg climbing, arm crank and wheelchair exercises, and **rowing** ergometry, have also been employed to achieve VO_2max. Regardless of exercise mode, variations in VO_2max typically reflect the quantity of muscle mass activated during exercise. Treadmill exercise generally elicits the highest VO_2max

values for the same untrained and/or recreationally trained individual performing different exercise mode VO_2max tests, although subject training specificity influences the magnitude of VO_2max values attained among different exercise modes. Elite-trained cyclists have similar treadmill and cycle ergometry VO_2max values. Likewise, untrained and trained collegiate swimmers achieve VO_2max values during swimming versus treadmill tests of 80% and 90%, respectively. Elite swimmers attain similar or greater VO_2max values.

Although genetics explain a considerable proportion of the variation in cardiorespiratory fitness, it is well known that VO_2max is higher in the majority of individuals who participate in regular and properly structured exercise programs. Physiological processes involving the cardiorespiratory system (heart, lungs, and blood vessels) and peripheral physiological functions (i.e., oxygen extraction at the skeletal muscle level) contribute to the overall magnitude of VO_2max. The ability of the **cardiovascular system** to transport oxygen to exercising skeletal muscles is referred to as the central component of VO_2max. The role of this component is to transport oxygen from the atmosphere and deliver it to the muscles where it is used in mitochondrial respiration to produce adenosine triphosphate (ATP). Oxygen delivery may be limited by maximal cardiac output, pulmonary diffusion, and blood volume and flow. The peripheral aspect of VO_2max involves the capacity for the exercising skeletal muscle to extract and use the oxygen delivered by the cardiovascular system. Peripheral factors that may hinder VO_2max are skeletal muscle diffusion capacity, capillary density, and mitochondrial enzyme levels.

Precautions

The risk of acute myocardial infarction or sudden death during vigorous exercise is higher in adults compared to their younger counterparts. The higher prevalence of **cardiovascular disease** in older adults is responsible for this elevated risk. Similarly, the risk of cardiac events associated with maximal exercise testing, during which cardiorespiratory fitness is frequently determined, is related to the incidence of cardiovascular disease. The overall risk remains relatively low; it has been reported that six cardiac events per 10,000 exercise tests can be expected. Measures taken to lower this risk include sufficient pre-testing screening to identify individuals with health conditions that could be affected by exercise testing, and determining an individual's risk stratification as either low, moderate, or high. The degree of monitoring and supervision

Adenosine triphosphate (ATP)—An adenosine-derived nucleotide that contains high-energy phosphate bonds. The hydrolysis of ATP to ADP and inorganic phosphate releases free energy that can be used for multiple physiological processes, most notably muscle contraction.

Capillary density—The quantity of minute blood vessels connecting the arterioles and venules, where oxygen and carbon dioxide exchange occur at the skeletal muscle tissue level, for a given surface area.

C_aO_2—Arterial blood oxygen content.

C_vO_2—Venous blood oxygen content.

Fick equation—A mathematical equation used to define maximal oxygen uptake: $VO_2max = Q(C_aO_2-C_vO_2)$. It reflects both the central component (i.e., Q or cardiac output) and peripheral component (i.e., difference between C_aO_2 or arterial blood oxygen content and C_vO_2 or venous blood oxygen content).

Indirect calorimetry—Measurement of oxygen consumption and carbon dioxide production; heat measurement is calculated using formula and energy expenditure can also be determined mathematically.

L/min—Liters of oxygen consumed per minute; the absolute expression of maximal oxygen uptake.

Maximal cardiac output—The highest blood volume pumped by the heart each minute.

Maximal oxygen uptake—The highest rate at which oxygen can be taken up and consumed by the body during intense exercise.

Metabolic equivalents (METs)—A single MET equates to the amount of energy expenditure during one minute of seated rest. In terms of oxygen uptake, 1 MET equates to 3.5 mL/kg/min.

Mitochondrial enzyme levels—The concentrations of those enzymes (i.e., biological catalysts) involved with aerobic respiration.

mL/kg/min—Milliliters of oxygen consumed per minute; the relative expression of maximal oxygen uptake.

Muscle diffusion capacity—Measure of the capability to exchange carbon dioxide and oxygen between skeletal muscle and the capillary bed.

Pulmonary diffusion—The volume of gases, principally carbon dioxide and oxygen, that diffuses across the membranes between the alveoli and lung capillaries per minute.

Rating of perceived exertion (RPE)—A subjective rating by an individual of their perception of exercise intensity.

Respiratory exchange ratio (RER)—The ratio of carbon dioxide production to oxygen consumption as measured from expired gas analysis during indirect calorimetry.

---

required before, during and after the maximal exercise test can be adjusted to suit the risk stratification of the individual.

Preparation

The most accurate method for determining individual cardiorespiratory fitness is through the measurement of VO_2max. This is generally accomplished during an incremental exercise test by using indirect calorimetry. Various protocols may be used for maximal exercise testing; however, the specific increases in workload at each stage vary considerably depending on the individual. In higher fit individuals and athletes it is common for the workload to be increased by two to three METs each stage. In contrast, for lower fit individuals or individuals with health complications (e.g., cardiac disease), the workload increment for each stage is 0.5 to 1.0 METs per stage.

Either continuous or discontinuous protocols may be employed during maximal exercise testing.

Continuous protocols call for the workload to be progressively increased over the course of the test until the individual being tested fatigues. Discontinuous protocols are intermittent in nature with workload stages separated by rest periods; each successive stage in a discontinuous protocol has a higher workload. The duration of each stage in either a continuous or discontinuous protocol stage can last from a few seconds to several minutes.

Oxygen consumption is determined by the collection and measurement of expired gases (i.e., indirect calorimetry) throughout maximal exercise testing. The relationship between oxygen consumption and workload is linear across the early part of an exercise test; however, the relationship becomes more curvilinear as an individual approaches **fatigue**. Near and at fatigue, many individuals exhibit a plateau in oxygen consumption; the plateau in VO_2max is one of the criteria frequently used in research to confirm VO_2max has been achieved. However, this phenomenon is not a consistent finding across all populations. Other criteria used to confirm the attainment of VO$_2$max include a heart rate within 10-15 beats per minute of age-predicted maximum, a respiratory exchange ratio value exceeding 1.10, and a rating of perceived exertion values of 18 or 19 on the 6 to 20 Borg Scale. Although it is the most precise method, direct measurement of VO$_2$max via indirect calorimetry may be unsuitable and unfavorable because the calorimetry equipment necessary for the measurement of VO$_2$max is expensive, requires trained laboratory personnel, and calls for maximal subject effort to ensure accurate testing results. Furthermore, the VO$_2$max testing procedures are time consuming, making the assessment less than ideal when testing a large number of individuals.

Researchers have looked to alternative methods for estimating VO$_2$max. In the 1920s, researchers at the Harvard Fatigue Laboratory began developing a submaximal test based on recovery heart rate in an effort to quantify individual fitness levels. The laboratory followed these initial efforts with the establishment of the well-recognized Harvard Step Test. Research has continued since this early pioneering work, resulting in various submaximal tests and prediction equations for different modes of exercise. Generally, exercise professionals select either treadmill exercise or cycle ergometry for submaximal exercise-testing assessments. Other exercise modes and field tests have also been used in the estimation of VO$_2$max, including bench stepping, rowing ergometry, stair climbing, track **walking**, track **running**, and swimming. Amongst the most common tests for predicting VO$_2$max are the Balke 15-minute run, the Bruce treadmill test, the Cooper 12-minute run, and the Rockport 1-mile (1.6 km) walk test.

Aftercare

Low cardiorespiratory fitness is exceptionally modifiable. Improvements in cardiorespiratory fitness are generally more favorable when compared to other risk factors. It has been has reported that following three months of **aerobic training** the typical improvement in cardiorespiratory fitness between 10-30%. These findings are comparable for both previously sedentary adults and older adults. These improvements in cardiorespiratory fitness pay big dividends in terms of long term health. Research suggests a 15% reduction in mortality for a 10% improvement in cardiorespiratory fitness.

Complications

Cardiorespiratory fitness has been coined the ultimate health outcome. Research has reported that low

---

QUESTIONS TO ASK YOUR DOCTOR

- What is the best method for testing my VO$_2$max?
- Are there health concerns that could impair my ability to perform the test?
- How can I use the test results to modify my current fitness program?

---

cardiorespiratory fitness is associated with premature mortality. Low levels of cardiorespiratory fitness are also linked to an increased risk of cardiovascular disease development and mortality from cardiovascular disease. It has been shown that low cardiorespiratory fitness accounts for more deaths in both men and women than any other cardiovascular disease risk factor, including smoking, **obesity**, **hypertension**, and hypercholesterolemia. In addition, individuals with poor fitness are less likely to be able to perform activities of daily living. Cardiorespiratory fitness tends to decline by approximately 10% per decade after the age of 25. Undeterred, these reductions in physiological functional capacity can eventually result in loss of independence.

Results

The magnitude of an individual's cardiorespiratory fitness level depends on variables including age, sex, race, training status, and genetics. Typical values for VO$_2$max with specific reference to age and sex are available at the Cooper Institute website (http://www.cooperinstitute. org). The proportion of low, moderate, and high cardiorespiratory fitness differs between race and race-sex groups. Low cardiorespiratory fitness is most prevalent in non-Hispanic black women. Nearly one of every three women is estimated to have low levels of fitness, while just over one of every 10 non-Hispanic white women is estimated to have low levels of cardiorespiratory fitness. Comparatively, the prevalence of high cardiorespiratory fitness is greatest amongst non-Hispanic men and lowest amongst non-Hispanic black women.

Resources

BOOKS

Ehrman, Jonathan K., editor. *ACSM's Resource Manual for Guidelines for Exercise Testing and Prescription.* Philadelphia: Lippincott Williams & Wilkins Health, 2010.

Heyward, Vivian, H., editor. *Advanced Fitness Assessment and Exercise Prescription.* Champaign, IL: Human Kinetics, Wilkins, 2010.

Katch, Victor L., William D. McArdle, and Frank I. Katch. *Essentials of Exercise Physiology*. Philadelphia: Wolters Kluwer/Lippincott Williams & Wilkins Health, 2011.

Thompson, Walter R., editor. *ACSM's Guidelines for Exercise Testing and Prescription*. Philadelphia: Lippincott Williams & Wilkins Health, 2010.

WEBSITES

Calculation maximum oxygen consumption. Runningtools. com. (June 13, 2010). http://www.runningtools.com/vo2max.htm (accessed August 23, 2011).

Fitness Testing. ExRx.net. (June 23, 2008). http://www.exrx.net/Testing.html (accessed August 23, 2011).

Mackenzie, Brian. *VO2max*. (June 8, 2011). http://www.brianmac.co.uk/vo2max.htm (accessed August 23, 2011).

ORGANIZATIONS

American College of Sports Medicine, 401 W. Michigan St., Indianapolis, IN, 46206-1440, (317) 637-9200, Fax: (317) 634-7817, http://www.acsm.org.

Centers for Disease Control and Prevention, 1600 Clifton Rd., Atlanta, GA, 30333, (800) 232-6348, cdcinfo@cdc.gov, http://www.cdc.gov.

The Cooper Institute, 12330 Preston Rd., Dallas, TX, 75230, (972) 341-3200, Fax: (972) 341-3227, (800) 635-7050, http://www.cooperinstitute.org.

Lance C. Dalleck, BA, MS, PhD

Men's fitness

Definition

Men's fitness includes nutrition and **exercise** that pertain to males, both teenagers and adults. It also includes mental and sexual health.

Description

Men have different physiology than women and generally have different fitness goals and nutritional needs. For example, men have a higher risk of heart disease than women so regular cardiovascular (cardio or aerobic) exercises are especially important for males. Men's fitness can include a wide range of topics, including exercise, nutrition, **mental health**, sports, **bodybuilding**, and sexual health. Research shows that regular physical activity, even **walking** for 30 minutes a day, may lower the risk of erectile dysfunction (impotence).

There are real differences between men and women when it comes to exercise and fitness. Men are more likely than women to concentrate on the upper body and less likely to spend time warming up and cooling down. Men are also less likely to do **stretching**, even though men generally are less flexible than women because of natural body structure.

Function

Regular exercise and proper nutrition is essential for men of all ages, from teenagers to seniors. In the United States, less than 10% of high school boys met the minimum requirements of physical activity, according to the U.S. Centers for Disease Control and Prevention (CDC). The CDC recommends teenage males get at least an hour of aerobic exercise a day and a minimum of three hours a week of muscle-strengthening exercise. For middle-age men, at least 45 minutes of moderate aerobic activity a day and 45 minutes three times a week should be spent on resistance or strength training. Research shows that men slowly start to lose muscle mass and strength beginning at about **age** 30. In middle age men, **metabolism** also slows, allowing fat to accumulate, especially around the abdomen. In men age 65 and older, physical fitness is important to help maintain muscle tone, stamina, flexibility, and balance. Exercise for seniors should include 30 minutes a day of light to moderate aerobics (such as walking briskly) and 30 minutes two or three times a week of resistance exercise, including 5-10 minutes each of warmup and cooldown exercises that includes stretching.

Nutrition is an important component of men's fitness. Men have a higher metabolism than women and thereby burn more **calories** when doing the same or similar activities. Active males ages 14 to 18 need 2,400 to 2,800 calories a day, ages 19 to 30 need 3,000 calories daily, men ages 31 to 50 require 2,800 to 3,000 calories a day, and men age 51 and older require about 2,400 to 2,800 calories a day. "Active" means physical activity equal to walking briskly at least 3 mi. (5 km) a day in an hour or less. Moderate activity means activity that equals 1–3 mi. (1.6–5 km) a day in an hour or less. Moderately active males require the following amounts of calories per day: ages 14 to 18, 2,400 to 2,800; ages 19 to 30, 2,600 to 2,800; ages 31 to 50, 2,400 to 2,600; and age 51 and older, 2,200 to 2,400. For males who engage in light activity associated with daily living, the daily calorie needs are: ages 14 to 18, 2,200; ages 19 to 30, 2,400; ages 31 to 50, 2,200; and age 50 and older, 2,000, according to the U.S. Department of Health and Human Services (HHS).

Role in human health

The benefits of proper nutrition and fitness for men is enormous, including reducing the risks of heart disease, stroke, cancer, diabetes, high **blood pressure**, and high **cholesterol**.

Men vary greatly in their physical fitness levels and goals. A workout routine for a young, healthy male, often for improved athletic or sports performance, is different than an exercise program for a middle-aged, out-of-shape man. Men's fitness includes all levels of activity, depending on age, ability, and health, from mild aerobic (walking briskly), to **weightlifting** that builds muscle mass and strength. There are also various levels of moderate exercises, including aerobic and weight-bearing routines.

A general basic exercise routine for men ages 18 to 50 includes five areas of physical fitness: muscle strength, muscle endurance, cardiovascular endurance, flexibility, and maintaining a healthy body weight and composition. To improve these five areas, three physical fitness routines are needed: strength or weight training, cardiovascular (aerobic) exercise, and stretching.

Obesity and men

Obesity, once only a problem in the industrialized nations of North American and Europe, is now a world-wide problem, with obesity rates among men increasing rapidly in India, China, Japan, Russia, and South America. Being overweight, obese, or severely obese has more serious health consequences on men than women, according to studies by the CDC. Specific risks caused by obesity include heart disease, stroke, colon cancer, lung disease, diabetes, erectile dysfunction, and sleep disorders. Studies show that otherwise physically fit men who were overweight live shorter lives than fit and lean or muscular men. Obesity is best targeted with a two-part approach of a proper but reduced-calorie diet and regular exercise. Building muscle also helps burn extra calories (fat) so a strengthening routine should be included with aerobics.

Obesity is a much bigger problem among men than women, statistics show. In the United States, More than 72% of American men age 20 and older are either overweight or obese. One third of all U.S. males age 20 and older are considered obese and nearly 6 % are extremely obese, according to the National Institute of Diabetes and Digestive and Kidney Diseases (NIDDKD). In Canada, the obesity rate for males ages 20–24 is 12% and for men ages 55–64, the rate is 22%, according to the Public Health Agency of Canada.

Common diseases and disorders

The most common sports and fitness injuries for men are ankle sprain, groin pull, hamstring strain, shin splints, anterior cruciate ligament (ACL) tear in the

---

KEY TERMS

Aerobic exercise—A type of exercise of brisk or vigorous activity that requires the heart and lungs to work harder to supply oxygen to the body.

Cardiovascular—Relating to the heart and blood vessels (circulatory system).

Erectile dysfunction—A medical condition, formerly called impotence, that prevents a male from getting and maintaining an erection.

Ligament—A band of strong, fibrous tissue that connects bones to joints.

Tendon—A cord of strong tissue that connects muscles to bones.

---

knee, and rotator cuff strain, according to the American College of Sports Medicine.

Sprains and strains

A sprain is a stretch or tear of a ligament, the band of connective tissues that joins the end of one bone with another. Sprains are caused by trauma such as a fall or blow to the body that knocks a joint out of position and, in the worst case, ruptures the supporting ligaments. Sprains can range from Grade I (minimally stretched ligament) to Grade III (a complete tear). Areas of the body most vulnerable to sprains are ankles, knees, and wrists. A strain is a twist, pull, or tear of a muscle or tendon, a cord of tissue connecting muscle to bone.

Knee injuries

Knee injuries can range from mild to severe. Some of the less severe, yet still painful and functionally limiting, knee problems include runner's knee (pain or tenderness close to or under the knee cap at the front or side of the knee), iliotibial band syndrome (pain on the outer side of the knee), and tendonitis, also called tendinosis (marked by degeneration within a tendon, usually where it joins the bone). More severe injuries include bone bruises or damage to the cartilage or ligaments.

Fractures

A **fracture** is a break in the bone that can occur from either a quick, one-time injury to the bone (acute fracture) or from repeated stress to the bone over time (stress fracture). Acute fractures can be simple (a clean break with little damage to the surrounding tissue) or compound (a break in which the bone pierces the skin). Most fractures are emergencies and require prompt medical attention. A fracture that breaks the skin is especially dangerous because there is a high risk of infection. Stress fractures occur largely in the feet and legs and are common in sports that require repetitive impact, primarily running/jumping activities such as jogging and **basketball**. **Running** creates forces two to three times a person's body weight on the lower limbs.

Other sports injuries

Other men's fitness injuries include achilles tendon injuries, compartment syndrome, and shin splints. In many parts of the body, muscles (along with the nerves and blood vessels that run alongside and through them) are enclosed in a "compartment" formed of a tough membrane called fascia. When muscles become swollen, they can fill the compartment to capacity, causing interference with nerves and blood vessels as well as damage to the muscles themselves. The resulting painful condition is referred to as compartment syndrome.

Shin splints are primarily seen in runners. While the term "shin splints" has been widely used to describe any sort of leg pain associated with exercise, the term actually refers to pain along the tibia or shin bone, the large bone in the front of the lower leg. This pain can occur at the front outside part of the lower leg, including the foot and ankle (anterior shin splints) or at the inner edge of the bone where it meets the calf muscles (medial shin splints).

Achilles tendon injuries can be sudden and agonizing. Achilles tendon injuries include a stretch, tear, or irritation to the tendon connecting the calf muscle to the back of the heel. Achilles tendon injuries are

common in older people who may not exercise regularly or do not take time to stretch properly before an activity.

Resources

BOOKS

Ellsworth, Pamela. *100 Questions & Answers About Men's Health*. Sudbury, MA: Jones & Bartlett Publishers, 2010.

Spinelli, Frank. *The Advocate Guide to Gay Men's Health and Wellness*. Los Angeles: Alyson Books, 2008.

Villepigue, James, and Hugo Rivera. *The Body Sculpting Bible for Men (Third Edition)*. Long Island City, NY: Hatherleigh Press, 2011.

Weber, Joel, and Mike Zimmerman. *The Men's Health Big Book of Food & Nutrition* Emmaus, PA: Rodale Books, 2010.

PERIODICALS

Bornstein, Adam. "The No-Fail Workout." *Men's Health* (June 2010): 46.

Clouatre, Dallas. "The Special Nutritional Needs of Men." *Total Health Online* (April 2011): 19.

Martin, Peter. "Extreme Health." *Esquire* (April 2011): 88.

Smith, Ian. "The Man Workout." *Jet* (June 14, 2010): 22.

Wilkinson, John. "Man Medicine." *Redbook* (September 2011): 100.

WEBSITES

Cleveland Clinic Health. "Minority Men's Health: Know Your Numbers." http://cchealth.clevelandclinic.org/multimedia/slideshows/minority-mens-health (accessed September 15, 2011).

LiveStrong.com. "Men's Fitness." http://www.livestrong.com/mens-fitness/ (accessed September 15, 2011).

Men's Fitness & Health. "Men's Fitness and Health: Fact Not Hype." http://www.mens-fitness-and-health.com/ (accessed September 15, 2011).

MSN. "Men's Health." http://health.msn.com/mens-health/ (accessed September 15, 2011).

WebMD. "Men's Health: Fitness & Exercise." http://men.webmd.com/guide/mens-health-fitness (accessed September 15, 2011).

ORGANIZATIONS

American College of Sports Medicine, PO Box 1440, Indianapolis, IN, 46206, (317) 637-9200, Fax: (317) 634-7817, http://www.acsm.org.

American Council on Exercise, 4851 Paramount Dr., San Diego, CA, 92123, (858) 576-6500, Fax: (858) 576-6564, (888) 825-3636, support@acefitness.org, http://www.acefitness.org.

Canadian Association of Fitness Professionals, 110-255 Consumer Rd., Toronto, Canada, ON, M2J 1R4, 1 (416) 493-3515, Fax: 1 (416) 493-1756, (800) 667-5622, info@canfitpro.com, http://www.canfitpro.com.

Men's Health Network, PO Box 75972, Washington, DC, 20013, 1(202) 543-6461, info@menshealthnetwork.org, http://www.menshealthnetwork.org.

Native American Fitness Council, PO Box K, Flagstaff, AZ, 86002, (928) 774-3048, Fax: (928) 774-5753, info@nativeamericanfitnesscouncil.com, http://www.nativeamericanfitnesscouncil.com.

Ken R. Wells

Mental health and exercise

Definition

Exercise directly benefits mental health, above and beyond the mental health benefits of exercise-derived improvements in physical health.

Purpose

Exercise helps relieve tension, anxiety, stress, anger, and depression, and enhances one's sense of well-being. Exercise and improved physical fitness build self-confidence, enhance self-image and self-esteem, and contribute to a positive outlook. Sports and other physical activities can be exhilarating and provide emotional release from anxieties and frustrations. Exercise increases **energy** levels and mental alertness and improves sleep, all of which contribute to good mental health. Exercising outdoors in the sunlight—so-called "green" activities—can help overcome seasonal affective disorder (SAD) or the "winter blues." Many people find exercise to be an enjoyable form of relaxation and an opportunity for socializing. This can be especially important for patients dealing with isolation and loneliness due to a mental health condition.

Over the long term, regular exercise benefits physical health, contributing to improved mental health. Weight gain is both a common cause and a common result of depression and other mental health problems. Weight gain can also be a side effect of some medications used to treat mental disorders. Exercise can slow or halt weight gain. It can also relieve stress and tension that can lead to overeating. Aging often has a negative impact on mental health; however, physical activity can help seniors continue to enjoy activities and remain independent—both important contributors to good mental health.

For many people, the effects of exercise on mental health go beyond improving mood and preventing "the blues." Research and clinical experience indicate that exercise can be an effective treatment for more serious mental disorders, including severe depression, anxiety disorders, substance dependence, and even schizophrenia. Physicians and psychologists commonly prescribe exercise for a range of mental health conditions, in place of, or in addition to, medications and counseling or psychotherapy. Some research suggests that the effects of exercise on mild depression may be longer lasting than the effects of antidepressants.

Whereas studies and experience have consistently demonstrated that exercise can benefit mental health, the reverse also appears to be true: lack of regular exercise is associated with symptoms of depression and anxiety. The numerous benefits of exercise on mental health are hardly surprising, since the human brain most likely evolved to cope emotionally and psychologically under much more physically demanding conditions than are common today.

Demographics

According to the World Health Organization, 450 million people globally have mental disorders in both developed and developing countries. Of these, 154 million have depression, 25 million have schizophrenia, 91 million have alcohol use disorder and 15 million have drug use disorder. Approximately 26% of Americans and 20% of Canadians experience a mental illness at some point in their lives. According to the National Institute of Mental Health, more than 4% of Americans have a serious mental illness, including about 6% of females and nearly 8% of young adults between the ages of 18 and 25. Among Americans over age 65, 14% demonstrate significant depressive symptoms. Men over age 75 have the highest overall suicide rate. Serious mental illness is somewhat more common among whites than among blacks, Hispanics, and Asian Americans. Mixed-race Americans have the highest rates of serious mental illness.

Regular physical activity is important for the mental health of most people. With the increase in sedentary employment and entertainment via television, video games, and the Internet, activity levels have decreased in recent decades among all age groups. During the same period, the incidence of mental health disorders has risen sharply. Although some of this increase is attributable to greater awareness of mental health issues and improved diagnoses, reduced activity levels may share some of the blame.

Any condition that limits physical activity can have a negative impact on mental health. Physical illnesses and conditions—such as **arthritis**, **cardiovascular disease**, stroke, cancer, and HIV/AIDS—are often accompanied by depression or other mental problems. Anxiety, fear, or stress can be secondary to such conditions, resulting from concern about the future or restriction of normal activities. Other times, a disease, physical condition, or medication used to treat a condition directly cause depression or other mental problems. For example, depression is the most common psychiatric diagnosis among HIV/AIDS patients, especially women. In addition to causing anxiety and fear, HIV/AIDS and HIV-related medications can contribute directly to depression.

Description

Origins

During the 1970s and 1980s, clinicians began to realize that people who exercised regularly were less likely to experience depression and were less likely to become depressed in the future. A trial conducted in 1999 demonstrated that an aerobic exercise plan was as effective in treating depressed adults as the antidepressant sertraline (Zoloft), a drug that earned its manufacturer more than $3 billion annually before its patent expired in 2006. Most subsequent studies have confirmed that regular aerobic exercise can be as effective as medication for treating depression and preventing the recurrence of depressive symptoms.

Effects of exercise

The effects of exercise on mental health are emotional, psychological, and physical. Exercise relaxes the mind and body. Physical activity provides a positive means of coping with stress, anxiety, sadness, and depression. It provides a distraction that can break cycles of negative thinking that increase anxiety and depression. In contrast, trying to wait out a depression or attempting to cope with drugs or alcohol often makes symptoms worse. Exercise also can improve self-esteem and self-confidence through a sense of achievement and improved body image and by encouraging social interaction.

Exercise may relieve muscle tension, burn off stress hormones, and increase blood flow to the brain. It may lower **immune system** chemicals that can worsen depression. Exercise also increases body temperature, which may have a calming effect.

Neuroscientists are beginning to understand the ways in which exercise alters brain chemistry. Exercise stimulates the production of endorphins—so-called pleasure hormones that improve mood and relieve stress. It appears that exercise functions in much the same way as antidepressant medications, by regulating the key neurotransmitters, serotonin and norepinephrine. Over a period of several weeks, regular exercise appears to turn on specific genes that increase the levels of galanin in the brain. Galanin is a neurotransmitter that reduces the body's stress response by regulating norepinephrine.

This means that new stimuli or negative events—such as a parking ticket or missed appointment—have less effect on emotions.

Exercise also may have a direct effect on nerve cells in the hippocampus—a part of the brain involved in regulation of mood and responses to antidepressants. In animals, exercise increases the production of brain-derived neurotrophic factor (BDNF), which is necessary for the growth and maintenance of brain cells and can relieve depressive symptoms in humans. Studies in animal models of human depression have found that exercise-induced symptom alleviation depends on the growth of new adult neurons in the brain and may involve the enhanced activity of a nerve growth factor.

Exercise as treatment

Exercise has several advantages as a mental health treatment. It is usually viewed in a positive light, without the stigma that is sometimes still associated with medication or psychotherapy. The mood-enhancing effects of exercise are quickly apparent—much faster than the physical benefits of exercise. This immediate effect encourages more exercise. This is particularly important for people with depression, which is characterized by a chronic lack of motivation. Unlike other treatments for mental disorders, exercise provides significant physical health benefits, is inexpensive or free, and without the side effects that limit the use of many medications.

Experts generally recommend at least 30 minutes of moderate-intensity aerobic exercise—such as walking—at least five times per week, or 30 minutes of high-intensity aerobic exercise at least three times per week. These are similar to physical fitness recommendations. As little as 30–45 minutes of **walking** three times per week has been associated with a reduction or alleviation of depressive symptoms. Even small increments of exercise—climbing stairs, walking the dog, or gardening for 10–15 minutes at a time—can have a significant effect. However, more vigorous exercise, such as **running** or playing a sport, may work faster. Anaerobic exercise, such as **weightlifting**, may have many of the same mental health benefits as aerobic exercise. Some types of exercise—such as **yoga**, **pilates**, and tai chi—are geared specifically toward improving mental as well as physical health.

Preparation

Sedentary individuals and those with health problems should always consult their physician before embarking on a new exercise program. Physicians or mental health professionals can prescribe exercise regimens that take into account pain, physical limitations,

KEY TERMS

Aerobic exercise—Activity that increases the body's requirement for oxygen, thereby increasing respiration and heart rate.

Antidepressant—A drug used to prevent or treat depression.

Anxiety disorder—A group of disorders characterized by anxiety, including panic disorder and post-traumatic stress disorder (PTSD).

Brain-derived neurotrophic factor (BDNF)—A brain protein that helps maintain nerves and promotes the growth of new nerve cells (neurons).

Depression—A mental condition of extreme sadness and loss of interest in life, including problems with appetite, sleep, concentration, and daily functioning; severe depression can lead to suicide attempts.

Eating disorders—Conditions, such as anorexia nervosa and bulimia nervosa, that are characterized by abnormal attitudes toward food, altered appetite control, unhealthy eating habits, and sometimes compulsive exercise; particularly common in young women.

Endorphins—A class of peptides in the brain that are produced during exercise and bind to opiate receptors, resulting in pleasant feelings and pain relief.

Galanin—A neurotransmitter with roles in various physiological processes, including regulation of the stress response.

Hippocampus—A part of the brain that is involved in forming, storing, and processing memory, and in regulating mood.

Hormone—A substance, such as a protein, that is produced in one part of the body and travels through the bloodstream to affect another part of the body.

Neurotransmitter—A chemical—such as norepinephrine or serotonin—that transmits impulses across synapses between nerves.

Norepinephrine—Noradrenaline; a neurotransmitter in the sympathetic nervous system and some parts of the central nervous system, as well as a blood-pressure-raising (vasoconstricting) adrenal hormone.

Pilates—An exercise regimen specifically designed to improve overall physiological and mental functioning.

Schizophrenia—A psychotic disorder characterized by loss of contact with one's environment, deterioration of everyday functioning, and personality disintegration.

Serotonin—A neurotransmitter located primarily in the brain, blood serum, and stomach.

Stroke—A sudden diminishing or loss of consciousness, sensation, or voluntary movement, due to the rupture or obstruction of a blood vessel in the brain.

Tai chi—An ancient Chinese discipline involving controlled movements specifically designed to improve physical and mental well-being.

and mobility issues. It is important to start slowly, gradually increasing exercise intensity and duration as strength and stamina improve.

Regardless of apparent mental health benefits, sticking with an exercise program is a challenge for many people. Therefore, it is important to choose activities that are both appropriate and enjoyable. Exercise should be something to look forward to each day. Goals should be reasonable and achievable, so as not to set oneself up for failure. Some people prefer to exercise at home, because of self-consciousness or financial considerations. Others find that exercising with companions is more motivating and enjoy the social aspect.

Risks

Although exercise can ease symptoms of anxiety, depression, or another mental disorder, it is not necessarily a substitute for psychotherapy, medication, or other treatment. Appropriate activities and intensity levels should be chosen in consultation with a physician, to avoid the risk of injury.

Compulsive exercise is sometimes a symptom of a mental health disorder, particularly **eating disorders** such as anorexia or bulimia. People with anorexia may exercise compulsively to lose weight inappropriately. Those with bulimia, which is characterized by episodes of uncontrollable binge eating, may engage in compulsive exercise to prevent weight gain from overeating.

Results

As little as 30 minutes or less of moderate-intensity exercise that raises the heart rate can result in noticeable mood enhancement and anxiety reduction. Many studies have shown that routine exercise can be as effective as medication at relieving depressive symptoms. However, some research suggests that psychological responses to exercise have a genetic component. A large, long-term study of identical twins, published in

2008, found that twins who exercised more had no fewer anxious or depressive symptoms than their identical siblings who exercised less. It is possible that some types of exercise have more effect on mental health in some people than in others. It is also unclear whether exercise is as effective for treating severe depression as it is for treating mild to moderate depression.

Research and general acceptance

The relationship between mental health and exercise is an area of active research. Studies have extended the mental health benefits of exercise to patients with schizophrenia and schizophrenia-like illnesses, bipolar disorder, major depression, and other mental disorders. Exercise has been found to relieve depressive symptoms in adult stroke patients and stroke patients who exercise are much less likely to report depressive symptoms. Studies published in 2010 reported that the amount of exercise by undergraduate students correlated positively with their ratings on mental health scales and that just five minutes of outdoor or "green" activity—walking or gardening—has noticeable mental health benefits, including improved mood and self-esteem. A study published in 2011 found conclusive evidence that tai chi improves mental health in seniors, as well as providing general health benefits and reducing the risk of falls.

A study published in 2010, involving more than 40,000 Norwegians, reported that those who engaged in even small amounts of light, regular exercise were less likely to have depressive symptoms—as long as it was leisure-time exercise rather than physical activity at work. Socializing during exercise was an important beneficial factor. Those who were not active during their free time were almost twice as likely to have depressive symptoms. Exercise intensity did not appear to influence the results.

Schools and hospitals are increasingly using yoga to help children relax and focus and to improve behavior, self-esteem, and academic performance, as well as physical health. Some schools use yoga before statewide tests to help children relax and concentrate. Over the long term, yoga has been found to reduce aggression and improve emotional balance in children. It appears to be particularly helpful for children with special needs, as well as those with eating and mood disorders and autism.

Resources

BOOKS

Amen, Daniel G. *Magnificent Mind at Any Age: Natural Ways to Unleash Your Brain's Maximum Potential.* New York: Harmony, 2009.

Carless, David, and Kitrina Douglas. *Sport and Physical Activity for Mental Health.* Ames, IA: Wiley-Blackwell, 2010.

Emmons, Henry. *The Chemistry of Calm: A Powerful, Drug-Free Plan to Quiet Your Fears and Overcome Your Anxiety.* New York: Simon & Schuster, 2010.

Friedman, Peach. *Diary of an Exercise Addict: A Memoir.* Guilford, CT: GPP Life, 2009.

Kemper, Kathi. *Mental Health, Naturally: The Family Guide to Holistic Care for a Healthy Mind and Body.* Elk Grove Village, IL: American Academy of Pediatrics, 2010.

Larsen, Laura. *Fitness and Exercise Sourcebook.* 4th ed. Detroit: Omnigraphics, 2011.

Otto, Michael W., and Jasper A.J. Smits. *Exercise for Mood and Anxiety Disorders: Workbook.* New York: Oxford University Press, 2009.

PERIODICALS

Dang, Michelle T. "Walking Away the Blues: Exercise for Depression in Older Adults." *Nursing* 40, no. 11 (November 2010): 33.

Demissie, Zewditu, et al. "Physical Activity and Depressive Symptoms Among Pregnant Women: The PIN3 Study." *Women's Mental Health* 14, no. 2 (April 2011): 145–57.

Harvey, William J., et al. "Physical Activity, Leisure, and Health for Persons with Mental Illness." *Palaestra* 25, no. 2 (2010): 36–41.

Lister, Sam. "Lift Your Mood with a Little Leisure-Time Exercise; But Exertion at Work 'Makes No Difference.'" *Times (London)* (November 1, 2010): 17.

Lowry, C.A., S.L. Lightman, and D.J. Nutt. "That Warm Fuzzy Feeling: Brain Serotonergic Neurons and the Regulation of Emotion." *Journal of Psychopharmacology* 23, no. 4 (June 2009): 392–400.

Tyson, Philip, et al. "Physical Activity and Mental Health in a Student Population." *Journal of Mental Health* 19, no. 6 (December 2010): 492–99.

Van Citters, Aricca D., et al. "A Pilot Evaluation of the In SHAPE Individualized Health Promotion Intervention for Adults with Mental Illness." *Community Mental Health Journal* 46, no. 6 (December 2010): 540–52.

WEBSITES

Blue, Laurie. "Is Exercise the Best Drug for Depression?" *Time Health*. June 19, 2010. http://www.time.com/time/health/article/0,8599,1998021,00.html (accessed July 18, 2011).

Cassels, Caroline. "Exercise Beneficial for Physical and Mental Health Outcomes in Schizophrenia." Medscape Medical News. May 12, 2010. http://www.medscape.com/viewarticle/721652 (accessed July 18, 2011).

Mayo Clinic Staff. "Depression and Anxiety: Exercise Eases Symptoms." Mayo Clinic. October 23, 2009. http://www.mayoclinic.com/health/depression-and-exercise/MH00043 (accessed July 18, 2011).

National Institute of Mental Health. "Novel Model of Depression from Social Defeat Shows Restorative Power of Exercise." Science Update. April 13, 2010. http://www.nimh.nih.gov/science-news/2010/novel-model-of-depression-from-social-defeat-shows-restorative-power-of-exercise.shtml (accessed July 18, 2011).

National Institute of Mental Health. "Stress-Defeating Effects of Exercise Traced to Emotional Brain Circuit." Science Update. June 9, 2011. http://www.nimh.nih.gov/science-news/2011/stress-defeating-effects-of-exercise-traced-to-emotional-brain-circuit.shtml (accessed July 18, 2011).

Preidt, Robert. "Tai Chi Prevents Falls, Boosts Mental Health in Seniors: Study." *HealthDay*. May 17, 2011. http://www.nlm.nih.gov/medlineplus/news/fullstory_112150.html (accessed July 17, 2011).

ORGANIZATIONS

Mental Health America, 2000 North Beauregard Street, 6th Floor, Alexandria, VA, 22311, (703) 684-7722, Fax: (703) 684-5968, (800) 969-6642, infoctr@mentalhealthamerica.net, http://www.mentalhealthamerica.net.

Mental Health America (formerly the National Mental Health Association) is the country's major nonprofit dedicated to mental health. It consists of more than 320 affiliates nationwide, whose members include patients, families, advocates, mental healthcare professions, primary-care professionals, researchers, school officials, and others. MHA provides support for the more than 60 million individuals and their families living with mental health and substance abuse problems.

National Institute on Aging, Building 31, Room 5C27, 31 Center Drive, MSC 2292, Bethesda, MD, 20892, (301) 496-1752, Fax: (301) 496-1072, (800) 222-2225, http://www.nia.nih.gov.

The NIA is the agency within the U.S. National Institutes of Health that provides research, training, health information dissemination, and other programs related to aging and older people. It is the primary federal agency for Alzheimer's disease and publishes research and information on mental health and exercise for seniors.

National Institute of Mental Health, Science Writing, Press, and Dissemination Branch, 6001 Executive Boulevard, Room 8184, MSC 9663, Bethesda, MD, 20892-9663, (301) 443-4513, Fax: (301) 443-4279, (866) 615-6464, nimhinfo@nih.gov, http://www.nimh.nih.gov.

The NIMH is the agency within the U.S. National Institutes of Health with primary responsibility for understanding and treating mental illnesses through basic and clinical research, with the goal of prevention, recovery, and cures.

Substance Abuse and Mental Health Services Administration, Health Information Network, P.O. Box 2345, Rockville, MD, 20847-2345, Fax: (240) 221-4292, (877) SAMHSA-7 (726-4727), SAMHSAInfo@samhsa.hhs. gov, http://www.samhsa.gov.

SAMHSA's mission is to reduce the impact of substance abuse and mental illness on American communities. Its work focuses on eight strategic initiatives for improving lives impacted by substance abuse and mental illness.

Margaret Alic, Ph.D.

Metabolic equivalent of tasks

Definition

Metabolic equivalent of tasks (METS), which is sometimes shortened to metabolic equivalents, is a standard measure in physiology used to denote the physical intensity involved while exercising at different intensities for various physical activities. METS are calculated as the ratio of the work metabolic rate (rate of energy consumption during a specific physical activity) to the resting metabolic rate (rate of energy consumption while sleeping). This plural form is sometimes stated in its singular form: metabolic equivalent of task (MET).

Purpose

METS are measures of the amount of oxygen used by the body during various types of activities or exercises. The term MET is used to express an individual's metabolic rate while performing some type of task based on that person's resting metabolic rate. The resting MET is measured as 1. That is, 1 MET is the amount of energy (as determined from the mount of oxygen inhaled) used by the body at rest. Activities considered to be resting include sitting quietly on a chair and reading a book while lying on a bed.

However, when more strenuous (non-resting) activities are pursued, such as walking at about 3 mi. (4.8 km) per hour, **bicycling** on flat terrain, and mowing the grass with a push mower, more energy is expended by the body and, thus, more oxygen is inhaled by the body. Then, when such activities occur, MET values are higher. The METS for various non-resting tasks range from 1.5 to 18.0.

KEY TERMS

Calorie—A unit used to indicate the potential to produce energy within the human body; although the term "calorie" (small calorie) is used commonly, it actually refers to "kilocalorie" (large calorie), where one kilocalorie is equal to 1,000 calories.

Carbon dioxide—A chemical compound composed of two oxygen atoms bonded to a single carbon atom; with chemical formula CO_2.

Energy—The ability (capacity) to do work.

Ergometer—A device for measuring work performed.

Metabolic—Referring to the processes in which nutrients are converted into energy for a living organism to sustain life.

Oxygen—An odorless, colorless gas and an element with the symbol "O" (atomic number 8 and chemical formula O_2), which is essential for respiration within most living beings, such as humans.

Demographics

Anyone can use METS to determine the intensity of a workout or for everyday activities around the house. When METS are used, calories per hour can be determined for a weight-loss program or to gauge intensity levels for a particular fitness level desired.

Description

The various values for METS were first standardized within the *Survey of Activity, Fitness, and Exercise (SAFE Study—1987 to 1989)*. Called the Compendium of Physical Activities, they were developed by Dr. Bill Haskell, from Stanford University (California). Originally, Dr. Haskell created a five-digit code that identified the category (heading) of physical activity (the first two digits) and the type of activity (the last three digits). For example, "01010" referred to "01" for "bicycling" and "010" stood for "bicycling at less than 10 miles per hour, leisure, to work or for pleasure." The first version of the Compendium was published in 1993 and the last update to it was published in 2011.

The MET is a unit of standard metabolic equivalent used to estimate an individual's metabolic rate while performing some type of task based on that person's resting metabolic rate (RMR). Two well known measures of RMR, which is also denoted as 1 MET, are the consumption of (1) 1 kilocalorie (kcal) per kilogram (kg) of body weight per hour (h) and (2) 3.5 milliliters (ml) of oxygen (O_2) per kilogram (kg) of body weight per minute (min). MET values range from 0.9 MET when sleeping to 18.0 MET when running at 10.9 mi. (17.5 km) per hour.

The value of 1 MET is the base metabolic equivalent of task, or the metabolic rate of a person who is at rest. The amount of energy expended for any activity is measured in METS, which are multiples of a person's base metabolic rate (1 MET).

A value of 3 MET to 6 MET is considered to be "moderate" physical activities. Moderate (low-intensity) physical activity is generally determined to be any activity that causes the heart rate or breathing to increase. Such activities usually burn 3.5 to 7.0 calories (cal) per minute (kcal/min).

Any MET values from 7 to 18 are considered "vigorous" physical activities. Examples of vigorous (high-intensity) activities are playing a strenuous game of tennis, doing demanding calisthenics, snow skiing down a hill, water skiing on a lake, and swimming competitive laps in a pool. When such levels are attained breathing and heart rates are rapid and the body is forced to expend quite a bit of energy to perform such activities. Vigorous physical activities expand 8.0 or more calories per minute, however this value may vary depending on fitness level, weight, age, and other such factors.

For instance, a man who is horse riding has a MET of about 3.5, meaning that his metabolic rate is 3.5 times than his resting metabolic rate. A woman who is backpacking, and has a 7 MET, means that her metabolic rate is seven times higher than her resting rate. METS for other activities include:

- active skindiving, 16.0 MET
- rigorous pedaling a stationary bicycle, 12.5 MET
- running at a pace of 8 mi. (12.9 km) per mile, 12.5 MET
- running at 12 mi. (19.4 km) per hour, 8.5 MET
- playing racquetball, 8.0 MET
- jogging at 6 mi. (9.7 km) per hour, 8.0 MET
- playing a game of basketball, 7.0 MET
- aerobic dancing, 6.0 MET
- performing gymnastics, 5.5 MET
- walking at 4 mi. (6.5 km) per hour on level, firm surface, 5.0 MET

- bicycling at 24 mi. (38.7 km) per hour, 5.0 MET
- doing calisthenics, 4.5 MET
- playing volleyball, 4.0 MET
- walking at 2 mi. (3.2 km) per hour on level, firm surface, 2.0 MET
- resting, 1.0 MET
- sleeping, 0.9 MET

Preparation

An Exercise Metabolic Test is one way to determine factors relating to MET. During the test, a person will exercise on a treadmill or a bicycle that is attached to an ergometer (a device for measuring work performed). The participant is hooked to a breathing device and gas analyzer. The operator of the equipment has the participant increase their level of exercise intensity, which causes the consumption of oxygen to increase. When the oxygen level does not rise further, but the exercise intensity level continues to increase, then the gas analyzer will determine the VO_2max, or the maximum (max) volume (V) of oxygen (O_2).

The test shows how an individual responds to physical activity at different levels of intensity. The equipment also produces some of the following statistics: calories burned per minute while exercising; percent of calories from fat, carbohydrates, and protein; volume (V) of carbon dioxide (CO_2) exhaled (VCO_2); and heart rate. The test is used for people who have breathing concerns such as shortness of breath, desire to lose (or gain) weight, or want to know their peak performance level.

Risks

There are no known medical risks for using metabolic equivalent of tasks. However, MET values are based on a large sample of people representing an even much larger population. Therefore, these values are average values and may vary depending on differences within individuals, such as fitness level; age; speed, intensity, and conditions while exercising; and other such factors.

Results

By knowing one's MET value for a particular exercise, it is possible to estimate the number of calories that will be burned while participating in physical activities. To calculate the number of calories burned: multiply the BMR by the activity's MET value. For instance, a man (11) who weighs 170 lb. (77 kg) and is walking at 2 mi. (3.2 km) per hour on a level surface

(2.0 MET) would expend the following number of calories for this activity each hour (24 hours per day): 170 x 11 ÷ 24 x 2.0 = 155.8 (77 x 11 ÷ 24 x 3.2 = 112.9), or this man will burn approximately 156 (113) calories per hour.

Resources

BOOKS

Bernhardt, Gale. *Training Plans for Multisport Athletes.* Boulder, CO: VeloPress, 2007.

Cheetham, Norman W. H. *Introducing Biological Energetics: How Energy and Information Control the Living World.* Oxford: Oxford University Press, 2011.

Katch, Victor L., William D. McArdle, Frank I. Katch. *Essential of Exercise Physiology.* Philadelphia: Wolters Kluwer/Lippincott Williams & Wilkins Health, 2011.

Meyerhof, Wolfgang, Ulrike Beiseigel, and Hans-Georg Joost, editors. *Sensory and Metabolic Control of Energy Balance.* Dordrecht: Springer, 2010.

Roth, Ruth A. *Nutrition & Diet Therapy.* Clifton Park, NY: Delmar Cengage Learning, 2011.

WEBSITES

The Compendium of Physical Activities. University of South Carolina. http://prevention.sph.sc.edu/tools/compendium.htm (accessed June 17, 2011).

Exercise Metabolic Test: VO2MAX Consumption Test. Rockwell Fitness. http://rockwellfitness.com/?page_id=1106 (accessed June 17, 2011).

Metabolic Equivalents (METs). American Heart Association. http://www.americanheart.org/presenter.jhtml?identifier=3046878 (accessed June 17, 2011).

ORGANIZATIONS

American Dietetic Organization, 120 South Riverside Plz., Ste. 2000, Chicago, IL, 60606-6995, (312) 899-0040, (800) 877-1600, http://www.eatright.org.

American Heart Association, 7272 Greenville Ave., Dallas, TX, 75231, 90245, (301) 223-2307, (800) 242-8721, http://www.americanheart.org.

William A. Atkins, BB, BS, MBA

Metabolism and energy

Definition

Metabolism refers to all of the chemical reactions that take place in a living body to keep that body alive. Metabolic reactions are of two general kinds: catabolic and anabolic reactions. Catabolic reactions are chemical reactions by which nutrients are broken down to produce the energy needed to keep a body alive and active. Anabolic reactions are chemical reactions that result in the formation of complex chemical compounds used to build body parts and for other purposes.

Description

The human body makes use of three types of nutrients in the metabolic reactions it performs: **carbohydrates**, proteins, and lipids. Carbohydrates are complex chemical compounds that consist of carbon, hydrogen, and oxygen, the latter two in the proportion of about two to one (as in H_2O), thus accounting for the expression "hydrate." Starches and sugars are the most common kind of carbohydrates included in the human diet. Starches are large, more complex compounds, accounting for their designation as complex carbohydrates. Sugars are simpler carbohydrates, hence the name simple carbohydrates. The body requires other types of nutrients, such as vitamins and minerals, although these compounds are used primarily as catalysts for catabolic and anabolic reactions, and are not used up in those reactions.

When a person eats carbohydrates, they pass through the **digestive system** into the stomach, where they are broken down into simple sugars, primarily the sugar known as glucose ($C_6H_{12}O_6$). Glucose, also known as "blood sugar," then passes through the stomach walls into the bloodstream, where it is transported to cells throughout the body. The primary means by which the human body produces energy is the breakdown of glucose within cells, a process known as glycolysis. When glucose breaks down, it produces carbon dioxide and water, as indicated by the following equation:

$$C_6H_{12}O_6 > 6\ CO_2 + 6\ H_2O$$

glucose   carbon   water
           dioxide

This equation is somewhat deceptive since the breakdown of glucose does not occur in a single step. Instead, the process involves a complex series of more than 30 individual reactions. In the first set of those reactions, the six-carbon glucose molecule is broken down into a three-carbon molecule called acetyl coenzyme A (CoA). Acetyl CoA then feeds into a series of reactions known as the Krebs cycle or the tricarboxylic acid cycle, a series of reactions that produce an energy-rich compound known as adenosine triphosphate (ATP). ATP is the key chemical compound that stores and provides energy for many chemical reactions needed to keep a human body alive and active. Energy is provided by the breakdown of ATP molecules to adenosine diphosphate (ADP). ATP is a very unstable molecule that spontaneously breaks down into ADP and a burst of energy very rapidly, the human body must produce ATP continuously in order to keep up with its energy needs.

Under most circumstances, the process of glycolysis depends on the availability of oxygen, accounting for the fact that these reactions are aerobic (with oxygen) reactions. On occasion, the body is not able to obtain oxygen fast enough for these reactions to continue. On such occasions, a back-up mechanism is available by which the body can continue to produce energy using substances other than oxygen. These reactions are known as anaerobic (without oxygen) reactions. Anaerobic metabolism is truly an emergency form of energy production for the human body for two reasons. First, the energy yield from anaerobic metabolism is much less than it is for aerobic metabolism, two molecules of ATP for each molecule of glucose for anaerobic metabolism versus 36 molecules of ATP per molecule of glucose for aerobic metabolism. Also, the main by-product of anaerobic metabolism is a compound called lactic acid or lactate. Lactic acid irritates human muscle tissue, so the longer anaerobic metabolism continues, the more lactic acid builds up in muscles, and the greater the discomfort associated with any form of activity. The sore muscles a person experiences in association with various types of **exercise** are caused by the action of lactic acid on muscle tissue.

The human body can obtain energy from nutrients other than carbohydrates. The next most important source of energy in the body is the family of compounds known as lipids, primarily **fats** and oils. When a person ingests fats and oils, they pass through the digestive system into the small intestine, where they are broken down into simpler compounds known as fatty acids and glycerol. These compounds then pass through cell walls into the bloodstream, where they are carried to cells for metabolism. As with carbohydrates, fatty acids go through a complex series of reactions that result in the formation of acetyl CoA and ATP. Lipids are actually a much richer source of energy than are carbohydrates, providing more than twice as much energy per gram than do carbohydrates. The body relies on its lipid sources of energy for long-term sources of energy compared to its carbohydrate sources, which are used for short-term energy needs. Proteins can be metabolized to produce energy also. **Protein** oxidation normally only contributes a small amount to whole body substrate oxidation (less that 5%) but may increase up to 10% depending on duration of activity and energy balance. Protein oxidation will be greater as the duration of exercise increases, particularly when there is low carbohydrate availability. Amino acid oxidation can be influenced by training and nutritional status. The branch chain amino acids are catabolized as a fuel source by contracting skeletal muscle. They are oxidized to form acyl CoA that can be converted to acetyl CoA for entry into the TCA cycle and respiratory chain.

Function

The course of metabolic reactions has significance for exercise and sport activities. The breakdown of ATP provides an immediate burst of energy over a very short period of time, usually no more than about three seconds. At that point, a secondary metabolic reaction takes over in which a substance known as creatine phosphate (CP) begins to produce additional ATP. That reaction lasts a very short period of time, no more than about seven seconds. When supplies of both ATP and CP become insufficient, another source of energy is required. Because the total time during which ATP and CP are available is so short, they provide the energy needed for very short exercises, such as a 100-m dash. A runner who continues beyond 100 m relies on the body to move to the next source of energy.

Anaerobic glycolysis is the next source of energy. During this process glucose is converted to carbon dioxide, water, and energy. This process is not very efficient, but it is available quickly, usually within a matter of seconds. Anaerobic metabolism continues until a point is reached at which lactic acid is being produced more rapidly by muscle cells than it can be removed by the blood. This point is known as the lactate threshold (LT), or lactate inflection point (LIP). Beyond the lactate threshold, lactic acid begins to accumulate in the blood, an event that not only causes discomfort for the athlete, but also interferes with efficient functioning of muscle tissue. Anaerobic metabolism is able to provide the energy required for activities that involve short bursts of energy, such as the brief shifts of about 60 seconds expected of **ice hockey** players. After a brief rest (for hockey players, about three or four minutes), their bodies have recovered sufficiently to allow aerobic metabolism to take over energy production once more.

QUESTIONS TO ASK YOUR DOCTOR

- Is there a special kind of diet you recommend for someone participating in sports that require short, intense bursts of energy, such as ice hockey and sprint racing?
- What exercises can you recommend for improving a person's lactate threshold?
- What view do you hold about the use of an exercise program in improving one's overall metabolic rate?

The energy needed for longer, more sustained exercise comes primarily from aerobic metabolism. Aerobic metabolism is a very efficient method for producing energy, especially compared to anaerobic metabolism. However, it takes much longer to develop, primarily because the oxygen needed by cells for aerobic metabolism must be transported from the lungs to the cells, a process that can take a few minutes. Aerobic metabolism is the primary (but not exclusive) method of energy production used by athletes who must continue to function over long periods of times, such as long distance runners.

Trainers and conditioners take into consideration known scientific information about metabolism to develop exercises that help athletes improve their bodies' ability to function at maximum efficiency. For example, **interval training** involves a sequence of exercises that push the body to its lactate threshold, provide a short period of rest, and then repeat an exercise. The purpose of this exercise is to improve the body's ability to exceed the lactate threshold and produce a burst of energy for a somewhat longer period of time before a rest period is needed.

Role in human health

Discussions of metabolism focus on two different aspects of the topic. First, the human body has to process nutrients at some given rate simply to stay alive. That is, cells, tissues, and organs need a constant supply of energy just to keep fundamental chemical reactions going in the body. The rate at which metabolism must occur for this basic level of functioning is known as the basic metabolic rate (BMR). Scientists measure a person's BMR by determining the rate at which oxygen is consumed or carbon dioxide is produced when a person is completely at rest. Any activity performed by a person

KEY TERMS

Aerobic—Reactions that occur in the presence of oxygen.

Anabolism—Chemical reactions that occur in cells by which new body parts are constructed.

Anaerobic—Reactions that occur in the absence of oxygen.

Basal metabolism rate—The rate of metabolism needed just to keep a body alive and functioning.

Catabolism—Chemical reactions in cells by which compounds are broken down to produce energy.

Complex carbohydrates—Chemical compounds consisting of carbon, hydrogen, and oxygen of high molecular weight, such as starch and cellulose.

Glycolysis—The series of reactions by which glucose is broken down to produce carbon dioxide, water, and energy.

Inborn errors of metabolism—Metabolic disorders caused by a genetic error.

Lactate threshold—The point in aerobic metabolism at which lactic acid is being produced more rapidly by muscle cells than it can be removed by the blood.

Simple carbohydrates—Chemical compounds consisting of carbon, hydrogen, and oxygen or lower molecular weights, such as disaccharide and monosaccharide sugars.

beyond this most fundamental resting level requires an increased rate of metabolism. For example, a person playing tennis for an hour will need to increase her or his metabolic rate far beyond the basal metabolic rate.

A team of researchers led by Edward Melanson at the University of Colorado at Denver in 2009, studied the effects on the BMR of a group of 65 volunteers who engaged in various forms of exercise. The group included moderately active people who engaged in both low intensity and high intensity cycling; endurance athletes, such as competitive runners and triathletes; sedentary individuals, both obese and of normal weight; and older men and younger men. The results obtained for all experimental groups were essentially the same: Beyond the immediate increase in BMR as a direct result of the exercise, no effects on BMR beyond a 24-hour period could be detected. Therefore, exercise is not an effective means for increasing an individual's BMR beyond its current level.

This information is important because many people try to lose weight by finding a way to use up one's food stores (the fat in one's body) faster than they are replenished. Experts who advise people about losing weight almost always suggest that they increase their level of exercise. A regular program of exercise makes a person healthier overall; but it is increasingly clear that just exercising by itself has limited effect on one's weight, because it does not affect one's BMR. Some weight may be lost during an exercise, but the weight will not continue to be lost because of an increased metabolic rater after the exercise has been completed. The key to **weight loss** is to reduce the intake of

nutrients, so that excess nutrients are not stored in the body as fatty tissue.

Common diseases and disorders

Any medical condition that occurs because of an error in metabolism is called a metabolic disorder. Some metabolic disorders occur because of genetic factors and are known as inborn errors of metabolism. Others develop as the result of disease or damage to the body after birth. Most metabolic disorders occur because an excess of some critical chemical is produced in the body or because an insufficient amount of a chemical is produced. An example of an inborn error of metabolism is the condition known as phenylketonuria (PKU). Children born with PKU lack an enzyme normally present in the body that breaks down the amino acid phenylalanine. Lacking that enzyme, phenylalanine begins to accumulate in the body, where it damages brain tissue, leading to mental retardation and related issues. Fortunately, PKU can be controlled rather easily by excluding from an affected person's diet any foods that may contain phenylalanine. Diabetes is a disorder that results when the pancreas does not produce sufficient amounts of insulin or the body does not properly respond to insulin that is available. Other familiar metabolic disorders include:

- hyperthyroidism
- hyperthyroidism
- hypogylcemia
- Cushing's syndrome
- glucose intolerance
- lactose intolerance

- galactosemia
- hyperlipidemia
- hypolipidemia
- gout
- cystic fibrosis
- homocystinuria

Resources

BOOKS

Lamb, David R., and Carl V. Gisolfi. *Energy Metabolism in Exercise and Sport*. Traverse City, MI: Cooper Publishing Group, 2003.

Wolinsky, Ira, and Judy A. Driskell. *Sports Nutrition: Energy Metabolism and Exercise*. Boca Raton, FL: CRC Press, 2008.

PERIODICALS

Bassami, Minoo, et al. "Effects of Mixed Isoenergetic Meals on Fat and Carbohydrate Metabolism during Exercise in Older Men." *Journal of Nutrition and Metabolism* (2011).

Griffin, Bruce A. "Lipid Metabolism." *Surgery* 27, no. 1 (January 2009): 1–5

WEBSITES

Freeman, Scott. "Activity 6.1: Glucose Metabolism." *Biological Science*. Prentice-Hall, 2003. http://wps.prenhall.com/esm_freeman_biosci_1/0,6452,498583-,00.html (accessed November 23, 2011).

Ophardt, Charles E. "Overview of Metabolism." *Metabolism/Energy Overview*. Virtual Chembook, 2003. http://www.elmhurst.edu/~chm/vchembook/5900verviewmet.html (accessed November 23, 2011).

ORGANIZATIONS

American College of Sports Medicine, 401 W. Michigan St., Indianapolis, IN, 46202-3233, (317) 637-9200, Fax: (317) 634-7817, http://www.acsm.org/AM/Template.cfm?Section = Contact_ACSM&Template = /Custom Source/Department/index.cfm&area = general, http://www.acsm.org.

David E. Newton, AB, MA EdD

METS *see* **Metabolic equivalent of tasks**

Military fitness tests

Definition

Military fitness tests are tests used by the United States armed forces to assess the physical fitness of individuals in the military.

Description

Military fitness tests are used by the armed forces to monitor the physical fitness of their forces and ensure a minimum level of fitness for all individuals in the military. Each branch of the military has its own set of requirements for the test, and each has a separate set of passing scores. Passing scores are different for men and women, and are broken down by **age** group. For example, a 50 year-old woman would need to do fewer sit-ups to receive a passing score than a 20-year-old man.

Each of the branches of the military: the Army, Navy, Air Force, and Marines, has a slightly different set of requirements for their military fitness test. Special elite units such as the Army Rangers or the Navy Seals often have higher threshold criteria required for passing scores on the tests. Typically, if an individual does not pass the fitness test, he or she is required to do additional physical training and may not be eligible for promotion.

Military fitness tests typically consist of push-ups, sit-ups, and a timed distance run. The number of sit-ups and push-ups, and the minimum time for the run vary by branch, age, and gender. Individuals are awarded points for the number of repetitions completed in a certain amount of time, and for the speed of completion of the run. In some cases, individuals must get a minimum score on each section, and in others, they must achieve an average minimum score to pass.

Some branches require additional sections for their fitness tests. The Navy requires a 1,476-ft. (450-m) swim in addition to curl ups, pull-ups, and a 1.5-mi. (3.3-km) run. In some cases a timed period on a stationary bike or elliptical machine during which a minimum number of **calories** must be burned can be substituted for the run portion of a test.

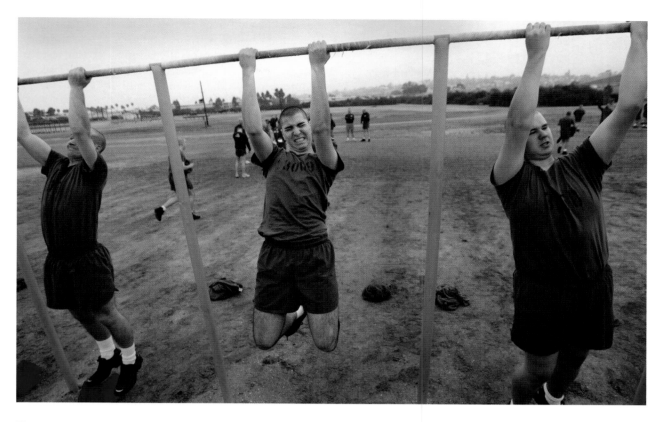

Three men do pull-ups as part of a fitness test. (© *Huy Nguyen/Dallas Morning News/Corbis*)

Purpose

The purpose of military fitness tests is to determine the fitness level of individuals in the military. When used by non-military individuals the tests have two main purposes. The first is to determine fitness level in a way that allows the individual to compare him or herself to the members of the military. The second use of a military fitness test by non-military individuals is as a goal. Passing a military fitness test requires a moderate-to-high level of physical fitness. Having a goal of passing such a test gives the individual a specific and concrete goal to work towards.

Risks

Military fitness tests are very strenuous. It is extremely important that individuals do not undertake a military fitness test if they are not in good physical health or do not have a high level of fitness. Anyone considering attempting a military fitness test should first consult a physician. Beginning a strenuous **exercise** regime can increase the chance of a heart attack or stroke, especially in individuals with a sedentary lifestyle. Beginning a new fitness regimen slowly and

incrementally increasing the duration or strenuousness of the physical activity over time can reduce these risks.

Military fitness tests require a variety of different athletic activities. Many of these have their own risks. These include risks of strains and sprains, especially of the ankle and knee during the **running** portions of the tests. As with all strenuous physical activity, there is a risk of **dehydration** if adequate fluid consumption is not maintained for the duration of the test.

Benefits

Military fitness tests have a variety of benefits. They allow individuals to compare their fitness level to the fitness levels of individuals in the armed forces. Military fitness tests also provide a concrete fitness goal. Having a concrete goal can make it easier to maintain an exercise regime over time.

Anyone who can successfully complete a military fitness test is in excellent shape. Being fit and exercising regularly has a wide variety of health benefits. Regular exercise has been found to decrease the risk of heart disease, high **blood pressure**, and type 2 diabetes. It has even been found to reduce the risk of some cancers and decrease the likelihood that an individual develops dementia, such as Alzheimer's, later in life.

Preparation

Preparation for a military fitness test is similar to preparation for any very strenuous athletic activity. It is important to stretch all major muscle groups prior to beginning the test, to help reduce the risk of strains and sprains. The individual should make sure to have plenty of water to drink prior to the test.

When training for a military fitness test, it is recommended that the individual begin by doing a few of each required activity, and slowly build up stamina over time. It is generally more effective to work a little on each activity, instead of focusing on one activity at a time. For example, it would be more effective to run a short distance, and do some pull-ups and some sit-ups each day, instead of just running or just doing pull-ups.

Aftercare

Aftercare for a military fitness test is similar to that for any other strenuous workout. The individual should **cool down** slowly and make sure to stretch every major muscle group. It is important to make sure to drink enough fluids after extreme exertion such as when completing a military fitness test. Water is excellent for **hydration**. Commercial products such as Gatorade contain electrolytes that can help restore balance to the body by replacing electrolytes lost through sweat. **Energy drinks** and drinks with added sugars should be avoided.

Certification and training

Only a specially trained member of the armed forces can officially administer a military fitness test. However, because the guidelines for passing are made available to the public by the various branches of the military, individuals can unofficially administer the tests to themselves and compare their results to the scores required to pass the test in the military.

Resources

BOOKS

Porterfield, Jason. *Your Career in the Army*. New York: Rosen, 2012.

Reiman, Michael P., and Robert C. Manske, *Functional Testing in Human Performance*. Champaign, IL: Human Kinetics, 2009.

Thompson, Walter R., ed. *ACSM's Guidelines for Exercise Testing and Prescription*. Philadelphia: Lippincott Williams and Wilkins, 2010.

PERIODICALS

Swain, David P., et al. "Effect of Training With and Without a Load on Military Fitness Tests and Marksmanship." *Journal of Strength and Conditioning Research* 25, no. 7 (July 2011): 1857–1865.

WEBSITES

Smith, Stew. "Ace Any Military PFT." http://www.military.com/military-fitness/fitness-test-prep/physical-fitness-test-standards (accessed August 1, 2011).

Tennent, Jeremy. "Soldiers Prepare for New Army Physical Fitness Test." http://www.army.mil/article/62578/ (accessed August 1, 2011).

ORGANIZATIONS

Aerobics and Fitness Association of America, 15250 Ventura Boulevard, #200, Sherman Oaks, CA, 91403, (877) 968-7263, http://www.afaa.com.

American Council on Exercise, 4851 Paramount Dr., San Diego, CA, 92123, (888) 825-3636, http://www.acefitness.org.

Tish Davidson, AM

Mindful eating

Definition

Mindful eating is an approach to food and nutrition that is one of several applications of mindfulness practice to health issues. One group of contemporary psychologists has defined mindfulness as "a kind of nonelaborative, nonjudgmental, present-centered awareness in which each thought, feeling, or sensation that arises in the attentional field is acknowledged and accepted as it is." Mindfulness has two dimensions: a focus on immediate experience rather than past or future issues; and an attitude of curiosity, openness, and acceptance of the present moment rather than a judgmental attitude. Applied to food and eating, mindfulness implies learning to detach from the strong emotions associated with specific foods, dieting, weight control, and body image, and making conscious choices about eating rather than falling back into reactive, emotion-driven, or automatic eating patterns.

Some dietitians describe mindful eating as focusing on the actual acts involved in food preparation and meal consumption rather than multitasking while cooking or eating. The theory underlying this definition of mindful eating is that distractions caused by such other activities as reading, watching television, or working at the computer while eating interfere with the body's messages to the brain about satisfaction with the food and fullness, thus, increasing the risk of overeating.

Purpose

Mindful eating grew out of research carried out since 1980 of the effects of mindfulness practice on a range of health issues, including stress-related illness, depression, anxiety, chronic pain, and heart disease. As of 2011, mindful eating is considered a complementary alternative medicine (CAM) approach to the treatment of **obesity**, type 2 diabetes, and **eating disorders**.

Demographics

There are no statistics available as of 2011 as to how many people in North America have tried or presently practice mindful eating, most likely because the approach is still relatively new.

History

Mindfulness as a meditative practice originated in Buddhism, and has been taught in the West by such psychologists as Jack Kornfield (1945–) and Joseph Goldstein (1944–). The application of mindfulness practice to clinical illness, however, is usually credited to Jon Kabat-Zinn (1944–), the founding director of the Stress Reduction Clinic and the Center for Mindfulness in Medicine, Health Care, and Society at the University of Massachusetts Medical School. Kabat-Zinn's 1991 publication of *Full Catastrophe Living: Using the Wisdom of Your Body and Mind to Face Stress, Pain, and Illness*, a paperback book intended for the general public, aroused interest in the application of mindfulness practice to such concerns as eating disorders and obesity as well as chronic pain and traumatic injury, Kabat-Zinn's original focus.

Description

There is no single overall program for mindful eating. The practice of mindful eating involves a combination of approaches including research, support, and communication with support professionals and peers.

General principles

In general, mindful eating is based on the following components:

- listening to the body's internal cues about hunger and satiety
- identifying personal triggers for mindless eating, such as social pressures, strong emotions, and particular foods
- paying attention to the quality rather than the quantity of one's food
- an appreciation of the sensual or pleasurable as well as the nutritional qualities of food
- an attitude of gratitude for, and appreciation of food

Mindful eating is also individualistic. People who take this approach to food and nutrition are invited to trust their own inner wisdom about food likes and dislikes; to choose foods that are pleasing to their senses as well as nourishing to their bodies; to accept their particular food preferences without judgment; to practice awareness of their body's specific signals to begin eating and stop eating; and to understand that their food preferences and eating experiences are unique to them.

The CAMP system

The CAMP system is a more structured approach to weight management that incorporates mindful eating within a larger framework of self-help psychology and specific strategies for coping with temptations to mindless eating. It places greater emphasis on control and power issues than most other discussions of mindful eating.

CAMP is an acronym for Control, Attitudes, Mindful eating, and Portion Control. Together, these components can help an individual to regain control over food.

- Control: This is based on the assumption that most people have given up control over their food choices and eating habits, allowing outside influences (people, events, emotions) to control how food is consumed and used. For example, how much is eaten, how fast it is eaten, etc.
- Attitudes: Changing the following attitudes can help in regaining control over eating: first, people should see food as a great gift and have respect for it; second,

they should recognize that eating more than they want dishonors food; third, they should not set themselves up for bingeing or overeating by depriving themselves of the foods they really enjoy; fourth, they should stop seeing food as an "enemy" and understand that there are no "bad" foods.

- Mindful eating: Mindful eating has four stages: arriving (noticing that one is in the presence of food and simply observing it); awakening (noticing every aspect of the food—color, texture, smells—before, during, and after eating it; tuning into the body (noticing the movements of hands, mouth, tongue, etc., as well as the level of hunger); and food as service (observing and paying attention to all the activities connected with food purchase, preparation, and serving.

- Portion control: This aspect includes paying attention to the size of each mouthful as well as to the total amount of food on the plate. It includes such strategies for portion reduction as saving half of the food on the plate for later and intentionally leaving some of the food on one's plate rather than eating it.

An exercise in mindful eating

A common way to introduce the concept of mindful eating to people who are new to it (or to mindfulness practice in general) is an **exercise** in consuming food mindfully. The following exercise is to be done with a friend; one person reads the instructions while the other carries out the steps in the exercise. Participants need two small slices of apple, one for each person.

- Take one bite of the apple slice and close the eyes. Do not begin to chew.
- Focus on the apple rather than on any ideas or thoughts that may be going through the mind. Notice the texture, taste, temperature, and any other sensations in the mouth.
- Begin chewing; chew slowly, paying attention to each small movement of the jaw.
- Try to avoid swallowing the apple; remain in the present moment and focus on the transition from chewing to swallowing.
- Prepare to swallow the apple and notice it moving from the tongue to the back of the throat. Swallow the apple and follow the sensations of the food moving down the esophagus until there are no more sensations of the food remaining.
- Take a deep breath and exhale.

The point of this exercise is not to consume all meals this carefully, but rather to learn more about a person's own eating habits and attitudes toward food.

Other exercises that can be done to practice mindfulness while eating include:

- Eating with chopsticks rather than the usual Western knife, fork, and spoon.
- Chewing each bite of food 30–50 times.
- Eating with the left hand if right-handed, with the right hand if left-handed.
- Eating while sitting down at a table rather than eating while standing up or while driving a car.
- Trying to make the meal last at least 20 minutes.
- Eating without looking at a book, magazine, television, or computer.

Preparation

Preparation for mindful eating requires a basic understanding of mindfulness practice in general and mindful eating in particular. It also involves practicing mindfulness during all activities involved in food purchasing, storage, cooking, and service, as well as mindfulness during the meal itself.

Risks

There are no known risks to practicing mindful eating, and no reports of malnutrition or other health problems arising from this approach as of 2011.

As with any CAM therapy or treatment, people considering mindful eating should consult their primary care physician. They may also wish to consult a dietitian, as the public health/community nutrition dietetic practice group (DPG) of the American Dietetic Association (ADA) has recommended that its members incorporate mindful eating into their nutritional counseling.

A person under medical supervision for type 2 diabetes, eating disorders, or obesity should consult their doctor while practicing mindful eating. A dietitian knowledgeable about this approach to food and nutrition may provide additional nutritional education and counseling.

Results

Research studies on mindful eating report that it is helpful in treating some obese patients seeking to lose weight, some older adults diagnosed with binge eating disorder, and some college students diagnosed with eating disorders. There are, however, no large population studies that have reported on the effectiveness of mindful eating compared to **weight loss** surgery or other mainstream approaches to weight management as of 2011.

Fewer than two dozen articles about mindful eating have been published in mainstream medical journals as of 2011, probably because this approach to eating and nutrition is considered a CAM form of therapy and is less than 20 years old. As of 2011, there are two clinical studies of mindful eating seeking participants. One is for pregnant women surrounding behaviors relating to healthy weight gain during pregnancy. The other, is a study examining small changes and lasting effects on eating behavior for overweight or obese individuals. Individuals who wish to participate or learn more about these clinical trials can find more information at http://clinicaltrials.gov. There is no cost to the patient to participate in a clinical trial.

Mindful eating is intended to be a lifelong approach to food and nutrition that can be extended to other aspects of a person's life.

Resources

BOOKS

Albers, Susan. *Eat, Drink, and Be Mindful: How to End Your Struggle with Mindless Eating and Start Savoring Food with Intention and Joy.* Oakland, CA: New Harbinger Publications, 2008.

Bays, Jan Chozen. *Mindful Eating: A Guide to Rediscovering a Healthy and Joyful Relationship with Food.* Boston, MA: Shambhala, 2009.

Cheung, Lilian W.Y. *Mindful Eating, Mindful Life: Savour Every Moment and Every Bite.* New York: Hay House Publishing, 2011.

Gauding, Madonna. *The Mindfulness Diet: Using Mindfulness Techniques to Heal Your Relationship with Food.* East Sussex, UK: Ivy Books, 2010.

Hanh, Thich Nhat, and Lilian Cheung. *Savor: Mindful Eating, Mindful Life.* New York: HarperOne, 2011.

Somov, Pavel G. *Eating the Moment : 141 Mindful Practices to Overcome Overeating One Meal at a Time.* Oakland, CA: New Harbinger Publications, 2008.

PERIODICALS

Framson, C., et al. "Development and Validation of the Mindful Eating Questionnaire." *Journal of the American Dietetic Association* 109 (August 2009): 1439–44.

Hammond, M. "Mindful Eating: Tuning In to Your Food." *Diabetes Self-Management* 24 (March-April 2007): 36–40.

Lavender, J.M., et al. "Bulimic Symptoms in Undergraduate Men and Women: Contributions of Mindfulness and Thought Suppression." *Eating Behaviors* 10 (December 2009): 228–31.

Mathieu, J. "What Should You Know about Mindful and Intuitive Eating?" *Journal of the American Dietetic Association* 109 (December 2009): 1982–87.

WEBSITES

Beck, Melinda. "Putting an End to Mindless Munching." *Wall Street Journal* (May 13, 2008): D1. http://online.wsj.com/public/article/SB121062985377986351-L2sPVaRuoMPJ_RQV6vkIKsr5AA8_20080611.html?mod=tff_main_tff_top (accessed November 13, 2011).

Bishop, Scott R., et al. "Mindfulness: A Proposed Operational Definition." *Clinical Psychology: Science and Practice* 11 (Fall 2004): 230–241. http://www.personal.kent.edu/~dfresco/mindfulness/Bishop_et_al.pdf (accessed November 13, 2011).

Bly, Terri, et al. "Exploring the Use of Mindful Eating Training in the Bariatric Population." *Bariatric Times* (December 2007). http://bariatrictimes.com/2007/12/10/exploring-the-use-of-mindful-eating-training-in-the-bariatric-population/ (accessed November 13, 2011).

Fred Hutchinson Cancer Research Center. "Regular Yoga Practice Is Associated with Mindful Eating." *Science News Daily* (August 3, 2009). http://www.sciencedaily.com/releases/2009/08/090803185712.htm (accessed November 13, 2011).

Hammond, Megrette. "Ways Dietitians Are Incorporating Mindfulness and Mindful Eating into Nutrition

Counseling." *The Digest* (Fall 2007). http://www.tcme.org/documents/PH_Fall2007_Final.pdf (accessed November 13, 2011).

Principles of Mindful Eating. The Center for Mindful Eating. http://www.tcme.org/principles.htm (accessed November 13, 2011).

Vangsness, Stephanie. "Mastering the Mindful Meal." Brigham and Women's Hospital. (October 2009). http://www.brighamandwomens.org/healththeweightfor women/special_topics/intelihealth0405.aspx (accessed November 13, 2011).

ORGANIZATIONS

American Dietetic Association, 120 South Riverside Plz., Ste. 2000, Chicago, IL, 60606-6995, (800) 877-1600, http://www.eatright.org.

American Society for Metabolic and Bariatric Surgery (ASMBS), 100 SW 75th St., Ste. 201, Gainesville, FL, 32607, (352) 331-4900, Fax: (352) 331-4975, info@asmbs.org, http://www.asmbs.org.

CAMP System, c/o DayOne Publishing, PO Box 676, Charlotte Hall, MD, 20622, (301) 753-DAY1, DayOnePublishing@aol.com, http://www.mindfuleating.org.

Center for Mindful Eating, http://www.tcme.org.

Center for Mindfulness in Medicine, Health Care, and Society, University of Massachusetts Medical School, Chang Building, 222 Maple Ave., Shrewsbury, MA, 01545, (508) 856-2656, Fax: (508) 856-1977, mindfulness@umassmed.edu, http://www.umassmed.edu.

National Institute of Diabetes and Digestive and Kidney Diseases (NIDDK), Bldg. 31, Rm 9A06, 31 Center Dr., MSC 2560, Bethesda, MD, 20892-2560, (301) 496-3583, http://www2.niddk.nih.gov.

National Institutes of Health (NIH), 9000 Rockville Pike, Bethesda, MD, 20892, (301) 496-4000, http://www.nih.gov.

U.S. National Library of Medicine, 8600 Rockville Pike, Bethesda, MD, 20894, http://www.nlm.nih.gov/medlineplus/medlineplus.html.

Rebecca J. Frey, PhD
Laura Jean Cataldo, RN, EdD

Moderate vs. vigorous intensity training

Definition

Numerous health organizations, including the World Health Organization, American Heart Association, and the American College of Sports Medicine endorse a minimum of 30 minutes of moderate-intensity aerobic activity on most days of the week, or 20 minutes of vigorous-intensity activity on three days of the week, or a combination of both. In healthy adults aged 18-65 years of **age**, moderate-intensity aerobic activity commonly equates to a brisk walk and should noticeably increase heart rate. Comparatively, in older adults (i.e., men and women age 65 years and older and adults age 50-64 years with clinically significant chronic conditions and/or functional limitations) moderate-intensity aerobic activity corresponds to a 5 or 6 on a 10-point scale, where 0 equates to **sitting** and 10 equates to an all-out physical effort. The physiological symptoms associated with 5 or 6 (i.e., moderate-intensity **exercise**) include a modest, but noticeable, increase in heart rate and breathing. In healthy adults vigorous-intensity aerobic activity generally includes activities such as jogging and should elicit marked increases in heart rate and rapid breathing. By comparison, for older adults, vigorous-intensity activity corresponds to a 7 or 8 on a 10-point scale. Vigorous-intensity activities in the older adult segment of the population produce large increases in breathing and heart rate.

Purpose

Exercise prescription is founded upon the F.I.T.T. principle; this acronym stands for exercise frequency, exercise intensity, exercise time, and exercise type. The most critical component of the exercise prescription model is arguably exercise intensity. Failure to meet minimal threshold values may result in lack of a training effect, while too high of an exercise intensity could lead to over-training and negatively impact adherence to an exercise program. Moreover, moderate- and vigorous-intensity exercise stress physiological systems differently; it is to be expected that training adaptations vary depending on the type of exercise intensity being performed. Accordingly, the goals of an exercise program should factor into the target exercise intensity—moderate, vigorous, or a combination of both.

Demographics

In 2009, just over one-third (35%) of American adults met current physical activity recommendations with 33% reporting no leisure-time activity. The prevalence of adults fulfilling physical activity guidelines is higher in non-Hispanic whites compared to non-Hispanic blacks, Hispanics, or other racial/ethnic groups. The prevalence of both moderate-intensity physical activity and vigorous-intensity physical activity is higher in men compared to women. Older men and women are less active in terms of either moderate- or vigorous-physical activity compared to their younger counterparts.

Description

Target ranges for moderate- and vigorous-intensity exercise can be established using several methods; these include percentage of maximal heart rate (HR_{max}), percentage of heart rate reserve (HRR), metabolic equivalents (METS), rating of perceived exertion (RPE), and percentage of maximal oxygen uptake reserve (VO_2R). The ranges for the different classifications of moderate-intensity exercise are:

• HR_{max}: 64-76%
• HRR: 40-59%
• METs: 3-6 METs
• RPE: 5 to 6 on a 10-point scale
• VO_2R: 40-59%

Common activities that are usually classified as moderate-intensity include **bicycling** on even terrain at 10 mph (16 km/h), **walking** at 3.0 mph (4.8 km/h), carrying/stacking wood, mowing the lawn with a push mower, and **golf** (walking and carrying own clubs).

The ranges for the different classifications of vigorous-intensity exercise are:

• HR_{max}: 77-93%
• HRR: 60-84%
• METs: <6 METs
• RPE: 7 to 8 on a 10-point scale
• VO_2R: 60-84%

Common activities that are usually classified as vigorous-intensity include **bicycling** on even terrain at 12-14 mph (19-22 km/h), walking at 4.5 mph (7 km/h), carrying heavy loads such as bricks, playing a **basketball** game, and competitive **volleyball** (gym or beach).

Preparation

Participation in either moderate- or vigorous-intensity exercise is relatively safe for most individuals. Nevertheless, older individuals and/or those with chronic diseases may be at increased risk for an adverse event during exercise. The incorporation of health assessments and medical history questionnaires can be useful in identifying conditions, risk factors, signs, and symptoms that are coupled with an increased risk of a cardiac event during exercise. In particular, risk stratification schema is beneficial in identifying those individuals who require further medical screening and exercise testing prior to engaging in vigorous-intensity exercise. The process of risk stratification assigns individuals into one of three risk categories (low, moderate, or high) based on the following factors:

• presence or absence of known cardiovascular, pulmonary, and/or metabolic disease
• presence or absence of signs or symptoms suggestive of cardiovascular, pulmonary, and/or metabolic disease
• presence or absence of cardiovascular disease risk factors

Individuals categorized as low risk are have no signs or symptoms of, nor have they been diagnosed with, cardiovascular, pulmonary, and/or metabolic disease. These individuals also possess no more than one **cardiovascular disease** risk factor. Low risk-stratified individuals have minimal risk for an acute cardiovascular event during exercise. This population can safely participate in either moderate-intensity or vigorous-intensity exercise.

Individuals categorized as moderate risk are those who have no signs or symptoms of, nor have they been diagnosed with, cardiovascular, pulmonary, and/or metabolic disease. However, these individuals possess two or more cardiovascular disease risk factors. Moderate risk-stratified individuals have an elevated risk for an acute cardiovascular event during exercise. Although it is appropriate for these individuals to begin a moderate-intensity exercise program, prior to engaging in vigorous-intensity exercise it is recommended that they first undergo a medical examination and complete a physician supervised exercise test.

Individuals categorized as high risk are those who have one or more signs or symptoms of, or have been diagnosed with, cardiovascular, pulmonary, and/or metabolic disease. High risk-stratified individuals have a substantial risk for an acute cardiovascular event during exercise. It is strongly recommended that prior to engaging in either a moderate-intensity or vigorous-intensity exercise program these individuals first undergo a medical examination and complete a physician supervised exercise test.

Risks

Despite the fact that regular exercise confers numerous health benefits and protects against various age-related chronic diseases, an increased risk of both cardiac and muscle-skeletal complications is associated with vigorous-intensity exercise. It is important to understand the risks related with exercise and how they can be reduced. The most common exercise-related complication is muscle-skeletal injury. The incidence of injury increases with exercise intensity. There is a minimal risk of muscle-skeletal complications linked to walking and other types of moderate-intensity physical activities. Conversely, risk of injury is elevated during vigorous-intensity activities such as

Autonomic control—The combined influence from the sympathetic and parasympathetic nervous system on controlling involuntary functions of the body; for example, heartbeat.

Cardiovascular disease risk factors—Physiological parameters whereby exceeding threshold values places one at an increased risk for developing cardiovascular disease. The specific risk factors used for risk stratification by the American College of Sports Medicine include age, family history for heart disease, high cholesterol, hypertension, obesity, physical inactivity, pre-diabetes, and smoking.

Co-morbidities—The presence of one or more disorders or diseases in addition to the primary disease; for instance an individual with cardiovascular disease and hypertension, obesity, and Parkinson's disease.

Cool down—A 5 to 10 minute period of low-intensity activity following the conditioning phase.

Energy expenditure—The collective energy cost for maintaining constant conditions in the human body plus the amount of energy required to support daily physical activities.

F.I.T.T. principle—An acronym that represents exercise frequency, exercise intensity, exercise time, and exercise type.

Heart rate reserve (HRR)—The difference between maximal heart rate and resting heart rate.

Insulin resistance—A condition where normal physiological concentrations of insulin become insufficient at lowering and maintaining normal blood sugar levels.

Maximal heart rate (HR$_{max}$)—The maximal heart rate that can be elicited in an individual during intense exercise or exertion. This value can either be estimated

(most commonly using 220-age) or directly measured from a maximal exercise test.

Maximal oxygen uptake reserve (VO$_2$R)—The difference between maximal oxygen uptake and resting oxygen uptake.

Metabolic equivalents (METs)—A single MET equals the amount of energy expenditure during one minute of seated rest. In terms of oxygen uptake, 1 MET equates to 3.5 mL/kg/min.

Myocardial infarction—A heart attack. Refers to changes to the heart tissue, with tissue death the principal one, due to sudden disruptions in oxygenated blood flow.

Rating of perceived exertion (RPE)—A subjective rating by an individual of their perception of exercise intensity.

Risk stratification—A pre-exercise screening process by which individuals at increased risk for an acute cardiac event are identified and subsequently referred for additional medical screening prior to starting an exercise program.

Sympathetic drive—The influence of increased impulses from the sympathetic nervous system.

Sudden cardiac death—Abrupt and unexpected death due to cardiac causes; usually death occurs within one hour of the onset of symptoms.

Thrombosis—The formation or presence of a blood clot in the vasculature.

Vagal tone—The impulses from the vagus nerve that contributes to a reduced heartbeat.

Warm up—A 5 to 10 minute period of low-intensity activity preceding the conditioning phase.

jogging. Similarly, muscle-skeletal problems are more pronounced with those individuals who participate in competitive sports.

There is an increased risk of myocardial infarction (heart attack) and sudden cardiac death that may be prompted by sudden and unfamiliar vigorous-intensity exercise. The most at-risk individuals include sedentary men and women with underlying clinical conditions or known heart disease; in particular this risk is exacerbated in individuals with co-morbidities (i.e., multiple chronic conditions such as **hypertension** and Type 2 diabetes) and when severe environmental conditions (e.g., hot and humid) are present. Vigorous-intensity

activities such as racquet sports, **running**, and strenuous sporting endeavors are linked with a greater incidence of cardiovascular events. Overall risk is diminished in these instances when the individual performs greater volumes of regular exercise. Numerous strategies may be employed to further attenuate risk; these include performing an exercise warm up and **cool down**, **stretching**, and gradual progression of exercise intensity from moderate-intensity to vigorous-intensity.

Results

It is appropriate for an individual to participate in either moderate-intensity exercise, vigorous-intensity exercise, or a combination of both in an effort to fulfill current physical activity guidelines. It is also important to consider whether participation in vigorous-intensity exercise yields greater benefits compared to moderate-intensity exercise. In order to address this issue, the total volume of exercise **energy expenditure** is controlled when comparing the difference in health outcomes between moderate- and vigorous-intensity exercise training programs. Reports that have examined the vigorous vs. moderate topic, while simultaneously controlling for **energy** expenditure, conclude that vigorous-intensity exercise is superior in terms of risk reduction for cardiovascular disease and mortality from all causes. Furthermore, important cardiovascular disease risk factors, including insulin resistance and low cardiorespiratory fitness, respond more favorably to vigorous-intensity aerobic exercise compared to moderate-intensity aerobic exercise.

It is unclear what exact physiological mechanisms are responsible for the more beneficial effects of vigorous-intensity exercise. The greatest benefit accrued from vigorous-intensity exercise may be the larger improvements in cardiorespiratory fitness. It has been proposed that for each 1 MET increase in cardiorespiratory fitness there is an accompanying reduction in mortality from cardiovascular disease and all-causes by 8–17%. The fact that vigorous-intensity exercise produces more favorable changes in cardiorespiratory fitness relative to moderate-intensity exercise would help to explain why vigorous-intensity exercise would be more cardio-protective. It has been suggested that autonomic control is improved following vigorous-intensity exercise training compared to moderate-intensity exercise training. Enhanced autonomic control would result in decreased sympathetic drive coupled with increased vagal tone at rest. Collectively, these physiological adaptations positively impact **blood pressure**, thrombosis, and additional features linked to heart risk.

Resources

BOOKS

Ehrman, Jonathan K., editor. *ACSM's Resource Manual for Guidelines for Exercise Testing and Prescription.* Philadelphia: Lippincott Williams & Wilkins Health, 2010.

Katch, Victor L., William D. McArdle, Frank I. Katch. *Essentials of Exercise Physiology.* Philadelphia: Wolters Kluwer/Lippincott Williams & Wilkins Health, 2011.

Thompson, Walter R., editor. *ACSM's Guidelines for Exercise Testing and Prescription.* Philadelphia: Lippincott Williams & Wilkins Health, 2010.

PERIODICALS

Garber, C.E., et al. "Quantity and Quality of Exercise for Developing and Maintaining Cardiorespiratory, Musculoskeletal, and Neuromotor Fitness in Apparently Healthy Adults: Guidance for Prescribing Exercise." *Medicine and Science in Sports and Exercise* 43, no. 7 (July 2011): 1334–59.

WEBSITES

Compendium of Physical Activities. Arizona State University, Healthy Lifestyles Research Center. http://www.sites.google.com/site/compendiumofphysical activities/home (accessed August 20, 2011).

Physical Activity Fact Sheets. National Coalition for Promoting Physical Activity. http://www.ncppa.org/resources/factsheets/ (accessed August 20, 2011).

ORGANIZATIONS

American College of Sports Medicine, 401 W. Michigan St., Indianapolis, IN, 46206-1440, (317) 637-9200, Fax: (317) 634-7817, http://www.acsm.org.

American Heart Association, 7272 Greenville Ave., Dallas, TX, 75231, (301) 223-2307, (800) 242-8721, http://www.heart.org.

Centers for Disease Control and Prevention, 1600 Clifton Rd., Atlanta, GA, 30333, (800) 232-6348, cdcinfo@cdc.gov, http://www.cdc.gov.

National Coalition for Promoting Physical Activity, 1100 H St., NW, Ste. 510, Washington, DC, 20005, (202) 454-7521, Fax: (202) 454-7598, http://www.ncppa.org.

Lance C. Dalleck, BA, MS, PhD

Muscle cramp

Definition

A muscle cramp is an involuntary contraction or spasm occurring suddenly to one or more skeletal muscles. They usually occur after exercising or during the night and can last anywhere from a few seconds to several minutes.

Description

A muscle cramp often occurs after long periods of **exercise** or other physical activity, especially in hot weather. Although muscle cramps are generally harmless, they can make it impossible to use the affected muscle for a temporary period of time. Muscle cramps may affect any muscle, but are most common in the calves, feet, and hands. They usually disappear on their own and rarely require medical attention. However, you should seek medical care if they happen frequently, do not improve with self-care, cause severe pain and discomfort, or are not associated with exercise.

The terms cramp and spasm are vague for most, and they are sometimes used to include types of abnormal muscle activity other than sudden painful contraction, including slow muscle relaxation, stiffness at rest, and spontaneous contractions of a muscle at rest or fasciculation. A muscle spasm is different than a muscle twitch. A muscle twitch or fasciculation is uncontrolled fine movement of a small segment of a larger muscle that can be seen under the skin. Fasciculation is a type of painless muscle spasm, marked by rapid, uncoordinated contraction of many small muscle fibers. Distinguishing the different meanings and symptoms allows the patient to describe the problem to their physician for a better diagnosis.

Types of muscle cramps

There are four types of skeletal muscle cramps: true cramps, tetany, contractures, and dystonic cramps:

- True cramps involve part or all of a single muscle or a group of muscles that generally act together, such as the muscles that flex several adjacent fingers. Most researchers agree that true cramps are caused by hyperexcitability of the nerves that stimulate the muscles. They are overwhelmingly the most common type of skeletal muscle cramps.

- Tetany occurs when all of the nerve cells in the body are activated, which then stimulate the muscles. This reaction causes spasms or cramps throughout the body. The name tetany is derived from the effect of the tetanus toxin on the nerves. However, the name is now commonly applied to muscle cramping from other conditions, such as low blood levels of calcium and magnesium. Oftentimes, tetanic cramps are indistinguishable from true cramps

- Contractures occur when the muscles are unable to relax for an even more extended period than a common muscle cramp. The constant spasms are caused by a depletion of adenosine triphosphate (ATP), an energy chemical within the cell. This prevents muscle fiber relaxation. The nerves are inactive in this form of muscle spasm.

- Dystonic cramps occur when muscles that are not needed for the intended movement are stimulated to contract. Muscles that are affected by this type of cramping include those that ordinarily work in the opposite direction of the intended movement, and/or others that exaggerate the movement. Some dystonic cramps usually affect small groups of muscles (eyelids, jaws, neck, larynx, etc.). The hands and arms may be affected during the performance of repetitive activities such as those associated with handwriting (writer's cramp), typing, playing certain musical instruments, and many others. Each of these repetitive activities may also produce true cramps from muscle fatigue. Dystonic cramps are not as common as true cramps.

Demographics

Muscle cramps or spasms can occur at any **age** but they are more common in older children and teenagers who are young (adolescent age) participating in organized, competitive sports and strenuous aerobic activities and older (over 65) people. Just about everyone will experience a muscle cramp sometime in life. It can happen while playing **tennis**, **golf**, **swimming** or exercising. It can also occur while you sit, walk, or even just sleep. Often the slightest movement that shortens a muscle can trigger a cramp.

Some people are predisposed to muscle cramps and get them regularly with physical exertion. Those at greatest risk for cramps and other ailments related to excess heat include infants and young children, people over age 65, and those who are ill, overweight, overexert during work or exercise, or take drugs or certain medications.

Muscle cramps are very common among endurance athletes, including **marathon** runners and triathletes, as well as older people who perform strenuous physical activities. Athletes are more likely to get cramps in the preseason when the body is not conditioned and, therefore, more subject to **fatigue**. Cramps often develop near the end of intense or prolonged exercise, or 4-6 hours later. Older people are more susceptible to muscle cramps due to normal muscle loss (atrophy) that begins in the mid-40s and accelerates with inactivity. As the body ages, muscles cannot work as hard or as quickly as they used to. The body also loses some of its sense of thirst and its ability to sense and respond to changes in temperature.

Causes and symptoms

Although the exact cause of muscle cramps is unknown, some researchers believe inadequate **stretching** and muscle fatigue leads to abnormalities in mechanisms that control muscle contraction. Other factors may also be involved, including poor conditioning, exercising, or working in intense heat.

Muscle cramps can be caused by the overuse of a muscle, **dehydration**, pregnancy, heavy exercise, **muscle strain**, a lack of minerals in the diet or the depletion of salt and minerals in the body, not enough blood getting to the muscles, or simply holding the same position for an extended period of time. They can also be caused by a sudden involuntary contraction of a muscle or muscles. It is uncommon for cramps to be due to a serious underlying disorder. In most cases, the cramp goes away within a few minutes. Some rare causes of muscle cramps are drugs such as lithium, alcohol, and inflammatory disorders such as polymyositis, and tetanus. Muscle cramps are also part of certain conditions such as nerve, kidney, thyroid or hormone disorders; diabetes; hypoglycemia; and anemia.

Symptoms of muscle cramps include intense, localized, and often debilitating pain that comes on quickly and may last for seconds or minutes, fading gradually. Another symptom is a hard lump of muscle tissue that can be felt or is visible beneath the skin. Contractures develop more slowly, over days or weeks, and may be permanent if untreated. Fasciculation may occur at rest or after muscle contraction and may last several minutes.

Muscle cramps may accompany other symptoms that vary depending on the underlying disease, disorder or condition. Symptoms that frequently affect the muscles may also involve other body systems. Exercising in high temperatures can lead to dehydration, another symptom of muscle cramps. Dehydration symptoms include dry mouth or tongue, increased or excessive thirst, few or no tears when crying, decreased urination, dark yellow urine, irritability, low **energy**, lightheadedness or fainting, severe weakness, and sunken abdomen, eyes and cheeks. Muscle cramps may accompany other symptoms affecting the muscle including, burning feeling, lump in the cramping muscle, **muscle pain** that may be severe and sharp, muscle weakness, and twitching.

Diagnosis

A usual bout of muscle cramps should not require a visit to the doctor. However, medical treatment is

---

KEY TERMS

Charley horse—A common name for a muscle spasm, usually occurring in the leg.

Contraction—The shortening and thickening of a functioning muscle or muscle fiber.

Contracture—A tightening or shortening of muscles that prevents normal movement of the associated limb or other body part.

Dehydration—Excessive loss of water from the body or from an organ or body part, as from illness or fluid deprivation.

Electrolytes—The ionized salts present in body fluids that play an important role in functioning of the human body. Electrolyte levels in blood plasma and urine are often used as diagnostic tools.

Fasciculation—Involuntary contractions or twitchings of groups of muscle fibers. Fasciculations can occur in normal individuals without an associated disease or condition and can also occur as a result of illness, such as muscle cramps, nerve diseases, and metabolism imbalances.

Motor neuron—A nerve cell that specifically controls and stimulates voluntary muscles.

Muscle spasm—Localized muscle contraction that occurs when the brain signals the muscle to contract.

Myotonia—The inability to normally relax a muscle after contracting or tightening it.

Nocturnal leg cramps—Cramps that may be related to exertion and awaken a person during sleep.

---

essential if any symptoms of dehydration are associated with the muscle cramps. In addition, any abnormal contractions or frequent muscle cramps or spasms that cause concern should be evaluated by a physician. Abnormal muscle contractions are diagnosed through a careful medical history, as well as a physical and neurological examination. In some cases, when a structural abnormality is suspected, x rays may be performed. The medical history helps the physician to evaluate the presence of other conditions or disorders that might contribute to or cause the abnormal contractions. Records of previous diagnoses, surgeries, and treatments will also be reviewed. The family medical history is evaluated to determine if there is a history of muscular or neurological disorders.

Treatment

Most cases of simple cramps require no treatment other than patience and stretching. When heat cramps occur, stop the activity, move to a cool or shady place, remove excess clothing, drink cool water or a sports drink with electrolytes, such as Gatorade, and rest. If nausea or dizziness occur, lie down, with feet slightly elevated. Gently and gradually stretching and massaging the affected muscle may ease the pain and hasten recovery. Briefly applying cold packs to cramped muscles, for about ten minutes, may also help ease pain. Acetaminophen (such as Tylenol) or ibuprofen (such as Advil or Motrin) should be used sparingly for relief of discomfort. If prolonged or recurrent cramps that disturb sleep occur, medication to relax the muscles can be prescribed by a doctor.

Cramps may be treated or prevented with gingko (*Ginkgo biloba*) or Japanese quince (*Chaenomeles speciosa*). Supplements of vitamin B_{12}, folate, vitamin E, niacin, calcium, and magnesium may also help. Taken at bedtime, they may help to reduce the likelihood of night cramps

Prognosis

In most cases, muscle cramps are relatively mild and resolve within a few minutes. Despite being a temporary discomfort, they are a benign condition. Their importance is limited to the discomfort and inconvenience they cause, or to the diseases associated with them. Careful attention to them will greatly diminish the problem of cramps for most individuals. Those with persistent or severe muscle cramps should seek medical attention.

Prevention

The best way to prevent muscle cramps is avoid dehydration by drinking plenty of liquids daily. The exact amount will depend on an individual's diet, sex, level of activity, the weather, health, age, and any medications currently being taken. Fluids help muscles contract and relax and keep muscle cells hydrated and less irritable. Fluids should be replenished after physical activity. Stretching muscles before and after use is another way to prevent muscle cramps. If cramps occur at night, stretch before bedtime. Stretching is recommended before and after for cramps that are caused by vigorous physical activity. An adequate **warm-up** and cooldown before and after activity can help prevent muscle cramps. Adequate **hydration** before, during, and after physical activity is important, especially if the duration exceeds one hour, and replacement of electrolytes (especially sodium and potassium, which are major components of perspiration) can also be helpful. Excessive fatigue, especially in warm weather, should be avoided. Supplemental calcium and magnesium have each been shown to help prevent cramps associated with pregnancy. Drinking water before bedtime can also alleviate night cramps.

QUESTIONS TO ASK YOUR DOCTOR

- What causes muscle cramps?
- Does metformin cause severe muscle cramps, especially in the legs and feet?
- Is there a difference between muscle contractions and muscle spasms?
- What is the best treatment for muscle cramps?
- Can poor circulation cause muscle cramps?
- How can I prevent muscle cramps from occurring?

Resources

BOOKS

Brinker, M.R., et al. "Basic Science and Injury of Muscle, Tendon, and Ligament." In *DeLee and Drez's Orthopaedic Sports Medicine*, 3rd ed., edited by J.C. DeLee, D. Drez Jr., and M.D. Miller. Philadelphia Saunders Elsevier; 2009.

Fauci, Anthony S., et al. *Harrison's Principles of Internal Medicine.* 17th ed. United States: McGraw-Hill Professional, 2008.

Filho, J.A.F., and A. Pestronk. "Chapter 28: Muscle Pain and Cramps." In *Neurology in Clinical Practice,* 5th ed., edited by Walter G. Bradley, et al. Philadelphia: Butterworth-Heinemann.

PERIODICALS

Schwellmus, M.P. "Muscle Cramping in Athletes: Risk Factors, Clinical Assessment, and Management." *Clinics in Sports Medicine* 27 (2008): 183.

ORGANIZATIONS

American Academy of Orthopaedic Surgeons, 6300 North River Rd., Rosemont, IL, 60018-4262, (847) 823-7186, http://www.aaos.org.

National Institute of Arthritis and Musculoskeletal and Skin Diseases (NIAMS), Fax: 301-718-6366, 877-226-4267, 1 AMS Circle, Bethesda, MD, 20892-3675, (301) 495-4484, http://www.niams.nih.gov.

Karl Finley

Muscle hypertrophy

Definition

Muscle hypertrophy is the increase in size (mass and cross-sectional area) of muscle cells. Muscle hypertrophy is different from muscle hyperplasia, which refers to an increase in the number of muscle cells.

Description

Skeletal muscles have two primary functions in the body: (1) to move bones in order to walk, run, turn around, wink, smile, lift objects, push objects away, and perform other functions, and (2) to maintain posture. All skeletal muscles are composed of bundles of muscle fibers (muscle cells) which, in turn, consist of hundreds or thousands of smaller structures called myofibrils. A single myofibril is a long, thin, spaghetti-like thread consisting of alternating sections called sacromeres. Myofibrils are composed of other long, thin filaments made of two different kinds of **protein**, actin and myosin. Actin filaments are thinner than myosin filaments. The arrangement of myosin and actin filaments is such that they are able to slide back and forth next to each other. When they slide in one direction, the myofibril contracts, pulling opposite ends of the muscle fiber toward each other. As they contract, the muscle fibers also pull the bones to which they are attached, making possible some type of motion. When myosin and actin filaments slide in the opposite direction, the myofibril expands to its original size, allowing the bones to which they are attached to return to their original position.

Muscle cells are genetically programmed to increase in size to adjust to additional stresses placed upon them. Individual skeletal muscle cells accustomed to lifting no more than 44 lb. (20 kg) have a particular size and shape. If those muscle cells were then used to lift somewhat heavier masses, such as a 55-lb. (25-kg) mass the cells grow in mass and cross-sectional area in an amount proportional to the new stress placed upon them. This process is known as hypertrophy. Scientists do not yet understand all the details as to how these changes in muscle cells occur. It appears that additional stress on muscle fibers triggers a change in the rate at which actin and myosin proteins are formed in muscle cells. The additional actin and myosin proteins formed by this process add to existing myofibrils, increasing either their width or length, or

KEY TERMS

Actin—A protein that occurs in muscle fibers.

Atrophy—Wasting away of tissues.

Myofibrillar hypertrophy—An increase in muscle size because of the addition of actin and myosin proteins to myofibrils.

Myofibril—A long, thin, spaghetti-like strand of actin and myosin that constitutes the basic structure of muscle tissue.

Myosin—A protein that occurs in muscle fibers.

Sarcoplasmic hypertrophy—An increase in muscle size resulting from an accumulation of fluid in the interior of muscle cells.

both. The larger muscle fibers thus formed are able to exert greater forces of contraction than were their predecessors.

Some authorities believe that damage to muscle fibers is an essential part of hypertrophy. They point to the fact that muscle tissue contains a number of biological and chemical agents, such as various types of growth hormone and steroid hormones, that are programmed to respond to torn or damaged muscle fibers. If a person intentionally damages muscle tissue by exercising it too much, those natural agents respond by building new muscle tissue that results in bulkier muscles. The extent to which tissue damage is a necessary component of muscle hypertrophy is still a matter of some dispute.

Function

Participants in almost every sport are interested in increasing their strength, although that objective differs among sports. For **football** and **ice hockey** players, for example, strength is an essential part of being a top-notch player. Although strength is important in other sports, such as **golf** and **tennis**, it probably does not rank as high as in contact events. For this reason, muscle hypertrophy exercises are an important aspect of training and conditioning regimes in most sports. The precise exercises included in such a regime are, however, important. The reason is that some forms of **exercise** result in tissue damage that leads to an accumulation of the cytoplasmic fluid within muscle cells called sarcoplasm. Sarcoplasmic hypertrophy, then, occurs when muscle cells swell up because they contain more fluid, not because their structure has changed to increase muscle strength. Sarcoplasmic hypertrophy is common among bodybuilders whose regime consists of many lifts in a single session. After the first few lifts, protein production has already increased to its maximum level for some given lift mass, and continuing to lift only increases muscle damage associated with the accumulation of fluid. By contrast, limiting lifts to just the number of repetitions required to initiate additional protein synthesis results in an actual increase in muscle size, a process known as myofibrillar hypertrophy.

Role in human health

Many discussions of muscle hypertrophy focus on its role in training and conditioning for individual and team sports. But hypertrophic training can be of considerable value to individuals of almost any **age** and physical condition. For the average person, even a marginal increase in muscle strength can have many advantages that lead to a healthier, more productive life. Increased muscle strength improves one's balance, endurance, and work capacity as well as increasing one's overall strength. Having a more sculptured body may also increase one's self-esteem.

Hypertrophic training is recommended for the elderly. As a person grows older, his or her muscles have a tendency to atrophy, decrease in size. Loss of muscular strength has some real disadvantages, such as reducing one's ability to maintain a stable posture, which can lead to falls and other accidents. Muscular atrophy can also lead to a kind of series of health problems as one is less able to move about and care for herself or himself easily, leading to further atrophy of muscles. Trainers do not generally expect that the elderly will become enthusiastic body builders or

weight lifters, but even modest levels of hypertrophic activities can lead to significant improvement in muscle strength that contribute to leading a healthier and longer life.

Common diseases and disorders

There appear to be no significant health risk associated with the proper execution of a well designed hypertrophic exercise program. Individuals who go beyond the limitations of a hypertrophic plan, however, may experience problems resulting from over exertion of their bodies.

Resources

BOOKS

Poliquin, Charles. *Modern Trends in Strength Training*. San Diego: QFAC Bodybuilding, 2001.

Tsatsouline, Pavel. *Power to the People: Russian Strength Training Secrets for Every American*. St. Paul, MN: Dragon Door Publications, 2000.

PERIODICALS

Ahtiainen, et al. "Muscle Hypertrophy, Hormonal Adaptations and Strength Development During Strength Training in Strength-trained and Untrained Men." *European Journal of Applied Physiology* 89, no. 6 (2003): 555-563.

Goto, K., et al. "Muscular Adaptations to Combinations of High- and Low-intensity Resistance Exercises." *Journal of Strength & Conditioning Research* 18, no. 4 (2004): 730-737.

Schoenfeld, B. J. "The Mechanisms of Muscle Hypertrophy and Their Application to Resistance Training." *Journal of Strength & Conditioning Research* 24, no. 10 (2010): 2857-2875.

West, D., N. Burd, A. Staples, and S. Phillips. "Human Exercise-mediated Skeletal Muscle Hypertrophy Is an Intrinsic Process." *The International Journal of Biochemistry & Cell Biology* 42, no. 9 (2010): 1371-1375.

WEBSITES

Hernandez, Joshua, and Len Kravitz. "The Mystery of Skeletal Muscle Hypertrophy." http://www.unm.edu/~lkravitz/Article%20folder/hypertrophy.html (accessed August 14, 2011).

"Muscular Hypertrophy." **Personal Evolution**. Endless Human Potential. http://www.endlesshumanpotential.com/muscular-hypertrophy. html (accessed August 14, 2011).

ORGANIZATIONS

American College of Sports Medicine, 401 West Michigan St., Indianapolis, IN, 46202-3233, (317) 637-9200, Fax: (317) 634-7817, http://www.acsm.org/.

David E. Newton, AB, MA, EdD

Muscle pain

Definition

Muscle pain is a general term that applies to achiness, soreness, and pain of a muscle or muscle group that may range from mild to severe and that may last from a few days to many months. The technical name for muscle pain is myalgia. The term myositis is used to describe inflammation of muscle tissue specifically.

Description

The biochemistry and pathophysiology of muscle pain is complex and not totally understood. Stress on muscle tissue, such as that caused by inflammation, trauma, or overuse, can produce changes in the physical structure and biochemical sensitivity of nociceptors, receptor sites on nerve cells that respond to pain signals. Both the damaged muscle tissue and its associated nerve cells begin to release a number of chemical agents, such as potassium ions, prostaglandins, bradykinin, serotonin, ATP, and substance P that stimulate nociceptors and reduce their sensitivity to additional pain signals. Muscle pain is reduced as the stress causing the pain is eliminated and muscle tissue and nerve cells are allowed to heal and return to their pre-stress status.

The most common type of muscle pain is localized muscle pain, which affects a single muscle or muscle group. Systemic muscle pain is muscle pain that appears to affect all or most of the muscles in a person's body. Systemic muscle pain is usually caused by factors other than trauma or overuse, often by an infection such as fibromyalgia or the use of certain types of drugs, such as statins. For example, the achiness that one often associates with an attack of influenza is not caused by stress on the muscles, but by the infectious agent that causes the flu. By contrast with localized muscle pain, which often resolves relatively easily on its own, systemic muscle pain may be an indication of a more serious medical problem and should prompt a visit to a medical professional.

Demographics

Statistics on the incidence and demographics of muscle pain worldwide are not generally available. The best source of such information on residents of the United States comes from the U.S. Centers for Disease Control and Prevention's (CDC) annual National Health Interview Survey (NHIS). Some of the demographic patterns reported in the most recent version (2009) of that survey include:

- More than a quarter of the adults interviewed (28%) had experienced lower back pain in the three months preceding the survey, compared to 15% who had experienced neck pain during that time and 5% who had experienced face or jaw pain.
- Women were more likely to experience all forms of pain than were men.
- The incidence of pain does not seem to be linearly related to age. For example, neck pain was most common among the 45-64 age group and least common among the 18-44 age group. Lower back pain was most common among those 75 years and older, and least common among the 18-44 age group. Face or jaw pain was most common among the 45-64 age group and least common among those over the age of 75.
- Adults over the age of 44 were more likely to have experienced muscle pain than were respondents under the age of 44.
- The ethnic group reporting the lowest rates of muscle pain in the survey were Asian Americans, followed by American Indian and Alaskan Natives; Whites; Blacks or African Americans; and Native Hawaiians or other Pacific Islanders.
- Adults in families classified as "poor," or "near poor" were significantly more likely to report neck, lower back, and face or jaw pain than were those in higher economic classes.
- Adults with a college degree were less likely to report having muscle pain than were those who had not graduated from high school.
- Adults of all ages who were covered by Medicaid and/or Medicare reported having more episodes of lower back, neck, and face or jaw pain than did those who were covered by private insurance.

Causes and symptoms

The most common causes of localized muscle pain are damage to a muscle, which may include a sprain, strain, or tear of the muscle; overuse of a muscle, as in many types of occupational and recreational activities; and tension or stress, which may cause a person to consciously or unconsciously tighten his or her muscles more frequently and more severely than is normal.

Among the infections and other medical conditions that may cause systemic muscle pain are the following:

- chronic fatigue syndrome
- claudication, a condition caused by a reduction in peripheral blood flow that may occur, especially during exercising and athletics

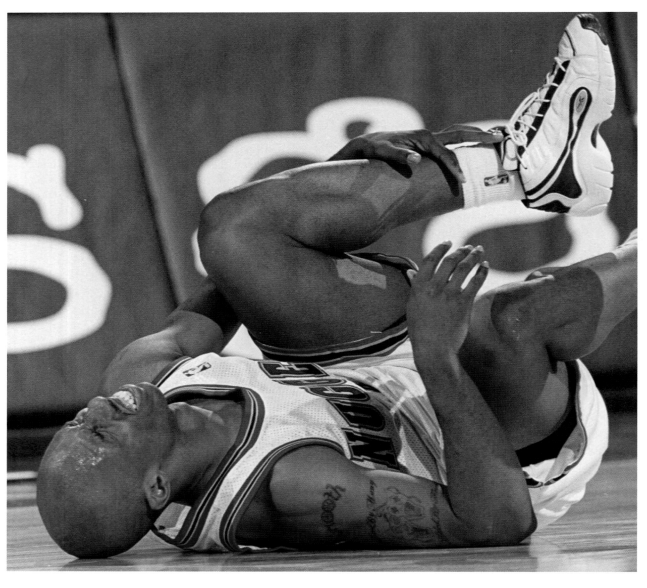

Chauncey Billups, a professional basketball player, experiences the pain of a sprained ankle. (© *AP Images/David Zalubowski*)

- dermatomyositis, a condition whose cause is not known characterized by inflammation of muscle tissue
- lupus, an autoimmune disorder in which the body's immune system attacks its own tissues
- polymyositis, a disease of unknown origin that results in inflammation of muscle tissue
- rhabdomyolysis, a potentially life-threatening condition in which muscle tissue breaks down, releasing harmful products to the kidney
- Rocky Mountain spotted fever
- Staph infections
- viral infections

Diagnosis

Diagnosis for muscle pain begins with a patient medical history that allows a medical professional to determine whether the condition is likely to be a localized or systemic issue. If the patient reports a recent injury to the body area in question or a history of repetitive use for that area, a localized pain issue may be indicated. The medical professional will also ask about other symptoms that may be present in association with the muscle pain, such as chills, fever, sweats, **weight loss**, or nausea, indicating that more serious underlying problems may be involved. Questions

KEY TERMS

ATP—An acronym for adenosine triphosphate, a molecule that provides the energy needed for many biochemical reactions that occur in the body.

Bradykinin—A peptide that causes dilation of blood vessels.

Fibromyalgia—A medical condition characterized by widespread musculoskeletal aches, pain and stiffness, soft tissue tenderness, general fatigue and sleep disturbances.

Myalgia—The technical name for muscle pain.

Myositis—Inflammation of muscle tissue.

Nociceptors—Receptor sites on nerve cells that respond to pain signals.

Prostaglandin—One of a family of lipid compounds that have a variety of functions in the body.

Serotonin—A neurotransmitter that has a variety of effects on a person's physical and mental states.

Substance P—A neuropeptide that functions as a neurotransmitter in the transmission of pain signals in the body.

regarding neurological symptoms, such as tingling, numbness, vision problems, or ringing in the ears may also help determine the precise nature of the pain problem.

A general physical examination may be indicated. In the examination, the medical professional will palpate the body, looking for tender or sore points that may be associated with the pain, and may determine the patient's general muscle tone. Abnormalities in a patient's gait, obvious changes in muscle size, swelling and redness of joints, and coordination problems may be indications of underlying issues related to pain. Finally, blood tests and a variety of imaging tests can be used to further narrow down the range of diseases and disorders that may be responsible for systemic pain symptoms. These tests may include x rays; CAT, MRI, and bone scans; and muscle biopsies.

Treatment

Most cases of localized muscle pain resolve fairly easily with simple home treatment that involves the following elements:

• Application of ice for the first 24–72 hours following onset of the pain. After that period of time switch to heat applied to the sore muscles.

• Use of over-the-counter medications to reduce pain and inflammation associated with muscle damage. Aspirin, acetaminophen, and ibuprofen are the usual drugs of choice.

• Gentle exercising of the sore muscles may help them heal more quickly. Massage is a related form of exercising muscles that is often helpful.

• Adequate amounts of rest and sleep are essential to allow muscle tissue to heal from damage that is causing the pain.

• As healing progresses, the assistance of a physical therapist may help complete the process and, at the same time, provide information about preventing the injury from reoccurring.

• Reduce stress and tension to the degree possible within your life.

Home treatment may be inadequate in dealing with muscle pain, or the conditions associated with the pain may indicate the need for professional medical care. A person should seek immediate care as soon as muscle pain occurs if there is:

• severe muscle pain every time a particular part of the body is used.

• a tick bite or rash associated with the pain.

• reason to believe that serious muscle damage occured, such as a muscle tear or sprain.

• an increase or decrease in muscle pain associated with changes in the use of a medication.

• a stiff neck, a high fever, or vomiting.

• a problem moving any part of the body.

• trouble swallowing or shortness of breath.

Other symptoms that may suggest the need for a visit to a health professional, although not on an emergency basis, include:

• muscle pain lasting more than a week

• swelling or redness in the vicinity of a sore muscle

• weakness or poor circulation in the vicinity of a sore muscle

Prognosis

Because muscle pain has a variety of possible causes, prognosis differs considerably from case to case. Localized muscle pain caused by stress or trauma generally resolves on its own or with simple home treatment in a matter of days. Muscle pain that results from an infection disappears when the underlying infection is itself cured. Muscle pain associated with other causes, such as rhabdomyolysis goes away only when the condition is cured. The corollary to this fact is that pain associated with certain types of diseases and disorders are a part of those conditions and remain as long as the condition itself remains.

Prevention

To the extent that muscle pain is associated with some other underlying condition, such as an infectious disease or reaction to a medication, the pain itself can be prevented only by avoiding the underlying condition, a situation that is often beyond control of an individual. The risk of localized muscle pain caused by stress or trauma, such as that encountered during **exercise** or sporting activities, however, can often be reduced by simple steps. **Stretching** exercises prior to an exercise or athletic event, warming up in other ways before the event and cooling down after the event, and drinking plenty of fluids while participating in the event or the exercise all help to minimize pain from exercise. People who live more sedentary lives, such as those who sit at a desk all day long, can reduce the risk of muscle pains simply by standing and moving about on a regular basis and, where possible, performing some simple stretching exercises.

Resources

BOOKS

Graven-Nielsen, Thomas, Lars Arendt-Nielsen, and Siegfried Mense. *Fundamentals of Musculoskeletal Pain.* Seattle: IASP Press, 2008.

Mense, Siegfried, and Robert Gerwin. *Muscle Pain: Understanding the Mechanisms.* Heidelberg, Germany: Springer, 2010.

PERIODICALS

Cheung, Karoline, Patria Hume, and Linda Maxwell. "Delayed Onset Muscle Soreness: Treatment Strategies and Performance Factors." *Sports Medicine* 33, no. 2 (2003): 145-164.

Whayne, Thomas. "Statin Myopathy: Significant Problem With Minimal Awareness by Clinicians and No Emphasis by Clinical Investigators." *Angiology* 62, no. 5 (2011): 415-421.

WEBSITES

"Myalgia and Myositis." NMIHI.com. July 12, 2011. http://www.nmihi. com/m/myalgia.htm (accessed August 26, 2011).

Vorvick, Linda. "Muscle Aches." MedLine Plus. May 1, 2011. http://www.nlm.nih.gov/medlineplus/ency/ article/003178.htm (accessed August 26, 2011).

ORGANIZATIONS

National Pain Foundation, 300 E. Hampden Ave., Ste. 100, Englewood, CO, 80113, (303) 783-8899, Fax: (303) 692-8414, npf@nationalpainfoundation.org, http:// www.NationalPainFoundation.org.

David E. Newton, AB, MA, EdD

Muscle strain

Definition

A muscle strain is a minor injury to a muscle or an attached tendon usually due to over-stretching, pulling, or tearing of the muscle. It is sometimes called a pulled muscle.

Description

A strain is a twist, pull, or tear of a muscle or tendon (a cord of tissue that connects muscle to bone). It is an acute, non-contact injury that results from over-stretching or putting undue pressure on a muscle. It is difficult to tell the difference between mild and moderate strains but severe strains are more painful and greatly impair the use of that muscle. General muscle aches and pains are normal when starting a new activity or increasing the intensity or duration of **exercise**. This soreness usually lasts one or two days. A muscle strain expresses itself in the same way, only the soreness or pain is stronger and lasts beyond two days. People who engage in sports or fitness activities are especially at risk of muscle injury.

A muscle strain is often classified by physicians based on the severity of the damage:

- Mild strain: Only a few muscle fibers are overstretched or torn; and although the strain may feel sore or painful, the muscle has normal strength.

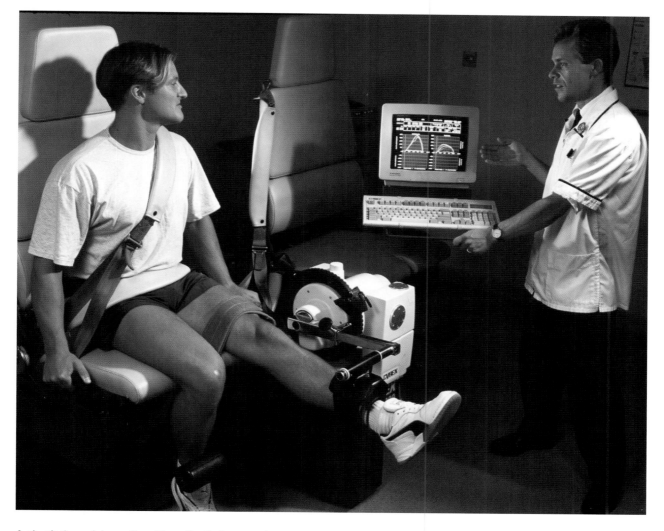

A physiotherapist monitors his patient's leg exercises with a computer generated assessment. *(© Geoff Tompkinson/Photo Researchers, Inc.)*

- Moderate strain: A larger number of fibers are damaged and there is increased pain and soreness, along with mild swelling, occasional bruising, and a noticeable loss of strength.

- Severe strain: An injury that tears through the muscle, sometimes causing a popping or cracking sound or sensation in the muscle. These are serious strains that can cause substantial or complete loss of muscle function along with pain, swelling, bruising, and soreness. There may be an indentation or small dent in the skin where the pieces of injured muscle have torn apart.

Demographics

More than nine million muscle strains occur in the United States each year, half of them requiring doctor visits. More than one-third of muscle strains occur in people ages 25 to 44. Men are 30% more likely to be injured than women. The most common muscle strain is to the ankle; the second most common strain is to the wrist, according to the National Institute of **Arthritis** and Musculoskeletal and Skin Diseases (NIAMS). The most common sports-related strain is to the thumb. Other common strains are to the back, neck, arms, groin, legs, abdomen, and shoulders. Muscle strains are more common in people over age 55 than in younger people, according to the American Association of Retired People (AARP). Nearly all fitness activity, even **walking**, carry some risk of muscle strain. However, they occur most commonly in sports, including **football**, **basketball**, **baseball**, **softball**, **soccer**, **volleyball**, and **tennis**. They occur less frequently in people doing general exercise programs at home or in fitness centers.

Causes and symptoms

Causes

Reasons for muscle strains include excessive physical activity, improper **warm-up** before exercise, and poor flexibility. Muscle strains occur when a muscle is stretched too far and too quickly, causing a slight tear to the muscle and surrounding tissue. Wrist strains usually occur when a person falls and lands on one or both outstretched hands. Leg and ankle strains often come from walking, jogging, **running**, and roller blading. Shoulder strains frequently occur with weight-lifters, and volleyball, tennis and **golf** players.

Symptoms

Signs of a muscle strain include pain, inflammation, swelling, bruising, redness, muscle weakness, or inability to use the muscle at all. Other symptoms include hearing a popping sound when the injury occurs, fever, an open wound caused by the injury, and a lack of pain relief after several days of using over-the-counter pain and anti-inflammation medicines.

Diagnosis

Mild muscle strains are often self-diagnosed while moderate and severe strains are generally diagnosed by a doctor, often a sports medicine or orthopedic specialist. A general examination of the sore or painful area by the doctor is often enough to diagnose mild or moderate muscle sprains. If the doctor suspects a severe strain or other damage, x rays or a magnetic resonance imaging (MRI) scan may be ordered. In Canada, all patients must be referred to an orthopedic surgeon or other specialist by a family physician.

Treatment

Mild strains heal on their own in a few days. Moderate and severe strains usually take several weeks to heal. The first line of strain treatment is rest, ice, compression, and elevation (R.I.C.E.). The affected area should be rested for at least two days and up to a week. If possible, elevate the sprained muscle, such as propping up a leg or arm with pillows, to reduce swelling. Ice, placed in a plastic bag or wrapped in a towel, should be applied to the sprained area for 20 minutes at a time several times throughout the day for up to three days. Compress the strain or sprain by wrapping the sore area with an elastic bandage to give the muscle added support and minimize swelling. Avoid using the strained muscle until the pain or soreness is gone. Over-the-counter, non-steroidal anti-inflammation medications can also be used for pain. These drugs include aspirin, ibuprofen (Advil and Motrin), naproxen (Aleve),

---

and acetaminophen (Tylenol). If the soreness does not improve in a few days or worsens, seek prompt medical treatment. In the most severe cases, surgery to repair the damage may be needed.

Alternative medicine

Alternative medicine treatments for muscle strains include: applying a topical solution of ice cold tofu and rice vinegar; the Chinese herbs yu nan bai yao and shang shi zhi tong gao; using acupressure, acupuncture, and topical treatment with Himalayan crystal salt; and various topical oils, including such as lemon grass, birch, marjoram, and lavender. These treatments are lacking in credible scientific evidence; however, many of them have been used for hundreds of years in Asia.

Prognosis

The duration of a muscle strain or other injury depends on its severity. Symptoms of a mild back strain, such as pain or soreness, usually improve in one to two weeks and should be gone altogether within six weeks. Muscle strains in the legs may take ten weeks or longer to heal. A severe strain may last until it is repaired by an orthopedic surgeon, followed by at least eight weeks of recovery and rehabilitation. A torn rotator cuff muscle can take months to heal, especially if surgery is required. Most muscle strains heal with rest or can be repaired.

Prevention

Stretching plays a vital role in keeping muscles and joints strong and pliable so they are less susceptible to injury. It is an important part of warming up before physical activity and cooling down afterwards to prevent muscle strains. A stretching routine is beneficial

QUESTIONS TO ASK YOUR DOCTOR

- Is my strain or sprain mild, moderate, or severe?
- What type of over-the-counter pain or anti-inflammation medicine do you recommend?
- How long can I expect the soreness or pain to last?
- What treatment options do I have?
- Are there any alternative medicine treatments that you can recommend or suggest?

even if no other exercise or physical activity is done. Preventative measures include:

- Spending at least five to ten minutes warming up and stretching before beginning a sports or fitness activity.
- Designing an exercise program that strengthens and stretches the muscles.
- Increasing the intensity of a sport or activity gradually, giving the muscles time to adapt to the extra work.
- Maintaining a healthy body weight. Being overweight or obese can place too much stress on your muscles when involved in a sport or fitness activity, especially to the leg and back muscles.
- Maintaining good posture while sitting and standing throughout the day, whether at home, work, or the gym.
- Using proper lifting techniques when picking up heavy items, including barbells, dumbbells, and heavy household items.

Resources

BOOKS

Brumfield, Theresa L. *Guide to Muscular Healing.* Bloomington, IN: AuthorHouse, 2010.

Bundy, Mike, and Andy Leaver. *A Guide to Sports and Injury Management.* Burlington, MA: Churchill Livingstone, 2011.

Kovacs, Mark. *Dynamic Stretching: The Revolutionary New Warmup Method to Improve Power, Performance, and Range of Motion.* Berkeley, CA: Ulysses Press, 2009.

Mense, Siegfried, and Robert D. Gerwin. *Muscle Pain: Diagnosis and Treatment.* New York: Springer, 2010.

Wiesel, Sam W., and John N. Delahay. *Essentials of Orthopedic Surgery.* New York: Springer, 2010.

PERIODICALS

Degon, Ryan, and David Wilkenfeld. "Keeping the Shoulder Safe: Protect Your Athletes from Throwing Injuries." *Coach and Athletic Director* (November 2009): 10.

Helland, Lee. "Ache? Pain? Sprain?" *Self* (February 2010): 96.

O'Conner, John. "Inflammation Helps Wounds Heal Faster, Investigators Find." *McKnight's Long-Term Care News* (November 2010): 8.

Rubina, Jessica. "Muscle Pain and Injuries." *Delicious Living* (February 2010): 16.

WEBSITES

Anderson, Owen. "Muscle Soreness & Overuse Injury: Do Questions About Muscle Soreness Hold the Key to Quicker Recoveries?" *Sports Injury Bulletin.* http://www.sportsinjurybulletin.com/archive/muscle-soreness-overuse.html (accessed October 30, 2011).

Gulotta, Lawrence V. *Muscle Injuries: An Overview.* Hospital for Special Surgery. (October 27, 2009). http://www.hss.edu/conditions_muscle-injuries-overview.asp (accessed October 30, 2011).

How Muscles Heal & Recover From Injury. Body In Balance. (December 9, 2010). http://www.bodyinbalance.com/856/muscular-injury-pain-muscle-healing/ (accessed October 30, 2011).

Muscle & Connective Tissue Injuries. Sharecare. http://www.sharecare.com/topic/muscle-connective-tissue-injuries (accessed October 30, 2011).

Muscle Strain. WebMD. http://www.webmd.com/fitness-exercise/muscle-strain (accessed October 30, 2011).

ORGANIZATIONS

American Academy of Orthopaedic Surgeons, 6300 N. River Rd., Rosemont, IL, 60018-4262, (847) 823-7186, Fax: (847) 823-8125, (800) 346-2267, orthoinfo@aaos.org, http://www.orthoinfo.aaos.org.

American Physical Therapy Association, 1111 N. Fairfax St., Alexandria, VA, 22314-1488, (703) 684-2782, Fax: (703) 684-7343, (800) 999-2782, memberservices@apta.org, http://www.apta.org.

Canadian Orthopaedic Association, 4150 St. Catherine St. West, Suite 450, Westmount, Canada, QC, H3Z 2Y5, 1 (514) 874-9003, Fax: 1 (514) 874-0464, (800) 461-3639, mailbox@canorth.org, http://www.coa-aco.org.

National Athletic Trainers' Association, 2952 Stemmons Fwy., Suite 200, Dallas, TX, 75247, (214) 637-6282, Fax: (214) 637-2206, http://www.nata.org.

National Institute of Arthritis and Musculoskeletal and Skin Diseases, 1 AMS Circle, Bethesda, MD, 20892-3675, (301) 495-4484, Fax: (301) 718-6366, (877) 226-4267, NIAMSinfo@mail.nih.gov, http://www.niams.nih.gov.

Ken R. Wells

Muscle toning

Definition

Muscle toning, which is also known as strength training, is a form of **exercise** that increases lean muscle and trains the muscles to work harder. Toning with equipment or body weight causes the body to use **calories** more efficiently, helping a person to control weight.

Purpose

The saying "use it or lose it" is often used in reference to muscle toning. A person's muscles are naturally toned, but muscle function is lost when an individual is **physically inactive**. In addition, there is an increase in body fat. The medical name for this condition is disuse atrophy. Muscle tone is lost through lack of use.

The aging process also brings a loss in muscle strength and flexibility.

The primary remedy for this muscle loss is muscle toning, an activity that is also known as strength training, resistance training, and weight training.

Muscles are bundles of fibers or tissues that contract and expand to produce body movements. Lean muscle is related to body mass, the part of the body that is not fat. Muscle toning focuses on skeletal muscles, which are exercised through resistance training that forces the muscles to contract.

Toning involves repetitions of an exercise while using equipment such as body weight, handheld weights called free weights, weight machines, and resistance bands. The repeated movements are frequently called reps.

Muscle toning is called strength training because the repetitions help to maintain and improve muscle mass. The toning allows the muscles to support the joints. This helps to prevent injuries, strengthen the bones, and provide better balance.

Strength training also helps with **bone health** because aging also brings a loss in bone mass (thickness). In women, menopause causes a rapid decrease in bone density. This places women at risk of **osteoporosis**, a condition characterized by low bone mass and the deterioration of bone tissue. The condition increases the risk of bone fractures. Osteoporosis affects about 25% of women age 60 and older.

In addition, strength training is also known as toning because the activity causes the body to burn calories more efficiently, and body fat is replaced with muscle. This usually produces a **weight loss** as the body becomes toned and firm. The toning is usually first seen in the loss of body fat in the upper arms.

Muscle toning is not body building

Muscle toning differs from muscle building in the goals set and the types of activity performed to reach the goals. Toning increases the tightness of existing muscles and keeps from losing their elasticity.

Muscle building, which is also known as **bodybuilding**, is the process of creating newer, stronger muscles. Toning and bodybuilding involve similar equipment, but the bodybuilder generally uses heavier weights and works out for a longer time than the person who does strength training.

Both people increase the number of reps or use heavier weights to reach their goals. However, women who do muscle toning should not worry about getting bulky muscles. Women do not have enough testosterone, the male hormone that builds bulky muscles.

Furthermore, some people are afraid that muscle toning will cause them to gain weight. The fear is often based on the fact that toning causes the body to use calories more efficiently. When a weight loss results, the toned person may start consuming more calories. Generally, a weight gain occurs only when the individual stops muscle toning and does not reduce the intake of calories.

Demographics

People of all ages can do muscle training activities. For children, the toning is part of physical activities such as climbing on playground equipment. Older children may workout with equipment such as resistance bands.

While strength training should be a regular part of exercise for all people, most adults can begin muscle toning at any age and benefit from improved muscle mass.

History

Throughout history, people did activities to gain muscle strength. Since ancient times, people in Greece and other countries demonstrated their strength at competitions. In the centuries that followed, **weightlifting** competitions were a popular form of entertainment as spectators watched men lift barbells and heavy weights.

Strength was also a matter of survival that kept people physically active. In early times, people actively hunted and gathered food. Over the centuries, families worked on farms; fishermen went to sea and returned with large catches.

During the 20th century, strength training became associated with fitness and health. Much of the credit for this goes to Jack LaLanne, a fitness enthusiast described by *The New York Times* as the "Father of the Modern Fitness Movement." Born in 1914, LaLanne worked out with weights and opened a business in 1936 with a gym, juice bar, and spa in Oakland, California.

His efforts were not well received. Doctors cautioned that working out with weights would result in heart attacks and loss of the sex drive. He found a more receptive audience when the "The Jack LaLanne Show" began airing in San Francisco in 1951. The daytime television program was broadcast nationally from 1959 through 1985.

In 1959, LaLanne successfully marketed the Glamour Stretcher, a rubber stretch cord that was the forerunner of the resistance band. The stretch cord sold with a phonograph album, *Glamour Stretcher Time*. The album provided a workout for women, with LaLanne' instructions accompanied by organ music.

Description

The American College of Sports Medicine (ACSM) recommends that people do strength-training exercises at least two days each week. A workout should consist of 8 to 12 repetitions of from 8 to 10 exercises that target all major muscle groups. The muscle groups that are exercised are the:

- Upper body. Reps work on the front and back of the arms, shoulders, chest, and upper back.
- Torso. Reps focus on the abdominals, the sides of the torso, and lower back.
- Legs. Reps work on the front and back of the thighs, calves, and buttocks.

Muscle toning may be done at home or a gym. Workouts should start with a warm up. Before lifting weights, a 5–10 minute warmup is recommended doing an aerobic activity such as **walking** briskly. Toning movements should be done slowly, and people should remember to breathe when lifting.

Bodyweight or equipment is used for this training. The body is used for exercises such as push-ups, abdominal crunches, and leg crunches.

Free weights

Free weights are hand-held weights that weigh from 3 lb. (1.4 kg) to 150 lb. (68 kg). The barbell is a bar that is from 4 ft. to 6 ft. (122 cm to 183 cm) long. Weights are attached to the ends, or there are slots where weight plates are attached. The barbell is lifted with two hands.

The dumbbell is a single weight that is held in one hand. Some people work out with two weights. A beginner may tone muscles at home with a pair of 3 lb. (1.4 kg) weights. The person could then advance to 5 lb. (2.3 kg) weights.

Weight machine

The weight machine has a bar or handles that are connected to weight plates. The plates weigh from 5 lb. (2.3 kg) to 20 lb. (9 kg), and the person installs a peg in the machine to select the amount of weight that will be lifted. The person sits at the machine and pushes or pulls on the bar or handles to lift the weights. Machines are designed to work on a certain part of the body, so one machine may be used for chest, and another one works on the abdominals.

Resistance bands

Resistance bands made of rubber or elastic work on the same principle as the rubber band. The band is flexible, and does not give any resistance until it is stretched as far as possible. The process is reversed as the stretched band returns to the flexible state. Some bands consist of long sheets of rubber; others have handles on them. The ACSM recommends using bands made of natural rubber latex.

Unlike weights that are measured in pounds or kilograms, there is no set standard of resistance measurement for the bands. Band resistance is usually described in terms of the thickness.

Some exercises involve standing on the bands and pulling on them.

Muscle-toning schedule

People who are new to muscle toning should set up a training schedule with a trainer or fitness professional. The fitness expert will give advice about technique, posture, and proper use of equipment. A workout of 20 to 30 minutes is sufficient.

The trainer will set up a schedule so that muscles are challenged. For toning, the person may start with medium weights and do 20 repetitions. Once a person is comfortable with this routine, the next challenge could be to add five more reps to the workout. Another challenge could be to add another weight plate when using a weight machine.

For people who do **balance training** and muscle training on the same day, the balance training should be done first so that muscles are not fatigued.

Furthermore, muscles need to rest, so the same muscle group should not be exercised two days in a row. Some people exercise all muscle groups twice a week. Others target one muscle group per day.

Preparation

Before beginning any exercise program, people should consult with their doctors. The healthcare professional will advise them about whether any health condition would limit the type of muscle toning they can do, what type of equipment to use, and what goals to set for training. Some older adults may find it easier to work with resistance bands while others are able to lift heavy weights.

Preparation also includes deciding upon the type of weights to use for this training. People who choose to use free weights or a weight machine may decide to do their toning workout at a gym. Those who decide to purchase weights or a home gym should consult with a trainer or other fitness professional before buying the equipment. This person will give advice about the appropriate amount of weight for the person's strength and strength goals.

People who work out with heavy weights should work with a spotter. This person watches the person lifting weights. If the spotter sees the person struggle or the individual asks for help, the spotter will take the weights so the lifter is not injured.

Risks

In any muscle-toning program, people should avoid lifting too much weight or overdoing repetitions until they are physically able to do these activities. Doing too much too soon could result in a muscle overload injury.

In addition, care should be taken when using free weights because movement is not restricted as it would be when the weights are attached to an exercise machine. It is important to have a good grip on handheld weights and use good technique and form.

Free weights require more muscular coordination than that needed when working out on a weight machine. There is more of risk of injury when using free weights, and most injuries occur when a weight plate drops or a dumbbell falls out of a person's hand.

In addition, when picking up weights, people must use leg muscles and avoid straining back muscles.

Furthermore, caution should be taken so that resistance bands do not slip and hit the person.

Results

A regular muscle-toning workout usually produces visible results within several weeks. Calories burn more efficiently, helping a person lose or control weight. The activity firms and shapes the body, and posture improves. Strength training also helps to reduce **fatigue**.

Long-term effects of muscle toning include reducing the risk of injury and preventing muscle loss. In addition, strengthening the bones increases bone density and reduces the risk of osteoporosis.

Resources

BOOKS

Caviano, D. Christine. *Strength Training Over 50*. New York: Barron' Education Series, Inc., 2005.

Gavin, Mary L., Steven A. Downshen, and Neil Izeneberg. *FitKids*. New York: DK Publishing, Inc., 2004.

PERIODICALS

WEBSITES

Goldstein, Richard. "Jack LaLanne, Founder of Modern Fitness Movement Dies at 96." *The New York Times*. (January 23, 2011). NYTimes.com. http://www.nytimes.com/2011/01/24/sports/24lalanne.html (accessed October 12, 2011).

ORGANIZATIONS

American College of Sports Medicine, 401 West Michigan Street, Indianapolis, IN, 46202-3233, (317) 637-9200, Fax: (317) 634-7817, http://www.acsm.org.

Liz Swain

Muscular strength and endurance tests

Definition

Muscular strength and endurance tests assess the ability of muscles and muscle groups to work against resistance with repeated muscular contractions. Muscular strength is the maximum force that a muscle or muscle group can exert in a single effort. Muscular endurance is the ability of a muscle or muscle group to perform repeatedly at submaximal force for a defined period of time. Thus, muscular strength and endurance tests measure two different types of ability and some tests may be referred to as muscular strength endurance tests.

Purpose

Muscular strength and endurance are important both for good health and for performing daily activities, including household chores, such as cleaning and yard work, and job-related duties, such as lifting and carrying. Muscular strength and endurance are especially important for weight training and for sports that put muscles under tension for longer periods of time, such as distance **running**, biking, **swimming**, skating, or climbing. Muscular strength and endurance testing is performed as a component of an overall fitness evaluation, as well as for guidance in developing individualized resistance training programs and monitoring progress over time. The tests can be strong motivators for improving muscular strength and endurance.

Description

Muscular strength and endurance tests assess muscle strength and **fatigue**, in contrast to **cardiorespiratory fitness tests** that measure the amount of oxygen supplied to and utilized by muscles. Muscular strength and endurance depend on the physical condition of the muscles, the number and size of the muscles involved in the work, the proportion of muscle fibers that are involved, coordination between muscle groups, and any contribution from mechanical leverage. Because these properties differ among the various muscle groups, there is no single muscular strength and endurance test. Rather, each test is specific for the muscle group or groups, the type and speed of muscular contraction, and the angles of the joints involved in the particular action. Most muscular strength and endurance tests are similar or identical to components of a muscle fitness training regimen.

Muscular strength and endurance tests are often performed using free weights or resistance machines. Although resistance machines are safer and easier to use, free weights require more motor coordination and better balance, and thus involve more muscle groups, particularly stabilizing muscles. Free weights also allow more varied testing protocols. However, there are many muscular strength and endurance tests that do not require weights or machines. The

Shape Up America! program uses push-ups to test muscular strength and endurance. The **President's Challenge** Adult Fitness Test uses half-sit-ups and push-ups.

Abdominal-muscle tests

Among the muscles of the body core, the abdominals are most frequently tested for strength and endurance. Weak abdominal muscles can cause poor posture, muscle fatigue, and **low back pain** and injury. There are various tests of abdominal strength, including straight leg lifts and four-stage and seven-stage tests that involve progressively more difficult sit-ups. However, half-sit-up or curl-up tests are the most common.

The YMCA half-sit-up test is used by the President's Challenge to assess abdominal muscle strength and endurance, although it also uses other muscle groups. It is considered a curl-up test because the trunk is only partially lifted from the floor. Curl-ups are often preferred to sit-ups because they do not involve the hip flexors. The test requires a mat or rug with two parallel strips of tape 3.5 in (9 cm) apart, which are placed perpendicular to the body and can be felt with the hands. The starting position is with the back on the mat, the knees bent to 90°, the feet flat on the floor, and the palms on the mat with the fingers just touching the upper tape. The lower back is flattened to the mat and the trunk is lifted so that the fingers move to the second tape. The fingers, feet, and buttocks remain on the mat. To complete the half-sit-up, the shoulders lower to the mat, although the head does not need to touch. The score is the number of half-sit-ups completed in one minute. Pacing should be such that the full minute can be completed. Alternatively, curl-ups are performed at a pace of 50 beats per minute and continued for 80 repetitions or until the pace or proper technique cannot be maintained.

Upper-body tests

Shoulder pain in middle-aged and older people is often caused by reduced strength and endurance in the upper body and shoulder muscles. These muscles are often tested with push-ups or pull-ups.

The starting position for push-ups is the elevated or up position. In a standard push-up test, performed by males in the President's Challenge and Shape Up America!, the hands are shoulders-width apart and flat on the floor and the arms are fully extended directly below the shoulders. The back and legs form a straight line, with the toes curled under, and all of the weight is on the hands and feet. The body is held rigid and pushed up and down using the muscles of the arms, shoulders, and chest, with the feet as the pivot point, so the workload is the body weight. The modified push-up is used for females and males who cannot perform at least eight standard push-ups. The hands are flat on the floor and slightly in front of the shoulders, to place them correctly for the downward motion. The knees are bent on the floor and the feet are in the air and crossed at the ankles. Thus, the knees form the pivot point and the workload is reduced to the upper body. In the President's Challenge, the chest is lowered to 2 in. (5 cm) from the floor on an inhale and raised back up on an exhale. For Shape Up America!, the chest touches the floor. Push-ups are continued for as long as possible. It is important to maintain a rigid position with a flat back and to fully straighten the arms in the up position. In the President's Challenge, a brief rest is permitted in the up position.

Pull-up or chin-up tests require a horizontal overhead or pull-up bar from which the subject can hang with the arms fully extended and the feet above the ground. The bar is grasped either overhand (palms away from the body) or underhand (palms toward the body). The body is raised until the chin clears the bar and then released back to the fully extended position in a smooth motion. Swinging, bending, or kicking the legs and jerky movements are not allowed. As many pull-ups as possible are completed.

Other upper-body muscular strength and endurance tests include:

- flexed-arm or bent-arm hang tests that measure time hanging with the chin above an overhead bar

- arm curl or biceps tests that count the number of arm curls with weights completed in 30 seconds

- dips tests that count the number of times the body is lowered and raised on parallel bars in one minute

- various types of bench-press and bench-pull tests

Lower-body tests

Squat tests assesses hip and lower-leg function, balance, and the strength of the quadriceps, gluteals, and hip stabilizers. Squat tests can be either single-leg or two-legged. For a two-legged squat test, standing with the back to a chair, hands on hips, and feet shoulders-width apart, the subject squats, lightly touching the chair, and stands back up as many times as possible.

For the chair-stand test, the subject sits in the middle of a chair, with feet flat on the floor and shoulders-width apart, arms crossed at the wrists and close to the chest. The score is the number of times the subject can stand up and sit down completely in 30 seconds.

The wall sit assesses lower-body strength, especially the quadriceps. Standing against a wall with the feet about shoulders-width apart, the subject slides down the wall until both knees and hips are at a 90° angle. One foot is lifted off the ground and held for as long as possible. After resting, the test is repeated with the other foot.

Several lower-body tests involve jumping. The 30-second endurance jump counts the number of jumps over and back a 12-in. (30-cm) hurdle—taking off and landing with both feet—in 30 seconds. Other tests include the multistage hurdle jump test and the 45-second agility hurdle jump test.

Other tests

Other muscular strength tests include:

- the one repetition maximum (1RM) test or 1RM bench press that measures the maximum weight that can be lifted or pressed once

- isokinetic strength tests that use specialized equipment to provide variable resistance at a constant speed

- handgrip strength tests that measure maximum strength of the hand and forearm muscles

- trunk-lift tests that test the ability of the back muscles to lift the upper body off the floor

- isometric back-strength tests

- isometric leg-strength tests, which require a strength dynomometer

- isometric leg-extension tests to measure lower-body strength

- the NHL push-and-pull strength test, which also requires a dynomometer

Other muscular strength and endurance tests include:

- a leg-raise machine test

- a side-ramp test, in which the body is held in a rigid elevated position by one elbow and forearm for as long as possible

- the ins-and-outs core-strength test, in which the subject sits with knees bent, raises the knees toward the chest, straightens the legs out, and bends them back to the chest without touching the ground, for as many repetitions as possible

Precautions

There are specific precautions for different muscular strength and endurance tests. For example, sit-ups and curl-ups must always be performed with the lower back flat on the mat, since arching the back can cause injury. Increased **blood pressure** is a normal consequence of resistance **exercise**. Exhaling on

KEY TERMS

Biceps—The large flexor muscle of the front of the upper arm.

Concentric phase—Muscle contraction in which the muscles shorten while generating force, as when lifting a weight.

Curl-up—A half-sit-up that does not involve the hip flexors.

Dynamometer—A device for measuring force, such as the strength of the back, grip, arms, or legs.

Eccentric phase—The phase of an exercise in which the muscles elongate under tension because the opposing force is greater than that generated by the muscles.

Gluteals—The gluteus muscles of the buttocks.

Hip flexors—The group of muscles that flex the thigh bone toward the pelvis to pull the knee up.

President's Challenge—America's primary physical activity and fitness initiative, which includes muscular strength and endurance tests.

Pull-up—An exercise or test of upper-body strength in which the suspended body is pulled up by the arms.

Push-up—Press-up; a test or exercise in which the body is lowered and pushed up with the arms.

Quadriceps—The large muscle of the front of the thigh.

Resistance exercise—Strength training; exercise performed with weights or other resistance to muscle contraction.

Shape Up America!—A public education initiative about the importance of achieving and maintaining a healthy weight through physical activity and healthy eating.

Sit-up—A common test or exercise for strength and endurance of the abdominal muscles.

the concentric phase—when the muscles are shortening, as in the up movement of a push-up—and inhaling during the eccentric phase when the muscles are lengthening under tension—as in lowering during a push-up—can help keep blood pressure within a safe range. Push-ups and pull-ups may aggravate pre-existing shoulder, elbow, or wrist pain. Finally, spotters are essential whenever using heavy free weights.

Preparation

Muscular strength and endurance tests should take place in a quiet environment at a comfortable temperature. Subjects should be carefully instructed in the proper exercise techniques, including body position and starting and ending points. Protocols should be followed carefully, so that the results on future tests are comparable. Although sit-up and push-up tests may not require a **warm-up**, other types of muscular strength and endurance tests do require warming up prior to testing.

Aftercare

Muscular strength and endurance test results can be improved by repeating the exercises frequently or increasing the workload for the same number of repetitions. Exercises should be performed at least three days each week. The half-sit-up load can be increased by folding the arms across the chest or placing them behind the head. Modified push-ups can be made

more difficult by switching from standard push-ups and made easier by performing them against a wall. The intensity should be increased only if proper posture and control can be maintained. Participants should work up to three sets of 25 half-sit-ups and three sets of ten to 20 push-ups, with short rests between each set. Once half-sit-ups and push-ups are mastered, additional exercises can be added, including equipment such as balance balls, weights, or elastic tubing.

Complications

Although any exercise can result in injury, there are generally no complications with muscular strength and endurance tests. However, they should always be conducted according to proper protocols and all precautions should be followed.

Results

Analysis and comparisons for individual muscular strength and endurance test results are available online. For the President's Challenge, the number of half-sit-ups performed in one minute and the total number of push-ups are entered into the online data analysis for the Adult Fitness Test. Scores depend on the subject's **age**. A "below average" to "very poor" rating on the half-sit-up indicates a need for improvement in abdominal-muscle strength and endurance. A "below average" to "poor" push-up score indicates the need for improved upper-body and shoulder-muscle strength and endurance. The normative data for standard and modified push-ups are based on a population aged 20 and older. The Shape Up America! website also uses the number of push-ups and the subject's age to assess upper-body strength.

Resources

BOOKS

Acevedo, Edmund O., and Michael A. Starks. *Exercise Testing and Prescription Lab Manual*. 2nd ed. Champaign, IL: Human Kinetics, 2011.

Coulson, Morc, and David Archer. *Practical Fitness Testing: Analysis in Exercise and Sport*. London: A. & C. Black, 2009.

Fahey, Thomas D., Paul M. Insel, and Walton T. Roth. *Fit & Well: Core Concepts and Labs in Physical Fitness and Wellness*. 8th ed. New York: McGraw-Hill Higher Education, 2009.

Plowman, Sharon A., and Denise L. Smith. *Exercise Physiology for Health, Fitness, and Performance*. 3rd ed. Philadelphia: Wolters Kluwer Health/Lippincott Williams & Wilkins, 2011.

WEBSITES

"Maximum Strength & Strength Endurance Tests." Topend Sports. June 16, 2011. http://www.topendsports.com/testing/strength-tests.htm (accessed August 8, 2011).

Mayo, Jerry J., and Len Kravitz. "Methods of Muscular Fitness Assessment." University of New Mexico. http://www.unm.edu/~lkravitz/Article%20folder/musassess.html (accessed August 8, 2011).

"Muscular Strength and Endurance." The President's Challenge Adult Fitness Test. http://www.adultfitnesstest.org/testInstructions/muscularStrengthAndEndurance/default.aspx (accessed August 8, 2011).

"The Muscular Strength and Endurance Test." Shape Up America! http://www.shapeup.org/fitness/assess/strength1.php (accessed August 8, 2011).

ORGANIZATIONS

American College of Sports Medicine, P.O. Box 1440, Indianapolis, IN, 46206-1440, (317) 637-9200, Fax: (317) 634-7817, http://www.acsm.org.

Cooper Institute, 12330 Preston Rd., Dallas, TX, 75230, (972) 341-3200, Fax: (972) 341-3227, (800) 635-7050, fitnessgram@cooperinst.org, http://www.cooperinstitute.org.

President's Challenge, 501 North Morton St., Ste. 203, Bloomington, IN, 47404, Fax: (812) 855-8999, (800) 258-8146, preschal@indiana.edu, http://www.presidentschallenge.org.

YMCA of the USA, 101 North Wacker Dr., Chicago, IL, 60606, (312) 977-0031, (800) 872-9622, fulfillment@ymca.net, http://www.ymca.net.

Margaret Alic, PhD

Muscular system

Definition

The muscular system is the body's network of tissues for both voluntary and involuntary movements. Muscle cells are specialized for contraction.

Description

Body movements are generated through the contraction and relaxation of specific muscles. Some muscles, like those in the arms and legs, bring about such voluntary movements as raising a hand or flexing the foot. Other muscles are involuntary and function without conscious effort. Voluntary muscles include the skeletal muscles, of which there are about 650 in the human body. Skeletal muscles are controlled by the **somatic nervous system**; whereas the **autonomic nervous system** controls the involuntary muscles. Involuntary muscles include muscles that line the internal organs and the blood vessels. These smooth muscles are called visceral and vascular smooth muscles, and they perform tasks not generally associated with voluntary activity. Smooth muscles control several automatic physiological responses such as pupil constriction, which occurs when the muscles of the iris contract in bright light. Another example is the dilation of blood vessels that occurs when the smooth muscles surrounding the vessels relax or lengthen. In addition to the categories of skeletal (voluntary) and smooth (involuntary) muscle, there is a third category, cardiac muscle, which is neither voluntary nor involuntary. Cardiac muscle is not under conscious control, and it can also function without regulation from the external nervous system.

Smooth muscles derive their name from their appearance under polarized light microscopy. In contrast to cardiac and skeletal muscles, which have striations

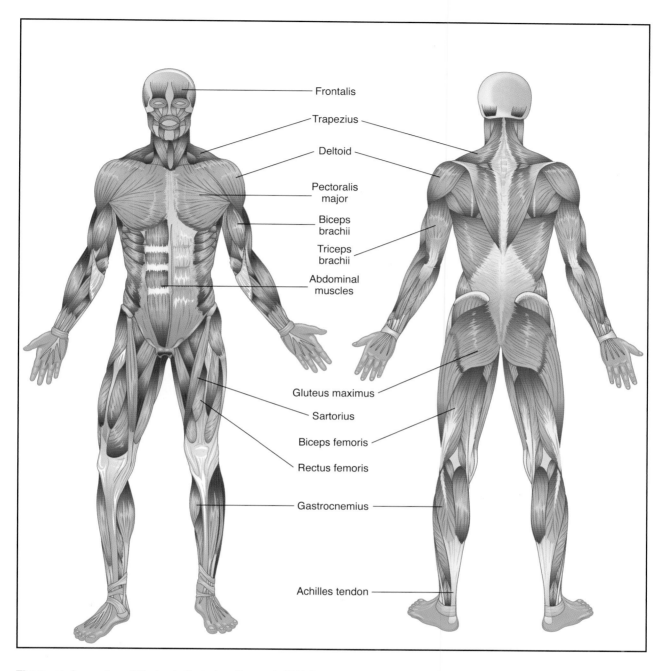

The muscular system. *(Electronic Illustrators Group. © 2012 Cengage Learning.)*

(appearance of parallel bands or lines), smooth muscle is unstriated. Striations result from the pattern of myofilaments, which are very fine threads of **protein**. There are two types of myofilaments, actin and myosin, which line the myofibrils within each muscle cell. When many myofilaments align along the length of a muscle cell, light and dark regions create a striated appearance. This microscopic view of muscle reveals that muscles alter their shape to produce movement. Because muscle cells are usually elongated, they are often called muscle fibers. Compared to other cells in the body, striated muscle cells are distinctive in shape, protein composition, and multinucleated structure.

Skeletal muscles

Skeletal muscles are what most people think of as muscle. Skeletal muscles are the ones that ache when someone goes for their first outdoor run in the spring after not **running** regularly during the winter. Skeletal muscles are also involved when someone carries heavy grocery bags, practices a difficult musical passage, or combs their hair. **Exercise** may increase the size of muscle fibers, but the number of fibers generally remains constant. Skeletal muscles take up about 40% of the body's mass, or weight. They also consume large amounts of oxygen and nutrients from the blood supply. Multiple levels of skeletal muscle tissue receive their own blood supplies.

GROSS ANATOMY OF STRIATED MUSCLE. At the macroscopic level, skeletal muscles usually originate at one point of attachment to a tendon (a band or cord of tough, fibrous connective tissue) and terminate at another tendon at the other end of an adjoining bone. Tendons are rich in the protein collagen, which is arranged in a wavy pattern so that it can stretch out and provide additional length at the junction between bone and muscle.

Skeletal muscles usually act in pairs, such that the flexing (shortening) of one muscle is balanced by a lengthening (relaxation) of its paired muscle or group of muscles. These antagonistic (opposite) muscles can open and close such joints as the elbow or knee. Muscles that cause a joint to bend or close are called flexor muscles, and those that cause a joint to expand or straighten out are called extensors. Skeletal muscles that support the skull, backbone, and rib cage are called axial skeletal muscles; whereas the skeletal muscles of the limbs are called distal. Several skeletal muscles work in a highly coordinated manner in such activities as **walking**.

Skeletal muscles are organized into extrafusal and intrafusal fibers. Extrafusal fibers are the strong, outer layers of muscle. This type of muscle fiber is the most common. Intrafusal fibers, which make up the central region of the muscle, are weaker than extrafusal fibers. Skeletal muscle fibers are additionally characterized as fast or slow according to their activity patterns. Fast or "white" muscle fibers contract rapidly, have poor blood supply, operate anaerobically (without oxygen), and tire easily. Slow or "red" muscle fibers contract more slowly, have a more adequate blood supply, operate aerobically (with oxygen), and do not **fatigue** as easily.

The skeletal muscles are enclosed in a dense sheath of connective tissue called the epimysium. Within the epimysium, muscles are sectioned into columns of muscle fiber bundles called primary bundles or fasciculi. Each fasciculus is covered by a layer of connective tissue called the perimysium. An average skeletal muscle may have 20–40 fasciculi, which are further subdivided into several muscle fibers. Each muscle fiber (cell) is covered by connective tissue called endomysium. Both the epimysium and the perimysium contain blood and lymph vessels to supply the muscle with nutrients and oxygen, and to remove waste products. The endomysium has an extensive network of capillaries that supply individual muscle fibers. Individual muscle fibers vary in diameter from 10–60 micrometers and in length from a few millimeters in the smaller muscles to about 12 in (30 cm) in the sartorius muscle of the thigh.

MICROANATOMY OF STRIATED MUSCLE. At the microscopic level, a single striated muscle cell has several hundred nuclei and a striped appearance derived from the pattern of myofilaments. Long, cylindrical muscle fibers are formed from several myoblasts in fetal development. Multiple nuclei are important in muscle cells because of the tremendous amount of activity. The two types of myofilaments, actin and myosin, overlap one another in a very precise arrangement. Myosin is a thick protein with two globular head regions. Each myosin filament is surrounded by six actin (thin) filaments. These filaments run along the length of the cell in parallel. Multiple hexagonal arrays of actin and myosin exist in each skeletal muscle cell.

Each actin filament slides along adjacent myosin filaments with the help of other proteins and ions present in the cell. Tropomyosin and troponin are two proteins attached to the actin filaments that enable the globular heads on myosin to instantaneously attach to the myosin strands. The attachment and rapid release of this bond induces the sliding motion of these filaments that results in muscle contraction. In addition, calcium ions and ATP (adenosine triphosphate, the source of cellular **energy**) are required by the muscle cell to process this reaction. Numerous mitochondria (organelles in a cell that produce enzymes necessary for energy **metabolism**) are present in muscle fibers to supply the extensive ATP required by the cell.

The system of myofilaments within muscle fibers are divided into units called sarcomeres. Each skeletal muscle cell has several myofibrils, long cylindrical columns of myofilaments. Each myofibril is composed of myofilaments that interdigitate to form the striated sarcomere units. The thick myosin filaments of the sarcomere provide the dark, striped appearance in striated muscle, and the thin actin filaments provide the lighter sarcomere regions between the dark areas. Muscle contraction creates an enlarged center region called the belly of the muscle. The flexing of a muscle—a bicep for example—makes this region anatomically visible.

Cardiac muscle

Cardiac muscle makes up the muscular portion of the heart. While almost all cardiac muscle is confined to the heart, some of these cells extend for a short distance into the cardiac vessels before tapering off completely. Heart muscle is also called myocardium. The myocardium has some properties similar to skeletal muscle tissue, but it also has some unique features. Like skeletal muscle, the myocardium is striated; however, the cardiac muscle fibers are smaller and shorter than skeletal muscle fibers. Cardiac muscle fibers average 5–15 micrometers in diameter and 20–30 micrometers in length. In addition, cardiac muscles align lengthwise more than they do in a side-by-side fashion, compared to skeletal muscle fibers. The microscopic structure of cardiac muscle is distinctive in that these cells are branched in a way that allows them to communicate simultaneously with multiple cardiac muscle fibers.

Smooth muscle

Smooth muscle falls into three general categories: visceral smooth muscle, vascular smooth muscle, and multi-unit smooth muscle. Visceral smooth muscle fibers line such internal organs as the intestines, stomach, and uterus. Vascular smooth muscle forms the middle layer of the walls of blood and lymphatic vessels. Arteries generally have a thicker layer of vascular smooth muscle than veins or lymphatic vessels. Multi-unit smooth muscle is found only in the muscles that govern the size of the iris of the eye. Unlike contractions in visceral smooth muscle, contractions in multi-unit smooth muscle fibers do not readily spread to neighboring muscle cells.

Smooth muscle is innervated by both sympathetic and parasympathetic nerves of the autonomic nervous system. Smooth muscle appears unstriated under a polarized light microscope, because the myofilaments inside are less organized. Smooth muscle fibers contain actin and myosin myofilaments that are more haphazardly arranged than their counterparts in skeletal muscles. The sympathetic neurotransmitter, Acetylcholine (Ach), and parasympathetic neurotransmitter, nor-epinephrine, activate this type of muscle tissue.

Smooth muscle cells are small in diameter, about 5–15 micrometers, but they are long, typically 15–500 micrometers. They are also wider in the center than at their ends. Gap junctions connect small bundles of cells which are, in turn, arranged in sheets.

Within such hollow organs as the uterus, smooth muscle cells are arranged into two layers. The cells in the outer layer are usually arranged in a longitudinal fashion surrounding the cells in the inner layer, which are arranged in a circular pattern. Many smooth muscles are regulated by hormones in addition to the neurotransmitters of the autonomic nervous system. Moreover, the contraction of some smooth muscles is myogenic or triggered by **stretching**, as in the uterus and gastrointestinal tract.

Function

Skeletal muscles

Skeletal muscles function as the link between the somatic nervous system and the **skeletal system**. Skeletal muscles carry out instructions from the brain related to voluntary movement or action. For instance, when a person decides to eat a piece of cake, the brain tells the forearm muscle to contract, allowing it to flex and position the hand to lift a forkful of cake to the mouth. But the muscle alone cannot support the weight of the fork; the sturdy bones of the forearm assist the muscles in completing the task of moving the bite of cake. Hence, the skeletal and muscular systems work together as a lever system, with the joints acting as a fulcrum to carry out instructions from the nervous system.

The somatic nervous system controls skeletal muscle movement through motor neurons. Alpha motor neurons extend from the spinal cord and terminate on individual muscle fibers. The axon, or signal-sending end, of the alpha neuron branches to innervate multiple muscle fibers. The nerve terminal forms a synapse, or junction, with the muscle to create a neuromuscular junction. The neurotransmitter ACh is released from the axon terminal into the synapse. From the synapse, the ACh binds to receptors on the muscle surface that trigger events leading to muscle contraction. While alpha motor neurons innervate extrafusal fibers, intrafusal fibers are innervated by gamma motor neurons.

Voluntary skeletal muscle movements are initiated by the motor cortex in the brain. Signals travel down the spinal cord to the alpha motor neuron to result in contraction. Not all movement of skeletal muscles is voluntary, however. Certain reflexes occur in response to such dangerous stimuli as extreme heat or the edge of a sharp object. Reflexive skeletal muscular movement is controlled at the level of the spinal cord and does not require higher brain initiation. Reflexive movements are processed at this level to minimize the amount of time necessary to implement a response.

In addition to motor neuron activity in the skeletal muscles, a number of sensory nerves carry information to the brain to regulate muscle tension and contraction. Muscles function at peak performance when they are not overstretched or overcontracted. Sensory neurons within the muscle send feedback to the brain with regard to muscle length and state of contraction.

Cardiac muscle

The heart muscle is responsible for more than two billion beats in the course of a human lifetime of average length. Cardiac muscle cells are surrounded by endomysium like the skeletal muscle cells. The autonomic nerves to the heart, however, do not form any special junctions like those found in skeletal muscle. Instead, the branching structure and extensive interconnectedness of cardiac muscle fibers allows for stimulation of the heart to spread into neighboring myocardial cells. This feature does not require the individual fibers to be stimulated. Although external nervous stimuli can enhance or diminish cardiac muscle contraction, heart muscles can also contract spontaneously. Like skeletal muscle cells, cardiac muscle fibers can increase in size with physical conditioning, but they rarely increase in number.

Smooth muscle

The concentric arrangement of some smooth muscle fibers enables them to control dilation and constriction in the blood vessels, intestines, and other organs. While these cells are not innervated on an individual basis, excitation from one cell can spread to adjacent cells through the nexuses that join neighbor cells. Multi-unit smooth muscles function in a highly localized way in such areas as the iris of the eye. Visceral smooth muscle facilitates the movement of substances through such tubular areas as blood vessels and the small intestine. Smooth muscle differs from skeletal and cardiac muscle in its energy utilization as well. Smooth muscles are not as dependent on oxygen availability as are cardiac and skeletal muscles. Smooth muscle uses glycolysis (the breakdown of **carbohydrates**) to generate much of its metabolic energy.

Role in human health

Building and maintaining muscle is important for everyone. The American Council on Exercise notes that most adults lose up to a half-pound of muscle per year after age 25 due to minimal exercise. With a slowdown of metabolism beginning around the same age as losing muscle mass, comes inevitable weight gain.

Maintaining a good fitness regimen is important to counter this reality. A fitness program should include strength training to improve balance and energy, prevent or minimize bone loss, and to minimize weight gain. Strength training also helps build lean muscle.

It is important to use weights in a progressive manner, increasing the amount of weight and the number of repetitions gradually. Strenuous or overzealous weight lifting can lead to muscle injury and early fatigue. It is best to have a goal in mind and work slowly and methodically toward that goal. Many individuals like to focus on one body part, whereas others choose to engage in an all-over body workout. Either way, one should ensure that all muscle groups are included for overall fitness.

An exercise routine should include not only aerobic and strength training, but a warm up period as well. Doing so gives muscle groups added flexibility for use during more intense activity, and helps to prevent muscle injury. Stretching after a workout is needed to move muscles through an increased range of motion and allow tissues to **cool down** gradually. Most experts agree that holding time for each stretch pose should last about 15–30 seconds.

A good workout keeps the heart strong and flexes cardiac muscle to help deliver blood throughout the circulatory system and bring oxygenated blood to cells and tissues throughout the body, as well as to all muscle groups. Exercise helps the **digestive system** by contracting muscles in the stomach and intestines, moving food along the digestive tract. It also strengthens the **respiratory system** by increasing tidal volume (the volume of air intake) and the delivery of oxygen in and out of the lungs. Adhering to a fitness program helps maintain a healthy back by sustaining strong muscle tone and good posture.

Both anaerobic and aerobic exercise activity benefit the muscular system. Anaerobic exercises are short, intense exercises such as weight lifting or sprinting short distances. Many bodybuilders include the effects of anaerobic exercise in their resistance training routines to help build muscle mass. Aerobic exercises are generally longer lasting exercises such as running or cardio routines. Most cyclists and long distance runners incorporate aerobic exercise with **endurance training** to develop long, lean muscle for use over sustained periods of movement such as during marathons.

Acetylcholine (ACh)—A short-acting neurotransmitter that functions as a stimulant to the nervous system and as a vasodilator.

Actin—A protein that functions in muscular contraction by combining with myosin.

Adenosine triphosphate (ATP)—A nucleotide that is the primary source of energy in living tissue.

Anaerobic—Pertaining to or caused by the absence of oxygen.

Angina pectoris—A sensation of crushing pain or pressure in the chest, usually near the breastbone, but sometimes radiating to the upper arm or back. Angina pectoris is caused by a deficient supply of oxygenated blood to the heart.

Axial—Pertaining to the axis of the body, i.e., the head and trunk.

Axon—The appendage of a neuron that transmits impulses away from the cell body.

Cardiac muscle—The striated muscle tissue of the heart. It is sometimes called myocardium.

Distal—Situated away from the point of origin or attachment.

Dystrophy—Any of several disorders characterized by weakening or degeneration of muscle tissue.

Epimysium—The sheath of connective tissue around a muscle.

Extensor—A muscle that serves to extend or straighten a part of the body.

Fasciculus (plural, fasciculi)—A small bundle of muscle fibers.

Flexor—A muscle that serves to flex or bend a part of the body.

Multinucleated—Having more than one nucleus in each cell. Muscle cells are multinucleated.

Myasthenia gravis—A disease characterized by the impaired transmission of motor nerve impulses, caused by the autoimmune destruction of acetylcholine receptors.

Myosin—The principal contractile protein in muscle tissue.

Parasympathetic—Pertaining to the part of the autonomic nervous system that generally functions in regulatory opposition to the sympathetic system, as by slowing the heartbeat or contracting the pupil of the eye.

Sarcomere—A segment of myofibril in a striated muscle fiber.

Skeletal muscle—Muscle tissue composed of bundles of striated muscle cells that operate in conjunction with the skeletal system as a lever system.

Smooth muscle—Muscle tissue composed of long, unstriated cells that line internal organs and facilitate such involuntary movements as peristalsis.

Sympathetic—Pertaining to the part of the autonomic nervous system that regulates such involuntary reactions to stress as heartbeat, sweating, and breathing rate.

Synapse—A region in which nerve impulses are transmitted across a gap from an axon terminal to another axon or the end plate of a muscle.

Tendon—A cord or band of dense, tough, fibrous tissue that connects muscles and bones.

Nutrition plays an active role in a healthy muscular system. Muscles rely on glucose, protein, and carbohydrates to produce and sustain energy. It is important to refuel energy stores depleted during exercise, so individuals should drink plenty of water and eat healthy **fats**, carbohydrates, and protein to replenish what the body used during a workout.

Eating right and exercising regularly has the benefit of increasing body metabolism that, in turn, helps in weight management and aids in weight reduction. Staying fit helps to minimize abdominal fat, which is known to be associated with diabetes, heart disease, and high **cholesterol**. Eating nutritious food and adhering to a

regular exercise routine also helps decrease fat stores throughout the body, contributing to a healthy, leaner, and more fit body build.

Common diseases and conditions

Mechanical injury

Disorders of the muscular system can result from genetic, hormonal, infectious, autoimmune, poisonous, or neoplastic causes. But the most common problem associated with this system is injury from misuse. Sprains and tears cause excess blood to seep into skeletal muscle tissue. The residual scar tissue leads to a slightly shorter muscle. Muscular impairment and cramping can result from a diminished blood supply. Cramping can be due to overexertion. An inadequate supply of blood to cardiac muscle causes a sensation of pressure or pain in the chest called angina pectoris. Inadequate ionic supplies of calcium, sodium, or potassium can also affect most muscle cells adversely.

Immune system disorders

Muscular system disorders related to the **immune system** include myasthenia gravis and tumors. Myasthenia gravis is characterized by weak and easily fatigued skeletal muscles, droopy eyelids being one of the symptoms. Myasthenia gravis is caused by antibodies that a person makes against their own ACh receptors; hence, it is an autoimmune disease. The antibodies disturb normal ACh stimulation to contract skeletal muscles. Failure of the immune system to destroy cancerous cells in muscle can result in muscle tumors. Benign muscle tumors are called myomas, while malignant muscle tumors are called myosarcomas.

Disorders caused by toxins

Muscular disorders may be caused by toxic substances of various types. A bacterium called *Clostridium tetani* produces a neurotoxin that causes tetanus, a disease characterized by painful repeated muscular contractions. In addition, some types of gangrene are caused by clostridial toxins produced under anaerobic conditions deep within a muscle. A poisonous substance called curare, which is derived from tropical plants of the genus *Strychnos* blocks neuromuscular transmission in skeletal muscle, causing paralysis. Prolonged periods of ethanol intoxication can also cause muscle damage.

Genetic disorders

The most common type of muscular genetic disorder is muscular dystrophy, of which there are several kinds. Duchenne's muscular dystrophy is characterized by increasing muscular weakness and eventual death. Becker's muscular dystrophy is a less severe disorder than Duchenne's, but both can be classified as X-linked recessive genetic disorders. Other types of muscular dystrophy are caused by a mutation that affects a muscle protein called dystrophin. Dystrophin is absent in Duchenne's and altered in Becker's muscular dystrophies. Other genetic disorders, including glycogen storage diseases, myotonic disorders, and familial periodic paralysis,

---

QUESTIONS TO ASK YOUR DOCTOR

- What are the indications that I may have a problem with my muscular system?
- What kind of fitness program should I follow to improve my muscle strength?
- Do I have any physical or health limitations?
- What measures can be taken to prevent muscular system problems?

---

can affect muscle tissues. In glycogen storage diseases, the skeletal muscles accumulate abnormal amounts of glycogen due to a biochemical defect in carbohydrate metabolism. In myotonic disorders, the voluntary muscles are abnormally slow to relax after contraction. Familial periodic paralysis is characterized by episodes of weakness and paralysis combined with loss of deep tendon reflexes.

Resources

BOOKS

Katch, Victor L., William D. McArdle, and Frank I. Katch. *Essential of Exercise Physiology*. Philadelphia: Lippincott Williams & Wilkins Health, 2011.

Manocchia, Pat. *Anatomy of Exercise: A Trainer's Inside Guide to Your Workout*. Richmond Hill, ONT: Firefly Books, 2009.

Marcher, Lisbeth, and Sonja Fich. *Body Encyclopedia: A Guide to the Psychological Functions of the Muscular System*. Berkeley, CA: North Atlantic Books, 2010.

McDowell, Julie, ed. *Encyclopedia of Human Body Systems*. Santa Barbara, CA: Greenwood, 2010.

Murphy, Wendy. *Weight and Health*. Minneapolis, MN: Twenty-First Century Books, 2008.

Prentice, William. *Get Fit, Stay Fit*, sixth ed. Boston: McGraw-Hill College, 2011.

Rizzo, Donald C. *Introduction to Anatomy and Physiology*. Clifton Park, NY: Delmar, 2011.

PERIODICALS

Boskey, Adele L. "Musculoskeletal Disorders and Orthopedic Conditions." *Journal of the American Medical Association* 285, no. 5 (2001): 619-623. http://jama.ama-assn.org/content/285/5/619.full (accessed November 4, 2011).

ORGANIZATIONS

American Council on Exercise (ACE), 4851 Paramount Drive, San Diego, CA, 92123, (858) 279-8227, (888) 825-3636, http://www.acefitness.org.

National Center for Alternative and Complementary Medicine, 9000 Rockville Pike, Bethesda, MD, 20892, (888) 644-6226, http://www.nccam.nih.gov.

National Institute of Arthritis and Musculoskeletal and Skin Diseases (NIAMS) Information Clearinghouse, 1 AMS Circle, Bethesda, MD, 20892, (301) 495-4484, http://www.niams.nih.gov.

National Institutes of Health (NIH), 9000 Rockville Pike, Bethesda, MD, 20892, (301) 496-4000, http://www.nih.gov.

Crystal Heather Kaczkowski, MSc.
Laura Jean Cataldo, RN, EdD

N

Nerve entrapment

Definition

Nerve entrapment occurs when a nerve becomes compressed by muscles or tissues around it, resulting in pain, numbness, or loss of function.

Demographics

The incidence of nerve entrapment varies by the type of condition. Carpal tunnel syndrome, in which a nerve is compressed as it passes through a narrow space in the wrist, is the most common is newly diagnosed nerve entrapment syndrome. Each year in about three in every 1,000 individuals in the United States develop carpal tunnel syndrome and approximately 50 of every 1,000 individuals have carpal tunnel at any one time. Whites are more likely than African Americans to have carpal tunnel syndrome, and it is about three times more common in women than it is in men. It is most likely to develop in individuals between the ages of 45 add 60.

Estimates suggest that between 15% and 40% of individuals will experience sciatica, in which a nerve in the lower back is compressed, at some time in their life. Most of these cases, however, resolve without medical treatment. Each year between 1% and 5% of individuals will experience sciatica.

Description

Nerves run throughout the human body. The nervous system allows the human body to feel sensations such as heat, and control movements such as **walking** and grasping. The brain is the center of the nervous system, and all nerves lead to the spinal cord, and through the spinal cord to the brain. The brain processes the input it receives from all of the nerves in the body.

Nerve entrapment is a condition in which a nerve is compressed by bone, muscle, tendon, or other tissues that surround it. The compressed nerve cannot function and send electrical impulses correctly. This leads to a number of symptoms including numbness, weakness, and pain.

Some of the most common nerves that become entrapped are nerves of the hand (such as in carpal tunnel syndrome), the lower back (such as in sciatica) and the elbow. However, nearly any nerve in the body can become compressed. Athletes are more likely to experience compression of the nerves that are in areas subjected to repetitive movements or repeated trauma. For example, **tennis** players may be more likely to experience compression of nerves in the elbow due to the repeated friction caused when swinging a racket.

Risk factors

The risk factors for nerve entrapment vary somewhat by the location of the problem. Women are at greater risk for carpal tunnel syndrome than men. It is not entirely clear why this is the case, however some experts believe that it is due to women having a smaller carpal tunnel to begin with, making even small amounts of swelling more likely to cause symptoms.

Obese individuals are a higher risk for nerve entrapment. There is some debate over whether a job that requires repetitive movements or involves high levels of vibration (such as using a jackhammer) increases the risk of nerve entrapment. Athletes who participate in sports or recreational fitness activities that require repetitive movements such as tennis or ballet may be at an increased risk of nerve entrapment. Elite athletes who practice movements thousands of times may also be at increased risk. Some experts believe that repetitive tasks put individuals at greater risk of nerve entrapment, but others provide evidence that individuals who participate in these types of

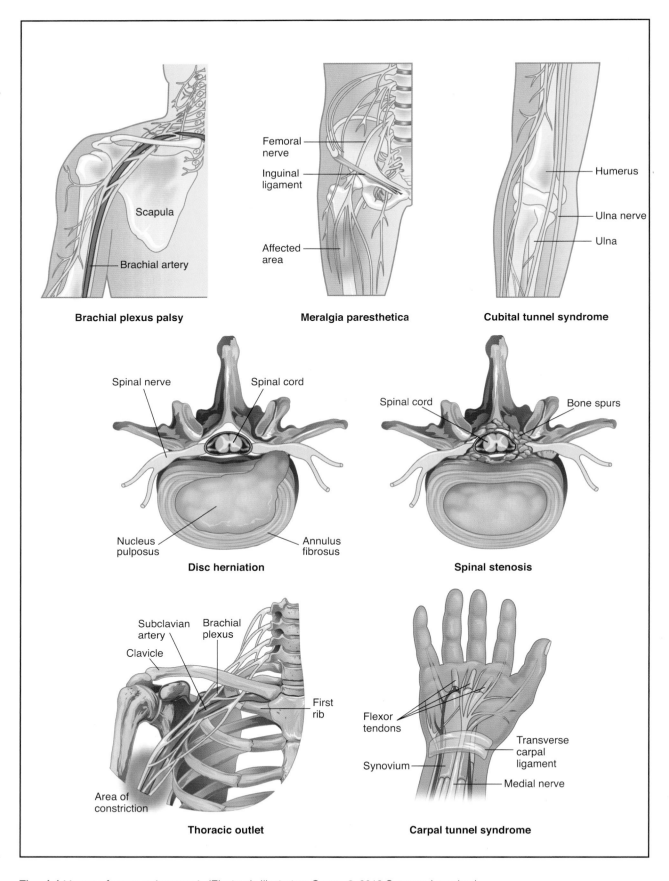

Brachial plexus palsy

Meralgia paresthetica

Cubital tunnel syndrome

Disc herniation

Spinal stenosis

Thoracic outlet

Carpal tunnel syndrome

The eight types of nerve entrapment. *(Electronic Illustrators Group. © 2012 Cengage Learning.)*

activities are at no greater risk than the general population. Research is ongoing to resolve this debate.

Causes and symptoms

Nerve entrapment is caused when tissues, bones, or muscles around a nerve push against the nerve and compressing it. This compression makes the nerve unable to function correctly. Nerve compression can occur for a number of reasons. In many cases, the cause is inflammation of the tissue in the surrounding area. When tissue is inflamed it expands or swells, and pushes against anything in the area. When a nerve is nearby, the inflamed tissue can press up against it, causing compression.

Tissue can become inflamed for many reasons. Overuse is one of the most common causes. Extremely repetitive movements can cause overuse of joints, tendons, and muscles, and the repeated friction between various internal structures can cause inflammation. Poor posture can also cause nerve entrapment, as this can causes areas of the body to move in ways that were not intended, causing stress to them.

The symptoms of nerve entrapment can vary somewhat depending on the nerve affected and the individual. In general, compression of a nerve causes feelings of tingling (similar to the "pins and needles's" feeling that occurs when a hand or foot "falls asleep"). A feeling of numbness is common, and the affected area may not be able to fully feel normal sensations. In many cases, the area will be weak, and in some cases, the compressed nerve may cause slight twitching movements. In many cases, nerve compression causes a moderate to severe level of pain. This pain may be worse at night or upon waking up in the morning.

Diagnosis

Nerve entrapment is diagnosed using a history of the symptoms present in conjunction with one or more diagnostic tests.

Magnetic Resonance Imaging (MRI) uses a large magnet and radio waves to create pictures of the internal structures of the body. This can help doctors look for various kinds of damage, and can help rule out other possible problems that have symptoms similar to nerve entrapment.

One common way to diagnose nerve entrapment is through tests that examine how well the nerve that is believed to be compressed is transmitting impulses. Compressed nerves do not transmit electrical signals as effectively as nerves that are not compressed. A

KEY TERMS

Corticosteroids—A group of hormones that are sometimes used as an injection to treat inflammation.

Magnetic resonance imaging (MRI)—MRI uses a large circular magnet and radio waves to generate signals from atoms in the body. These signals are used to construct images of internal structures.

Nonsteroidal anti-inflammatory drugs (NSAIDs)— A class of drugs that is used to relieve pain, and symptoms of inflammation, such as ibuprofen and ketoprofen.

nerve conduction study uses electrodes placed on the skin to send a test impulse through the nerve believed to be compressed. How quickly the impulse moves through the nerve is then measured.

Treatment

The majority of cases of nerve entrapment can be treated successfully with noninvasive interventions. The first treatment typically suggested for nerve entrapment is to rest the problem area. This can help reduce swelling that will, in turn, reduce the compression on the nerve. It is especially important to stop doing any of the activities that may have caused the nerve entrapment. For example, if the compressed nerve occurs in the elbow it is advisable to stop playing tennis to allow the area time to heal.

Physical therapy may be recommended, depending on the area of the compressed nerve. Physical therapy can provide strengthening exercises for the muscles around the compressed nerve that can take some of the pressure off the problem area. In some cases, posture can be improved through physical therapy, which may be able to help nerve entrapment that occurs in the back.

Non-steroidal anti-inflammatory medications (NSAIDs) such ibuprofen may help reduce the swelling and can treat any pain associated with the compressed nerve. For individuals who have a lot of pain caused by the nerve entrapment that is not adequately treated b NSAIDs, corticosteroid injections may be recommended. Corticosteroid injections are given directly to the site of the problem, and are very successful in reducing swelling.

If nonsurgical treatments are not successful at alleviating the symptoms associated with nerve entrapment, surgery may be indicated. Surgery for nerve entrapment focuses on reducing the pressure on the affected nerve. This can be done in a number of ways, depending on the specific nerve. For carpal tunnel syndrome, surgery is often used to enlarge the carpal tunnel, giving the nerve and surrounding tissue more room. In some cases, tissue around the nerve may be removed to reduce the compression.

Prognosis

The prognosis for nerve entrapment is generally quite good. The significant majority of individuals can find relief through a combination of rest, splinting, and anti-inflammatory medications. In a minority of cases, surgery is required. Surgery is generally quite successful at reducing the compression of the nerve and providing relief. In cases of nerve entrapment that are left untreated, or for which treatment was not successful, permanent nerve damage can occur.

Prevention

There is no certain way to prevent nerve entrapment. However, some things can help reduce the risk. Maintaining a healthy weight can help reduce the pressure on nerves. Regular strength training, especially for areas likely to be a problem such as the back, can help increase muscle tone, improve posture, and relieve pressure that may lead to nerve compression. Maintaining good posture in general can help prevent nerve entrapment in the spine. Avoiding doing repetitive activities and taking frequent breaks to stretch can help prevent some kinds of nerve entrapment, especially carpal tunnel syndrome.

Resources

BOOKS

Akuthota, Venu, and Herring, Stanley A., eds. *Nerve and Vascular Injuries in Sports Medicine.* New York: Springer, 2009.

Fonseca, David J., and Martins, Joanne L., eds. *Sciatic Nerve: Blocks, Injuries, and Regeneration.* Hauppauge, NY: Nova Science, 2011.

Michael-Titus, Adina, Revest, Patricia, and Shortland, Peter. *The Nervous System: Basic Science and Clinical Conditions,* 2nd ed. New York: Churchill Livingstone, 2010.

PERIODICALS

Atroshi, Isam, et al. "Incidence of Physician-Diagnosed Carpal Tunnel Syndrome in the General Population." *Archives of Internal Medicine,* (May 23, 2011) 171(10):943–944. (accessed).

Kovacevic, David, Mariscalco, Michael, and Goodwin, Ryan C. "Injuries About the Hip in the Adolescent Athlete." *Sports Medicine and Arthroscopy Review,* (March 2011) 19(1):64–74.

Kox, Ida K., and Mackinnon, Susan E. "Adult Peripheral Nerve Disorders: Nerve Entrapment, Repair, Transfer, and Brachial Plexus Disorders." *Plastic and Reconstructive Surgery* (May 2011) 127(5):105e–118e.

WEBSITES

Hanna, Amgad Saddik, et al. (Medscape Reference). "Nerve Entrapment Syndromes." http://emedicine.medscape.com/article/249784-overview (accessed August 21, 2011).

Mayo Clinic. "Pinched Nerve." http://www.mayoclinic.com/health/pinched-nerve/DS00879 (accessed August 21, 2011).

ORGANIZATIONS

American Medical Society for Sports Medicine, 4000 W. 114th St., Suite 100, Leawood, KS, 66211, (913) 327-1415, Fax: (913) 327-1491, office@amssm.org, http://www.amssm.org.

American Neurological Association, 5841 Cedar Lake Rd., Suite 204, Minneapolis, MN, 55416, (952) 545-6284, Fax: (952) 545-6073, ana@llmsi.com, http://www.aneuroa.org.

The American Orthopedic Society for Sports Medicine, 6300 N River Rd., Suite 500, Rosemont, IL, 60018, (847) 292-4900, Fax: (847) 292-4905, http://www.sportsmed.org.

Tish Davidson, AM

Nervous system, autonomic

Definition

The autonomic nervous system is a network of nerves that regulate involuntary control of cardiac muscle, organ smooth muscle, and glands such that

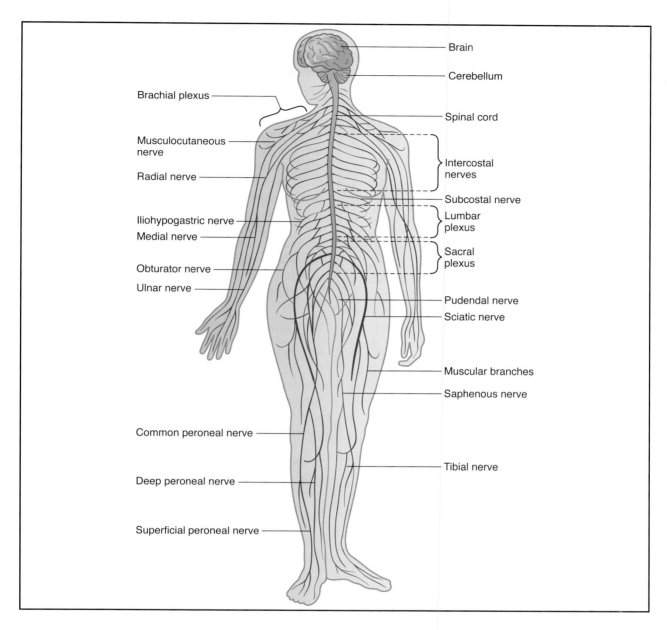

The nervous system. *(Electronic Illustrators Group. © 2012 Cengage Learning.)*

basic biological processes such as digestion and breathing can occur without conscious thought.

Description

The peripheral nervous system consists of nerves that must travel outside of the brain and spinal cord in order to contact organs, glands, and muscles. Under the umbrella of the peripheral nervous system are the somatic and autonomic nervous systems. The **somatic nervous system** is responsible for controlling voluntary movements during activities such as **walking**, while the autonomic nervous system regulates involuntary tasks such as food digestion. More specifically, the somatic division mediates voluntary or reflexive control of skeletal muscles, while the autonomic nervous system is responsible for the involuntary and reflexive control of glands, organ smooth muscle, and cardiac muscle.

The autonomic nervous system has three components:

- sympathetic nervous system
- parasympathetic nervous system
- enteric nervous system

The enteric nervous system is the less common of the three and is responsible for coordinating the digestive functions of the gastrointestinal tract, pancreas, and gall bladder. The two other subdivisions of the autonomic nervous system, parasympathetic and sympathetic, work in concert to subconsciously control other bodily functions, such as heart rate, **blood pressure**, digestion, **metabolism**, reproduction, breathing, excretion, sweating, and temperature.

The parasympathetic and sympathetic divisions have similar organizations but are distinguishable at the anatomical, biochemical, and functional levels. Both systems are organized into a two-neuron chain. The first neuron in this chain is referred to as a preganglionic neuron and the second as a postganglionic neuron. The nucleus containing cell bodies of preganglionic neurons are found in the brain and spinal cord of the central nervous system. The preganglionic neuron extends a fiber process, known as an axon, outside of the central nervous system to make contact with the cell body of the postganglionic neuron. The place where the axon of the preganglionic neuron meets the cell body of the postganglionic neuron is called a synapse. The synapses of the autonomic nervous system are outside of the brain and spinal cord of the central nervous system in specialized structures known as autonomic ganglia.

The preganglionic neurons of the parasympathetic nervous system originate in the brainstem and sacral spinal cord. These preganglionic neurons communicate with postganglionic neurons by extending very long axons that release the neurotransmitter, acetylcholine. The synapses of the parasympathetic ganglia are usually in or near the targeted organ. The postganglionic neuron expresses **protein** receptors on the surface that are capable of responding to acetylcholine. The postganglionic neurons have very short axons that release acetylcholine onto the targeted organ to modulate the intrinsic activity of that particular organ. These organs include the eye, lacrimal gland, salivary gland, heart, bronchi and lungs, small intestine, stomach, gallbladder, liver, pancreas, large intestine, rectum, genitalia, blood vessels, and bladder. Each of these targeted organs expresses acetylcholine receptors to respond to the parasympathetic nervous system.

The preganglionic neurons of the sympathetic nervous system originate in the thoracic and upper lumbar regions of the spinal cord. These preganglionic neurons send very short axons to synapse in the paravertebral or in the prevertebral ganglia. The paravertebral ganglia lie in close proximity to the spinal cord. The postganglionic neurons of the paravertebral ganglia send axons to the head, trunk, and limb regions. The other organs in the body receive inputs from the prevertebral ganglia which is further away from the spinal cord and closer to the target organ. An exception to organization is the adrenal gland which is directly contacted by preganglionic neurons of the sympathetic nervous system. Identical to the parasympathetic nervous system, the preganglionic neurons of the sympathetic nervous system communicate by releasing the neurotransmitter acetylcholine. However, the postganglionic neurons of the sympathetic nervous system differ in that they release norepinephrine onto the targeted organ. An exception to this is in the sweat glands where sympathetic postganglionic neurons release acetylcholine instead of norepinephrine. The target organs of the sympathetic nervous system include many of the same ones as the parasympathetic nervous system.

Function

The autonomic nervous system maintains internal balance (homeostasis) but also enables humans to respond to changes in the environment. This is achieved because the parasympathetic and sympathetic divisions of the systems are antagonistic. The parasympathetic and sympathetic nervous system usually have opposing effects on target organs. The predominate resting tone of an organ is established by either the sympathetic or parasympathetic system. For example, the predominate resting tone of the eye pupil is constriction, maintained by the parasympathetic nervous system. However, a fearful situation may induce pupil dilation, mediated by the sympathetic nervous system. In other words, the autonomic nervous system enables humans to deviate from normal functions to respond to changes in the environment. The parasympathetic nervous system is often referred to as "rest and digest" and the sympathetic nervous system as "fight or flight."

Each organ has a predominate resting tone that is influenced in a distinct way by the sympathetic and parasympathetic nervous systems. The sympathetic nervous system increases heart rate, while the parasympathetic slows it down. Likewise, the sympathetic system constricts blood vessels while the parasympathetic dilates them and therefore both systems influence blood pressure. The sympathetic nervous system reduces motility of the stomach and intestines while the parasympathetic increases motility. Most of the organs and glands controlled by the autonomic nervous system have this dual but opposing mechanism of regulation.

In some situations it is beneficial to override the autonomic nervous system. The postganglionic neurons and the targeted organs express protein receptors that sense and respond to the neurotransmitters acetylcholine and norepinephrine. The practice of autonomic pharmacology uses drugs to modify these receptors to override the existing setting. In this manner, dysfunctions such as high blood pressure can be treated and maintained.

The autonomic nervous system has a crucial role in human health because it maintains the internal balance as well as allows the individual to respond to environmental stimuli. Problems can arise when this system is over- or underactive. The autonomic nervous system is designed to respond to stress but too much stress can lead to abnormal resting organ tones. This is exemplified by heart disease and high blood pressure which can be treated by drugs that block the autonomic nervous system.

Common diseases and conditions

Holmes-Adie's syndrome

This is believed to be a disorder of the autonomic nervous system characterized by loss of the ability to constrict the eye pupil. This syndrome is also referred to as tonic pupil. The presenting patient maintains a dilated pupil and has decreased reflexes. The cililary ganglion, where the parasympathetic pre- and postganglion fibers meet, has been observed to degenerate. This loss of the parasympathetic tone renders the patient unable to constrict the pupil in response to light and nearby objects. The underlying cause is unknown but possibilities include viral infections that induce inflammation of the ciliary ganglion.

Familial dysautonomia

Familial dysautonomia is also referred to as Riley-Day syndrome and is an inherited disorder of the autonomic nervous system. The inheritance is autosomal recessive with widespread prevalence in patients of Ashkenazi Jewish decent. It is characterized by an increase in pain sensation, decreased lacrimation, an inability to regulate temperature, excessive sweating, and **hypertension**. It is usually diagnosed early in life and impairs development. There is evidence that there are a decreased number of sensory and autonomic nervous system neurons. Recently, the gene has been mapped to chromosome 9 and codes for a protein called IKAP. The function of IKAP is unknown, but it is hypothesized to be involved in gene activation mechanisms.

Horner's syndrome

Horner's syndrome is characterized by a lack of sympathetic tone to one side of the face. Therefore, symptoms that present are dropping eyelids, pupil constriction, and dryness to the face. The underlying cause of this is not clear but may originate within the spinal cord due to injury or tumor formation.

Shy-Drager syndrome

Patients with Shy-Drager syndrome have general autonomic nervous system dysfunction as well as parkinsonian-like symptoms. The autonomic symptoms included a decrease in blood pressure, orthostatic hypotension, constipation, urinary incontinence, and abnormal sweating. Some patients may also develop irregular heartbeats and have difficulty breathing. The parkinsonian-like symptoms included, tremor, slowness of movement, and problems maintaining balance. A key feature of the syndrome is dizziness or fainting due to the inability to maintain blood pressure. The underlying cause of the disease is unknown but neurons in the spinal cord have been observed to degenerate.

Effect of fitness and nutrition

The autonomic nervous system controls muscles of the internal organs and glands, affecting the heart, blood vessels, lungs, stomach, intestines, salivary glands and sweat glands. One part of this system helps the body relax and digest food, while another part of the system is geared toward quick reactions in an emergency.

As a result, the autonomic nervous system has a direct impact on organs and glands during **exercise**, as well as during ingestion and digestion of food. This system is constantly changing in response to physical activity and environmental changes.

When exercising, the autonomic nervous system balances fluctuations in respiration, blood pressure, digestion, and circulation of blood and hormones. All activity within the autonomic nervous system is involuntary and occurs in concert with ongoing physiological activities.

The mind body connection is prevalent when looking at functionality of the autonomic nervous system. The sympathetic portion of the autonomic nervous system responds readily to stress related situations, and parasympathetic portions of the autonomic nervous system maintain non–stress related bodily functions. Vital signs such as breathing, blood pressure and heart rate will increase or decrease accordingly, as the brain interacts with the autonomic nervous system, whether at rest or in a physically active situation.

During exercise the sympathetic portion of the autonomic nervous system is in control, increasing heart rate, heart contraction, muscle movement, and constriction of certain blood vessels. In addition, norepinephrine and **epinephrine** are released throughout the body, further assisting in the body's response to an exercise activity.

When at rest, the parasympathetic system takes over, allowing for a slower heart rate and dilation of blood vessels. In high stress situations or feeling stress over an extended period of time, the parasympathetic system is less engaged, so individuals feel minimally relaxed or rested. It is important then, that individuals pay attention to warning signs of stress such as insomnia, agitation, changes in appetite, muscle tension, and digestive problems. Exercise has long been known to aid in reducing stress and has the added benefit of increased confidence associated with feeling and looking physically fit.

Diets high in fat can create an imbalance in the autonomic nervous system by effecting changes in neurotransmitters. For reasons not yet clear, some chemicals in the body, such as dopamine, are impacted by a high fat diet, resulting in low levels of dopamine release and dopamine uptake, and disruption of autonomic nervous system balance. Studies show that low levels of dopamine fuel a desire toward overeating and a feeling of not being satiated after eating a meal. Studies suggest that there may be a correlation between **obesity** and imbalance in the autonomic nervous system with negative consequences in health and wellness, including insulin resistance. Nutrition, body weight, activity levels and

exercise play an important role in maintaining a healthy autonomic nervous system.

Resources

BOOKS

Aminoff, Michael J., ed. *Neurology and General Medicine,* 4th ed. New York: Churchill Livingstone, 2007.

McDowell, Julie., ed. *Encyclopedia of Human Body Systems.* Santa Barbara, CA: Greenwood, 2010.

Rizzo, Donald C. *Introduction to Anatomy and Physiology.* Clifton Park, NY: Delmar, 2011.

Upledger, John E., DO., OM. *A Brain Is Born: Exploring the Birth and Development of the Central Nervous System.* Berkeley, CA: North Atlantic Books, 2010.

PERIODICALS

Slaugenhaupt, Susan A., et. al. "Tissue-Specific Expression of a Splicing Mutation in the IKBKAP Gene Causes Familial Dysautonomia." *American Journal of Human Genetics* 68 (March 2001): 6803-6806.

ORGANIZATIONS

American Academy of Neurology. 1080 Montreal Ave. Saint Paul, MN 55116. (800) 879-1960. http://www.aan.com.

American Neurological Association. 5841 Cedar Lake Rd., Suite 204 Minneapolis, MN 55416. (952) 545-6284. http://www.aneuroa.org.

National Institutes of Health (NIH), 9000 Rockville Pike, Bethesda, MD, 20892, (301) 496-4000, http://www.nih.gov/index.html.

U.S. National Library of Medicine, 8600 Rockville Pike, Bethesda, MD, 20894, http://www.nlm.nih.gov/medlineplus/medlineplus.html.

Susan M. Mockus, PhD
Laura Jean Cataldo, RN, EdD

Nervous system, somatic

Definition

The somatic nervous system (SNS) is a division of the peripheral nervous system (PNS). The SNS controls voluntary activities, such as movement of skeletal muscles. It includes both sensory and motor nerves. Sensory nerves convey nerve impulses from the sense organs to the central nervous system (CNS), while motor nerves convey nerve impulses from the CNS to skeletal muscle effectors.

Description

Nervous tissue

All nervous tissue—including that of the SNS—consists of two main cell types: neurons and glial cells. Neurons transmit nerve signals and are surrounded by glial cells, which provide mechanical and physical support as well as electrical insulation between neurons.

Neurons

A neuron consists of a cell body, the soma, which contains the nucleus and surrounding cytoplasm; several short thread-like projections, called dendrites; and one long filament, called the axon. The dendrites receive information from other nearby cells and transmit the signals to the soma and the axon carries signals away from the neuron. Both axons and dendrites are surrounded by white protective coatings called myelin sheaths. The average adult brain contains about 100 billion neurons. Neurons are also the longest cells of the body, a single axon can be several feet long. There are two types of neurons found in the SNS: sensory neurons, which typically have long dendrites and short axons and carry messages from sensory receptors to the CNS, and motor neurons, which have a long axon and short dendrites and transmit signals from the CNS to muscles or glands.

The nervous system

The nervous system of the human body is divided into the central nervous system (CNS), consisting of the spinal cord and brain, and the peripheral nervous system (PNS), consisting of all the nerves that connect the CNS with organs, muscles, blood vessels, and glands. The PNS is subdivided into the somatic nervous system (SNS) and the **autonomic nervous system** (ANS). The ANS is further divided by function into sympathetic and parasympathetic systems.

The somatic nervous system (SNS)

The somatic nervous system (SNS) consists of sensory and motor nerve divisions. The sensory division, also called the afferent division, contains neurons that receive signals from the tendons, joints, skin, skeletal muscles, eyes, nose, ears and tongue, and many other tissues and organs. These signals are conveyed to the cranial and spinal nerves. The motor division, also called the efferent division, contains pathways that go from the brain stem and spinal cord to the lower motor neurons of the cranial and spinal nerves. When these nerves are stimulated, they cause the skeletal muscles to contract. This is called voluntary contraction of the skeletal muscles.

The nerves of the sensory-somatic system are:

THE CRANIAL NERVES (12 PAIRS).

- olfactory nerve, a sensory nerve for the sense of smell
- optic nerve, a sensory nerve for vision
- oculomotor nerve, a motor nerve for eyelid and eyeball muscle control
- trochlear nerve, a motor nerve for eyeball muscle control
- trigeminal nerve, a mixed nerve, the sensory part for facial and mouth sensation and the motor part for chewing
- abducens nerve, a motor nerve for eyeball movement control
- facial nerve, a mixed nerve, the sensory part for taste and the motor part for the control of facial muscles and salivary glands
- auditory nerve, a sensory nerve for hearing and balance control
- glossopharyngeal, a mixed nerve, the sensory part for taste and the motor part for the control of swallowing
- vagus, a mixed nerve, main PNS nerve that controls the gut, heart, and larynx
- accessory, a motor nerve for swallowing and moving the head and shoulders
- hypoglossal, a motor nerve for the control of tongue muscles

THE SPINAL NERVES (31 PAIRS). All of the spinal nerves are mixed nerves containing both sensory and motor neurons. They consist of eight cervical, 12 thoracic,

KEY TERMS

Axon—Long filament of a neuron that carries outgoing electrical signals from the cell body towards target cells. Each neuron has one axon, which can be longer than a foot. Neurons communicate with each other by transmitting signals from branches located at the end of their axons. At the end of the axons, nerve impulses are transmitted to other nerve cells or to effector organs.

Brachial plexus—A group of lower neck and upper back spinal nerves supplying the arm, forearm and hand.

Brain stem—Lowest part of the brain that connects with the spinal cord. It is a complicated neural center with several neuronal pathways between the cerebrum, spinal cord, cerebellum, and motor and sensory functions of the head and neck. It consists of the medulla oblongata, the part responsible for cardiac and respiratory control, the midbrain, which is involved in basic, involuntary body functions, and the pons, where some cranial nerves originate.

Central nervous system (CNS)—One of two major divisions of the nervous system. The CNS consists of the brain, the cranial nerves and the spinal cord.

Cranial nerve—In humans, there are 12 cranial nerves. They are connected to the brain stem and basically "run" the head as well as help regulate the organs of the thoracic and abdominal cavities.

Dendrites—Threadlike extensions of the cytoplasm of a neuron.

Effector—Any molecule, chemical, organ, structure or agent that regulates a pathway by changing the pathway's reaction rate.

Ganglia—A mass of nerve tissue or a group of neurons.

Mechanoreceptors—Receptors specialized to detect mechanical signals and relay that information centrally in the nervous system. Mechanoreceptors include hair cells involved in hearing and balance.

Myelin—The substance making up the protective sheath of nerve axons.

Nervous system—The entire system of nerve tissue in the body. It includes the brain, the brain stem, the spinal cord, the nerves, and the ganglia, and is divided into the peripheral nervous system (PNS) and the central nervous system (CNS).

five lumbar, five sacral, and one coccygeal. In spinal nerves, some nerves fibers are ascending, meaning that they carry messages to the brain, while others are descending, meaning that they carry messages from the brain.

Sensory input to the nervous system occurs through the senses, which are: vision, taste, smell, touch and hearing, also called the special senses. Additional input is provided by the somatic senses, which are pain, temperature, and pressure. This sensory input uses sensors, also called sensory receptors. The major sensory receptors are:

- mechanoreceptors that respond to hearing and stretching
- photoreceptors that are sensitive to light
- chemoreceptors that respond mostly to smell and taste
- thermoreceptors that are sensitive to changes in temperature
- electroreceptors that detect electrical currents in the environment

Function

The overall role of the nervous system is to act as an internal communications system that allows the body to react to environmental changes and to perform all activities required to maintain life. The PNS is the message carrier between the CNS and the rest of the body and it can not function with an impaired SNS. Thus, the role of the SNS in human health is crucial.

The major function of the SNS is the voluntary control of the muscle system of the body and the processing of sensory information to the CNS. All conscious knowledge of the external world and all the motor activity performed by the body to respond to it operates through the SNS.

Common diseases and conditions

Somatic nervous system diseases are diseases of the peripheral nerves that are external to the brain and spinal cord. Thus, they include diseases of the nerve roots, ganglia, sensory and motor nerves. A functional disorder and/or abnormal change that occurs in any region of the peripheral nervous system is called a neuropathy. If the involvement is in one nerve only, it is called a mononeuropathy, and if in several nerves, mononeuropathy multiplex or polyneuropathy. The most common disorders are the following:

Neurons—Cells of the nervous system. Usually consist of a cell body, the soma, that contains the nucleus and the surrounding cytoplasm; several short thread-like projections (dendrites); and one long filament (the axon).

Neuropathy—A general term describing functional disorders and/or abnormal changes in the peripheral nervous system. If the involvement is in one nerve it is called mononeuropathy, and if in several nerves, mononeuropathy multiplex.

Oculomotor nerve—Cranial nerve responsible for motor enervation of the upper eyelid muscle, the extraocular muscle and the eye pupil muscle.

Parasympathetic nervous system—One of the two divisions of the autonomic nervous system. Parasympathetic nerves emerge from the skull as fibres from the oculomotor, facial, glossopharyngeal and vagus nerves and from the sacral region of the spinal cord.

Peripheral nerves—The nerves outside of the brain and spinal cord, including the autonomic, cranial, and spinal nerves. These nerves contain cells other than neurons and connective tissue as well as axons.

Peripheral nervous system (PNS)—One of the two major divisions of the nervous system. The PNS consists of the somatic nervous system (SNS), which controls voluntary activities, and of the autonomic nervous system (ANS), which controls regulatory activities. The ANS is further divided into sympathetic and parasympathetic systems.

Plexus—A network or group of nerves.

Sensory cells—Cells that contain receptors on their surface.

Sensory nerve—A nerve that receives input from sensory cells, such as the skin mechanoreceptors or the muscle receptors.

Spinal cord—Elongated part of the central nervous system that lies in the vertebral column and from which the spinal nerves emerge.

Sympathetic nervous system—One of the two divisions of the autonomic nervous system. The sympathetic neurons have their cell bodies in the thoracic and lumbar regions of the spinal cord and connect to the paravertebral chain of sympathetic ganglia. They innervate heart and blood vessels, sweat glands, organs and the adrenal medulla.

- Brachial plexus neuropathies: Diseases of the peripheral nerve components of the brachial plexus, a group of lower neck and upper back spinal nerves supplying the arm, forearm and hand. Symptoms include local pain, muscle weakness, and decreased sensation (hypesthesia) in the upper extremity.

- Cranial nerve diseases: Disorders and diseases of the cranial nerves.

- Cranial nerve neoplasms: Benign or cancerous growth in cranial nerve tissues. Examples are: acoustic neuroma, optic nerve glioma, optic nerve meningioma.

- Diabetic neuropathies: Peripheral and cranial nerve disorders that are associated with diabetes. A common condition associated with diabetic neuropathy includes third nerve palsy, which affects the oculomotor nerve.

- Guillain-Barre syndrome: An acute inflammatory autoimmune neuritis caused by the body attacking the myelin coating of its own peripheral nerves. The syndrome often occurs as a result of viral or bacterial infection, surgery, immunization, lymphoma, or exposure to toxins.

- Mononeuropathies: Disease or trauma involving a single peripheral nerve. Mononeuropathies result from a wide variety of causes such as traumatic injury; nerve compression, and connective tissue diseases.

- Myasthenia gravis (MG): MG (and also the less common Lambert-Eaton syndrome) are neuromuscular junction diseases, that affect how nerve impulses are transmitted to muscle at the neuromuscular junction. They are autoimmune diseases, meaning that the body generates an immune system attack against its own skeletal muscles.

- Nerve compression syndromes: These syndromes are due to the compression of nerves or nerve roots from internal or external causes and result in the blocking of nerve impulses due to myelin sheath or axon damage.

- Neuralgia: Neuralgias are disorders of the cranial nerves that result in intense or aching pain occurring along a peripheral or cranial nerve. Neuralgias are associated with all of the cranial nerves: trigeminal neuralgia in the facial area, glossopharyngeal neuralgia in the throat, occipital neuralgia in the rear and side of the head, geniculate neuralgia in the ear, and vegal neuralgia in the jaw.

- Neuritis: Inflammation of a peripheral or cranial nerve.
- Peripheral nervous system neoplasms: Benign or cancerous growths that arise from peripheral nerve tissue. They include neurofibromas, granular cell tumors and malignant peripheral nerve sheath tumors.
- Trigeminal neuralgia (TN): Most common neuralgia. It affects the fifth cranial (trigeminal) nerve and causes episodes of intense, stabbing, electric shock-like pain in the areas of the face where the branches of the nerve are distributed, that is lips, eyes, nose, scalp, forehead, upper jaw, and lower jaw.

Effect of fitness and nutrition

The somatic nervous system is the portion of the peripheral nervous system where (together with motor neurons and the brain), an individual consciously decides to move a muscle and actually makes the muscle movement occur. This portion of the nervous system is considered "voluntary" in that individuals determine that they will enable whatever body movement needs to occur, in order to get out of bed, brush their teeth, sit on the sofa, etc. Although most of these types of movements occur in minute seconds and appear to be done without forethought, the somatic nervous system enables the necessary connections between the brain and spinal nerves, allowing skeletal muscles to perform these everyday movements.

The somatic system then, is the portion of the nervous system that enables individuals to participate in **exercise**. This system is responsible for motor (efferent) fibers to communicate between the brain and the muscles that are used during a workout. Motor neurons between the brain and muscles work in concert to allow the movement (contraction) of muscles when performing one's exercise routine. Motor neurons connect to multiple muscle fibers throughout the body.

This portion of the nervous system is directly responsible for enabling the body's control and response to exercise. Skeletal muscles need signals or "instruction" from motor neurons of the somatic nervous system in order to contract.

When exercising, the somatic nervous system "excites" a muscle or muscle group into action. As we incorporate fitness into our daily routine, these muscles increase in size, resulting in a body that is toned and strong. Resistance training is especially helpful in this regard however, both aerobic and anaerobic exercise has overall health benefits associated with more **energy**, stamina, strength, and endurance.

QUESTIONS TO ASK YOUR DOCTOR

- What are the indications that I may have a problem with my nervous system?
- What diagnostic tests are needed for a thorough assessment?
- What kind of fitness program should I follow?
- What dietary changes, if any, would you recommend for me?
- What tests or evaluation techniques can you perform to see if my fitness and nutritional choices promote a healthy condition?
- What treatment options do you recommend for me?
- What physical or health limitations do you foresee?
- What measures can be taken to prevent nervous system problems?
- How can my quality of life be improved?
- What symptoms are important enough that I should seek immediate treatment?

As noted previously, the somatic nervous system is also responsible for control of all five senses and as such, plays a major role in how individuals "relate" to food. All five senses come into play as we eat; while **sitting** down to a meal, we visualize and smell our food, we interpret the sound and feel of food while chewing and tasting our meal. The somatic nervous system is inherently associated with sensory perception, that is, how we perceive food and shape our nutritional habits. Through the somatic nervous system, our eyes, tongue, and even muscles of the jaw are part of the process involved with food intake, resulting in the sensation of enjoying the overall eating experience.

Resources

BOOKS

Aminoff, Michael J., ed. *Neurology and General Medicine,* 4th ed. New York: Churchill Livingstone, 2007.

McDowell, Julie., ed. *Encyclopedia of Human Body Systems.* Santa Barbara, CA: Greenwood, 2010.

Rizzo, Donald C. *Introduction to Anatomy and Physiology.* Clifton Park, NY: Delmar, 2011.

Upledger, John E., DO., OM. *A Brain Is Born: Exploring the Birth and Development of the Central Nervous System.* Berkeley, CA: North Atlantic Books, 2010.

PERIODICALS

Vaillancourt, P. D., and Langevin, H. M. "Painful peripheral neuropathies." *The Medical Clinics of North America* 83 (1999): 627-642.

WEBSITES

Kimball's Biology Pages. "The Sensory-Somatic Nervous System." http://www.ultranet.com/~jkimball/Biology-Pages/P/PNS.html#sensory-somatic (accessed December 28, 2011).

NINDS Peripheral Neuropathy Information Page. http://www.ninds.nih.gov/health_and_medical/disorders/peripheralneuropathy_doc.htm (accessed December 28, 2011).

ORGANIZATIONS

American Academy of Neurology. 1080 Montreal Ave. Saint Paul, MNm 55116, (800) 879-1960, http://www.aan.com.

American Neurological Association. 5841 Cedar Lake Rd., Suite 204 Minneapolis, MN, 55416, (952) 545-6284, http://www.aneuroa.org.

GBS/CIDP Foundation International. The Holly Building, 104 1/2 Forrest Ave., Narberth, PA, 19072, (610) 667-0131, http://www.gbs-cidp.org.

National Institute of Neurological Disorders and Stroke (NINDS), P.O. Box 5801, Bethesda, MD, 20824, (800) 352-9424, http://www.ninds.nih.gov/index.htm.

National Institutes of Health (NIH), 9000 Rockville Pike, Bethesda, MD, 20892, (301) 496-4000, http://www.nih.gov/index.html.

Neuropathy Association. 60 East 42nd St., Suite 942, New York, NY, 10165-0999, (212) 692-0662, (800)-247-6968. info@neuropathy.org. http://www.neuropathy.org.

U.S. National Library of Medicine, 8600 Rockville Pike, Bethesda, MD, 20894, http://www.nlm.nih.gov/medlineplus/medlineplus.html.

Monique Laberge, PhD
Laura Jean Cataldo, RN, EdD

Nutrition supplements

Definition

Nutritional supplements are substances designed to supplement an individual's diet to provide nutrients such as vitamins and minerals that might otherwise be missing from a diet or might be present in inadequate amounts. Nutritional supplements are also known as dietary supplements or food supplements. The precise definition of these terms varies from nation to nation and between national and international regulatory agencies. The legal definition of a nutritional supplement in the United States is provided in Section 3 of the Dietary Supplement Health and Education Act of 1994 (DSHEA) as including substances such as vitamins, minerals, herbs and other botanicals (except for tobacco), amino acids, and metabolites or concentrates of these substances.

Purpose

Nutritional supplements provide an individual with essential nutrients or active compounds that they might not otherwise get in their diets, or that they might receive in amounts less than those recommended for maintenance of good health or needed in higher doses to achieve a desired effect or response.

Description

About 100 substances listed as nutritional supplements are regularly sold in the United States in substantial quantities. A sampling of the substances found on any list of popular nutritional supplements includes:

- 5-HTP
- aloe
- beta carotene
- biotin
- calendula
- chondroitin sulfate
- devil's claw
- echinacea
- fish oil
- gingko
- ginseng
- lavender
- melatonin
- pantothenic acid
- red clover
- saw palmetto
- turmeric
- yohimbe

The market for nutritional supplements in many parts of the world is huge. According to the *Nutrition Business Journal*, sales of nutritional supplements in the United States increased in 2010 by 7%, the last year for which data are available, to a total of US$28.7 billion. That increase was somewhat surprising since experts had expected that the nation's economic downturn might prompt some users of supplements to cut back. In fact, supplement sales grew more than 5% every year during the nation's recession. According to one recent survey, 65% of all Americans regularly take at least one nutritional supplement, while many take a number of supplements. The most popular supplements sold in the United States are multivitamins, followed by meal replacements (such as Ensure and Slim Fast), sports and fitness supplements, calcium, and B vitamins.

Manufacturers make a number of health claims for their products, such as claims that the supplements can increase **energy**, lower the risk of certain diseases, boost the **immune system**, etc. The U.S. Food and Drug Administration (FDA), responsible for the oversight of both drugs and nutritional supplements, requires that every new drug that appears on the market be thoroughly tested to show that it is (1) safe and (2) effective. Drug manufacturers have to go through extensive testing of a new drug that may last many years and cost many millions of dollars to prove that the drug (1) will not kill or harm you and (2) will act the way the company says it will (e.g., cure cancer or reduce the symptoms of **asthma**).

Under provisions of the Dietary Supplement Health and Education Act (DSHEA) of 1994, the makers of nutritional supplements no longer have to provide that kind of evidence for their products. Any product that contains a new substance must undergo testing before it informs the FDA that it intends to start marketing the supplement. No matter what the manufacturer's tests show, the FDA can not prohibit production and sale of the supplement because supplements are not classified as drugs. The only role the FDA has in ensuring the safety of a product arises when evidence becomes available that a supplement may be harmful to a person or other animal. In that case, the FDA must undertake tests to determine the safety of the product and, if it turns out to be harmful, have it banned from the marketplace. That event has occurred only once to date, with regard to the herbal product called ephedra, which was found to be responsible for a number of human deaths.

Under DSHEA, the most effective tool available to the FDA is the requirement that manufacturers are not allowed to make claims for supplements for which there is no evidence. Thus, a manufacturer can not say, "Product X will prevent HIV," although it can say "Product X may contribute to a stronger immune system that may protect you against HIV." Supplement companies have become very skilled at promoting the supposed benefits of their products without making outright scientific claims. Consumers sometimes have difficulty recognizing the limitations of claims made for nutritional supplements by manufacturers.

The use of nutritional supplements, especially for essential nutrients, is necessary for some people and supported by the medical community. For example, people who have limited sun exposure may need additional vitamin D, pregnant women require higher levels of folic acid, and people who follow a vegan diet need vitamin B_{12}.

A central issue surrounding the sale and use of supplements has to do with the question as to whether they actually produce the results they claim. Some people are satisfied with anecdotal evidence provided by friends, family, or the media. Such individuals are not concerned that the best scientific evidence available indicates that any reasonably healthy person in any developed nation gets an adequate supply of essential nutrients in all but the worst of diets, and that the purchase of multivitamins may be the greatest unnecessary medical expense most people realize. For people who are interested in scientific evidence concerning the efficacy of supplements, that information may be difficult to obtain. Until fairly recently, there have been few, if any, controlled studies on how well substances in supplements produce the results claimed for them. Over the past decade, however, the National Center for Complementary and Alternative Medicine (CAM) has been accumulating data on the efficacy of various nutritional supplements. Those data are now available on CAM's website at http://nccam.nih.gov/. CAM has found that some claims for supplements do have some basis in scientific evidence, but many claims can not be confirmed or have not yet been adequately tested. For anyone interested in obtaining information about specific products, the CAM website is the best repository of data on these products.

Recommended dosage

The FDA has established certain recommended dosages, called Recommended Daily Intakes (RDIs) for vitamins and minerals. A chart listing those RDAs is available on the FDA website at http://www.fda.gov/Food/GuidanceComplianceRegulatoryInformation/GuidanceDocuments/FoodLabelingNutrition/FoodLabelingGuide/ucm064928.htm. Similar recommended dosages for most other supplements are not available because scientific studies have not shown the efficacy of particular products and, therefore, cannot specify the dosage recommended, if any amount of the product is useful. Nonetheless, manufacturers often suggest recommended dosages on the labels of their supplement products that are based more or less on whatever studies of the product may be available.

Precautions

An issue of some concern with regard to nutritional supplements is the lack of adequate information about possible harmful effects of these products on consumers. Since most nutritional supplements have not been exposed to the detailed testing process required of drugs, the information one needs about precautions is often not readily available. Nonetheless, a fair amount of anecdotal and circumstantial evidence is available about at least some of these supplements:

• The consumption of kava has been associated with a number of cases of liver disease, including cirrhosis, hepatitis, liver failure, and death.

- The use of gingko biloba has been associated with headaches, dizziness, excessive bleeding, rash, and stomach disorders.

- In 2001, the FDA issued a consumer advisory about possible liver damage resulting from the use of comfrey.

- A supplement commonly used by athletes, yohimbine, has been found to have a number of adverse effects, including high blood pressure, rapid heart rate, insomnia, headaches, dizziness, panic attacks, and hallucinations.

- The FDA banned the sale of ephedra in 2004 because of the substance's involvement in a number of deaths, perhaps the most famous of which was that of Baltimore Orioles pitcher Steve Bechler in 2003. Although the nutritional supplement industry contested this decision, the U.S. Court of Appeals for the Tenth District finally agreed with the FDA decision two years later.

This list of supplements and possible side effects should not be interpreted to suggest that the use of such products is dangerous across the board. Many nutritional supplements are perfectly safe to use or, at least, reasonably safe for most people most of the time. It is in a consumer's best interests, however, to obtain as much information as possible about a supplement before beginning to use that product on a regular basis.

Individuals should also be cautioned against taking supplements in excessive, or megadoses. Taking more than the RDI may lead to side effects that could be harmful to one's health. Also, women who are pregnant should discuss the use of nutrition supplements with her physician before taking them. Consuming additional vitamin A during pregnancy, for example, should be avoided.

Interactions

Potentially dangerous interactions can occur between nutritional supplements and prescription and over-the-counter (OTC) drugs or other products ingested by people. Interactions identified so far include:

- The herbal supplement St. John's wort may reduce the concentration of certain drugs, such as the protease inhibitor indinavir and the heart medication digoxin, in the blood; thus, reducing the drugs' efficacy.

- Kava may interact with alprazolam (Xanax), a drug used to control anxiety attacks, producing lethargy and disorientation.

- Ginseng has been found to interact with more than 100 drugs and other supplements to produce a variety of potentially harmful side effects.

- Ginger, goldenseal, and a number of other supplements may interact with anticoagulants to increase the potential of uncontrolled bleeding.

- Echinacea may interact with immunodepressant drugs, such as cyclosporine, methotrexate, and asathioprine; and with steroidal medicines, such as cortisone, hydrocortisone, and prednisone.

- A number of supplements, such as valeian, ginger, goldenseal, and chamomile, may interact with sedatives (such as barbiturates and alcohol) to increase the sedative effects of those substances.

- The herbal supplement dong quai may interact with warfarin and other anticoagulants to further decrease the rate of blood clotting, leading to potentially serious bleeding problems.

- Interactions between the supplement 5-HTP and medications for the treatment of depression, such as fluoxetine (Prozac) and sertraline (Zoloft) may occur since both act to suppress the neurotransmitter serotonin. Taking a combination of the substances may cause heart problems and anxiety.

This list should not be taken as a prescription not to use dietary supplements, but to use them cautiously. A study completed in 1999 found that 18% of all adults in the United States were simultaneously taking prescription medications and nutritional supplements, placing an estimated 15 million people at risk for potentially dangerous supplement-drug interactions.

Prevention

Many people choose to take nutritional supplements to increase their strength, mental ability, or some other trait. To the extent that a supplement does have these effects, and assuming that one observes all necessary cautions with their use, there is no reason not to use nutrition supplements. A larger number of people take supplements for the reason for which they are designed, to provide a daily intake of some vital nutrient that they would not otherwise be getting. For people who take supplements for this reason, an option to dietary supplements is a more nutritious diet that includes adequate amounts of **carbohydrates**, **fats**, **protein**, vitamins and minerals. Eating such a diet in any developed nation is not a problem except for individuals who are surviving in dire poverty. Even then, a variety of government programs are available (such as food stamps) that make it relatively easy for a person to get all the nutritious food necessary.

Resources

BOOKS

Hendler, Sheldon, and David Rorvik. *PDR for Nutritional Supplements*, 2nd ed. Montvale, NJ: PDR Network, 2008.
Sarubin-Fragakis, Allison, and Cynthia Thomson. *The Health Professional's Guide to Popular Dietary Supplements*, 3rd ed. Chicago: American Dietetic Association, 2007.

PERIODICALS

Denham, B. E. "Dietary Supplements—Regulatory Issues and Implications for Public Health." *Journal of the American Medical Association* 306, no. 4 (July 25, 2011): 428–9.
Grigg, William Norman. "Globalist Threat to Vitamins: Bureaucrats Attached to the United Nations Are Seeking to Deprive Millions Worldwide of Access to Nutritional Supplements." *The New American* 21, no. 18 (September 5, 2005): 31 +.

WEBSITES

Background Information: Dietary Supplements. Office of Dietary Supplements. (June 24, 2011). http://ods.od.nih.gov/factsheets/DietarySupplements/ (accessed November 15, 2011).
Dietary Supplements. U.S. Food and Drug Administration. (October 6, 2011). http://www.fda.gov/Food/DietarySupplements/default.htm (accessed November 15, 2011).

ORGANIZATIONS

Office of Dietary Supplements, National Institutes of Health, 6100 Executive Blvd., Room 3B01, MSC 7517, Bethesda, MD, 20892-7517, (301) 435-2920, Fax: (301) 480-1845, ods@nih.gov, http://ods.od.nih.gov.

David E. Newton, AB, MA EdD

Nutrition timing

Definition

Nutrition timing is a program for providing the body with the proper nutrients in the proper amounts at the appropriate time before, during, and after an **exercise** workout or a sports event.

Description

Virtually all athletes and trainers have long been aware that individuals who engage in vigorous exercise require a sound program of nutrition to perform at maximum efficiency. Further, almost all also recognize that timing is an important factor in maintaining the proper nutritional schedule. For example, **marathon** runners have traditionally eaten a dinner heavy in **carbohydrates** on the night before a race, a process known as "carbo loading," on the presumption that a huge store of carbohydrates will help provide the runners with a store of **energy** to get them through the event.

Over the last decade, researchers have been looking more carefully at the details of nutrition timing. A leading scholar in this field has been John Ivy, chairperson of the Department of **Kinesiology** and Health Education in the College of Education at The University of Texas at Austin. Ivy has now written three popular books on his findings about nutrition timing and how they apply to anyone who engages in vigorous exercise or sports event. Ivy has based his findings on a general review of the biological and biochemical changes that take place in the human body before, during, and after exercise, three periods that he classifies as the energy phase, the anabolic phase, and the growth phase. The energy phase is that period of time during which a person is actively engaged in an exercise or sports: **running**, jumping, lifting weights, cycling, or **rowing**, for example. During this stage, the body focuses on providing the energy needed to complete these activities. Specifically, hormones (in particular, glucagon, cortisol, and catecholamine) increase in number to make possible a more rapid rate of the catabolism (breakdown) of glycogen to glucose in the liver, muscle cells, and adipose (fat) cells.

The anabolic phase begins toward the end of an exercise and continues at a more rapid rate as soon as the exercise has been completed. Anabolism is the process by which cells use raw materials such as glucose and amino acid to build larger, more complex compounds, such as glycogen ("stored energy") and proteins. The catabolic reactions that dominate the energy phase do

BRIAN MAXWELL (1953–2004)

Brian Maxwell was a long-distance runner who struggled with stomach pains during a 1983 marathon, inspiring him to create a more appropriate fitness food. The goal—a nutritious and highly digestible food high in carbohydrates and low in fat.

In 1986, with a US$55,000 budget, Maxwell founded PowerBar Inc. He refined the energy bars based on feedback received from runners and athletes. The 1987 U.S. Tour de France team swore that the PowerBar was their "secret weapon" and this caused sales to quickly accelerate.

1998 was a watershed year for the company. PowerBar had almost 40% of the market share, earning US$120 million annually. The company also branched into sponsorship—sponsoring almost 2,500 events in 1998.

In 1998, PowerBars were available for purchase in health clubs and certain specialty stores. The company ranked 22nd on the *Inc.* 500 list of the fastest-growing, privately held companies.

Though an avid athlete his whole life, Maxwell died on March 19, 2004, of a heart attack.

not automatically come to a halt when an exercise has been completed and, in fact, will continue unless something happens to turn them off and shift cells into an anabolic mode. The "something" that is necessary is an infusion of proteins which, when broken down, provide the amino acids needed to drive anabolic reactions in cells. The growth phase is, in a word, everything else, from an hour following completion of an exercise to the beginning of the next exercise period. During this period of time, muscle cells are most active in repairing damage produced during the exercise stage and in building new muscle tissue.

A nutrition program based on this line of cellular functioning focuses on the types of nutrients needed to maximize the efficiency of each step. The specifics of such a program depend on some factors other than cellular biochemistry, such as the type of exercise or sport involved and the specific characteristics of a participant's body. But some general recommendations can be made about a nutrition timing program that can be beneficial to any athlete:

First, unrelated to Ivy's three phase theory of conditioning, adequate **hydration** is essential at all stages of any physical activity. The physical consequences of **dehydration** are now well known, ranging from increased strain on the heart at body water loss of only 0.5% to reduced muscular endurance at body water loss of 3% to cramping, **heat exhaustion**, and reduced mental capacity at body water loss of 5%. To reduce the possibility of dehydration, then, Ivy recommends that athletes drink 14–20 ounces of water of sports drink 30 minutes before exercise or an event.

Hydration continues to be the primary concern during the energy phase of exercise. It is during this period that the body is losing water through perspiration and using up glucose for the production of energy. Again, the

specific nutritional recommendation for this depends somewhat on the type of exercise or the sport involved, but generally speaking, rehydration with 200–300 milliliters of a drink that contains electrolytes and four to six percent carbohydrate and two to four percent **protein**. Some sports nutritionists are doubtful about the protein component of this rehydration process, but Ivy believes that small amounts of protein may help the body start to repair damaged muscle tissue produced during an exercise and may prevent post-exercise muscle soreness.

Research studies suggest that the body begins to prepare itself for a recovery phase even before an exercise has been completed. For example, cells begin making changes that replenish the supplies of essential biochemicals depleted in an exercise workout. Molecules used to transport glucose to muscle cells for conversion to glycogen start to relocate in such a way as to make them more efficient in carrying out this process. Also, enzymes needed for the conversion of amino acids to proteins become more abundant and more active, increasing the rate at which new protein is being produced in cells. The anabolic reactions needed to restore the body to its pre-exercise state do not actually begin to function efficiently, however, until they have the essential raw materials, the nutrients that must be ingested to get the process going. Ivy says that this "window of opportunity" during which a person can provide his or her body with exactly the right nutrients is very narrow, probably no more than 30 to 45 minutes. An athlete who has waited two hours after an exercise for a nutritious meal has probably waited too long. The body has probably switched over to its anabolic phase, although at a much less efficient pace that would otherwise have been possible. Ivy's recommendations for the first

KEY TERMS

Anabolism—The process by which cells use simple molecules, such as simple sugars and amino acids, to build more complex molecules, such as glycogen and proteins.

Carbo loading—The process by which a person eats relatively large amonts of complex carbohydrates (such as starches) with the aim of building up a large supply of energy-releasing compounds needed for endurance events, such a marathon races.

Catabolism—The process by which cells breakdown molecules, such as glycogen, glucose, proteins, and amino acids into simpler molecules, such as carbon dioxide and water, accompanied by the release of energy.

Catecholamines—So-called "fight or flight" hormones released during times of stress.

Cortisol—A hormone involved in the breakdown of carbohydrates and proteins.

Glucagon—A hormone produced in the pancreas that breaks down glycogen to glucose.

QUESTIONS TO ASK YOUR DOCTOR

• What are you views in general on nutrition timing?

• What recommendations would you make for a program of modest exercise for me that includes a program of nutrition timing?

• Given the intense program of exercise that I follow regularly, what specific nutritional timing recommendations you can make to increase the efficiency of that program of exercise?

---

post-exercise meal is one that contains 1.0–1.5 grams of carbohydrate and 0.3–0.4 grams of protein per kilogram of body weight, again depending on the type and intensity of workout.

Ivy's recommendations for the post-exercise growth stage do not differ significantly from those made by most nutrition experts. Athletes should continue to eat at regular intervals (every few hours), following a diet that is rich in carbohydrates, proteins, and other essential nutrients. This kind of diet supplies the basic raw materials the body needs to get through its continuing period of sustained growth that follows completion of an exercise or sports event.

Function

The nutrition timing program outlined here is intended specifically for individuals who engage regularly in exercises of some intensity, usually with the goal of improving their overall physical strength or conditioning in some way or another. The program has no specific application for individuals who are not involved in such activities.

Resources

BOOKS

Portman, Robert, and John Ivy. *Hardwired for Fitness.* Laguna Beach, CA: Basic Health Publications, 2011.

Seebohar, Bob. *Nutrition Periodization for Athletes: Taking Traditional Sports Nutrition to the Next Level.* Boulder, CO: Bull Publishing Company: 2011.

Skolnik, Heidi, and Andrea Chernus. *Nutrient Timing for Peak Performance.* Champaign, IL: Human Kinetics, 2010.

PERIODICALS

Millard-Stafford, Melinda, et al. "Recovery Nutrition: Timing and Composition after Endurance Exercise." *Current Sports Medicine Reports.* 7(4; July/August 2008): 193–201.

Ulrich, Laura. "Timing is Everything." *Coaching Management.* 16(1; 2008): 29–33.

WEBSITES

Paczosa, Adrien. "Get the Most from Your Workout: Nutrient Timing. Austin Simply Fit." http://www. austinsimplyfit. com/Nutrition.html?entry = get-the-most-from-your and http://www.austinsimplyfit.com/ Nutrition.html? entry = get-tthe-most-oout-of (accessed on August 17, 2011).

Randall, Kay. "Timing Is Everything." University of Texas at Austin. http://www.utexas.edu/features/archive/ 2004/nutrition.html (accessed on August 17, 2011).

ORGANIZATIONS

American College of Sports Medicine, 401 West Michigan St., Indianapolis, IN, 46202-3233 (317) 637-9200, Fax: (317) 634-7817, http://www.acsm.org/AM/Template.cfm? Section = Contact_ACSM&Template = /CustomSource/ Department/index.cfm&area = general, http://www. acsm.org/.

International Society of Sports Nutrition, 600 Pembrook Dr., Woodland Park, CO, 80863, Fax: (719) 687-5184, (866) 740-4776, issn.sports.nutrition@gmail.com.

David E. Newton, AB, MA, EdD

Obesity

Definition

Obesity is a medical condition in which there is an excessive accumulation (storage) of body fat resulting in a **body mass index** (BMI) that is significantly above the norm. It is associated with increased risk of illness, disability, and death. Medical professionals generally consider obesity, or being excessively overweight, to be a chronic illness requiring lifelong treatment and management. It is often grouped with other chronic conditions—such as high **blood pressure** and **diabetes**—that can be controlled but not cured.

Description

The human body is composed of bone, muscle, specialized organ tissues, and fat. Together these comprise the total body mass, measured in pounds (lb) or kilograms (kg). Fat, or adipose tissue, is a combination of essential and storage **fats**. Essential fat is an **energy** source for the normal physiologic function of cells and organs, it protects and insulates internal organs, and it is an important building block for all cells of the body. Storage fat is a reserve supply of energy. It accumulates in the chest and abdomen and, in much greater volume, under the skin. When the amount of energy consumed as food exceeds the amount of energy expended in the maintenance of life processes and physical activity, storage fat accumulates in excessive amounts.

The human body needs fat for good health. However, sometimes the body accumulates too much fat. Thus, obesity is excessive body weight that develops over time as people consume more **calories** than they expend in energy over their daily lives. As excess energy accumulates in the body, people first become overweight, then obese (excessively overweight).

In times of famine, the ability of the human body to store energy can mean the difference between life and death. This protective mechanism becomes a potential problem when food is readily available in unlimited quantities. This is evident in the increasing prevalence of obesity in modern society, particularly in the developed world. For instance, in the early 2010s, the United States and Australia are considered to have two of the largest percentages of obese people in the world. Too much food, especially those high in sugar and fat content, and not enough **exercise** are reasons why people are becoming obese in these two countries and in other regions of the world. In fact, the U.S. Centers for Disease Control and Prevention (CDC) states that obesity levels in the United States has doubled for adults and tripled for children over the past few decades. As obesity rates have increased, bariatrics—the branch of medicine that studies and treats obesity—has become a separate medical and surgical specialty.

Guidelines

Obesity was originally defined as body weight that was at least 20% above one's ideal weight, defined as the weight at which individuals of the same height, gender, and **age** had the lowest rate of death. Mild obesity was defined as 20–40% over ideal weight, moderate obesity as 40–100% over ideal, and gross or morbid obesity 100% over ideal weight.

Current guidelines use the body mass index (BMI) to define obesity. The BMI utilizes height and weight to compare the ratio of body fat to total body mass. To calculate BMI using metric units, weight in kilograms is divided by height in meters squared. To calculate BMI in English units, weight in pounds is divided by height in inches squared and then multiplied by 703. This calculated BMI is compared to the statistical distribution of BMIs for adults aged 20–29 to determine whether an individual is underweight, average, overweight, or obese. The 20- to 29-year age group was chosen as the standard because it represents fully developed adults at the point in their lives when they have the least amount of body fat. Ideally, body fat is

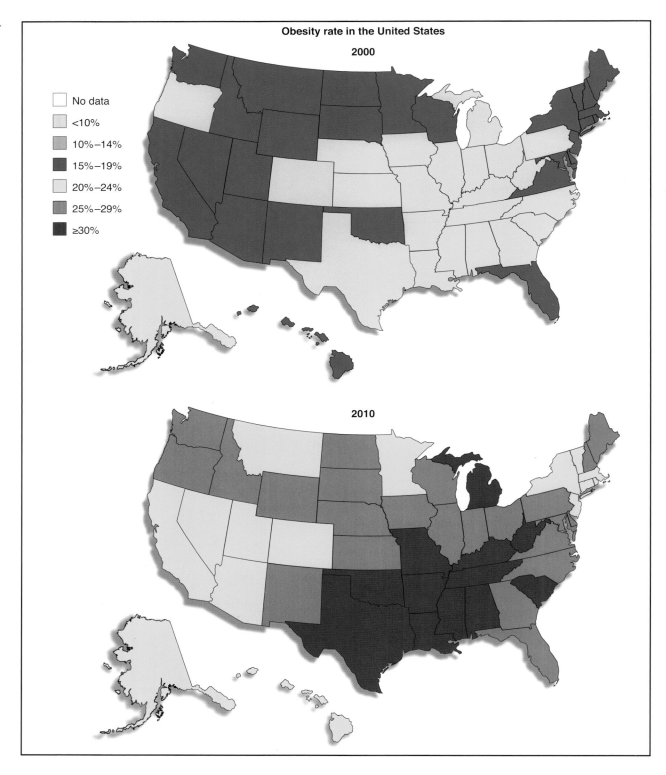

Obesity rate in the United States

2000

2010

No data
<10%
10%–14%
15%–19%
20%–24%
25%–29%
≥30%

Two color-coded maps show the growing obesity problem in the United States. *(Electronic Illustrators Group. © 2012 Cengage Learning.)*

about 15% of total body mass for adult males and about 20–25% for adult females. A simple BMI calculator is available at http://www.nhlbisupport.com/bmi. BMI does not distinguish between fat and muscle.

Adult BMIs are age- and gender-independent. All adults 20 years of age and older are evaluated on the same BMI scale:

- underweight: BMI below 18.5
- normal weight: BMI 18.5–24.9
- overweight: BMI 25.0–29.9
- obese: BMI 30 and above

Research has shown that adults with BMIs within the normal weight range live the longest and enjoy the best health. For a healthy life and a fit body, it is important that a normal weight is maintained consistently throughout one's life.

The BMI for children and teens is calculated in the same way as for adults, but the results are interpreted differently. A child's BMI is compared to those of other children of the same age and gender and assigned to a percentile. For example, a girl in the 75th percentile for her age group weighs more than 74 of every 100 girls her age and less than 25 of every 100 girls her age. The following is a guide to use for children and teens:

- underweight: below the 5th percentile
- healthy weight: 5th percentile to below the 85th percentile
- at risk of overweight: 85th percentile to below the 95th percentile
- overweight: 95th percentile and above

The CDC does not use the term obese for children and teens because the proportion of body fat fluctuates during growth and development and is slightly higher than in mature adults.

Problems of obesity

Obesity places stress on the body's organs and puts people at higher risk for many serious and potentially life-threatening health problems. Problems caused by obesity include:

- fatigue
- joint problems
- poor physical fitness
- digestive disorders
- dizzy spells
- rashes
- hypertension (high blood pressure)
- menstrual disorders

- complications during childbirth and surgery
- type 2 diabetes mellitus (non-insulin dependent)
- heart disease
- unexplained heart attack
- gallstones
- breathing problems
- hyperlipidemia
- infertility
- colon, prostate, endometrial, and breast cancers
- premature aging
- Alzheimer's disease.

Obese individuals have a shorter life expectancy than people of normal weight. Many diseases, especially degenerative diseases of the joints, heart, and blood vessels, tend to be more severe in obese individuals, increasing the need for some surgical procedures. Obesity is directly related to the increasing prevalence of type 2 diabetes in the United States and for the appearance of type 2 diabetes in children, previously a rarity.

Although acute complications of obesity are rare in children, childhood obesity is a risk factor for insulin resistance and type 2 diabetes, **hypertension**, hyperlipidemia, liver and renal disease, and reproductive dysfunction. Childhood obesity increases the risk of deformed bones in the legs and feet, and it can result in emotional disorders such as depression caused by social isolation and negative comments by peers. Childhood obesity also increases the risks of adult obesity and **cardiovascular disease**.

According to a CDC study completed in 2009, the direct and indirect cost of obesity to the U.S. economy in 2006 was estimated as high as US$147 billion. The study found that obese people spend an average of US$1,429 more each year for their medical care than did people with a normal weight range. This comparison finds that obese people have a 42% higher cost for medical care than do normal-weighted people. The increasing prevalence of obesity and diabetes in children and young adults heralds spiraling healthcare costs in the future. The social costs of obesity, including decreased productivity, discrimination, depression, and low self-esteem, are less easily measured.

Benefits of losing weight

In 1995 the Institute of Medicine (IOM) of the U.S. National Academies published a report describing obesity as a "complex, multifactorial disease of appetite regulation and energy metabolism." The report cited the following outcomes from even relatively modest **weight loss**:

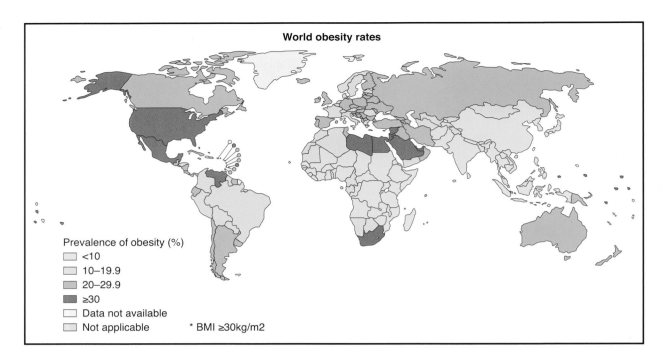

World obesity rates

Prevalence of obesity (%)
- <10
- 10–19.9
- 20–29.9
- ≥30
- Data not available
- Not applicable   * BMI ≥30kg/m2

Worldwide obesity rates have also risen, making obesity a global health issue. *(Electronic Illustrators Group. © 2012 Cengage Learning.)*

- lower blood pressure (and lower risk of heart attack and stroke)
- reduction of abnormally high levels of blood glucose
- lower blood levels of cholesterol and triglycerides (and lower risk of cardiovascular disease)
- lower incidence of sleep apnea
- lower risk for osteoarthritis in weight-bearing joints
- lower incidence of depression
- improved self-esteem

Since that year, the IOM has continued to emphasize the adverse consequences that obesity has on adults and children.

Risk factors

Obesity tends to run in families. Children of obese parents are about 13 times more likely than are other children to be obese. Additional obese family members, including siblings and grandparents, greatly increase the likelihood of childhood obesity. The tendency toward a body type with an unusually high number of fat cells—termed endomorphic—appears to be inherited. Other genetic factors influence appetite and the metabolic rate at which food is transformed into energy.

Family eating habits are major contributors to the development of obesity. Although the majority of adopted children have patterns of weight gain that more closely resemble those of their birth parents than those of their adoptive parents, normal-weight children adopted into obese families are more likely than other children to become obese. Longitudinal studies of juvenile-onset obesity have demonstrated parental and peer encouragement of overeating and even deliberate overfeeding of obese children.

Low socioeconomic status is also a risk factor for adult-onset obesity.

Demographics

Obesity is a serious public-health problem that affects both sexes and all ethnic, racial, age, and socioeconomic groups in the United States and around the world. According to the CDC, 34% of adults (about 103 million in a total population of 304 million) in the United States are obese, as of 2007–2008. As of 2009, approximately 440,000 deaths a year are attributed to obesity, prompting public-health officials such as former Surgeon General C. Everett Koop to label obesity "the second leading cause of preventable deaths in the United States." Smoking tobacco is the number one cause of preventable deaths in the United States.

As of 2008, according to the National Institute of Diabetes and Digestive and Kidney Diseases, slightly more women than men are obese in all adult age groups—36% of women and 32% of men. The highest percentage of obesity is in the over 65 age group, the 45–64-year age group is a close second. Approximately

50% of non-Hispanic black women and 43% of Hispanic women are obese, compared with about 33% of non-Hispanic white women of the same age. Among men, non-Hispanic black men have a rate of obesity of 37% while Hispanic men have a rate of 34% and non-Hispanic white men a rate of 32%, all of the same age bracket.

Obesity is the most common nutritional disorder among U.S. children and teens. African-American and Hispanic children are considerably more likely to be overweight than Caucasian-American children.

According to the CDC, childhood obesity has more than tripled from 1980 to 2008. For children between ages 6 and 11 years of age, the rate of obesity has gone from 6.5% in 1980 to 19.6% in 2008. For adolescents from the age of 12 to 19 years, the rate increased from 5.0% to 18.1% in this age group.

Similar trends are reported by the World Health Organization (WHO), an organization that refers to the escalating global epidemic of obesity as "globesity." WHO estimated that in March 2011, the worldwide obesity level has more than doubled since 1980. In addition, WHO states that, in 2008, 1.5 billion people over age 20 were overweight, and of these people, 200 million are obese. The organization further found that, in 2010, almost 43 million children under five years of age were overweight.

Causes and symptoms

Causes

Obesity is caused by the consumption of more calories than the body uses for energy. The excess calories are stored as adipose tissue. Although inheritance may play a role, a genetic predisposition toward weight gain does not in itself cause obesity. Hormonal and genetic disorders account for less than 10% of obesity in children. Eating habits, physical activity, and environmental, behavioral, social, and cultural factors all contribute to the development of obesity.

Sometimes obesity does have a purely physiological cause. Some of the physiological causes are:

• Cushing's syndrome, a disorder involving the excessive release of the hormone cortisol

• hypothyroidism caused by an under-active thyroid gland, resulting in low levels of the hormone thyroxin and the slow metabolism of food, causing excess unburned calories to be stored as fat

• some cases of hypoglycemia, or low blood sugar, due to a metabolic disorder that results in carbohydrates being stored as fat

• neurological disturbances, such as damage to the hypothalamus, a structure located deep within the brain that helps regulate appetite

• certain drugs such as steroids, antipsychotic medications, and antidepressants

Some researchers have suggested that low levels of the neurotransmitter serotonin increase cravings for **carbohydrates**. In addition, a combination of genetics and early nutritional habits may result in a higher "set point" for body weight that causes obese individuals to feel hunger more often than others. Recent obesity research has focused on two peptide hormones, leptin and ghrelin. Leptin produced by fat cells affects hunger and eating behavior and an insensitivity to leptin may contribute to obesity. Ghrelin is secreted by cells in the lining of the stomach and is important in appetite regulation and maintaining the body's energy balance.

However, most obesity is caused by overeating. During the past several decades American eating habits have changed significantly, with many people consuming larger meals and more high-calorie processed foods. School and **workplace** cafeterias often have a poor selection of nutritional food offerings. Furthermore, it is estimated that in a given six-month period, 2–5% of Americans binge eat. It has been estimated that approximately 15% of the mildly obese participating in weight-loss programs have binge-eating disorder and that the percentage is much higher among the morbidly obese.

Some recent studies suggest that the amount of fat in a person's diet may have a greater impact on weight than the total number of calories. Carbohydrates from cereals, breads, fruits, and vegetables, and **protein** from fish, lean meat, turkey breasts, and skim milk are converted into fuel almost as soon as they are consumed. In contrast, most fats are immediately stored in fat cells that multiply and expand, adding to the body's weight and girth. Current evidence indicates that weight gain depends primarily on total calories consumed, rather than the amount from carbohydrates versus fats, and that low-fat diets are no more effective for weight reduction than low-calorie diets.

Sedentary lifestyles that are particularly prevalent in affluent societies such as the United States, also contribute to obesity. Rather than physical labor on farms and in factories, people are now employed at sedentary jobs in post-industrial service industries. Calorie-saving; machines and devices—cars, computers, remote control devices, household electric appliances, and power tools—have become standard equipment. One study found that the average Western European adult walks about 8,000–9,000 steps daily. In contrast, among the Amish of Pennsylvania who do not use cars or electricity, men accumulate 18,425 steps daily and have no obesity. Amish women walk 14,196 steps daily and have an obesity rate of only 9%.

Psychological factors, such as depression and low self-esteem, can contribute to overeating and obesity. People may eat compulsively to overcome fear or social maladjustment, express defiance, or avoid intimate relationships.

Some babies are born obese. This can be caused by excessive insulin production in the fetuses of diabetic mothers or excess trans-placental nutrients in the case of obese mothers or those who gain excessive weight during pregnancy.

Babies can become obese because they are overfed. Grandmothers may value a "nice plump baby" or care-givers may use a bottle to quiet an infant or to demonstrate their own competence as child-rearers. Because obese one-year-olds may be physically delayed in crawling and **walking**, they become less active toddlers, burning fewer calories. By the age of ten years, obese boys and girls are taller than their peers by as much as 3.9 in (10 cm). Their skeletal maturation, called "bone-age," is also accelerated, so they stop growing earlier. Sexual maturation is advanced. It is not uncommon for obese girls to experience precocious menarche (early onset of menstruation), sometimes even before the age of ten years. Parental separation and divorce or other psychological stresses may stimulate compensatory overeating in children. Obese teenagers and, increasingly, obese preteens may combine periods of binge eating and caloric deprivation, leading to bulimia or anorexia nervosa.

In developed countries people generally experience increased BMI with age. The proportion of intra-abdominal fat that correlates with disease and death increases progressively with age. There is also a progressive decline in daily total **energy expenditure**, associated with decreased physical activity and lower metabolic activity, especially in those with chronic disabilities and diseases.

Symptoms

The major symptoms of obesity are excessive weight and large amounts of fatty tissue. Common secondary symptoms include shortness of breath and lower back pain from carrying excessive body weight. Obesity can also give rise to secondary conditions including:

- arthritis and other orthopedic problems
- hernias
- heartburn
- adult-onset asthma
- gum disease
- high cholesterol levels
- gallstones
- high blood pressure
- menstrual irregularities or cessation of menstruation (amenorhhea)
- decreased fertility and pregnancy complications
- incapacitating shortness of breath
- sleep apnea and sleeping disorders
- skin disorders from the bacterial breakdown of sweat and cellular material in thick folds of skin or from increased friction between folds
- emotional and social difficulties

Diagnosis

Examination

Obesity is usually diagnosed by observation of excessive storage fat and by calculating BMI from weight and height. Physicians observe how the excess weight is carried by comparing waist and hip measurements: "apple-shaped" patients—who store most of their weight around the waist and abdomen—are at greater risk for cancer, heart disease, stroke, and diabetes than "pear-shaped" patients whose extra pounds settle primarily in their hips and thighs.

Procedures

BMI and other measurements do not necessarily accurately reflect body composition and muscle mass. A heavily muscled **football** player may weigh far more than a sedentary man of similar height, but have significantly less body fat. Chronic dieters, who have lost significant muscle mass during periods of caloric deprivation, may look slim and weigh little, but have elevated body fat. Direct measurements of body fat are obtained using calipers to measure skin-fold thickness at the back of the upper arm and other sites that distinguishes between muscle and adipose tissue.

The most accurate means of estimating body fat is hydrostatic weighing—calculating the volume of water displaced by the body. The patient exhales as completely as possible and is immersed in water and the relative displacement is measured. Women whose body fat exceeds 30–32% of total body mass by this method and men whose body fat exceeds 25–27% are generally considered obese. Since this method is unpleasant and impractical, it is usually used only in scientific studies.

Treatment

Traditional

Treatment of obesity aims at reducing weight to a BMI within the normal range (below 25). The best way to achieve weight loss is to reduce dietary caloric intake and increase physical activity. However, obesity will return unless the weight loss includes life long behavioral changes. "Yo-yo" dieting, in which weight is repeatedly lost and regained, has been shown to increase the likelihood of fatal health problems even more than no weight loss at all.

Behavioral treatment for obesity is goal-directed and process-oriented and relies heavily on self-monitoring, with emphasis on:

- Food intake: This may involve keeping a food diary and learning the nutritional value, caloric content, and fat content of foods. It may involve changing shopping habits, such as only shopping on a certain day and buying only what is on the grocery list, timing meals and planning frequent small meals to prevent hunger pangs, and eating slowly to allow for satiation.
- Response to food: This may involve understanding psychological issues underlying eating habits. For example, some people binge eat when under stress, whereas others use food as a reward. By recognizing psychological triggers, alternate coping mechanisms that do not focus on food, can be developed.
- Time usage: Integrating exercise into everyday life is a key to achieving and maintaining weight loss. Starting slowly and building endurance keeps patients from becoming discouraged. Varying routines and trying new activities keeps interest high.
- Stimulus control: This may involve removing environmental cues for inappropriate eating.
- Contingency management: A system of positive and negative reinforcements may help with behavioral modification.

Most mildly obese patients can make lifestyle changes independently with medical supervision. Others may utilize a commercial weight-loss program such as Weight Watchers or Jenny Craig. The effectiveness of these programs is difficult to assess, since they vary widely, dropout rates are high, and few employ medical professionals. Programs that emphasize realistic goals, gradual progress, sensible eating, and exercise can be very helpful and are recommended by many physicians. Programs that promise instant weight loss or utilize severely restricted diets are not effective and, in some cases, can be dangerous.

Moderately obese patients require medically supervised behavior modification and weight loss. A realistic goal is a 10% weight loss over a six-month period. Most doctors use a balanced, low-calorie diet of 1,200–1,500 calories a day. Certain patients may be put on a medically supervised very-low 400–700 calorie liquid protein diet, with supplementation of vitamins and minerals,

for as long as three months. This therapy should not be confused with commercial liquid-protein diets or weight-loss shakes and drinks. Very-low-calorie diets must be designed for specific patients who are monitored carefully and are used for only short periods. Physicians also refer patients to professional therapists or psychiatrists for help in changing eating behaviors. Without changing eating habits and exercise patterns, the lost weight will be regained quickly.

For morbidly obese patients, dietary changes and behavior modification may be accompanied by bariatric surgery. Gastroplasty involves inserting staples to decrease the size of the stomach. Gastric banding is an inflatable band inserted around the upper stomach to create a small pouch and narrow passage into the remainder of the stomach. Although bariatric surgery has become less risky in recent years with innovations in equipment and surgical techniques, it is still performed only on patients for whom supervised diet and exercise strategies have failed, who are at least 100 lb (45 kg) overweight or twice their ideal body weight, and whose obesity seriously threatens their health. Risks and possible complications include infections, hernias, and blood clots. Overall, 10–20% of patients who undergo weight-loss surgery require additional operations to correct complications, more than 33% develop gallstones, and 30% develop nutritional deficiencies such as anemia, **osteoporosis**, or metabolic bone disease.

Other bariatric surgical procedures—including liposuction (a purely cosmetic procedure in which a suction device removes fat from beneath the skin), and jaw wiring that can damage gums and teeth and cause painful muscle spasms—have no place in obesity treatment.

Weight loss is recommended for obese children over age seven and for obese children over age two who have medical complications. Weight maintenance is an appropriate goal for children over the age of two who have no medical complications. Most treatment approaches to childhood obesity involve a combination of caloric restriction, physical exercise, and behavioral therapy. Bariatric surgery is considered as a last resort only for adolescents who are fully grown.

Drugs

The short-term use of prescription medications may assist some individuals in managing their condition, but it is never the sole treatment for obesity, nor are drugs ever considered as a cure for obesity. Diet drugs are designed to help medically at-risk obese patients "jump-start" their weight-loss effort and lose

10% or more of their starting body weight, in combination with a diet and exercise regimen. Prescription weight-loss drugs are approved by the U.S. Food and Drug Administration (FDA) only for patients with a BMI of 30 or above or a BMI of 27 or above and an obesity-related condition such as high blood pressure, type 2 diabetes, or dyslipidemia (abnormal amounts of fats in the blood). The weight is usually regained as soon as the drugs are discontinued, unless eating and exercise habits have changed.

Most appetite-suppressants are based on amphetamine. They increase levels of serotonin or catecholamine, brain chemicals that control feelings of fullness. Serotonin also regulates mood and may be linked to mood-related eating behaviors. Prescription weight-loss medications include:

- diethylpropion (Tenuate, Tenuate Dospan)
- mazindol (Mazanor, Sanorex)
- phendimetrazine (Bontril, Melfiat)
- phentermine (Adipex-P, Ionamin)
- sibutramine (Meridia)

Sibutramine should be taken only under close medical supervision. It can significantly elevate blood pressure and should not be used by patients with a history of congestive heart failure, heart disease, stroke, or uncontrolled high blood pressure.

While most of the immediate side effects of appetite suppressants are harmless, their long-term effects may be unknown. Dexfenfluramine hydrochloride (Redux), fenfluramine (Pondimin), and the fenfluramine-phentermine combination (Fen/Phen) were taken off the market after they were shown to cause potentially fatal cardiac effects. Phenylpropanolamine, a component of many nonprescription weight-loss and cold and cough medications (Acutrim, Dex-A-Diet, Dexatrim, Phenldrine, Phenoxine, PPA, Propagest, Rhindecon, Unitrol) was removed from shelves because of an increased risk of stroke. Appetite-suppressants can be habit-forming and have the potential for abuse. Appetite suppressants should not be used by patients taking monoamine oxidase inhibitors (MAOIs) and are not recommended for children.

Side effects of prescription and over-the-counter weight-loss products may include:

- constipation
- dry mouth
- headache
- irritability
- nausea
- nervousness
- sweating

Unlike appetite suppressants, orlistat is a lipase inhibitor that reduces the breakdown and absorption of dietary fat in the intestines. It is available in both prescription (Xenical) and non-prescription (alli) forms. Side effects of orlistat may include abdominal cramping, gas, fecal urgency, oily stools, frequent bowel movements, and diarrhea.

Other drugs are sometimes prescribed off-label for treating obesity. For example, fluoxetine (Prozac) is an antidepressant that sometimes aids in temporary weight loss. Side effects of this medication include diarrhea, **fatigue**, insomnia, nausea, and thirst.

Alternative

Functional food diets are newer, as yet unproven, approaches to weight loss. These include:

- carbohydrates with a low glycemic index that may help suppress appetite
- green tea extract that may increase the body's energy expenditure
- chromium that may encourage the burning of stored fat rather than lean muscle tissue

Various herbs and supplements are promoted for weight loss. Some of these include:

- Diuretic herbs that increase urine production, can result in short-term weight loss, but do not help with lasting weight control. Increased urine output increases thirst to replace lost fluids and patients who use diuretics for an extended period of time eventually start retaining water anyway.
- In moderate doses, psyllium, a mucilaginous herb available in bulk-forming laxatives like Metamucil, absorbs fluid and provides a feeling of fullness.
- Red peppers and mustard may help encourage weight loss by accelerating the body's metabolic rate. They also cause thirst, so patients crave water instead of food.
- Walnuts can be a natural source of serotonin for providing a feeling of satiation.
- Dandelion (*Taraxacum officinale*) can increase metabolism and counter a desire for sugary foods.
- The amino acid 5-hydroxytryptophan (5-HTP) that is extracted from the seeds of *Griffonia simplicifolia* is thought to increase serotonin levels in the brain. Patients should consult with their healthcare provider before taking 5-HTP, as it may interact with other medications and can have potentially serious side effects.

Acupressure and acupuncture can suppress food cravings. Visualization and meditation can create and reinforce a positive self-image that can enhance a patient's determination to lose weight. By improving physical strength, mental concentration, and emotional serenity, **yoga** can provide the same benefits. Patients who play soft slow music during meals often find that they eat less food but enjoy it more.

Home remedies

Eating the correct ratios of protein, carbohydrates, and high-quality fats are important for weight loss. Support and self-help groups—such as Overeaters Anonymous and TOPS (Taking Off Pounds Sensibly)—that promote nutritious, balanced diets can help patients maintain proper eating regimens.

Fad dieting can have harmful health effects. Weight should be lost gradually and steadily by decreasing calories while maintaining an adequate nutrient intake and level of physical activity. A daily caloric intake of 1,000–1,200 calories for women and 1,200–1,600 for men enables most people to lose weight safely. A loss of about 2 lb (1 kg) per week is recommended. Diets of less than 800 calories a day should never be attempted unless prescribed and monitored by a physician.

At least 60–90 minutes of daily moderate-intensity physical activity is recommended to maintain weight loss. Obese people who have led sedentary lives may need monitoring to avoid injury as they begin to increase their physical activity. Exercise should be increased gradually, perhaps starting by climbing stairs instead of taking elevators, followed by walking, biking, or **swimming** at a slow pace. Eventually, 15-minute walks can be built up to brisk, 45–60-minute walks.

The American Academy of Family Physicians offers advice for families with children who need to maintain or lose weight. This advice includes:

• Weight-loss interventions should begin as soon as possible in children over two years of age.

• The family must be ready for change; if not, the program is likely to fail.

• The physician should educate the family as to the medical complications of obesity.

• All family members and caregivers should be involved in the treatment program.

• The physician should encourage the child and family, not criticize them.

• The treatment program should institute permanent changes in eating habits and other behaviors.

• The program should help the family to make small gradual changes.

• The program should include learning ways to monitor eating and exercise.

• Goals should be realistic; even a 5% weight loss, if maintained, can reduce risks to health.

Prognosis

The primary factor in achieving and maintaining weight loss is a lifelong commitment to sensible eating habits and regular exercise. As many as 85% of dieters who do not exercise on a regular basis regain their lost weight within two years and 90% regain it within five years. Short-term diet programs and repeatedly losing and regaining weight encourage the storage of fat and may increase the risk of heart disease.

Prudent dieting and exercise are not quick cures for obesity. With decreased caloric intake, the body breaks down muscle for carbohydrates. Much of the early weight loss on a very low-calorie diet represents loss of muscle tissue rather than fat. Similarly, fat is not easily accessed as fuel for exercise.

The chronically or habitually obese tend to come from families with a larger number of risk factors for obesity and have a much more difficult time losing weight than the newly obese. Likewise, previously obese people have a high probability of reverting to obesity.

When obesity develops in childhood, the total number of fat cells increases (hyperplastic obesity), whereas in adulthood the total amount of fat in each cell increases (hypertrophic obesity). Patients who were obese as children may have up to five times as many fat cells as a patient who became obese as an adult. Decreasing the amount of energy (food) consumed or increasing the amount of energy expended reduces the amount of fat in the cells—but does not reduce the number of fat cells already present—and this process is slow, just like the accumulation of excess fat.

Neonatal obesity does not necessarily translate into childhood or adult obesity, but there is an increased probability if the child is born or adopted into a family with multiple obese members. Likewise, excess weight in a child under age three does not necessarily predict adult obesity unless one of the parents is obese.

Summer camps specializing in habitually obese children, especially girls, have little long-term success in reducing obesity and a high degree of recidivism for habitual overeating and under-exercising. About 30% of overweight girls eventually develop **eating disorders**.

According to the Obesity Prevention Center at the University of Minnesota, obesity-control programs that rely on educational messages encouraging greater physical activity and a healthier diet have been only modestly successful. The best outcomes have been with children's programs that have high levels of physical activity.

KEY TERMS

Adipose tissue—Fat tissue.

Anemia—Red blood cell deficiency.

Appetite suppressant—A drug that reduces the desire to eat.

Bariatrics—The branch of medicine that deals with the prevention and treatment of obesity and related disorders.

Binge-eating disorder—A condition characterized by uncontrolled eating.

Body Mass Index (BMI)—A measure of body fat: the ratio of weight in kilograms to the square of height in meters.

Calorie—A unit of food energy.

Carbohydrate—Sugars, starches, celluloses, and gums that are a major source of calories from foods.

Catecholamines—Hormones and neurotransmitters including dopamine, epinephrine, and norepinephrine.

Eating disorder—A condition characterized by an abnormal attitude towards food, altered appetite control, and unhealthy eating habits that affect health and the ability to function normally.

Epidemic—Affecting many individuals in a community or population and spreading rapidly.

Fat—Molecules composed of fatty acids and glycerol; the slowest utilized source of energy, but the most energy-efficient form of food. Each gram of fat supplies about nine calories, more than twice that supplied by the same amount of protein or carbohydrate.

Gastroplasty—A surgical procedure used to reduce digestive capacity by shortening the small intestine or shrinking the side of the stomach.

Ghrelin—A peptide hormone secreted primarily by the stomach that has been implicated in the control of food intake and fat storage.

Hyperlipidemia—Abnormally high levels of lipids in the blood.

Hyperplastic obesity—Excessive weight gain in childhood, characterized by an increase in the number of fat cells.

Hypertension—Abnormally high arterial blood pressure that can lead to heart disease and stroke if untreated.

Hypertrophic obesity—Excessive weight gain in adulthood, characterized by expansion of pre-existing fat cells.

Ideal weight—Weight corresponding to the lowest death rate for individuals of a specific height, gender, and age.

Leptin—A peptide hormone produced by fat cells that acts on the hypothalamus to suppress appetite and burn stored fat.

Metabolic activity—The sum of the chemical processes in the body that are necessary to maintain life.

Metabolic bone disease—Weakening of bones due to a deficiency of certain minerals, especially calcium.

Normal weight—A BMI of less than 25.0.

Obesity—An abnormal accumulation of body fat, usually 20% or more above ideal body weight or a BMI of 30.0 or above.

Osteoporosis—A disease characterized by low bone mass and structural deterioration of bone tissue, leading to bone fragility.

Overweight—A BMI between 25.0 and 30.0.

Serotonin—A neurotransmitter located primarily in the brain, blood serum, and stomach membrane.

Prevention

Prevention is far superior to any available treatment for obesity. Obesity can be prevented by eating a healthy diet, being physically active, and making lifestyle changes that help maintain a normal weight. Examples include:

• eating smaller portions of food

• taking the time to prepare healthy meals

• avoiding processed foods

• parking farther away from a store

• walking or **bicycling** instead of driving

• walking the dog instead of just letting it out

Obesity experts suggest that monitoring fat consumption, as well as counting calories, is a key to preventing excess weight gain. The National **Cholesterol** Education Program of the National Heart, Lung, and Blood Institute maintains that only 30% of calories should be derived from fat and only one-third of those should be saturated fats. High concentrations of saturated fats are found in meat, poultry, and dairy products. Fat replacers or substitutes are now added to many foods. They reduce the amount of fat and usually reduce the number of calories. It is not clear what effect these will have on the long-term battle against obesity.

Total caloric intake cannot be ignored, since it is usually the slow accumulation of excess calories, regardless of the source, that results in obesity. A single daily cookie providing 25 excess calories will result in a 5-lb weight gain by the end of one year. Because most people eat more than they think they do, keeping a detailed and honest food diary is a useful way to assess eating habits. Eating three balanced, moderate-portion meals a day—with the main meal at midday—is a more effective way to prevent obesity than fasting or crash diets that trick the body into believing it is starving. After 12 hours without food, the body has depleted its stores of readily available energy. It then begins to protect itself for the long term. Metabolic rate starts to slow and muscle tissue is broken down for the raw materials needed for energy maintenance.

The U.S. Department of Agriculture (USDA) recently introduced, on June 2, 2011, the *MyPlate* program to replace the long-time food pyramid called *MyPyramid*. Although the new symbol looks very different than the old one, it still contains recommendations on diet based on the *Dietary Guidelines for Americans 2010*, tailored for an individual's BMI. It includes recommendations on physical activity and in five food categories (and their associated approximate percentages to be consumed each day): grains (30%), vegetables (30%), fruits (20%), protein (20%), and dairy (without a percentage).

It has been suggested that there may be little benefit in encouraging weight loss in older people, especially when there are no obesity-related complications or when promoting changes in lifelong eating habits creates stress. However, studies have shown that weight loss in seniors can lower the incidence of **arthritis**, diabetes, and other conditions, reduce cardiovascular risk factors, and improve well-being. Increased physical activity in the elderly also improves muscle strength and endurance.

The poor prognosis for reversing adult obesity makes childhood prevention imperative. Unhealthy eating patterns and behaviors associated with obesity can be addressed by programs in nutrition, exercise, and stress management involving the entire family.

Resources

BOOKS

Adolfsson, Birgitta, and Marilynn S. Arnold. *Behavioral Approaches to Treating Obesity*. Alexandria, VA: American Diabetes Association, 2006.

Apovian, Caroline M., and Carine M. Lenders, editors. *Clinical Guide for Management of Overweight and Obese Children and Adults*. Boca Raton, FL: Taylor and Francis, 2006.

Apple, Robin F., James Lock, and Rebecka Peebles. *Is Weight Loss Surgery Right for You?* New York: Oxford University Press, 2006.

Duyff, Roberta Larson. *ADA Complete Food and Nutrition Guide*, third ed. Chicago: American Dietetic Association, 2006.

Finkelstein, Eric A., and Laurie Zuckerman. *The Fattening of America: How the Economy Makes Us Fat, If It Matters, and What To Do About It*. New York: John Wiley & Sons, 2008.

Flamenbaum, Richard K., editor. *Childhood Obesity and Health Research*. New York: Nova Science Publishers, 2006.

Hassink, Sandra Gibson. *Guide to Pediatric Weight Management and Obesity*. Philadelphia: Lippincott Williams and Wilkins, 2007.

Marcovitz, Hal. *Diet Drugs*. Farmington Hills, MI: Lucent Books, 2007.

PERIODICALS

Birch, Leann L. "Child Feeding Practices and the Etiology of Obesity." *Obesity* 14, no. 3 (March 2006): 343–344.

Chen, H., and X. Guo. "Obesity and Functional Disability in Elderly America." *Journal of the American Geriatric Society* 56, no. 4 (April 2008): 689–694.

Fabricatore, Anthony N., and Thomas A. Wadden. "Obesity." *Annual Review of Clinical Psychology* 2 (2006): 357–377.

Johannsen, Darcy L., Neil M. Johannsen, and Bonny L. Specker. "Influence of Parents' Eating Behaviors and Child Feeding Practices on Children's Weight Status." *Obesity* 14, no. 3 (March 2006): 431–439.

Masi, C. M., et al. "Respiratory Sinus Arrhythmia and Diseases of Aging: Obesity, Diabetes Mellitus, and Hypertension." *Biological Psychology* 74, no. 2 (February 2007): 212–223.

Ogden, C., et al. "High Body Mass Index for Age Among U.S. Children and Adolescents, 2003–2006." *Journal of the American Medical Association* 299 (2008): 2401–2405.

WEBSITES

Assessing Your Weight and Health Risk. National Heart, Lung, and Blood Institute. http://www.nhlbi.nih.gov/health/public/heart/obesity/lose_wt/risk.htm (accessed November 6, 2011).

Body Percentile Calculator for Child and Teen. Centers for Disease Control and Prevention. http://apps.nccd.cdc.gov/dnpabmi/Calculator.aspx (accessed November 6, 2011).

Bridging the Evidence Gap in Obesity Prevention: A Framework to Inform Decision Making. Institute of Medicine. (April 23, 2010). http://www.iom.edu/Reports/2010/Bridging-the-Evidence-Gap-in-Obesity-Prevention-A-Framework-to-Inform-Decision-Making.aspx (accessed November 6, 2011).

Calculate Your BMI. National Heart, Lung, and Blood Institute. http://www.nhlbisupport.com/bmi/ (accessed November 6, 2011).

Childhood Obesity Facts. Centers for Disease Control and Prevention. (September 15, 2011). http://www.cdc.gov/healthyyouth/obesity/ (accessed November 6, 2011).

Choose My Plate. U.S. Department of Agriculture. (September 30, 2011). http://www.choosemyplate.gov/ (accessed November 6, 2011).

Dietary Guidelines for Americans, 2010. Health.gov, U.S. Department of Health & Human Services. (September 13, 2011). http://www.health.gov/dietaryguidelines/2010.asp (accessed November 6, 2011).

Obesity and Overweight. World Health Organization. (March 2011). http://www.who.int/mediacentre/factsheets/fs311/en/index.html (accessed November 6, 2011).

Overweight, Obesity, and Weight Loss Fact Sheet. Office on Women's Health, Women's Health.gov. (March 6, 2009). http://www.womenshealth.gov/publications/our-publications/fact-sheet/overweight-weight-loss.cfm (accessed November 6, 2011).

Prescription Medications for the Treatment of Obesity. Weight-control Information Network, National Institutes of Health and Department of Health and Human Services. (December 2010). http://win.niddk.nih.gov/publications/prescription.htm (accessed November 6, 2011).

ORGANIZATIONS

American Academy of Family Physicians, 11400 Tomahawk Creek Parkway, Leawood, KS, 66211-2680, (913) 906-6000, Fax: (800) 274-2237, (800) 274-2237, http://www.aafp.org.

American Council on Exercise, 4851 Paramount Dr., San Diego, CA, 92123, (888) 825-3636, http://www.acefitness.org.

American Council for Fitness and Nutrition, 1350 I St., Suite 300, Washington, D.C., 20005, http://www.acfn.org.

American Dietetic Association, 120 South Riverside Plaza, Suite 2000, Chicago, IL, 60606-6995, (312) 899-0040, (800) 877-1600, http://www.eatright.org.

American Society for Metabolic and Bariatric Surgery, 100 SW 75th St., Suite 201, Gainesville, FL, 32607, (352) 331-3900, Fax: (352) 331-4975, info@asmbs.org, http://www.asbs.org.

Centers for Disease Control and Prevention, 1600 Clifton Rd., Atlanta, GA, 30333, (800) 232-4636, odcinfo@cdc.gov, http://www.cdc.gov.

National Heart, Lung, and Blood Institute, NHLBI Health Information Center, P.O. Box 30105, Bethesda, MD, 20824-0105, (301) 592-8573, Fax: (240) 629-3246, nhlbiinfo@nhlbi.nih.gov, http://www.nhlbi.nih.gov.

Obesity Prevention Center, University of Minnesota, 1300 S. Second St., Suite 300, Minneapolis, MN, 55454, (612) 625-6200, umopc@epi.umn.edu, http://www.ahc.umn.edu.

The Obesity Society, 8758 Georgia Ave., Suite 1320, Silver Spring, MD, 20910, (301) 563-6526, Fax: (301) 563-6595, http://www.obesity.org.

Overeaters Anonymous, P.O. Box 44020, Rio Rancho, NM, 87174-4020, (505) 891-2664, Fax: (505) 891-4320, http://www.oa.org.

Weight-Control Information Network (WIN), 1 WIN Way, Bethesda, MD, 20892-3665, 32607, Fax: (202) 828-1028, (877) 946-4627, win@info.niddk.nih.gov, http://win.niddk.nih.gov.

Rosalyn Carson-DeWitt, MD
William Atkins, BB, BS, MBA

Ocean sports

Definition

For the purpose of this essay, the term ocean sports is taken to refer to sporting activities involving a single individual in some portion of a deep body of water (such as a sea or ocean) requiring only a minimal amount of equipment. Sports included in this definition include scuba diving, snorkeling, surfing, and windsurfing.

Purpose

The primary purpose of all ocean sports is usually recreational, the personal enjoyment that comes from participating in such sports. In some cases, competitions are held in a sport, in which case the purpose becomes one of achieving some goal (such as completing a given course) in a faster time and/or with greater artistic skill than other competitors.

Demographics

Some of the best available data on participation in ocean sports can be found in the annual report of the Outdoor Foundation. The organization's 2011 report provided the following statistics on the four ocean sports covered here:

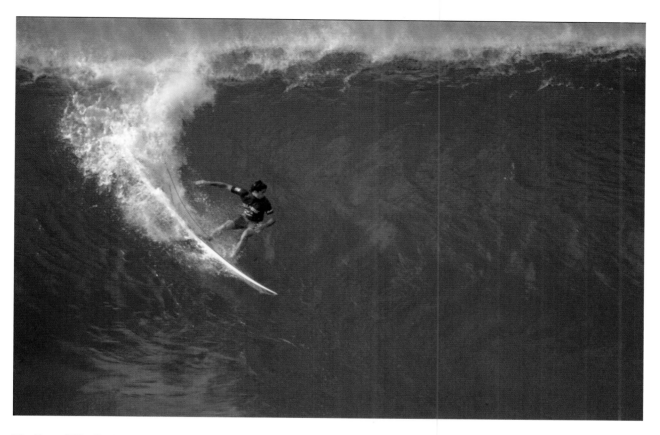

The Banzai Pipeline is a set of vicious waves that entice surfers to test their skills on the waters of Waimea in Oahu. *(© Corel Corporation)*

• An estimated 2,767,000 individuals participated in surfing during 2010. That made the sport the fifth most popular among young people age six to 24, who reported an average of 21.9 outings per surfer, for a total of 25 million total outings for the sport. The sport showed an increase in popularity in one year of 15.1 percent.

• An estimated 1,617,000 individuals above the age of six engaged in windsurfing or boardsailing during 2010. That number represented an increase of 43.4 percent over the 2009 figures.

• The number of people who engage in snorkeling has remained relatively constant over the period from 2006 to 2010 covered by the report. In 2010, the number of snorkelers was estimated at 9,305,000, a decrease of only 0.6 percent from 2009.

• The number of scuba divers in the United States tends to vary around the 3,000,000 mark, with the 2010 total estimated at 3,153,000, an increase of 15.8 percent over 2009. More detailed information on the demographics of ocean sports are available from other sources, including the Sporting Goods Manufacturers Association (http://www.sgma.com/reports/) and Statista (http://www.statista.com/).

History

Each of the ocean sports described here has its own unique history. Surfing is perhaps the oldest of these sports, with its origins dating at least to 1000 bce, and perhaps much earlier, along the coasts of northern Peru. The sport also has very ancient beginnings in the Polynesian culture, from which it was probably transplanted to the Hawaiian Islands in the period from about 300 to about 750 ce. Throughout history, the sport has, quite naturally, had its greatest popularity in regions where good surf is regularly available, such as Hawaii, Australia, and parts of the California coast. Modern surfing is often dated to the 1960s in the United States, when a series of movies ("Gidget" and the "Beach Party" films) and some popular music themes (for example, songs by the Beach Boys) popularized the sport, until it eventually reached its current appeal.

Compared to surfing, windsurfing is a much younger sport. Its origin can be dated to a 1948 invention by a

KELLY SLATER (1972–)

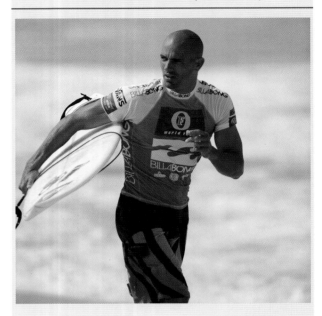

(© Jarvis Gray/ShutterStock.com)

Kelly Slater was born February 11, 1972, in Cocoa Beach, Florida, and is recognized around the world for his accomplishments in surfing. He has been the youngest and oldest surfer to win 11 world surfing titles. His accomplishments in surfing have allowed him to present himself on popular television shows and be the title character of a video game released in 2002.

20-year-old man by the name of Newman Darby, who designed the surfboard to which a sail was attached, the first windsurfing board. Although relatively simple in concept, the final design of a practical windsurfing board took almost twenty years. In fact, it was not until 1970 that the first patent for the board was approved. That patent was granted to Jim Drake, an aeronautical engineer, and his surfer friend, Hoyle Schweitzer. Some dispute still remains as to who it is that should receive credit for designed the first windsurfing board: Darby, Drake and Schweitzer, or Peter Chilvers, a 12-year-old English boy who, some claimed, built the first windsurfing board in 1958.

Like surfing, snorkeling has a very long history. At least three millennia before the birth of Christ, sponge farmers in Crete were using long, hollow reeds as breathing tubes during their deepest offshore dives. Almost certainly, people dwelling along the oceans in other parts of the world had developed similar technologies for breathing underwater. A bas relief dating to 900 bce, for example, shows Assyrian divers using air-filled animal bladders for deep dives. The snorkel tube and mask that are the only equipment used by many snorkelers today represent only a modest conceptual improvement over the equipment used by these earliest divers.

As with windsurfing, scuba diving also has a very short history, dating to the winter of 1942-43 when two Frenchmen, Jacques-Yves Cousteau and Émile Gagnan, invented the first "self contained underwater breathing apparatus" (SCUBA) that they called an Aqua-Lung. The device allowed a swimmer to remain underwater for extended periods of time with an easily controlled, long-term source of air. Although the Aqua-Lung has undergone a number of modifications, it still serves as the general model for underwater aids used by scuba devices.

Description

In order to surf, all one needs is a board on which to stand or lie down and waves of sufficient power to carry one towards the shore with some degree of speed. A form of surfing known as bodysurfing allows one to dispense with the surf board, producing a somewhat similar experience as that with the board itself.

A windsurfing board consists of a surfboard-type platform to which is attached a sail by means of a universal joint. The windsurfer stands on the board and pivots the sail in such a way as to catch the wind to propel the windsurfer across the water.

The sport of snorkeling is simply a modified form of **swimming** with the aid of goggles, to allow one to see underwater; a breathing tube, through which the diver can obtain air from just above the water' surface; and swim fins that allow one to propel himself or herself more easily. With these aids, a person can swim easily beneath the water and enjoy the scenery to be found there, usually beautiful coral formations and unusually colored and figured fish.

The most common scuba device today is a single line, two stage device in which compressed air (or oxygen-enriched air) is stored in a cylindrical tank at a pressure of about 200 atmospheres (200 times normal atmospheric pressure). The delivery tube contains two regulators that control the pressure of air leaving the tank. The first regulator is attached to the tank itself and reduces the air pressure from 200 atmospheres to about 10 atmospheres. The second regulator is connected to the opposite end of the hose, at the diver's mouth. It reduces air pressure a second time, to what it would be in the water surrounding the diver (about 1 to 5 atmospheres). Air exhaled by the diver passes directly into the water surrounding the diver.

Preparation

Unlike many sports, such as **baseball**, **football**, **tennis**, and **track and field**, ocean sports do not required much advance conditioning or training. Perhaps the most important form of preparation is ensuring that one has the necessary equipment in the best possible condition. Being aware of weather conditions that might promote or inhibit one's participation in a sport is also of some importance.

Equipment

Surfboards are commonly made of solid or hollow polyurethane or balsa wood. They are light, but strong enough to support the weight of the surfer. They take many different shapes, but are always elongated with a length ranging from six to 30 feet in length. Shorter boards are known as short boards, and longer boards as long boards. The specific board suitable for surfing depends on a person's weight, experience, and surfing objectives. Beginning surfers normally seek the advice of experts in the field to selected the board most appropriate for them.

The design of a windsurfing board is determined to a considerable extent on the purpose for which it is intended: beginning surfers, slalom racers, freestyle boards, recreational sailing, or racing. In general, most boards measure from six to 12 feet in length, powered by a sail that is anywhere from 20 square feet to 100 square feet in area. A measure often used in selecting the appropriate windsurfing board is board volume, since the board's volume determines the amount of weight the board can support and the extent to which it rides on top of, versus slicing through, the water.

Snorkeling requires only a face mask, a snorkeling tube, and fins. In the simplest possible cases, one can snorkel using only the tube itself.

Scuba diving requires a sophisticated and dependable apparatus that includes all the elements that store a supply of air (the "tank"), that deliver the air to the diver at the proper rate and pressure (the tube and regulators), and provides the diver with information about the amount of air left in the tank (indicated by a dial that reads the air pressure in the tank directly). A complete list of equipment needed in addition to the air system itself includes a number of items, such as

- wet suit
- mask
- fins

KEY TERMS

Aqua-Lung—The name of the original type of scuba diving device invented in the 1940s by Jacques-Yves Cousteau and Émile Gagnan.

decompression illness—A condition that develops when a diver ascends from a dive at two rapid a rate, resulting in the accumulation of gas bubbles in the bloodstream.

regulator—A device on scuba diving apparatus that controls air pressure within the apparatus.

- buoyancy vest
- depth gauge
- compass
- dive log book
- underwater light
- diving knife
- repair kit for damage incurred on any of the above items.

Risks

An estimate of the risk of surfing injury was reported in 2007 by a group of researchers at the Rhode Island Hospital. They studied injuries that had been incurred at 32 amateur and professional surfing competitions between 1999 and 2005. They recorded a total of 116 injuries, 89 of which occurred during the competition itself, for an injury rate of 5.7 injuries per 1000 athlete exposures. This number is relatively small, less than that of amateur **soccer** games. The greatest risk to surfers occurred when waves were over their heads or when they were surfing in water with a rocky ground. Sprains and strains to the lower extremities were the most common type of surfer injuries, with lacerations and contusions being the next most common injuries. Such injuries, found in other studies to be the most common surfer injuries, usually resulted from contact between a surfer and his or her own board or the board of another surfer.

A study reported in the British Journal of Sports Medicine in 2006 followed 107 recreational and competitive windsurfers over a period of two years. Researchers found that the average rate of injuries among windsurfers was 1.5 injury per person per year. The most common types of injury were muscle and tendon strains (accounting for about half of all new injuries), followed by ligament sprains. Cuts and abrasions were common, and a total of six concussions were reported among the experimental group. Researchers found a somewhat different pattern of injuries between recreational and competitive windsurfers and concluded that methods should be developed to reduce the most common types of injuries.

The most common injuries incurred by divers (either snorkeling or scuba diving) are scrapes, abrasions, and contusions resulting from rubbing against the sharp edges of coral and other rocks. While these injuries are not in and of themselves very serious, they may often lead to infections that are of much greater concern. Another category of injuries associated with diving sports are stings and bites resulting from contact with organisms such as jelly fish and the Portugese man-of-war. These stings and bites may range in severity from moderate pain to neuromuscular effects, such as anaphylactic shock and paralysis. More serious accidents, while not common, are hardly rare. Such accidents can result in death or permanent disability. The three most common causes of fatal diving accidents (each accounting for about a third of such accidents) are drowning, arterial gas embolism, and cardiac arrest. About ten percent of all fatalities during diving accidents results from other causes, such as decompression illness, trauma or loss of consciousness while diving. There is also some evidence that frequent diving can result in certain types of chronic health problems affecting the ears and circulatory system. These injuries are far more common among people who make their lives diving than those who dive less often for recreational purposes.

Resources

BOOKS

Collis, Jim, and Amanda van Santen. *RYA Start Windsurfing*. Hamble, UK: Royal Yachting Association, 2006.

Jennings, Gayle. *Water-based Tourism, Sport, Leisure, and Recreation Experiences*. Oxford; New York: Elsevier, 2007.

Robison, John. *Surfing Illustrated : an Illustrated Guide to Wave Riding*. Chicago: International Marine/McGraw-Hill, 2010.

WEBSITES

Scuba Diving Community - The Scuba Site. http://www.thescubasite.com/ (accessed October 19, 2011).

Snorkeling.info. http://www.snorkeling.info/ (accessed October 19, 2011).

Surfinghandbook.com. http://www.surfinghandbook.com/ (accessed October 19, 2011).

Windsurfing. http://windsurfingmag.com/ (accessed October 19, 2011).

ORGANIZATIONS

Professional Association of Diving Instructors, 30151 Tomas, Rancho Santa Margarita, CA, 92688-2125, (949) 858-7234, Fax: (949) 267-1267, (800) 729-7234, webmaster@padi.com, http://www.padi.com/scuba/.

International Surfing Association, 5580 La Jolla Blvd. #145, La Jolla, CA, 92037, (858) 551-8580, Fax: (858) 551-8563, surf@isasurf.org, http://www.isasurf.org/index.php.

International Windsurfing Association, Mengham Cottage, Mengham Lane, Hayling Island, Hampshire, United Kingdom, PO11 PJX, +44(0) 1983 854938, ceri@offshore-sports.co.uk, http://www.internationalwind surfing.com/.

David E. Newton, A.B., M.A., Ed.D

Olympics

Definition

The Olympic Games are an international sporting event that occurs every four years, once during the summer (the Summer Games) and once during the winter (the Winter Games). The 2012 Summer Games will be held in London, the 2016 Summer Games in Rio de Janeiro, the 2014 Winter Games in Sochi, Russia, and the 2018 Winter Games in Pyeongchang, South Korea. The Olympic Games are formally known as the Games of the XXX Olympiad, where "XXX" represents the Roman numeral representation of the event. The 2008 Summer Olympics, for examples, was formally known as the Games of the XXIX Olympiad.

Purpose

The purpose of the Olympic Games is to bring together the world's finest male and female athletes in some predesignated group of summer and **winter sports**. Winners in each of these contests are now

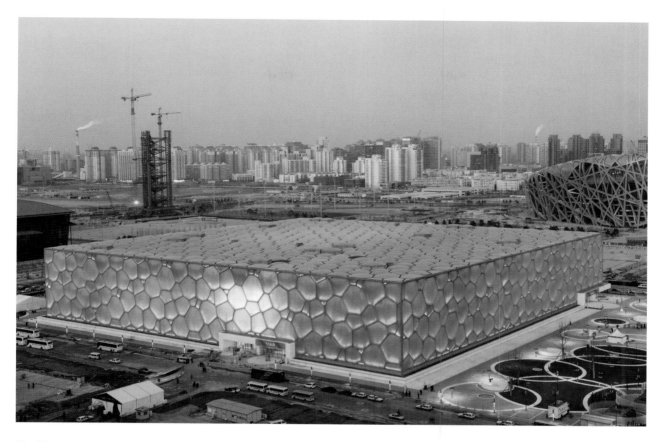

The Water Cube National Aquatics Center swimming arena and National Stadium at the Olympic Park, Beijing, China. *(© Robert Harding World Imagery/Alamy)*

generally regarded as the champions in their sport for the four-year period following their triumph.

Demographics

Both men and women can compete in the Olympic Games, with minimum and maximum **age** limits (if there are any) being established by the international governing bodies for the sports involved. In general, the minimum age for participation in most Olympic sports is 16, although that age varies for some sports. The minimum age for **marathon** competitors, for example, is 20. A new category of Olympic Games was introduced in 2010 with the Youth Olympic Games held in Singapore. The age limit for participants in those games was 14 to 18 years of age.

History

The first records of an Olympics game-like event date to the year 776 BCE at Olympia, Greece. Competitions were held among a number of city-states and kingdoms on the Greek peninsula in a number of athletic events. The original event consisted of a single race across the length of a stadium of 180 - 240 meters (one "stadion"). Over time, a number of other **running** and non-running events were added, and the games extended from a single day up to as many as five days. These events included not only longer running races, but additional contests in **boxing, wrestling,** equestrian events, javelin, discuss, and pentathlon (a group of five different athletic events). The ancient Olympic Games were brought to an end in 393 CE by edict of the Roman emperor Theodosius I. One reason for the emperor's decision was that contestants in the Olympic Games typically participated in the nude, apparently an affront to the most fervent of the early Christian emperors.

Sporadic attempts to revive Olympic-like contests occurred in the seventeenth and eighteenth century, with relatively few long-term results. The oldest of these events was the Cotswold Olympick Games, first held in 1612 in the English village of Chipping Camden. Those games have been held on an irregular basis ever since and are regarded by some observers as the progenitor of the modern Olympics games. A comparable event was introduced in France, *L'Olympiade de la République*, shortly after the French Revolution, although those games were short-lived. Enthusiasm for the restoration of the Olympic Games in their native land arose after the 1821–1832 Greek War of Independence , when the nation obtained its independence from the Ottoman Empire. A wealthy Greek philanthropist, Evangelis Zappas, volunteered to fund the first revival of the games, held in Athens in 1859. Zappas then provided funds for the restoration of the ancient Panathenaic stadium in Athens, where modern versions of the game were held in 1870 and 1875. Inspired at least in part by the 1875 games, French historian Baron Pierre de Coubertin founded the International Olympic Committee in 1890 with the objective of sponsoring a quadrennial modern version of the original Olympic Games, open to competitors in a number of sports from all over the world.

The first of the modern Olympic Games were held in Athens' Panathenaic stadium from April 6 - 15, 1896. A total of 241 athletes (all male) from 14 nations participated in 43 events in athletics (sprints and runs,discus and shot put, hurdles, jumps, and pole vault), cycling, **fencing**, **gymnastics**, shooting, **swimming**, **tennis**, **weightlifting**, and wrestling. The 1900 games were held in conjunction with the Paris Exposition and the 1904 games in association with the World's Fair in St. Louis. In both cases, the Olympic events were overshadowed by the main focus of the Exposition, in 1900, and the World's Fair, in 1904. Although no special stadium or other facilities were available at the 1900 games, they were marked by the first appearance of women athletes.

After an attempt to insert a so-called "intercalated" event in 1906 (in the middle of a four-year Olympiad, the games resumed their regular quadrennial schedule in 1908 with the London games, a pattern that has been followed every four years since then. The first winter games were introduced in 1924 in Chamonix, France, and the first Summer Youth Olympics, in Singapore, in 2010, and the first Winter Youth Olympics in Innsbruck, Austria, in 2012. In 1948, German neurologist Ludwig Guttmann recommended the inclusion of athletes with physical disabilities in a "parallel Olympics," or paralympics games. Such a competition was first held in conjunction with the 1960 games in Rome and has been a part of every Olympic competition since that time. The only years in which Olympic Games have not been held as scheduled were 1916, 1940, and 1944, all because of world wars.

The Olympic Games have changed substantially since they were first conceived by Baron de Coubertin as an amiable opportunity for the world's best amateur athletes to come together in friendly competition. Today, the Games are a huge commercial operation with venue costs easily exceeding the billion dollar mark and professional athletes as welcome as amateurs. The business now routinely endorses a large variety of commercial products (at a cost to the producers) and guards the use of its name against organizations it regards as unsuitable for the Olympics ideal (such as the use of its name in the "Gay Olympics"). The games themselves have also been saturated with political factors, most notably perhaps boycotts of the games on a number of occasions, including the 1936 games (Ireland), 1956 games (Cambodia, China, Egypt, Iraq, Lebanon, Netherlands, Spain, and Switzerland), 1980 games (a group of 65 nations objecting to the policies and actions of the Soviet Union), and 1984 games (Soviet Union and 14 sympathetic partners). Probably the saddest single day in the history of the Olympics occurred on September 5, 1972, when Palestinian terrorists kidnaped 11 members of the Israeli Olympic team, eventually killing all of them; this event is now widely known as the Munich Massacre (for the site of the event).

The 2008 Summer Olympics were held in Beijing, China. The event attracted 11,028 athletes from 204 nations who competed in 302 distinct events distributed among 28 sports. Although estimates vary, it seems likely that the games cost the host nation about US $40 billion to produce. The 2010 Winter Olympics were held in Vancouver, Canada, where about 2,600 athletes from 82 nations participated in 86 events in 15 sports. The final official cost of the games was announced by the organizing committee to have been US $1.84 billion.

Description

The sports included in an Olympics event vary from games to games. Five sports have been included in every Summer Olympic Games since 1896: athletics, cycling, fencing, gymnastics, and swimming. A few sports have been included in the Olympics schedule for almost all of that period, including weightlifting and wrestling. A number of sports have made brief appearances, and then disappeared from the games, including Basque pelota (1900 only), **cricket** (1900), rackets (1908), **rugby** sevens (2006), and water motorsports (1908). Seven sports have been included in all 21 Winter Olympic Games, including cross-country skiing, figure skating, **ice hockey**, Nordic combined, ski jumping, and speed skating. The two newest winter sports are freestyle skiing and short-track speed skating (both introduced in 1992).

KEY TERMS

Intercalated games—A proposed series of Olympic Games schedule in the even off years between regularly scheduled Olympic Games, always to be held in Athens. In fact, the intercalated games were held only once, in 1906.

Olympiad—The four-year period between Olympic Games. Also, a synonym for "Olympic Games."

Paralympics—An Olympics event designed for physically challenged men and women, first held officially in 1960, and since repeated every four years.

Venue—The physical location in which an Olympics event is held.

Preparation

Athletes who compete in the Olympics Games follow training and conditioning regimes appropriate for their individual sports.

Equipment

Each player who competes in the Olympics wears equipment required or recommended for the sport in which they are involved.

Training and conditioning

Olympic athletes are among the best trained athletes in the world, who follow the most recent and most highly approved methods of training and conditioning for their individual sports.

Risks

Olympic athletes are challenged by the specific risks and medical issues characteristic of the sports in which they compete.

Resources

BOOKS

Barney, Robert Knight, Stephen R. Wenn, and Scott G. Martyn. *Selling the Five Rings: The International Olympic Committee and the Rise of Olympic Commercialism.* Salt Lake City, UT: University of Utah Press, 2004.

Pound, Richard W. *Inside the Olympics: A Behind-the-scenes Look at the Politics, the Scandals, and the Glory of the Games Title.* Chichester, UK: Wiley, 2006.

Shaw, Christopher A. *Five Ring Circus: Myths and Realities of the Olympic Games.* Gabriola Island, BC: New Society Publishers, 2008.

Wallechinsky, David, and Jaime Loucky. *The Complete Book of the Olympics.* South Yarra, Victoria, Australia: Hardie Grant, 2008.

Wallechinsky, David, and Jaime Loucky. *The Complete Book of the Winter Olympics.* London: Aurum, 2010.

WEBSITES

The Ancient Olympics Perseus Digital Library Project. http://www.perseus.tufts.edu/Olympics/ (accessed August 18, 2011).

The Modern Olympic Games The Olympic Museum. http://multimedia.olympic.org/pdf/en_report_668.pdf (accessed August 18, 2011).

The Olympic Games ThinkQuest. http://library.thinkquest.org/27528/main.htm (accessed August 18, 2011).

ORGANIZATIONS

International Olympic Committee, Route de Vidy 9, 1001 Lausanne, 356, Switzerland, 4121 621 61 11, Fax: 4121 621 62 16, pressoffice@olympic.org, http://www.olympic.org/.

United States Olympic Committee, One Olympic Plaza, Colorado Springs, CO, 80909, (719) 632-5551, Fax: (719) 866-4654, media@usoc.org, http://www.teamusa.org/.

David E. Newton, A.B., M.A., Ed.D

Orienteering *see* **Adventure racing**

Orthotics

Definition

Orthotics are devices that attach to the body externally and are used to help improve function, restrict movement, correct alignment, reduce pain, or improve deformities.

Purpose

Orthotics are special devices worn on the outside of the body that are used to correct problems with posture, gait, body alignment, or to improve problems related to deformities. The devices are most frequently used with athletes to reduce pain associated with certain kinds of movements such as jumping or **running** and to help heal injuries that occurred in the course of athletic activity. Orthotics are frequently prescribed when an individual goes in to see the doctor because of recurring pain. Orthotics are also used to restrict movement in cases where such restriction is required for proper healing, such as after surgery. In some cases, orthotics may be prescribed prophylactically, to help prevent a problem that is likely to occur later in life.

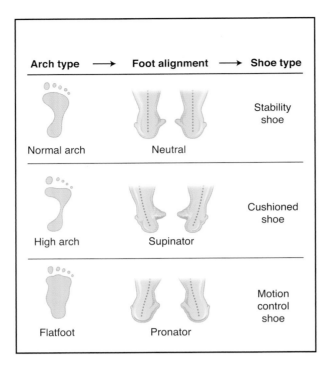

Arch type → **Foot alignment** → **Shoe type**

Normal arch — Neutral — Stability shoe

High arch — Supinator — Cushioned shoe

Flatfoot — Pronator — Motion control shoe

The type of foot arches dictates what kind of shoe to wear for the most support. *(Electronic Illustrators Group. © 2012 Cengage Learning.)*

Description

Orthotics can vary widely depending on the type of problem they are designed to correct. The three main types of orthotics are those designed for correcting the spine, those designed for correcting a lower limb, and those designed to correct an upper limb.

Orthotics are made out of a variety of different materials, including molded plastic and metal. The type of materials used depend on the type of orthotic device and to some extent the company that manufactures it. Orthotics are created by doctors who specialize in orthotics, many of whom also specialize in producing prostheses for individuals who are missing a body part.

Orthotics are specially shaped and molded to fit the individual who will be wearing them. They are adjusted to provide the correct alignment that the doctor feels will best improve the condition or alleviate the pain. Because orthotics are made to fit a specific individual, multiple trips to the doctor for consultations and fittings may be required.

Many insurance plans cover orthotics, although coverage varies depending on the type of plan and why the orthotic is required. Most insurance plans do not cover specially made shoe inserts unless rigid criteria are met.

Spinal orthotics

Spinal orthotics are typically used for individuals who have severe back pain, to manage scoliosis, or to immobilize the back after spinal surgery or because of a **fracture**. The spinal orthotic is a hard device, usually made of plastic, that fits around the individual's torso from just above the tail bone to the middle of the chest. It has straps that allow the individual to adjust the orthotic, and to remove it.

How long a spinal orthotic is required depends on the condition it is being used to treat. If it is being used to treat back pain, the device is only required until the individual can tolerate the amount of pain that occurs in the absence of the orthotic. If it is being used after spinal surgery, or to immobilize the spine so a fracture can heal, the device may be required for 6–12 weeks. When used to treat scoliosis, it may be required for even longer.

Upper limb orthotics

Upper limb orthotics are used to immobilize or restrict the motion of an upper limb or body part, commonly the hand, wrist, or shoulder. There are a variety of reasons that an upper limb orthotic may be indicated, most often trauma or injury to the body part. This is especially true for athletes who may require upper limb orthotics after injuring their hands and wrists during sports such as **basketball** or their shoulders pitching in **baseball**.

The materials out of which upper limb orthotics are made vary depending on the nature of the movement restriction necessary. Orthotics designed to hold the hand and wrist in place are typically made of hard plastic, molded to fit the lower arm, with straps to secure the hand or wrist in place. Orthotics designed for the shoulder are often made of a set of metal pins holding together straps that restrict the movement of the shoulder and provide additional support.

Lower limb orthotics

Lower limb orthotics are orthotics designed to correct position and provide support for the foot, ankle, and knee. The most familiar type of orthotic is the foot orthotic that inserts into the shoe. Shoe inserts are so common that some are sold in supermarkets, shoe stores, and other major retailers. Shoe insert orthotics work by adjusting the way that the foot is aligned when it hits the ground. Correctly aligning the foot can adjust the way that the ankles, hips, and even spine is aligned. Correct alignment can help reduce back, hip, ankle, knee and foot pain. Many doctors who make specially molded shoe inserts warn against using mass produced inserts sold in retail stores. These inserts have not been specially designed for the indivudal's specific foot issues, and can actually exacerbate problems with alignment, increasing pain rather than reducing it.

Sports orthotics

Sports orthotics typically refers to lower limb orthotics that are specially made for use during athletic activities. It can also refer to upper limb orthotics made for athletic use, although this is much less common. Individuals with a spinal orthotic device are typically not able to participate in athletic activities, and thus, sports orthotics does not usually encompass spinal orthotics.

Sports orthotics are usually shoe inserts made of more durable materials than typical shoe inserts. They may also be made of materials designed to better absorb the impact created by jumping or running. In many cases, sports orthotics are thicker than normal orthotics, and fit better in shoes designed for running or other athletic activities than daily wear shoes.

If an individual has sports orthotics made, they may be of a slightly different shape than his or her daily wear orthotics because the foot can fall differently while running or jumping than while **walking**. It is generally advisable for professional and serious athletes to have sports orthotics made and not use their daily wear orthotics while participating in athletic activities.

Precautions

Orthotics should be created and fitted specifically for each individual by a doctor, usually a podiatrist, who specializes in orthotics. Using orthotics designed for someone else can lead to misalignment, possibly causing serious consequences. Some orthotics, usually foot orthotics, are available in supermarkets, shoe stores, and general merchandise stores. Although these orthotics can sometimes offer relief, consumers should be wary. Each individual's foot is different, and orthotics should be specially molded to provide the best support possible. Using mass-produced orthotics can lead to misalignment. Misalignment can cause serious pain in the shins, ankles, calves, thighs, and lower back. It can put strain on the arches, knees, ankles and hips that can lead to joint pain and inflammation. Poorly fitted foot orthotics can also increase the risk of ankle sprain, as the foot may not land evenly when moving. Landing at the wrong angle can cause the ankle to twist or sprain.

Athletes should ensure that any orthotics used during sports or recreational fitness activities are designed

and manufactured as sports orthotics. Sports orthotics are made of more durable materials and are designed to provide support and alignment during athletic activity. Athletes should see a doctor who specializes in sports orthotics. The orthotic device should be designed to provide maximal benefit for the sport the athlete is planning to participate in while wearing it. Athletes should typically have two sets of orthotics, one for use during athletic activity, and one for day-to-day use.

Preparation

Prior to having an orthotic made, the patient must be examined by a medical professional, specifically one specializing in orthotics. The medical professional will evaluate the correction necessary to relive a specific type of pain, or to provide stabilization of a certain area. Multiple visits or consultations may be necessary to ensure proper form and fit of the orthotic.

Athletes should talk to their doctor about what sports and fitness activities can be done while wearing the orthotic. In some cases it may require a scaling back of training to learn correct movements with the orthotic in place. While this can be frustrating, it is important to prevent the strains and sprains that can occur when muscles are used to make new movements too quickly.

Aftercare

No aftercare is typically required for orthotics. For common orthotics such as shoe inserts no special training or practice is usually necessary to make full use of the orthotic correctly. For more specialized and complex orthotics such as spinal braces, practice may be required to learn to move effectively with the new device.

Complications

Complications from orthotics are typically caused by the realignment of body parts straining muscles or putting additional pressure on joints. This can cause pain, soreness, and discomfort. These complications typically resolve within a few weeks of beginning to wear the orthotic. If they do not resolve or there is significant pain the individual should consult the doctor who prescribed the orthotics or the clinic that created and fitted the device.

To reduce the chance of pain associated with wearing a new orthotic, it is recommended that the orthotic be introduced gradually. The individual begins by wearing the orthotic for a short time, often as little as one hour a day, and slowly increases the wearing time over a few weeks until the orthotic is worn all the time, or as often as prescribed.

Results

Many athletes find that a good pair of sports orthotics can improve foot, ankle, and even back comfort while running. In some cases, athletes may even find their performance enhanced due to the increased comfort and correct alignment of the spine and foot.

Resources

BOOKS

Curtin, Michael, Matthew Molineux, and Jo-Anne Supyk-Mellson, eds. *Occupational Therapy and Physical Dysfunction: Enabling Occupation,* 6th ed. New York: Churchill Livingstone/Elsevier, 2010.

Edelstein, Joan E., and Alex Moroz. *Lower-Limb Prosthetics and Orthotics.* Thorofare, NJ: Slack, 2011.

May, Bell J., and Margery A. Lockard. *Prosthetics and Orthotics in Clinical Practice: A Case Study Approach.* Philadelphia: F.A. Davis. 2011.

PERIODICALS

Hsu, Wellington, et al. "The Professional Athlete Spine Initiative: Outcomes After Lumbar Disc Herniation in 342 Elite Professional Athletes." *Spine Journal* 11, no. 3 (March 2011): 180–6.

McMillan, Andrew, and Craig Payne. "Immediate Effect of Foot Orthoses on Plantar Force Timing During Running: A Repeated Measures Study." *Foot* 21, no. 1 (March 2011): 26–30.

Yeung, Simon S., Ella W. Yeung, and Lesley D. Gillespie. "Interventions for Preventing Lower Limb Soft-Tissue Running Injuries." *Cochrane Database of Systematic Reviews* (2011).

WEBSITES

"Assistive Devices and Orthotics." WebMD. (April 17, 2009). http://arthritis.webmd.com/tc/assistive-devices-and-orthotics-topic-overview (accessed November 12, 2011).

Kulkarni, Shantanu S., et al. "Spinal Orthotics." Medscape Reference. (October 28, 2011). http://emedicine.medscape.com/article/314921-overview (accessed November 12, 2011).

ORGANIZATIONS

American Academy of Orthotists and Prosthetists, 1331 H St., NW, Suite 501, Washington, DC, 20005, (202) 380-3663, Fax: (202) 380-3447, http://www.oandp.org.

American Medical Society for Sports Medicine, 4000 W. 114th St., Suite 100, Leawood, KS, 66211, (913) 327-1415, Fax: (913) 327-1491, office@amssm.org, http://www.amssm.org.

American Orthotic and Prosthetic Association, 330 John Carlyle St., Suite 200, Alexandria, VA, 22314, (571) 431-0876, Fax: (571) 431-0899, info@aopanet.org, http://www.aopanet.org.

The American Orthopedic Society for Sports Medicine, 6300 N. River Rd., Suite 500, Rosemont, IL, 60018, (847) 292-4900, Fax: (847) 292-4905, http://www.sportsmed.org.

Tish Davidson, AM

Osteoporosis

Definition

Osteoporosis is a disease characterized by low bone mass and deterioration of bone tissues leading to bone fragility and an increase in **fracture** risk. The term osteoporosis comes from the Greek word *osteon,* meaning bone, and *porus,* meaning pore or passage. Osteoporosis literally makes bones porous. The amount of calcium stored in human bones decreases over time, causing the skeleton to weaken.

Description

Osteoporosis is a disorder that has no noticeable symptoms until the weakening of the bones leads to problems with posture, lower back pain, and brittle or easily broken bones. Although osteoporosis can appear at any **age**, it is most commonly a disease of older

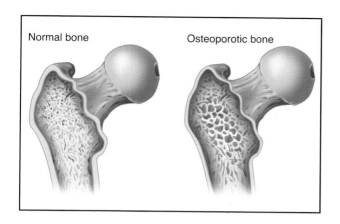

On the left, a healthy bone that has normal tissue and density. As one ages, calcium and phosphate are two minerals that are reabsorbed by the body, causing the bone to lose density as on the right. *(Electronic Illustrators Group. © 2012 Cengage Learning.)*

adults. It develops when the breakdown of old bone—a process known as resorption—outpaces the production of new bone tissue.

Bone is living material. It is constantly broken down by cells called osteoclasts and built up again by cells called osteoblasts. This process is called bone remodeling, and it continues throughout an individual's life. Normally, more bone is built up than is broken down from birth through adolescence. In the late teens or early 20s, people reach their peak bone mass—the most bone that they will ever have. For 20 or so years, bone gain and bone loss remain approximately balanced in healthy people with good nutrition. However, when women enter menopause, usually in their mid to late forties, for the first five to seven years bone loss occurs at a rate of 1–5% a year. Men tend to lose less bone, and the loss often begins later in life. Osteoporosis occurs when bone loss continues and bones become so thin and their internal structure is so damaged that they break easily.

Bone remodeling occurs because bone is made primarily of calcium and phosphorous. Calcium is critically involved in muscle contraction, nerve impulse transmission, and many metabolic activities within cells. To remain healthy, the body must keep the level of free calcium ions (Ca^{2+}) in the blood within a very narrow concentration range. Besides providing a framework for the body, bone acts as a calcium "bank." When excess calcium is present in the blood, osteoblasts deposit it into bones where it is stored. When too little calcium is present, osteoblasts dissolve calcium from bones and move it into the blood. This process is controlled mainly by parathyroid hormone

(PTH) secreted by the parathyroid glands in the neck. As people age, various conditions cause them to take more calcium out of the "bone bank" than they deposit, and osteoporosis eventually develops. A person's peak bone mass and the rate at which they lose it in later life affect their risk of developing osteoporosis; the higher the peak bone mass at age 30, the lower the risk of osteoporosis later on.

Doctors divide osteoporosis into three categories, or types. Types 1 and 2 are considered primary because they are not caused by other diseases or conditions. Type 3 osteoporosis is sometimes called secondary osteoporosis because it results from taking certain drugs or having other diseases.

- Type 1: This type occurs in women after menopause and results from declining levels of estrogen and other sex hormones in the body. Sometimes called postmenopausal osteoporosis, it is the most common type of the disease. Type 1 may also occur in older men due to low levels of the sex hormone testosterone.

- Type 2: Sometimes called senile osteoporosis, this type of osteoporosis occurs in elderly men as well as elderly women because of decreased bone formation due to aging.

- Type 3: Type 3 osteoporosis is caused by long-term use of certain medications, particularly steroids and drugs given to treat epilepsy, and by such conditions as malnutrition, Klinefelter syndrome, Turner syndrome, thyroid disorders, hemophilia, Marfan syndrome, rheumatoid arthritis, lupus, and lymphoma. Some studies indicate that people receiving chemotherapy for cancer are at increased risk for this type of osteoporosis.

Demographics

According to the National Osteoporosis Foundation (NOF), as of 2011 about 10 million people (8 million women and 2 million men) in the United States have osteoporosis, and another 34 million adults have low bone density, a condition called osteopenia. Osteopenia can develop into osteoporosis if it is not treated. Osteoporosis is responsible for more than 1.5 million fractures annually in the United States, including 300,000 hip fractures, 700,000 vertebral fractures, 200,000 wrist fractures, and more than 300,000 fractures in other parts of the body. The costs of treating osteoporosis and the fractures that it causes come to more than US$19 billion each year. An osteoporosis-related fracture occurs in one in two women and one in eight men over the age of 50.

Although osteoporosis is often thought of as a woman's disease, it affects men, too. Men who take certain medications, particularly cortisone and other steroid drugs, have the same risk of developing osteoporosis as women who take these medications. Each year, 80,000 American men with osteoporosis have a hip fracture, and one-third of them die within a year.

Worldwide, osteoporosis is estimated to affect one in three women and one in 12 men over the age of 50. It is the most common metabolic bone disease in the world.

Osteoporosis in children is very unusual. There is a rare condition called juvenile idiopathic osteoporosis. About 60 cases have been reported worldwide. Idiopathic means that the cause of the condition is unknown.

Risk factors

There are two basic categories of risk factors for osteoporosis. Some of these risk factors can be changed, while others cannot be altered. Risk factors that cannot be changed include:

- Sex. Women have four times the risk of the disease as men, particularly after the menopause.

- Race/ethnicity. Asian and Caucasian women have a higher risk of osteoporosis than African American or Hispanic women. Although their risk is smaller, African-American and Hispanic-American women should still take precautions against osteoporosis. An estimated 10% of African-American women over age 50 have osteoporosis and an additional 30% have low bone density that puts them at risk of developing osteoporosis.

- Body build. Small-boned people of either sex are at greater risk of osteoporosis than people with average or heavy bones.

- Age. Both men and women have an increased risk of osteoporosis as they get older. The highest incidence of the disease is found among those men and women aged 80 or older.

- Genetic factors. A tendency for bones to fracture easily is thought to run in some families.

Risk factors for osteoporosis that people can change include:

- Low sex hormone levels. These can be raised in both men and women by hormone replacement therapy.

- Eating disorders (particularly anorexia nervosa) and female triad syndrome.

- Depression. Emotional depression can be treated, most often with a combination of medication and psychotherapy.

- Low intake of calcium and vitamin D. People can change their eating habits and take vitamin or calcium supplements.

- Smoking and alcohol intake. People can quit smoking and drink in moderation.

- Getting the right amount of exercise. Bed rest or inadequate exercise can weaken bones, but so can too much exercise (such as marathon running).

- Medications. People who are taking medications that increase their risk of osteoporosis can ask their doctor about alternatives.

Certain diseases also increase a person's risk of developing osteoporosis:

- hyperthyroidism
- hyperparathyroidism
- celiac disease
- inflammatory bowel disease (IBD)
- cystic fibrosis
- diabetes
- chronic liver disease

Causes and symptoms

The basic cause of osteoporosis is that the loss of bone tissue occurs faster than the production of replacement bone. The increased rate of bone loss can be particularly critical if the person had a low or inadequate peak bone mass to begin with. A low peak bone mass can result from malnutrition in childhood; inadequate intake of calcium or vitamin D (Vitamin D is necessary for the body to make use of calcium in the diet.); an eating disorder in adolescence, when the body's need for calcium is at its height; or not getting enough **exercise**.

Genetic profile

Osteoporosis results from a complex interaction between genetic and environmental factors throughout life. Evidence suggests that peak bone mass is inherited, but current genetic markers are able to explain only a small proportion of the variation in individual bone mass or fracture risk. As of 2011, no specific mode of inheritance has been identified. Heritability of bone mass has been estimated to account for 60–90% of its variance. Studies have shown reduced bone mass in daughters of osteoporotic women when compared with controls, in men and women who have first-degree relatives (parents, siblings) with osteoporosis, and in perimenopausal women who have a family history of hip fracture. Body weight in infancy may be a determinant of adult bone mass.

Many candidate genes exist for osteoporosis; however, relatively few have been studied. The first candidate gene to be identified was the vitamin D receptor

(VDR) gene, and studies are ongoing as to how much this gene accounts for variance in bone mass. The response of bone mass to dietary supplementation with vitamin D and calcium is known to be dependent, in part, on VDR polymorphisms. Other genes may aid in establishing who would benefit from treatments such as drug therapy or exercise. Associations between bone mass and polymorphisms have also been found in the estrogen receptor gene, the interleukin-6 genes, the transforming growth factor beta, and a binding site of the collagen type I alpha1 (COLIA1) gene.

The risk of osteoporosis is greatly determined by peak bone mass, and any gene linked to fractures in the elderly may possibly be associated with low bone mass in children as well. Some scientists think that environmental influences during early life interact with the genome to establish the functional level of a variety of metabolic processes involved in skeletal growth.

Symptoms

Osteoporosis can proceed for a long time without any noticeable symptoms. Some older adults simply notice that their height is shrinking. This loss of height is caused by compression of the bones in the spinal column. Sometimes the vertebrae fracture as they come closer together; this type of injury is called a compression fracture.

Over many years, a sequence of spinal compression fractures may cause kyphosis, the bent-over posture known as dowager's or widow's hump. These fractures rarely require surgery, and they can range from causing minor discomfort to severe painful episodes of backache. In either case, pain generally subsides gradually over one to two months.

Another common symptom of osteoporosis is a fragility fracture. Fragility fractures occur when a person falls from a standing position or a low height and breaks a bone that would not break in a person with healthy bone. The most common locations of fragility fractures in people with osteoporosis are the wrists, the hips, and the vertebrae in the spine. The individual may experience vertebral pain in various ways; some describe it as sharp while others describe it as dull or nagging. In some cases the pain gets worse when the **walking** or moving around.

Diagnosis

Since osteoporosis can develop undetected for decades until a fracture occurs, early diagnosis is important. Osteoporosis is most likely to be diagnosed following a fragility fracture. The doctor will take a careful history of the patient's risk factors, including a possible family history of easily broken bones as well as a medication history and questions about such lifestyle factors as exercise, diet, smoking, and drinking.

Examination

The physical examination includes measurement of the patient's height, evaluation of possible loss of height, and assessment for evidence of kyphosis.

Tests

The doctor may order a blood test to rule out a thyroid disorder or to check the levels of sex hormones in the patient's blood.

A bone mineral density test (BMD) is the only way to diagnose osteoporosis and determine risk for future fracture. The painless, noninvasive test measures bone density and helps determine whether medication is needed to help maintain bone mass, prevent further bone loss, and reduce fracture risk. To take this test, the patient lies on an examination table while two x-ray beams of different intensities are aimed at the bones. The result is called a T-score. It is calculated by comparing the patient's bone mineral density to that of a healthy 30-year-old of the same sex and race. A T-score of -1.0 or higher is normal; a score between -1.0 and -2.5 indicates osteopenia; a score below -2.5 indicates osteoporosis.

Several different machines measure bone density. Central machines, such as the dual energy x-ray absorptiometry (DXA or DEXA) and quantitative computed tomography (QCT), measure density in the hip, spine, and total body. Peripheral machines, such as radiographic absorptiometry (RA), peripheral dual energy x-ray absorptiometry (pDXA), and peripheral quantitative computed tomography (pQCT), measure density in the finger, wrist, kneecap, shin bone, and heel.

A physician may be able to observe osteoporotic bone in a routine spinal x ray, however, BMD tests are more accurate and can measure small percentages of lost bone density. In an x ray, osteoporotic bone appears less dense and the image is less distinct, suggesting weaker bone.

As of 2011, the United States Preventive Services Task Force recommended using dual energy x-ray absorptiometry to screen all women 65 years and older and women 60–64 years of age who have increased fracture risk. Some physicians also recommend bone density testing at menopause at whatever age it occurs to begin preventive treatment, if necessary. The major risk factors are low body weight, low calcium intake, poor health, and a family history of osteoporosis.

Some health care organizations recommend screening all men 70 years and older, as well as men with one of the following risk factors: bone fracture, poor health, or low testosterone levels.

Treatment

Drugs

Medications are an important part of treatment for osteoporosis. Various drugs have been shown to be effective in preventing or slowing bone loss and increasing bone mass. These include:

- Raloxifene. One of a class of drugs called selective estrogen receptor modulators (SERMs) that appear to prevent bone loss, raloxifene (Evista) produces small increases in bone mass. It is approved for the prevention and treatment of osteoporosis. However, it carries a serious warning that it can increase the formation of blood clots in the legs and lungs. Women who have a history of blood clots are strongly discouraged from taking this drug.
- Alendronate. One of a class of medications called bisphosphonates, alendronate (Fosamax) may prevent bone loss, increase bone mass, and reduce the risk of fractures. Patients receiving any bisphosphonate should take calcium and vitamin D before and during treatment with a bisphosphonate to lower the risk of side effects from these drugs. Fosamax and other bisphosphonates have been associated with osteonecrosis of the jaw, a rare but serious condition in which the bones of the jaw die, causing severe pain and swelling. This side effect has mainly been found to occur in individuals undergoing chemotherapy and those who have jaw or mouth surgery while taking a bisphosphonate.
- Ibandronate. Also a bisphosphonate, ibandronate (Boneiva) is available as a one daily or once monthly pill. It has been shown to reduce the incidence of some bone fractures and to increase bone density. Possible side effects include osteonecrosis of the jaw, low blood calcium, and unusual fractures of the thigh bone.
- Risedronate. Also from the bisphosphonate family, risedronate (Actonel) has been shown to reduce bone loss, increase bone density, and reduce the risk of fractures.
- Calcitonin. A hormone that regulates calcium levels in the blood, calcitonin may prevent bone loss. It is approved for treatment of diagnosed osteoporosis.
- Denosumab. Approved by the U.S. Food and Drug Administration to treat osteoporosis in 2010, denosumab (Prolia) is a twice-annual injection given in the doctor's office that may prevent bone loss. It is generally recommended for individuals who have found

that other treatments for osteoporosis were not successful. It is not recommended for individuals with low blood calcium levels, and is not approved for use in pregnant women. Some serious side effects have been found to occur including hypocalcaemia (low blood calcium), serious infections, skin problems, and osteonecrosis of the jaw.
- Teriparatide. Teriparatide (Forteo) has been shown to increase bone growth when given intermittently. Teriparatide is synthetic parathyroid hormone (a hormone involved in regulating bone growth). Teriparatide is injected once daily by the patient into the thigh or lower stomach. Possible side effects include dizziness, difficulty breathing, and fainting. Studies have found that in lab rats teriparatide injections increase the risk of bone cancer. It is not clear if this risk is also increased in humans who use the drug.
- Hormone replacement therapy (HRT). Before 2002, many physicians encouraged women undergoing menopause to use hormone replacement therapy (HRT) to treat menopausal symptoms (e.g., hot flashes, mood changes). HRT treats these symptoms by increasing estrogen and progesterone levels enough to suppress symptoms. Estrogen is known to protect bone against resorption, so an added benefit of HRT was that increased levels of estrogen slowed bone loss and the development of osteoporosis. However, in the summer of 2002, a large Women's Health Initiative study was released that showed HRT could have significantly harmful effects such as an increased risk of heart attack, stroke, blood clots, and breast cancer. The risk was high enough that the study was stopped early. Because of increased risks, HRT is no longer a standard treatment for osteoporosis in postmenopausal women despite its positive effects on slowing bone loss.

Lifestyle changes

Recommended lifestyle changes that can reduce the rate of bone loss include regular exercise, particularly weight-bearing forms of exercise like walking, dancing, **treadmill** exercises, and jumping. Other measures include quitting smoking, taking supplemental vitamin D and calcium, and watching one's alcohol intake.

NUTRITIONAL THERAPY. A healthful diet low in **fats**, salt, sugar, and nutritionally inferior processed foods, and containing whole grains, fruits and vegetables, nuts and seeds and calcium-rich foods (particularly dairy products, dark-green leafy vegetables, sardines, salmon, and almonds), along with nutritional supplements (such as calcium, magnesium, and vitamin D) are important components of nutritional approaches to treating this disease. Calcium

KEY TERMS

Alendronate—A non-hormonal drug used to treat osteoporosis in postmenopausal women.

Bisphosphonates—Compounds that slow bone loss and increase bone density.

Calcitonin—A naturally occurring hormone made by the thyroid gland that can be used as a drug to treat osteoporosis and Paget's disease of the bone.

Compression fracture—A fracture caused by the collapse of a vertebra in the spinal column, usually caused either by trauma or by weakening of the bone in osteoporosis.

Fragility fracture—A fracture that occurs because of a fall from standing height or less. A person with healthy bones would not break a bone falling from a standing position.

Glucocorticoids—A general class of adrenal cortical hormones that are mainly active in protecting against stress and in protein and carbohydrate metabolism. They are widely used in medicine as anti-inflammatories and immunosuppresives.

Kyphosis—The medical term for curvature of the upper spine. Osteoporosis is a common cause of kyphosis in older adults.

Osteoblast—A type of bone cell responsible for bone formation. The number of osteoblasts in a person's body decreases with age.

Osteoclast—A type of bone cell that removes bone tissue.

Osteopenia—The medical name for low bone mass, a condition that often precedes osteoporosis.

Polymorphism—A change in the base pair sequence of DNA that may or may not be associated with a disease.

Resorption—The removal of old bone from the body.

T-score—The score on a bone densitometry test, calculated by comparing the patient's bone mineral density to that of a healthy 30-year-old of the same sex and race.

Vertebra (plural, vertebrae)—One of the segments of bone that make up the spinal column.

---

found in dairy products is well absorbed by the body making them a valuable source of calcium.

In addition, women should avoid foods that may accelerate bone loss. They should cut down on caffeinated beverages if their intake is excessive (more than five cups of coffee a day). Some studies have shown that high amounts of caffeine can decrease calcium absorption. Research is mixed on the impact of soda consumption on **bone health**. Some studies have suggested that the phosphoric acid found in many sodas can negatively affect bone health, while others have shown that it has no effect. What most experts do agree on is that caffeinated beverages and sodas should be consumed in moderation for good health.

Prognosis

The prognosis for osteoporosis depends on its type and cause; the patient's age, sex, and ethnicity; the presence of other diseases or disorders; and the patient's willingness to follow the doctor's recommendations about medications and lifestyle changes.

People do not die from osteoporosis itself, but from complications from bone fractures. These complications can include chronic pain, pneumonia, blood clots in the deep veins of the leg, or breathing disorders caused by the stooped posture resulting from compression fractures in the spine. The death rate within the first six months after a hip fracture is 14%. Even patients who survive often have a greatly lowered quality of life.

Prevention

People cannot change such risk factors for osteoporosis as age, sex, and race, but they can eat properly, exercise regularly, and ask their doctor about vitamin D and calcium supplements. Male and female adolescents should participate in sports and get adequate calcium in the diet in order to build up a high peak bone mass before midlife. Women who have not yet gone through menopause should get at least 1,000 milligrams (mg) of elemental calcium and a minimum of 800 international units (IU) of vitamin D every day; women who have completed menopause, anyone who must take steroid medications, and all men and women over 65 should aim for 1,500 mg of elemental calcium and at least 800 IU of vitamin D daily.

Other recommendations for lowering the risk of osteoporosis in older adults include:

- participating in regular weight-bearing exercise, such as walking, jogging, **tennis**, **weightlifting**, and cross-country skiing to strengthen bones

- stopping smoking

QUESTIONS TO ASK YOUR DOCTOR

- Will my insurance cover a bone mineral density test to determine if I have osteoporosis?
- Is there a nutritionist on your staff who could help me ensure I am getting a healthy diet with enough calcium and vitamin D?
- Could my fracture be related to low bone mineral density?
- How can I be sure my child athlete is not at risk for osteoporosis?

- reducing intake of caffeine to not more than three cups a day
- limiting alcohol intake to not more than two drinks per day
- avoiding excessive amounts of dietary fiber as it binds to calcium and may interfere with absorption

Older adults should try to reduce their risk of falls whether or not they have osteoporosis. There are balance and strength exercises that older adults can practice at home. In addition, such safety measures as wearing properly fitted shoes with non-slip soles, checking one's house for loose rugs, poor lighting, and other hazards, installing grab bars in shower stalls, and keeping a cordless phone within easy reach in case of an accident are all good forms of fall prevention.

Calcium and vitamin D are both essential to building and maintaining strong bones. Dairy products are a good source of these nutrients. Calcium supplements are recommended for many women who have difficulty getting enough calcium in their diet. Recommended dietary allowances (RDAs) and lists of foods that are high in calcium and vitamin D can be found in their individual entries. Fluoride also is needed to develop healthy bones and teeth.

Special concerns for athletes

Although good bone health is important for everyone, it is especially important for athletes and individuals who engage in recreational fitness activities. Weak bones can increase the likelihood of serious injury during participation in sports and fitness activities for athletes of all ages and skill levels.

Special concerns for elite athletes

Elite athletes can be at increased risk of osteoporosis. Extreme training regimens and diets that lack the required amounts of calcium and vitamin D can be problematic. It is especially important for elite athletes to have strong, healthy bones because of the repeated pressures and strains often put on them during training and competition.

Repetitive stress on the bones, such as **running** during marathons or **track and field** events, and repeated jumping during **basketball**, figure skating, or ballet can lead to fractures in athletes who do not have good bone health. Many sports involve sudden strains on bones, such as during **gymnastics**, **wrestling**, and **baseball**, that can lead to fractures and breaks if bones are brittle. These kinds of injuries, while painful and difficult for everyone, can be especially problematic for elite and professional athletes as serious injuries can lead to missing seasons, forgoing important competitions, and loss of income.

Female athletes are at special risk of the female athlete triad, which is the combination of disordered eating, **amenorrhea** (cessation of a normal menstrual period), and osteoporosis. This triad is often caused by **eating disorders** including anorexia and bulimia. Athletes are at increased risk for developing eating disorders, because of the focus on body shape and the perception that losing a few more pounds could provide a competitive edge.

Young people with the eating disorder anorexia nervosa are at especially high risk of developing osteoporosis later in life because they have poor, unbalanced diets. The menstrual cycle in girls with anorexia is often delayed in starting or if it has started, stops. In addition, people with anorexia almost never get enough calcium to build strong bones during adolescence and they make unusually larger amounts of cortisol, a corticosteroid made by the adrenal gland that causes bone loss. Although the effect of this eating disorder on bones will not be seen until the individual is older, failure to build strong, dense bones during the teen years substantially increases the risk of osteoporosis later.

Special concerns for young athletes

The bone health of young athletes is especially important because good bone health is required for normal growth and development. Children and adolescents who do not get enough calcium and vitamin D are at an increased risk for growth problems as well as bone fractures and breaks. Young female athletes are especially at risk for the female athlete triad. Parents of young athletes of both genders should be alert for signs of disordered eating, and work closely with their children to ensure that their children are eating a healthy, well-balanced diet.

Special concerns for older athletes

Regular exercise is important to good health, and can improve quality of life and bone health well into the later senior years. However, older athletes need to take precautions when exercising to help protect their bones. Because older people are more likely to have osteoporosis, and because bones generally weaken during the later years, older athletes are at increased risk for bone fractures and breaks. Working with a doctor and nutritionist is important to ensure a balanced diet that includes enough calcium and vitamin D. Participating in sports such as walking and low impact aerobics that have a reduced likelihood of causing sudden impacts to the bones is a good idea. Strength training can improve balance and help reduce the risk of falls that can reduce the risk of broken hips and wrists. With a few precautions, older athletes are often able to continue to engage in the sports and fitness activities they enjoy well into their senior years.

Resources

BOOKS

Saxton, John, ed. *Exercise and Chronic Disease: An Evidence-Based Approach.* New York: Routledge, 2011.

Whipple, Thomas J., and Robert B. Eckhardt. *The Endurance Paradox: Bone Health for the Endurance Athlete.* Walnut Creek, CA: Left Coast Press, 2011.

Yamaguchi, Masayoshi. *Nutritional Factors and Osteoporosis Prevention.* New York: Nova Science Publishers, 2010.

PERIODICALS

Croswell, Jennifer. "Screening for Osteoporosis." *American Family Physician* 83, no. 10 (May 15, 2011): 1201–1202.

Nichols, Jeanne F., and Mitchell J. Rauh. "Longitudinal Changes in Bone Mineral Density in Male Master Cyclists and Nonathletes." *Journal of Strength and Conditioning Research* 25, no. 3 (March 2011): 727–734.

Wentz, Laurel, et al. "Females Have a Greater Incidence of Stress Fractures than Males in Both Military and Athletic Populations: A Systemic Review." *Military Medicine* 176, no. 4 (April 2011): 420–430.

WEBSITES

Bone Up on Bone Health: Exercise to Build Healthy Bones. Eunice Shriver National Institute of Child Health & Human Development. http://www.nichd.nih.gov/publications/pubs/upload/boneup_boneloss1rev.pdf (accessed November 8, 2011).

Osteoporosis. The Mayo Clinic. (November 20, 2010). http://www.mayoclinic.com/health/osteoporosis/DS00128 (accessed November 8, 2011).

United States Centers for Disease Control and Prevention. "Calcium and one Health" http://www.cdc.gov/nutrition/everyone/basics/vitamins/calcium.html (accessed July 17, 2011).

ORGANIZATIONS

American Bone Health, 1814 Franklin St., Suite 620, Oakland, CA, 94612, (510) 832-2663, Fax: (510) 208-7174, (888) 266-3015, info@americanbonehealth.org, http://www.americanbonehealth.org.

National Association of Sports Nutrition, 7710 Balboa Ave., Suite 311, San Diego, CA, 92111, (888) 694-0317, http://nasnurtition.com.

National Institutes of Health Osteoporosis and Related Bone Diseases National Resource Center, 2 AMS Circle, Bethesda, MD, 20892-3676, (202) 223-0344, Fax: (202) 293-2356, (800) 624-2663(BONE), NIAMSBoneInfo@mail.nih.gov, http://www.niams.nih.gov/Health_Info/Bone.

National Osteoporosis Foundation, 1150 17th St. NW, Suite 850, Washington, DC, 20036, (202) 223-2226, Fax: (202) 223-2237, (800) 231-4222, http://www.nof.org.

Osteoporosis Canada, 1090 Don Mills Rd., Suite 301, Toronto Ontario, Canada, M3C 3R6, (416) 696-2663, Fax: (416) 696-2673, (800) 463-6842 (English), (800) 977-1778 (French), http://www.osteoporosis.ca.

Tish Davidson, AM

Overhydration

Definition

Overhydration is a serious, possibly fatal, problem within the brain caused when the normal balance of electrolytes in the body is altered due to an excessive amount of water being consumed over a short time period. This over consumption of water is also sometimes called **water intoxication**, water excess, hyper-hydration, or water poisoning. Normal **hydration** is important in the area of fitness and **exercise** because a proper water level within the body is an essential part of a healthy lifestyle. During strenuous physical activities, the body's water level can drastically change, leading to health issues.

Description

The consumption of water is a necessary function of life. Humans must drink water on a regular basis in order to stay alive. In fact, humans can live for only about a week without water, even less if they in a hot, dry environment. Hydration is the process by which humans take in and maintain a steady level of water in their tissues and organs down to the cellular level. During this process, adequate fluid levels in the body are in balance, what is called homeostasis. However, it is possible for people to become overhydrated from excessive fluid intake.

Too much water over a short period can be potentially dangerous, to the point of causing coma or death. Under normal circumstances, it is very unlikely that someone will accidently drink too much water. Usually, cases of overhydration occur when infants are fed too many fluids, adults have medical or mental problems related to water consumption, or people consume huge amounts of water while trying to stay hydrated during intense periods of physical activity or exercise. For instance, when **marathon** runners or bicyclists are competing during very hot conditions, they will drink large amount of water to replenish fluids lost to perspiration. The normal percentage of water that is daily replaced in healthy adults is between 5% and 10%. That percentage dramatically increases during physical activities and and/or during very hot climatic conditions. Thus, people participating in strenuous activities try to replenish those fluids lost through sweating. However, sometimes they drink too much water—much more than they actually lose.

In addition, cases have been documented where contests were held in which people won money or prizes for the most water drunk. For instance, in January 2007, Jennifer Strange, of Rancho Cordova, California, was found dead after participating in a radio contest called "Hold Your Wee for a Wii", in which the prize was a Nintendo Wii video game system. She drank a large amount of water while not urinating, and died from overhydration. Such contests are dangerous and should not be held due to the extreme danger involved in such actions.

When overhydration happens the normal balance of electrolytes in the body is altered. Electrolytes are chemical compounds that help to control bodily fluid levels that allow for the proper transmission of nerve signals throughout the body. When too much water and not enough electrolytes (especially sodium) are in the body, then the cells in the brain try to swell. However, they cannot expand because the brain is encased within a rigid skull called the cranium. This causes intracranial pressure, the first sign of overhydration. Other later symptoms of overhydration include seizures and, in some rare cases, death. Overhydration usually leads to **hyponatremia**, a condition in which the level of sodium, one type of electrolyte, in the blood plasma is too low.

Demographics

Overhydration can occur in anyone. However, it is more commonly found in infants under the age of six months. Often times infants may become overhydrated when drinking several bottles of water in a day or from drinking milk formula that has been diluted too much.

Athletes and others that exercise strenuously can also become afflicted with overhydration if they drink much more water than they lose to perspiration. When athletes sweat heavily, they lose both water and electrolytes. If water is consumed in large amounts during and after such strenuous exercise, then the balance of electrolytes can be altered. In such circumstances, people who drink liquids that contain electrolytes are less likely to become overhydrated, but are still at risk due to the excessive amount of liquid introduced into the body.

Other groups of people at increased risk for overhydration include those people who use excessive amount of alcohol or drugs, have medical problems such as diarrheal diseases, and have certain psychological disorders.

Causes and symptoms

Causes

Causes for overhydration include:

- cholera or severe gastroenteritis, especially in infants leading to dehydration through diarrhea that is countered with too much fluid intake
- drinking too much water during or after exercise, such as during endurance sports like marathons, without replacing electrolytes lost through sweating
- drug or alcohol intoxication
- low body mass, particularly in infants below six months of age
- medical conditions such as heart, liver, kidney diseases
- overexertion and heat stress
- psychiatric conditions such as psychogenic polydipsia in which patients intentionally drink large amounts of water
- water-drinking contests

Symptoms

Various symptoms that initially during overhydration include:

- confusion
- drowsiness
- headache
- inattentive
- irritability
- other various personality and behavioral changes

Later symptoms that occur after the initial symptoms of overhydration, include:

- blurred vision
- cramping
- difficulty breathing, especially during exertion
- digestive problems
- elevated blood pressure

- inability to perceive and interpret sensory information
- muscle twitching
- muscle weakness
- nausea
- poor coordination and balance
- rapid breathing
- sudden weight gain
- thirst
- vomiting

In the later stages of overhydration the following more dangerous symptoms occur:

- brain damage
- cerebral edema (excessive water accumulation in the intracellular and/or extracellular spaces of the brain)
- dysfunction to the central nervous system
- lowered heartbeat (what is called bradycardia)
- seizures
- widened pulse pressure (the increasing of systolic pressure and the decreasing of the diastolic pressure)

Finally, coma and death can occur.

Diagnosis

A medical professional will analyze the symptoms of the patient, along with his/her past history over the past few days to partially determine whether overhydration is the cause. However, symptoms of overhydration occur in many medical disorders, so this process only narrows down the exact problem. Consequently, the doctor will also use blood and urine tests to completely and properly diagnosis overhydration.

Treatment

Mild cases of overhydration can be generally alleviated by limiting fluid intake. However, in serious cases diuretics may be prescribed to quickly increase urination. In the most dangerous of overhydration cases, fluids to restore a normal balance of electrolytes will be administered quickly. After about half of the fluids have been introduced into the body, the rate of absorption is reduced to a more moderate rate.

Prognosis

Mild overhydration has a favorable outcome. However, moderate to serious cases can be fatal if not properly and quickly treated. In most circumstances, death is rarely the final outcome.

KEY TERMS

Electrolytes—Substances in the body that are able to conduct electricity. They are essential in the normal functioning of body cells and organs.

Gastroenteritis—A condition characterized by severe inflammation of the gastrointestinal tract, usually involving both the small intestines and the stomach; with main symptoms of diarrhea and vomiting.

Homeostasis (water)—A condition of adequate fluid level in the body in which fluid loss and fluid intake are equally matched and sodium levels are within normal range.

Hyponatremia—An abnormally low level of sodium in blood plasma.

Psychogenic polydipsia—A psychiatric disorder in which patients consume excessive amounts of water, sometimes going to great lengths to obtain it from any source possible.

Prevention

Never drink excessively large amounts of water over a short time period. The American College of Sports Medicine (ACSM) recommended in 2007 that proper hydration during exercise should be geared personally to each athlete rather than strictly associated with general guidelines. The ACSM states: "The goal of drinking during exercise is to prevent excessive (more than 2% body weight loss from water deficit) dehydration and excessive changes in electrolyte balance to avert compromised performance."

Because there is considerable variability in sweating rates and sweat electrolyte content between individuals, customized fluid replacement programs are recommended." The ACSM added in 2008: "Drink fluids before exercise and periodically during exercise, instead of practicing rapid fluid replacement in the middle of exercise. Drinking at intervals will provide more adequate hydration and urine production."

To prevent overhydration, never drink excessive amounts of water. A healthy adult would have to drink over 2 gal (7.6 L) of water in a day to develop overhydration. The medical community suggests that people drink at least 0.25–0.5 gal (1–2 L) of water per day. Specifically, the Food and Nutrition Board of the Institute of Medicine (IOM) recommended in 2004 (and is still accurate as of February 2011) that relatively inactive adult men take in about 125 oz (3.7 L, about 15 cups) of fluids daily and that women take in about 91 oz. (2.7 L, about 10 cups) to replace lost water. These recommendations are for total fluid intake from both beverages and food.

The World Health Organization (WHO) recommendations are slightly different: 98 oz. (2.9 L) for men and 74 oz. (2.2 L) for women (162 oz. [4.8 L] for pregnant women). Highly active adults and those living in very warm climates need more fluid; WHO recommends 152 oz. (4.5 L) per day for both men and women in these conditions. This amount may also vary depending on body mass. Overhydration will occur only at levels much higher than this amount.

Resources

BOOKS

Cook, Gregg, and Fatima d'Almeida-Cook. *The Gym Survival Guide: Your Road Map to Fearless Fitness.* New York: Sterling, 2008.

"Dehydration." *The Merck Manual of Diagnosis and Therapy,* Section 6, edited by R. S. Porter. White House Station, NJ: Merck Research Laboratories, 2007.

Dunford, Marie. *Fundamentals of Sport and Exercise Nutrition.* Champaign, IL: Human Kinetics, 2010

Isaac, Jeff. *Outward Bound Wilderness First-Aid Handbook,* revised and updated. Guilford, CT: Falcon Guides, 2008.

Knoop, Kevin J. et al., editors. *Atlas of Emergency Medicine,* 3rd ed. New York: McGraw-Hill Professional, 2009.

Micheli, Lyle J., editor. *Encyclopedia of Sports Medicine.* Thousand Oaks, CA: SAGE, 2011.

Moorman III, Claude T., and Donald T. Kirkendall, editors. *Praeger Handbook of Sports Medicine and Athlete Health.* Santa Barbara, CA: Praeger, 2011.

Plowman, Sharon A., and Denise L. Smith. *Exercise Physiology for Health, Fitness, and Performance.* Philadelphia: Wolters Kluwer Health/Lippincott Williams & Wilkins, 2011.

Rich, Brent E., and Mitchell K. Pratte. *Tarascon Sports Medicine Pocketbook.* Sudbury, MA: Jones and Bartlett Publishers, 2010.

Smolin, Lori A., and Mary B. Grosvenor. *Nutrition for Sports and Exercise.* New York: Chelsea House, 2010.

Sutton, Amy L, editor. *Fitness and Exercise Sourcebook.* Detroit: Omnigraphics, 2007.

WEBSITES

Fallon, Jr., L. Fleming. *Overhydration.* Healthline. (January 13, 2007). http://www.healthline.com/galecontent/over hydration#prognosis (accessed September 5, 2011).

Fit Facts: Healthy Hydration. American Council on Exercise. http://www.acefitness.org/fitfacts/fitfacts_display. aspx?itemid = 173 (accessed July 11, 2011).

Heat and Hydration: Important Concerns for Outdoor Workouts. American College of Sports Medicine. (March 25, 2008). http://www.acsm.org/AM/Template. cfm?Section = ACSM_News_Releases&TEMPLATE = / CM/ContentDisplay.cfm&CONTENTID = 9797 (accessed July 11, 2011).

Johnston, Brian D., and Paul L. Liebert. "Overview of Exercise." *Merck Manual for Medical Professionals.* http://www.merckmanuals.com/professional/sec22/ ch344/ch344a.html?qt = Hydration&alt = sh#v1116096 (accessed July 11, 2011)

Mark, David A. *How to Avoid Overhydration.* Ehow.com. http://www.ehow.com/how_6658002_avoid-overhydration. html (accessed September 5, 2011).

Water Requirements in Adults. Water U.K. (January 2007). http://www.water.org.uk/home/water-for-health/ medical-facts/adults (accessed July 7, 2011).

Woman Dies After Water-drinking Contest. MSBNC. (January 13, 2007). http://www.msnbc.msn.com/id/ 16614865/ns/us_news-life/t/woman-dies-after-water- drinking-contest/ (accessed September 5, 2011).

ORGANIZATIONS

American Alliance for Health, Physical Education, Recreation and Dance, 1900 Association Drive, Reston, VA, 20191-1598, (703) 476-3400, (800) 213-7193, http:// www.aahperd.org/.

American Council on Exercise, 4851 Paramount Drive, San Diego, CA, 92123, (888) 825-3636, support@ acefitness.org, http://www.fitness.gov/.

American College of Sports Medicine, P.O. Box 1440, Indianapolis, IN, 46206-1440, (317) 634-9200, Fax: (317) 634-7817, http://www.acsm.org/.

National Coalition for Promoting Physical Activity, 1100 H Street, N.W., Suite 510, Washington, DC, 20005, (202) 454-7521, Fax: (202) 454-7598, http://www.ncppa.org/ membership/organizations/.

National Strength and Conditioning Association, 1885 Bob Johnson Drive, Colorado Springs, CO, 80906, (719) 632-6722, Fax: (719) 632-6367, (800) 815-6826, http:// www.nsca-lift.org/.

President's Council on Fitness, Sports and Nutrition, 1101 Wootton Parkway, Suite 560, Rockville, MD, 20852, (240) 276-9567, Fax: (240) 276-9860, http://www. fitness.gov/.

William A. Atkins, B.B., B.S., M.B.A.

Overpronation *see* **Foot health; Orthotics**

Overtraining

Definition

Overtraining is a general term for the situation that can occur over time when the intensity and/or the duration of **exercise** someone does is more than what the individual can adequately recover from with respect to improved fitness. In other words, the person exercises so much—either the amount of time or the effort expended—that the muscles are unable to recover and actually lose strength rather than gaining it. Overuse of the muscles, or overtraining, can occur whenever sufficient time is not allowed between training sessions for the exercised muscles to recover.

Description

Exercising is a great way to maintain a good fitness level. It strengthens the muscles, joints, and bones of the body. However, too much exercising can sometimes be detrimental to fitness, conditioning, and strength. A good balance between exercise and rest is essential for overall health.

Several days of rest, or a few days of reduced activity, may be necessary if the exercise routine is very strenuous or of an extra long duration. If such rest is not provided to the affected muscles then they may not be able to completely regenerate. Over a long period of overtraining, this situation is likely to lead to a decline in overall fitness and health.

Demographics

Overtraining can occur to anyone that exercises too much. Its adverse effects can be behavioral, emotional, and/or physical in nature. Overtraining has been found to be especially frequent in bodybuilders because their main goal is to lift heavy weights, often on consecutive days, to build up muscle mass and strength. People who regularly exercise and are exposed to various situations can run the risk of overtraining. Some of these situations include poor nutrition, illness, overworking, mental disorders, menstruation (in women), and jet lag.

Causes and symptoms

Causes

The cause of overtraining is doing too much exercising and not allowing adequate rest for the exercised muscles. Muscles that are not given time to recover degrade over time. Rather than growing, muscles actually decrease in size when overtraining occurs over an extended period.

Poor nutrition and excessive exercising is a bad combination because overworked muscles are not given the necessary nutrients to grow and become stronger. A **protein** deficiency develops when essential amino acids (those that must be supplied in the diet because it cannot be synthesized internally) in the body are used faster than they can be produced (because of a diet poor in such nutrients).

Diets that restrict calorie intake make overtraining a much higher risk because the body has too few **calories** to expend (burn). Consequently, the body cannot supply sufficient **energy** to the muscles so they can properly grow and perform.

A mental condition, such as anxiety, can lead to higher than normal levels of cortisol. Cortisol is a steroid hormone produced by the adrenal gland. It is released in response to stress in the body, and can add risk to overtraining.

Other factors that may lead to overtraining are excessive use of alcohol, tobacco or drugs; certain personality types; the external environment, and quality and quantity of sleep.

Symptoms

Overtraining **fatigue** sets in when the muscles begin to feel sluggish in the middle of a workout. Fatigue may continue after the workout, and throughout the week. This sluggishness is usually the result of expending more calories than are taken into the body. It is important to maintain a well-balanced diet and consume energy sufficient foods before and after the workout.

Symptoms of overtraining may include any or all of the following:

- higher than normal number and/or severity of infections
- higher incidences of illnesses such as colds and influenza (flu)
- muscle soreness or pain
- joint achiness or pain
- dehydration (because excess water is lost from the body during exercise)
- higher frequency of injuries (because the muscles, tendons, and joints are being excessively worked)
- irritability
- depression
- mental problems such as mood disturbances, anxiety, depression

- excessive weight loss (excessive loss of body fat) and loss of appetite
- decreased muscular strength
- constipation or diarrhea
- fatigue; loss of energy
- reduced menstruation or loss of a menstrual cycle in women
- insomnia; change in sleeping habits
- heart palpitations; increased resting heart rate
- loss of enthusiasm, motivation, and competitive drive
- headaches

Diagnosis

A doctor is likely to diagnosis overtraining by carefully looking at a patient's past medical history (including a detailed review of exercise programs currently used) and performing a complete physical examination. Heart rate irregularities and **weight loss** are two key indicators of overtraining, as is the feeling of fatigue.

The medical professional is also likely to perform various tests to eliminate other causes such as **asthma** or allergies, cardiovascular problems, diabetes, metabolic or hormonal imbalances, muscle diseases, nutritional deficiencies and anemia, psychiatric conditions, and other such medical problems.

Treatment

When overtraining is mild, then resting for several days may be all that is needed to recover. Exercise can also be reduced in its intensity or duration. Alternating heat and cold compresses or other such devices can relieve sore and tired muscles. For instance, massaging the overtrained muscles may help in recovery. Additional sleep each night gives the muscles time to recover. Nutritional supplements (such as multivitamins) can increase nutrient deficiencies within the body. In addition, a nutritious and balanced diet is important during recovery.

If overtraining continues, then the condition may persist with increased fatigue and other more serious symptoms.

Prognosis

Short-term overtraining (STO) involves minor symptoms such as temporary fatigue while exercising. It usually can be resolved with a few days of rest.

Long-term overtraining (LTO) is likely to cause overtraining syndrome. With LTO, more serious symptoms are present, such as fatigue whether exercising or not, mood state disturbances, and muscle stiffness or

---

KEY TERMS

Anemia—An abnormal condition of the blood in which too few red blood cells are produced or adequate red blood cells are produced but they are lacking in hemoglobin.

Asthma—A disease of the respiratory system that is sometimes caused by allergies; its symptoms include coughing, tightness in chest, and difficulty breathing.

Cardiovascular—Relating to the heart and blood vessels.

Jet lag—A physiological condition that results when the body's circadian rhythm becomes disoriented by air travel from east to west or west to east across the Earth.

Menstruation—The approximate monthly discharge of blood and other bodily matter from the womb that occurs in female primates, such as humans, from puberty to menopause.

Overtraining syndrome—A state that occurs in athletes or people who exercise regularly when the exercise routine is very strenuous or lasts for excessive amounts of time and rest between exercise sessions is not sufficient for muscle recovery.

---

soreness. LTO is likely to require weeks or months before recovery is complete. Its prognosis is less favorable.

Prevention

Overtraining can be prevented by resting muscles after they are exercised. More time is necessary if the exercise is especially strenuous or extra long in duration. If an intense workout is performed on muscles in the upper body on one day, then make sure the muscles in the lower body are worked out the next day. A day of recovery, such as an easy walk in the park or a relaxing bike ride around the neighborhood will keep a person from overtraining their body.

If symptoms that lead to overtraining are present, then the amount of exercising should be reduced until the symptoms disappear. Get plenty of rest and make sure nutritious meals are eaten.

People who begin an exercise routine should do so gradually. The muscles are not used to exercise and need to become accustomed to the new physical activity. For example, if beginning to run, an individual should start by **walking**, gradually increasing the walking speed a little faster each day, until the body is ready to run without the muscles becoming overworked. The same thing applies when beginning a weight-lifting program. Start with light weights and work up to heavier weights over a gradual period. The number of repetitions and number of sets should also be progressed accordingly.

Overtraining can be minimized by:

- eating nutritious foods after exercising
- not exercising if pain is present; also not exercising when feeling tired
- getting proper sleep each night
- drinking plenty of water

Resources

BOOKS

Cook, Gregg, and Fatima d'Almeida-Cook. *The Gym Survival Guide: Your Road Map to Fearless Fitness.* New York: Sterling, 2008.

Plowman, Sharon A., and Denise L. Smith. *Exercise Physiology for Health, Fitness, and Performance.* Philadelphia: Wolters Kluwer Health/Lippincott Williams & Wilkins, 2011.

Schoenfeld, Brad. *Women's Home Workout Bible.* Champaign, IL: Human Kinetics, 2010.

Sutton, Amy L, editor. *Fitness and Exercise Sourcebook.* Detroit: Omnigraphics, 2007.

WEBSITES

Hanes, Tracii. *Risks of Overtraining.* LiveStrong.com. (May 12, 2011). http://www.livestrong.com/article/437775-risks-of-overtraining/ (accessed November 8, 2011).

Patterson, James. *Side Effects of Overtraining.* LiveStrong.com. (September 18, 2010). http://www.livestrong.com/article/282653-side-effects-of-overtraining/ (accessed November 8, 2011).

Waehner, Paige. *Are You Exercising Too Much?* About.com. (April 22, 2010). http://exercise.about.com/cs/exercisehealth/a/toomuchexercise_2.htm (accessed November 8, 2011).

Willey II, J. Warren. *Overtraining Syndrome.* BodyBuilding ForYou.com. http://www.bodybuildingforyou.com/articles-submit/j-warren-willey/overtraining.html (accessed November 8, 2011).

ORGANIZATIONS

American Alliance for Health, Physical Education, Recreation and Dance, 1900 Association Dr., Reston, VA, 20191-1598, (703) 476-3400, (800) 213-7193, http://www.aahperd.org.

American Council on Exercise, 4851 Paramount Dr., San Diego, CA, 92123, (888) 825-3636, support@acefitness.org, http://www.acefitness.org.

National Coalition for Promoting Physical Activity, 1100 H St., NW, Suite 510, Washington, DC, 20005, (202) 454-7521, Fax: (202) 454-7598, http://www.ncppa.org.

National Strength and Conditioning Association, 1885 Bob Johnson Dr., Colorado Springs, CO, 80906, (719) 632-6722, Fax: (719) 632-6367, (800) 815-6826, http://www.nsca-lift.org.

President's Council on Fitness, Sports and Nutrition, 1101 Wootton Parkway, Suite 560, Rockville, MD, 20852, (240) 276-9567, Fax: (240) 276-9860, http://www.fitness.gov.

William A. Atkins, BB, BS, MBA

Overuse injury

Definition

Overuse injuries are injuries that occur because of tissue damage caused by repetitive activities associated with occupational, recreational (including physical activity, **exercise**, and sport), or other types of habitual activities. Overuse injuries are also known as cumulative trauma disorders.

Description

Overuse injuries occur when a person places stress on some particular part of the body that has previously not been exposed to such a stress. For example, a person who is learning to play a new sport or an athlete who is working on a new training technique may place stress on fingers, toes, ankles, knees, shoulders, or other parts of the body unaccustomed to such stresses. The body's normal response to a new stress is to experience minor strains and tears that begins to heal through the repair of damaged tissue. As long as the repair process occurs at a rate at least as fast as damage occurs, no long-term effects are to be expected. But it often happens that such is not the case, and damage occurs more rapidly than the body can repair itself. In such cases, the trauma that has taken place begins to occur, manifesting itself as discomfort, achiness, and pain. These symptoms generally do not show up until some time after the new activity has begun, a matter of weeks or months.

Many specific examples of overuse injury are known by the location of the injury (knee or ankle, for example) and the activity responsible for the damage (typing or throwing for examples). Among the dozens of overuse injuries that have been given special names are:

- Blackberry thumb
- climber's finger
- computer vision syndrome
- golfer's elbow
- jumper's knee.
- Little League elbow
- Nintendo thumb
- runner's toe
- tennis elbow

A number of the most common overuse injuries are also well known by their medical names, including:

- Achilles tendinitis
- carpal tunnel syndrome
- median nerve palsy
- patellar tendinitis
- plantar fasciitis
- rotator cuff tear
- shin splints
- stress fracture
- ulnar nerve entrapment

Demographics

Data on the incidence of overuse injury among participants in a variety of occupation and sports and among the general public are widely available. Space limitations here permit a review of only a sample of those data.

- A survey of 4,358 joggers found that 46 percent of respondents have experienced at least one overuse injury from their activity during the preceding year, of whom 14 percent had sought medical assistance for their injury.

- Among 223 adventure racers studied in 2003, 73 percent had experienced at least one overuse injury in the preceding 16 months, the most common location of which was the ankle, followed by the knee, lower back, shin, and Achilles tendon.

- Among a population of 56 equestrian athletes, 79 percent reported injuries in the lower back or lower extremities and 70 percent in the neck

- A 2009 study of 398 elite junior rowers found that 74 percent of subjects reported at least one overuse injury, the most common site of which was the lower back, followed by the knee, forearm, and wrist. Women were more likely to experience such injuries than were men.

- Rotator cuff injuries are fairly common in the general population, with experts estimating that somewhere between 20 and 30 percent of all people experiencing some degree of the problem. Cadaver studies have found that 30 percent of subjects studied had complete rotator tears.

- A 2011 survey of 748 male and female runners age 13 to 18 found that 68 percent of all females and 59 percent of all males had experienced an overuse injury at some time in their running career, the most common injuries being tibial stress injury, ankle sprain, and patellofemoral pain.

- Overuse injuries are common in basketball also. A 2007 study of 164 Belgian senior men and women players (average age: 23.7 years) found a total of 87 overuse injuries that affected most commonly the knee.

Overuse injuries are hardly restricted to sports and other athletic events. Any person who uses the same mechanical motion over and over again is subject to overuse injury. For example, a 1992 study of 59 adult piano players found that over half (53.7 percent) experienced overuse injuries severe enough to interfere with their regular practice schedule.

Causes and symptoms

In general, overuse injuries are caused by one of two kinds of factors: intrinsic or extrinsic. Intrinsic factors are those that are part of an individual's basic physical make-up, his or her anatomical structure. Sometimes it is just not possible for a person to ask her or his body to perform certain types of functions: to throw a ball in a particular way, to clear a high hurdle properly, or to swing a **golf** club correctly. Anyone who forces his or her body to perform actions that are physically impossible or unsuitable is likely to develop an overuse injury as the person tries over and over again to get the action "right." No amount of training or expert advice can prevent overuse injuries in such cases.

Extrinsic factors are a different matter. Most experts divide extrinsic causes of overuse injury into one of two categories: lack of proper training or improper technique. It is not uncommon for a person to make a commitment to developing a skill as quickly as possible and forcing a training schedule that places too much strain on the body. That type of commitment is a certain recipe for overuse injury that is defined as placing more stress on body tissues than they are able to adapt to. Overuse injuries can also develop when a person performs an action improperly: swinging a golf club or **tennis** racket, throwing a **baseball** or discuss, or performing a **gymnastics** action incorrectly. Again, forcing one's arms, legs, knees, elbows, wrists, and ankles to perform actions that cause damage to tissue results in overuse injuries. Finally, using the wrong equipment or equipment that is not in proper condition can also lead to overuse injury.

Diagnosis

Overuse injuries are sometimes difficult to diagnose because they develop over a long period of time. An individual may feel for some time that a knee, ankle, shoulder, or other body part is just "sore" because of exercise and workouts. By the time a person recognizes that the problem may be more serious, the injury may be well developed. The first step in diagnosing any form of overuse injury is a medical history in which patient and doctor try to identify the specific physical actions that may have led to the problem. Often, this history in and of itself may be enough to identify the general type of injury involved. The medical worker may then follow up the patient history with a thorough physical examination that includes a biomechanical evaluation, that may identify the specific location of tissue damage. In some cases, imaging tests, such as x rays, CAT scans, or MRI scans may be needed to determine whether or not there has been a bone **fracture** or tissue tear, and the extent of that damage.

Treatment

Probably the most common treatment for overuse injuries is RICE. RICE is a term that refers to treatment that includes four elements:

- Rest: Simply stop doing whatever it is that caused the injury in the first place: swinging a tennis racket, throwing a softball, or running. Stop the activity entirely until the pain associated with the injury has gone away.
- Ice: Using an ice pack on an injured body part reduces blood flow to the body part, thus reducing swelling. The sooner one uses this technique after an injury has

---

occurred, the more successful it will be. Use ice treatment with care, however, never exceeding more than about 30 minutes at any one time.

- Compression: The use of any kind of bandage that exerts pressure on the injured body part also reduces blood flow and swelling, reducing pain associated with the injury.
- Elevation: Placing the injured body part above the heart is a third way of reducing blood flow and swelling of the injured body part.

RICE is largely an immediate, short-term approach to the treatment of overuse injuries. On a long-term basis, one may have to use medications that reduce the swelling that causes pain associated with overuse injuries, such as non-steroidal anti-inflammatory agents (NSAIDs). Physical therapy is often an essential element also in helping damaged tissues to repair themselves and muscle groups to regain their normal strength. Treatments such as hydrotherapy and ultrasound may also help tissues to heal.

Prognosis

Prognosis for full recovery of overuse injuries differs somewhat based on the severity of the injury and the type and location of injury. Generally speaking, however, most overuse injuries heal completely provided that a person (1) follows completely a recommended treatment regime and (2) corrects any training errors or errors in technique that led to the problem originally. On average, most overuse injuries improve in a matter of four to six weeks, although more difficult problems may take up to six months to get better.

Prevention

The most obvious way to prevent overuse injuries is to be aware of and to avoid their main causes, poor training programs and poor technique. Some specific recommendations that trainers make include the following:

- Start out with warm-up exercises, such as calisthenics and jogging, allowing the muscles to get ready for more active exercises.

QUESTIONS TO ASK YOUR DOCTOR

- What specific treatment recommendations would you make for the type of overuse injury I am experiencing?

- What training exercises do you recommend for my child that will reduce his/her chance of developing an overuse injury?

- How will I know that the pain and discomfort I'm experiencing in connection with an exercise is a symptom of an overuse injury and not just normal soreness?

- Include stretching exercises in your warm-up workout, since they also help muscles become more flexible and ready to go to work with the main exercise.

- Avoid overtraining that can lead to tissue damage and overuse injuries. Give your body time off between training sessions to let it recover from any damage that has occurred.

- Make use of periodization training, in which you take short breaks between exercise events, as another way of letting the body recover from damage incurred during an exercise.

- Organize practices so that athletes do not have to perform the same action over and over again. Instead of having a golfer hit 100 drives, let him or her hit a few drives, then a few chips, then a few putts.

- Increase the stress level of an exercise gradually. One of the ways overuse injuries develop is that an athlete may try to improve a particular skill more rapidly than his or her muscles can adapt to greater stress. Some trainers use the so-called "ten percent rule," according to which an athlete is never asked to do more than ten percent more work on day 2 than she or he did on day 1.

Resources

BOOKS

Bahr, Roald, and Lars Engebretsen. Sports Injury Prevention. Chichester, UK: Wiley-Blackwell, 2009.

Gorlin, Robert S. Sports Injuries Guidebook. Champaign, IL: Human Kinetics, 2008.

PERIODICALS

Berliner, M. An Ounce of Prevention: Physical Activity Plan Can Help Weekend Athletes Allay Overuse Injuries. Rehab Management. 24(3; April 2011): 18–19.

McLeod, Valovich, et al. National Athletic Trainers' Association Position Statement: Prevention of Pediatric Overuse Injuries. Journal of Athletic Training, 46(2; March 3, 2011): 206–220.

WEBSITES

Overuse Injuries. American Orthopaedic Society for Sports Medicine. http://www.sportsmed.org/uploadedFiles/Content/Patient/Sports_Tips/ST%20Overuse%20Injuries%2008.pdf (accessed on August 19, 2011).

Overuse Injuries. Healthcare South. http://www.healthcaresouth.com/pages/overuseinjuries.htm (accessed on August 19, 2011).

ORGANIZATIONS

American Orthopaedic Society for Sports Medicine, 6300 N. River Rd., Suite 500, Rosemont, IL, 60018, (847) 292-4900, Fax: (847) 292-4905, (877) 321-3500, info@aossm.org, http://www.sportsmed.org/.

David E. Newton, A.B., M.A. Ed.D.

P

Paddleboarding

Definition

Paddleboarding is a sport in which a person rides on the surface of the water, in a prone or kneeling position on a surfboard-like board (prone paddleboarding or kneeling paddleboarding) or standing and using an oar for propulsion (stand up paddleboarding or SUP).

Purpose

As a purely recreational sport, the purpose of paddleboarding is to enjoy the experience of traveling over the water by means of some system of self-propulsion. In competitive paddleboarding, the object of the sport is to cover some given distance on the water at a faster time than all of one's competitors.

Demographics

Paddleboarding is a sport that is available to individuals of both genders, all ages, and all ethnicities. Competitions recognize the wide reach of the sport's appeal by having a number of divisions in races. As an example, a race might have divisions for juniors (boys and/or girls) under the age of 16, men and women in various age groups (such as 17 to 39, 40 to 49, and 50 and over), and same-sex or coed teams in either or both forms of paddleboarding. (The number and type of divisions vary from race to race.)

History

Credit for the invention of the modern paddleboard is usually given to a California surfer from Wisconsin, Thomas Edward (Tom) Blake. At the age of 17, Blake moved to California, took a job as a lifeguard, and soon became fascinated by surfing. In 1924, Blake visited Hawaii, where he worked part-time at the Bishop Museum and became interested in Hawaiian culture. He learned about the surfboard-type devices used by early Hawaiian royalty known as the olo. Blake saw in the olo a possible solution for the biggest problem facing modern surfboarders, the heavy construction of their board. Blake spent many years trying to find ways to produce new kinds of surfboards that were lighter in weight and easier to handle. Eventually, he conceived of a way in which a person could travel on a surfboard not by standing on it, but by lying down on the board and paddling with a **swimming** motion. In 1932, Blake participated in the first recorded paddleboard competition, a race from the California mainland to Catalina Island, a competition he won over two friends in a time of 5 hours 53 minutes.

Some afficionados trace the beginning of stand-up paddleboarding (SUP) to a mode of transportation that has existed for centuries, in which a person stands on a flat piece of wood and paddles through calm waters to collect food, building materials, or other products. Others argue that stand-up paddleboarding was simply a natural development as the sport of prone and kneeling paddleboarding became more popular towards the end of the twentieth century. According to this line of argument, SUP became popular in the 1960s when young men in Hawaii stood on their surfboards on the water to take pictures of tourists learning how to surf. Before long, they were traveling on their surfboards while standing up and propelling themselves with long paddles. From that point, SUP rapidly became more popular. Today, it is probably even more popular among the general, non-competitive public than traditional paddelboarding.

Arguably the most famous paddleboard racing site in the world is the Ka'iwi Channel, the stretch of ocean between Molokai and Oahu in the Hawaiian Islands. That stretch of water was first navigated on paddleboard in 1938 by Californian Gene "Tarzan" Smith. It has been the site of the Molokai 2 Oahu race every year since 1997 when 44 paddleboarders covered

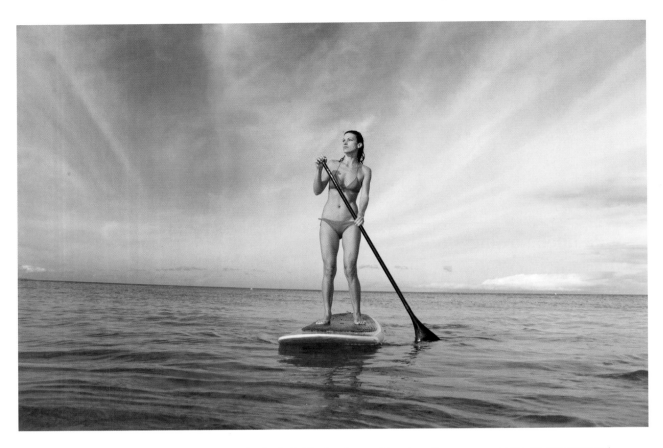

Paddleboarding is an activity gaining popularity for individuals who want to strengthen core muscles. *(© idreamphoto/ ShutterStock.com)*

the course. The fifteenth version of the race in 2011 saw more than 250 participants from 15 countries paddling or **rowing** the channel.

Description

The principles on which paddleboarding are based are simple. In the traditional form of the sport, one can lie prone (face down) on the board and paddle on either side of the board, much as one does during swimming. Alternatively, one can kneel on the board and paddle in much the same way. In SUP, one stands on the board and uses a single long paddle to propel oneself through the water, as one might do in a canoe or kayak.

Preparation

As with any sport, participation in paddleboarding is best done by those who are at least minimally physically fit for the sport. The participant should be able to swim and be comfortable in a water environment. One should also be familiar with general safety procedures and appropriate etiquette associated with the sport. Many experts recommend that a beginner have at least one instructional course to become familiar with these points and with the general skills and techniques involved in paddleboarding.

Equipment

Paddleboarding requires a minimum of personal equipment, including a shirt and shorts appropriate for the sport. Paddleboards come in a variety of sizes and shapes, but are classified into three general categories: Stock boards are boards less than 12 ft (3.6 m) in length; 14 boards are boards 14 ft (4 m) in length; and unlimited boards are boards longer than 14 ft (4 m), usually 16–19 ft (5–6 m) in length. Boards may have a variety of accessories to make their use safer, more comfortable, or more efficient, such as deck pads, hand grips, fins, leashes, and tie-downs. The paddle used in SUP is very similar to a canoe paddle with relatively few restrictions placed by governing bodies. For example, the World Paddle Association, the governing body for stand up paddleboarding requires only that a paddle be "a single blade design, with one blade on one end and a handle on the other end. The length of a paddle may be adjustable."

Additional recommended equipment includes life vests, helmets, and sun protection such as sunglasses and sunscreen.

Training and conditioning

Training and conditioning for recreational paddleboarding can reasonably be limited to the type of exercises one uses for any physical activity, such as **stretching** and simple **warm-up** exercises. To the extent that one chooses to become involved in competitive racing, a more intensive program of training designed to improve one's strength and endurance is recommended. The website YOLO Board, for example, recommends the whole range of strength and **endurance training** expected of any professional athlete, including weight training, **core training**, balance and coordination training, and **interval training**. This type of training and conditioning program makes sense for athletes who expect to spend five hours or more paddling across the open ocean in weather that may be less than conducive to an easy row on the water.

Risks

Given the vagaries of the weather and bodies of water in general, paddleboarders are subject to a number of risks inherent to the sport, such as body damage as a result of hitting the board and drowning as a result of falling off the board. Schools that teach paddleboarding skills and race officials commonly acknowledge risks such as these and require participants to sign waivers excusing them from any responsibilities for injuries that students or competitors may incur.

Relatively few studies have been conducted on the number and type of injuries suffered by paddleboarders. A study reported in 2010 found that more than half of the 88 respondents experienced some type of injury as a result of their sport; most of them were overuse or repetitive injuries. The body part most commonly involved in an injury was shoulder strain The researcher noted that shoulder strain was a problem primarily because people were using the wrong technique in their paddling.

Results

An important element in preventing injuries during paddleboarding is proper preparation that, at the minimum, means stretching and warm-up **exercise** prior to participating in the sport. In addition, one should become familiar with proper techniques to be used in prone, kneeling, and stand up paddleboarding to avoid injuries associated with improper procedures. There is a risk of repetitive motion injury (**overuse injury**) so breaks should be scheduled at appropriate times and of appropriate lengths to avoid such injuries. Individuals involved in competitive paddleboarding should consider more sophisticated training and conditioning programs that help strengthen the body and reduce injury risk.

Resources

BOOKS

Casey, Rob. *Stand Up Paddling: Flatwater to Surf and Rivers.* Seattle: Mountaineers Books, 2011.

Marcus, Ben. *The Art of Stand Up Paddling: A Complete Guide to SUP on Lakes, Rivers, and Oceans.* Guilford, CT: FalconGuides, 2012.

WEBSITES

Frey, Roch. *Paddleboard Tips from Roch Frey: Paddle Longer and Faster.* Watermans Applied Science. (February 28, 2010). http://watermansapphedscience.com/blog/?p = 2439 (accessed November 8, 2011).

General Information. Molokai2Oahu. http://www.molokai2oahu.com/event-info/about-race/general-info/ (accessed November 8, 2011).

Lynch, Gary. *Tom Blake.* HawaiiHistory.org. http://www.hawaiihistory.org/index.cfm?fuseaction = ig.page& PageID = 449 (accessed November 8, 2011).

ORGANIZATIONS

World Paddle Association, (888) 972-4959, info@worldpaddleassociation.com, http://worldpaddleassociation.com.

David E. Newton, AB, MA, EdD

Pain *see* **Muscle pain**

Paraplegic and quadriplegic athletes

Definition

Paraplegics are individuals who are paralyzed from the waist down, usually as the result of a lower spinal cord injury (SCI). Quadriplegics are individuals who have lost complete or partial use of all four limbs, usually as the result of an upper spinal cord injury.

Quadriplegia is also known as tetraplegia, meaning "four paralysis," or "paralysis of all four limbs." Individuals who have lost the use of their legs are generally confined to wheelchairs, so athletic events in which they may participate are sometimes referred to as wheelchair athletics or wheelchair sports. Paraplegics and quadriplegics are sometimes classified as "disabled" persons, although that term is obviously inappropriate for individuals who may be limited in some physical activities, but who are also clearly capable of very significant physical accomplishments in many areas, such as recreational sports and world-class athletics. Sports and other athletic events in which paraplegic, quadriplegic, and other disabled individuals compete are sometimes referred to as adapted sports.

Purpose

In spite of their physical limitations, paraplegics and quadriplegics are active in a wide variety of sports and recreational activities, often with the assistance of equipment and rules that are specially adapted to their specific needs.

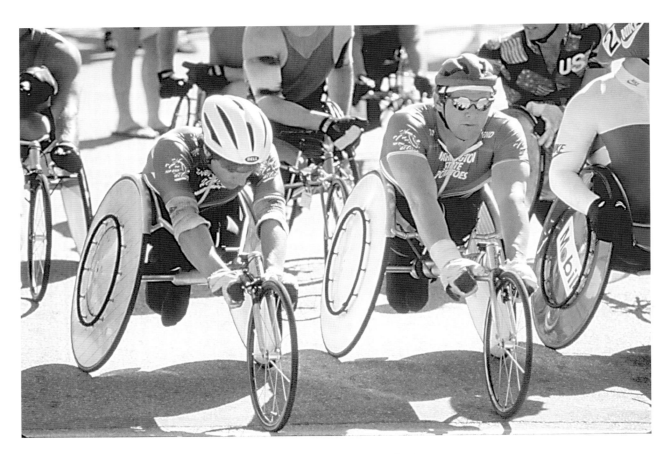

Racers prepare for a marathon in Los Angeles. *(© David Young-Wolff/PhotoEdit)*

Demographics

There appears to be no data or statistics on the number of paraplegic and quadriplegics who are actively engaged in recreational or sporting activities. Wheelchair & Ambulatory Sports, USA, the parent group for much of disabled athletics, had a membership in 2010 of just over 900 males and females, ranging in **age** from eight to 76. They classified themselves as recreational participants, active competitive athletes, coaches, and officials.

History

Special competitive athletic events designed exclusively for paraplegics and quadriplegics had their origin shortly after World War II, largely as a consequence of the many men and women who suffered physical injuries as a result of their military service. In 1948, Dr. Ludwig Guttmann at the Stoke Mandeville Hospital in Aylesbury, United Kingdom, organized an event designed to coincide with the Games of the XIV Olympiad, being held in London. Called the Stoke Mandeville Games for the Paralysed, the competition consisted of archery contests for 16 male and female veterans with spinal cord injuries incurred during the war. Some version of the Stoke Mandeville Games has been repeated almost every year since then, often with an expanded agenda of events. In 1952, a team from the Netherlands joined the games, making the event an international event for the first time. In 1960, the Ninth Annual International Stoke Mandeville Games were held in Rome in conjunction with the Games of the XVII Olympiad. The Ninth Stoke Mandeville Games later became known as the First Paralympics Games, a sporting event now held in association with the Summer and Winter Olympic Games, immediately following those events at the same location as the **Olympics**.

During this period, the formalization of sporting and athletic events for paraplegics and quadriplegics was also developing in other parts of the world. In 1946, two chapters of the Paralyzed Veterans of America, in California and New England, each played the first game of wheelchair **basketball** within two weeks of each other. Two years later, six wheelchair basketball teams were in existence, and they had begun playing each other in cross-country games. The National Wheelchair Basketball Association was formed in 1948, an association that currently has 22 conferences and 165 teams.

Over time, opportunities for paraplegics and quadriplegics were extended to more and more sports. For example, the National Foundation for Wheelchair Tennis was founded in 1980. The organization has grown in popularity and 112 players took part in the tennis portion of the 2008 Paralympics competition in Beijing. Opportunities for younger paraplegics and quadriplegics were first formalized in 1984 with the creation of the National Junior Disability Championships (NJDC), held in Delaware for contestants ages 7 to 19. The NJDC is held annually with competitions in archery, pentathlon, **swimming**, **table tennis**, three-on-three wheelchair basketball, and **track and field**. In 2011, more than 250 athletes aged 7 to 21 took part in the NJDC games in Saginaw, Michigan. Paraplegic and quadriplegic athletes can participate in a wide range of events, including archery, basketball, billiards, bowling, **fencing**, floor hockey (a form of **ice hockey**), **football**, handcycling, hang gliding, **racquetball**, **rock climbing**, sailing, scuba diving, shooting, skiing, **soccer**, swimming, table tennis, tennis, track and field, and **weightlifting**.

Description

Most sports and athletic events designed for paraplegics and quadriplegics involve modifications of the equipment or rules, or both, for the event. These modifications have been developed and codified by governing bodies in each sport, including Wheelchair Archery, USA; International Wheelchair Basketball Federation; American Wheelchair Bowling Association; Universal Wheelchair Football Association; American Wheelchair Table Tennis Association; International Wheelchair Tennis Federation; and Handicapped Scuba Association. Adaptations have been proposed and promulgated by groups with a general interest in disabled sporting events, such as America's Athletes with Disabilities; Disabled Sports, USA; International Wheelchair & Amputee Sports Federation; National Center on Physical Activity and Disability; and United States Paralympic Committee.

Some examples of the types of modifications used for paraplegic and quadriplegic athletes include:

- Archery: Wheelchair archery contestants use essentially the same equipment as non-disabled archers, except that they may use special equipment for specific physical disabilities. Some examples are an amputee adapter device that allows the archer to hold and release the bow string more easily; a bow sling that helps the archer to maintain control of the bow; an adaptive archery bow, for use with individuals who have severe disabilities and are unable to hold a bow at all; and a wheelchair bow stringer that can be used to assist in stringing the bow.

- Basketball: No special equipment is needed for the wheelchair version of the game, although a number of rule changes are necessary, such as the use of a basket at a lower elevation and prohibition on running, dribbling, and contact between players.

• Extreme sports: Many wheelchair participants can use special equipment that allows them to adapt to sports such as rock climbing, hang gliding, and surfing. Such equipment is designed to allow them to maintain balance and position while participating in such sports.

• Floor hockey: This version of ice hockey is played on a gymnasium floor with a felt disk and traditional hockey sticks or plastic versions of such sticks.

• Skiing: Depending on one's disability, a participant may use a three-ski (one ski and two outrigger boards) or a four-ski (two skis and two outrigger boards) for the sport.

• Table tennis: Disabled participants may perform with non-disabled colleagues, except that they may be provided with a floor lift to allow them to reach table height and a strap that allows them to hold the paddle more easily.

• Soccer: To a considerable extent, the rules for adapted soccer are the same as those for regular soccer, with the major differences having to do with the number of players on a team, the size of the playing field, and the size of the goal.

Preparation

Preparation for an adapted sport requires somewhat more preparation than would be needed for a non-adapted sport. Many governing organizations require that participants have a preparticipation examination (PPE) before they are allowed to take part in a sport. The PPE consists of a number of elements, one of which is confirmation that the athlete has completed acute rehabilitation from his or her injury, that is, they are no longer recovering from the specific event that result in his or her disability. The PPE should focus on being certain that the athlete understands the demands of the proposed sport or athletic event, with special recognition of the ways in which the sport might place demands on the body. In general, authorities recommend that disabled athletes develop and maintain a close relationship with a healthcare provider with whom they can discuss the demands of any given sport and the progress or problems one may be experiencing in taking part in that sport. In addition to these general expectations, prospective participants must be aware of and prepared for the special demands posed by any specific sport in which one hopes to participate.

KEY TERMS

Adapted sport—A sport whose equipment, rules, or other characteristics have been changed in some way or another to make it more amenable to play by a disabled person.

Paralympics games—An athletic competition held in connection with the Summer and Winter Olympics games designed for persons who are blind, deaf, or otherwise physically handicapped.

Paraplegic—An individual who is paralyzed from the waist down.

Preparticipation examination—A series of tests, inventories, and examinations recommended for a disabled person before she or he participates in a sporting or athletic event.

Quadriplegic—A person who has lost complete or partial use of all four limbs.

Wheelchair sport—A term often used to describe a sport or athletic event in which participants are confined to a wheelchair.

Equipment

Disabled athletes may, and sometimes are required to, use special equipment designed to protect them in the sport in which they have chosen to participate. This equipment should be used in addition to whatever basic equipment is a natural part of the sport.

Training and conditioning

The training and conditioning program that is best for any one athlete depends on a number of factors in addition to the general physical and mental skills that would be expected of any athlete engaged in a given sport. As part of a PPE, athletes are encouraged to work with their medical advisors to develop a specific training program that is appropriate to the sport being attempted as well as to one's own physical attributes. One common goal of a training program is to help an individual learn how to respond in case of an accident that may present problems not normally occurring with a non-disabled participant. For example, a physical therapist may be able to teach a person how to fall out of a wheelchair in the safest possible way, protecting the neck and head from damage; how to avoid falling out of the chair itself; and how most easily to get back into the chair if one does fall out.

Proper training for an athletic event may also involve preparation not directly related to the athlete's personal physical skills. For example, the participant should be provided with equipment suited to permit safe and enjoyable participation in a sport, such as extra padding in a wheelchair to protect against accidents that occur during play, or in case a person falls over in the chair. In addition, the prospective player may benefit from having a tour of the playing facility before an event begins so that she or he is aware of physical obstructions that may interfere with one's movement across the playing area. Any special equipment, especially the wheelchair, should be inspected in advance to make certain that it is in good condition and proper working order.

Risks

Individuals with spinal cord injuries are more subject to a variety of medical complications than are their non-injured colleagues. While these conditions are not necessarily aggravated by participation in sports and athletic events, participants and their medical advisors should be aware of such possible complications when they participate in an activity or event. Some common complications of spinal cord injury include temperature regulation disorders, pressure sores from **sitting** too long in a wheelchair, and urinary tract complications that often develop as a by-product of spinal cord injury.

In addition to these basic health issues, men and women who participated in adapted sports are also subject to injuries related to the sport in which they are engaged. Research suggests that the most common injuries are relatively mild, and seldom life-threatening. They include abrasions, **blisters**, cuts, lacerations, and soft-tissue damage. Other common injuries include:

- sprains, fractures, and contusions of the shoulder, elbow, and wrist
- blistering of the hands and fingers and finger injuries resulting from entrapment in the wheel of the chair
- muscular spasms resulting from overuse of trunk muscles in an effort to maintain posture
- pressure sores and ulcers on the buttocks from extended periods of sitting

Results

As with injuries that result from non-adapted games and sports, injuries like these can be avoided or reduced by proper training and conditioning procedures. For example, the athlete should perform **stretching** and **warm-up** exercises before beginning participation in an event and should be provided with some relief from

---

QUESTIONS TO ASK YOUR DOCTOR

- Can you recommend a sport in which my disabled child could easily participate?
- What special training and conditioning program would you recommend for my child for this sport?
- Are there serious risks associated with this sport about which I should become familiar?
- Can you recommend a professional organization or association that can provide additional information about the adapted form of this sport?

---

sitting whenever possible during an event. The participant should advise a colleague or medical advisor if a medical problem appears to be developing, so that it can be avoided if possible. Equipment should be provided to reduce injuries resulting from long periods of sitting in a chair, such as extra padding around the torso or on the seat. Padded wheel rims and the use of gloves can help reduce the risk of damage to fingers and hands during operation of a wheelchair.

Resources

BOOKS

Goosey-Tolfrey, Vicky. *Wheelchair Sport: A Complete Guide for Athletes, Coaches, and Teachers.* Champaign, IL: Human Kinetics, 2010.

Hayes, Sid, and Gary Stidder. *Equity and Inclusion in Physical Education and Sport: Contemporary Issues for Teachers, Trainees, and Practitioners Title.* New York: Routledge, 2003.

Rouse, Pattie. *Inclusion in Physical Education: Fitness, Motor, and Social Skills for Students of All Abilities Title.* Champaign, IL: Human Kinetics, 2009.

Winnick, Joseph P. *Adapted Physical Education and Sport,* fifth ed. Champaign, IL: Human Kinetics, 2011.

WEBSITES

AAASP, Inc. *AAASP Parents and Coaches Speak Out.* American Association of Adapted Sports Programs. March 25, 2011. http://www.adaptedsports.org/ (accessed September 29, 2011).

Malanga, Gerard A. *Athletes with Disabilities* Medscape Reference. April 9, 2008. http://emedicine.medscape.com/article/88304-overview#a1 (accessed September 29, 2011).

ORGANIZATIONS

International Paralympic Committee, Adenauerallee 212-214, 53113 Bonn, Germany, 49 228-2097-200, Fax: 49 228-2097-209, info@paralympic.org, http://www.paralympic.org.

Wheelchair & Ambulatory Sports USA, P.O. Box 5266, Kendall Park, NJ, 08824-5266, (732) 266-2634, Fax: (732) 355-6500, http://www.wsusa.org.

David E. Newton, AB, MA, EdD

Patellofemoral syndrome

Definition

Patellofemoral syndrome (PFS), sometimes referred to as patellofemoral pain syndrome and chondromalacia patella, is a disorder characterized by thinning, softening, and breaking down of the cartilage located on the back side of the patella (kneecap) and/or on the medial (inner) or lateral (side) femoral condyles; pain and inflammation from synovial fluid that lubricates the lining of the knee joint and its tendons; and general deterioration in the distal femur or patella. PFS is a condition involving damage to the cartilage under and around one or both kneecaps that becomes worse when active or when getting up after being sedentary for a long time. It is frequently the result of sports injuries.

Description

Patellofemoral is a term that incorporates the words patella, the medical name for the kneecap,

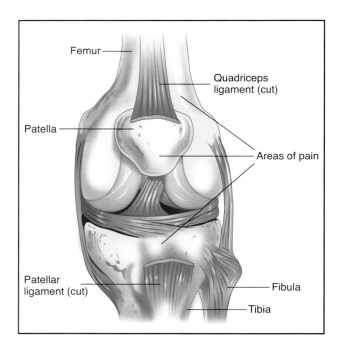

(Electronic Illustrators Group. © 2012 Cengage Learning.)

and femoral that refers to the thigh and, specifically, the femur (the main bone in the thigh). The patellofemoral joint is one of the joints of the knee. It is formed by the kneecap and the femur.

The main knee joint connects the thigh bone and the shin bone (tibia). The knee joint is surrounded by a capsule containing ligaments that loop around the inside and outside of the joint (collateral ligaments), along with cruciate ligaments that cross within the joint. These ligaments provide the knee joint with stability and strength.

The kneecap is positioned over the front of the knee joint. Tendons—specifically, the patellar tendon that attaches the kneecap to the shin and the quadriceps tendon that attaches the thigh muscles to the top of the kneecap—attach the kneecap to the bones and muscles that surround the knee. As the knee moves, the underside of the kneecap slides over the knee bones. PFS can occur then the kneecap loses this normal motion as it begins to grind against the lower part of the thigh bone.

Demographics

PFS is frequently diagnosed in people participating in sports that have high impact to the knees, such as **basketball**, **handball**, **racquetball**, and **volleyball**—specifically, sports that involve a lot of **running**, jumping, sudden stopping, and twisting. These activities place abnormally high stress onto the knees. A change of physical activity, such as its intensity or the sport itself, may also contribute to increased risk of PFS. PFS is most often found in adolescent and young adult athletes, and is more likely to occur in females than in males. The Mayo Clinic states that PFS is twice as likely to occur in women than it is in men—possibly because the wider pelvis in the female frame increases the angle in which the bones of the knee joint meet.

Causes and symptoms

Causes

The exact cause of PFS is not known. However, the medical community does know that abnormal forces on the knee joint, and/or prolonged repetitive stress on the knee joint (specifically, compressive or shearing stresses [forces]) can likely lead to the syndrome.

Abnormal forces can include excessive pulling of the lateral retinaculum (fibrous tissue on the outer side of the kneecap) with acute or chronic lateral patellofemoral subluxation (partial dislocation of the kneecap when it does not glide properly along a groove). Prolonged repetitive shearing or compressive forces of

KEY TERMS

Arthroscope—A type of endoscope (an instrument used to look inside a hollow cavity or organ of the body) inserted into a joint through a small incision on the surface of the body.

Articular cartilage—Cartilage that covers joint surfaces.

Cartilage—Strong, flexible tissue found throughout the body, such as in the nose, throat, ear, and knee.

Chondromalacia—Abnormal softening or degeneration of cartilage.

Condyle—A rounded end of a bone that forms a moving joint with a cup shaped cavity in another bone.

Distal—Referring to being away from a point of attachment.

Subchondral—Located beneath cartilage.

the joint are often the result of physical activities that include running, jumping, quickly stopping, and twisting.

PFS is often a frequent result of pain in the back of the knee (anterior knee pain). Causes of PFS include:

- incorrect alignment of the patellofemoral joint
- tightness and/or weakness of the front and/or back muscles of the thigh
- excessive stress on the kneecap
- arthritis of the kneecap
- previous dislocation, fracture, or other injury to the kneecap
- flat feet

Once one or more of these causes occur, the following can also result:

- internal knee derangement/misalignment
- difficulties performing routine physical activities such as climbing stairs and squatting
- further fractures, dislocations, and other injuries
- osteoarthritis of the knee
- bony tumors in or around the knee

Symptoms

Symptoms of PFS include a grating or grinding feeling when the knees are bent, along with a dull, aching pain in the front of the knee and tenderness around the knee. Swelling of the knee usually does not occur. The most common symptom is knee pain that increases when **walking** up or down stairs. Localized pain in the front of the knee often occurs when:

- squatting or kneeling
- the ankle is moved toward the back of the thigh
- standing after sitting long periods with bent knees
- the knee is straightened out

If such symptoms do not improve or go away after a few days of experiencing them, then a visit to the doctor is recommended. Upon an examination by a family doctor or other such general practitioner, a physical therapist, sports medicine specialist, or orthopedic surgeon may be recommended.

Diagnosis

A physical examination of the knee is performed by a physician. X rays, computerized tomography (CT) scans, or magnetic resonance imaging (MRI) scans may be taken of the knee. X-ray scanning effectively shows the bones, and to a lesser degree the tissues around the knee. CT scans involve X rays taken in many different angles to create a three-dimensional image of the knee"s structure. Such a technique is a much better way (when compared to x-ray scans) to visualize both bones and soft tissues. MRI scans use radio waves (a form of electromagnetic radiation) and a strong magnetic field to produce exact images of the bones and tissues of the knee.

During the exam, the doctor examines different parts of the knee and moves the leg into various positions to analyze the extent of the pain and other symptoms. Besides eliminating other problems, the examination, along with the various scans taken, help the physician understand how to better treat the injury if all the signs point to PFS.

Treatment

Initially, the knee should be rested until the pain disappears. Pain relievers, such as acetaminophen (Tylenol), and nonsteroidal anti-inflammatory drugs (NSAIDs), such as aspirin (acetylsalicylic acid) or ibuprofen (Advil, Motrin), should also be taken to reduce pain immediately after exercising. Apply ice for 10 to 20 minutes to reduce inflammation. The RICE treatment (Rest, Ice, Compression, and Elevation) reduces the pain and discomfort and helps to shorten the recovery process.

For those with worsening pain from **sitting** too long, periodically straighten the leg. Individuals who are overweight or extremely overweight (obese) should begin a **weight loss** program that will help to place less stress onto the knees.

Physical therapy may be recommended, including rehabilitation exercises. These exercises stretch and strengthen the muscles of the knees and help them to properly re-align themselves. Other exercises help areas positioned away from the knee but still important for knee health. Some of the recommended exercises include those for the quadriceps (especially the front quadriceps), back (hamstrings), calf, and hips (especially the hip abductor muscles, and the iliotibial band, near the hip joint). Strengthening the hip abductor muscle has been medically shown to decrease both pain and joint problems within the knee. In addition, strengthening the quadriceps helps to stabilize the kneecap. Overall, strong muscles help to correct problems with the knee. Proper flexibility of the muscles is also important to reduce the risk of getting PFS.

Exercise is important to strengthen muscles around the knee. Until symptoms disappear or reduce, stop performing high-impact exercises and physical activities such as running. Non-impact or low-impact exercises (sometimes called "knee-friendly" activities) such as aerobics, bicycling, **swimming**, and walking should be substituted. The use of elliptical trainers or similar machines are excellent ways to get a workout without introducing high forces onto the knees.

If running is continued, it is better to run on a smooth, soft surface (such as a running track) than on a hard surface (such as concrete or asphalt). It is also better to walk down slopes rather than running up them. Once the pain has subsided, slowly return to normal activities by increasing the amount of time by no more than about 20% per week.

Supportive braces, arch supports, custom **orthotics**, tape, and other external measures can be worn to help protect and stabilize the knee joint and improve the alignment of the kneecap. In addition, such external measures may help to prevent future injury. A physical therapist can provide proper instruction on how to use such devices. Shoe inserts help to provide extra support to cushion impacts onto the knees. This is especially true for people with flat feet. When exercising, especially for running and other high impact activities, make sure the athletic shoes are made of quality materials, fit comfortably, and have sufficient cushion. Discuss shoes and

---

QUESTIONS TO ASK YOUR DOCTOR

- What specific exercises should I do to strength my knees?
- What activities should I avoid when pain occurs?
- What medicines will best help me?
- Will I need surgery for my knee problems?
- Will my health insurance pay for surgery or rehabilitation?

---

shoe inserts with a doctor because proper footwear can reduce the impact on the knees.

Prognosis

PFS is difficult to treat and is usually not resolved in the short term. It may take six weeks or longer for the knee to improve to any noticeable degree. However, it usually improves with treatment in the long term. In a small percentage of cases—when symptoms and pain are not reduced or eliminated—surgery may be necessary.

Two types of surgery for the knee are arthroscopy and open surgery. Arthroscopic surgery involves the insertion of an arthroscope, a thin device with a camera and light that goes into the knee through a tiny incision in the skin. The surgery involves various procedures, such as removing fragments of damaged cartilage, that improve the condition of the knee. Open surgery may be performed in more serious cases, such as when the knee must be realigned. When performed, surgery usually resolves the problem. However, in a small number of surgical cases, infection may occur, along continuation of the pain, or even a worsening of the symptoms.

Prevention

The knee is less likely to be injured with PFS if the entire body is in good shape and muscles remain strong. Attention to strong muscles, in order to keep the knee properly balanced and aligned during exercise, resides primarily with the hip abductor muscles and quadriceps. Asking a family doctor of physical therapist for a list of recommended exercises that can build flexibility and strength into the muscles, especially those that are used for running, jumping, moving from side to side, squatting, and stepping down will help minimize the potential for injuries. Regular exercise is a good preventive measure to avoid hurting the knee.

Always **warm-up** with light exercises (walking, **stretching**, etc.) for at least five minutes before doing any type of exercises or activities. Stretching is important to add flexibility to the muscles before exerting them. Caution should be used when performing high-impact sports. Overexertion in such sports or making, drastic changes in the intensity of workouts should be avoided. Instead, if changes occur, do them gradually over a long period. Make sure proper footwear is used, and that shoes fit well and provide adequate shock absorption.

Resources

BOOKS

Feagin, Jr., John A., J. Richard Steadman, and Karen Briggs, editors. *The Crucial Principles in Care of the Knee.* Philadelphia: Wolters Kluwer/Lippincott Williams & Wilkins, 2008.

Katch, Victor L., William D. McArdle, Frank I. Katch. *Essentials of Exercise Physiology.* Philadelphia: Wolters Kluwer/Lippincott Williams & Wilkins Health, 2011.

LaPrade, Robert F. *Posterolateral Knee Injuries: Anatomy, Evaluation, and Treatment.* New York: Thieme, 2006.

Noyes, Frank R, and Sue D. Barber-Westin, editors. *Noyes' Knee Disorders: Surgery, Rehabilitation, Clinical Outcomes.* Philadelphia: Saunders/Elsevier, 2010.

WEBSITES

Chondromalacia Patella. Mayo Clinic. (August 7, 2010). http://www.mayoclinic.com/health/chondromalacia-patella/DS00777 (accessed November 13, 2011).

"Patellofemoral Pain Syndrome." *American Family Physician* (November 1, 1999). http://www.aafp.org/afp/991101ap/991101b.html (accessed November 13, 2011).

Shiel Jr., William C. *Chondromalacia Patella (Patellofemoral Syndrome).* MedicineNet.com. (June 13, 2010). http://www.medicinenet.com/patellofemoral_syndrome/article.htm (accessed November 13, 2011).

Vorvick, Linda J., and C. Benjamin Ma. *Chondromalacia Patella.* MedlinePlus. (June 13, 2010). http://www.nlm.nih.gov/medlineplus/ency/article/000452.htm (accessed November 12, 2011).

ORGANIZATIONS

American Association of Orthopaedic Surgeons, 6300 N. River Rd., Rosemont, IL, 60018-4262, (847) 823-7186, Fax: (847) 823-8125, http://www.aaos.org.

American Pain Society, 4700 West Lake Avenue, Glenview, IL, 60025, (847) 375-4715, Fax: (847) 375-6479, info@ampainsoc.org, http://www.ampainsoc.org.

William A. Atkins, BB, BS, MBA

Pedometer

Definition

A pedometer is an electronic device that senses movement to count and display the number of steps taken or the distance traveled.

Description

A pedometer is a small device usually worn attached to the belt or pants. It counts each time an individual takes a step and displays the total number of steps taken. Pedometers have become increasingly complex in recent years, with pedometers now available that analyze data, upload to computers, or can integrate with applications on smartphones.

Pedometers work by recording movements. Most pedometers work by recording the movement of the hips. Each time a step is taken, the hips move slightly. This shifts the mechanism inside the pedometer, which records the step. Pedometers on the belt should be worn vertically for highest accuracy. Some, usually higher end, pedometers attach to the shoe instead of the belt. These pedometers work by sensing the vibration that is created with the foot hits the ground. Pedometers cannot tell what is causing the movement they sense. This means that if an individual shakes a pedometer back and forth the pedometer will count it as steps taken. Pedometers do not work accurately if placed in backpacks, purses, or pockets.

Types of pedometers

There are many different types of pedometers. Most pedometers cost between US$10 and US$30 dollars, but they can cost upwards of US$100 for very accurate high-tech versions. Pedometers vary greatly in the type of options included and in accuracy. Some pedometers have been shown to misestimate the number of steps taken by as much as 50%. After purchasing a pedometer, it may be helpful to count a specified number of steps (e.g., 100) while taking them, and then check the pedometer readout for accuracy. No pedometer is completely accurate, but some come quite close.

Some pedometers simply count steps. Others provide information about **calories**, distance, or speed. Some reset automatically each day or week, others must be reset by hand. Pedometers with a reset button that is covered by a closed case are generally considered preferable, as those with an exposed reset button may be reset accidently if the pedometer is bumped.

Many newer models of pedometers can integrate with a computer or smartphone to store performance data and provide graphs and other performance feedback. These types of pedometers are usually more expensive than similar pedometers that do not provide this type of integration. Although such data analysis can be fun and helpful, a lower cost traditional pedometer is usually just as effective.

The type of pedometer that is right for a given individual depends on a variety of factors including budget, interest in technology, what kind of functions are desired, and fitness activities. Some types of pedometers are better calibrated for **walking**, and others for **running** or jogging. Reading reviews of pedometers can help determine the pedometer that is the right fit with an individual's goals and lifestyle.

Using a pedometer to improve health

How many steps each day are right for an individual depend on a number of factors, including **age**, health, and fitness level. However for most individuals in good health 10,000 steps a day (about 5 miles or 8 kilometers) is recommended.

When beginning to use a pedometer to lose weight or improve health, the first few days should be used to get a baseline reading. The pedometer should be used all day while doing usual daily activities. This will allow the individual to determine how many steps he or she is taking in an average day. After determining this number, weekly or monthly goals can be determined. It is a good idea to increase the number of steps being taken in small increments each week. For example, an individual who starts out taking 2,500 steps a day may decide to try to add 150 more steps each week.

Below are some easy ways to increase the number of steps taken each day:

- take the stairs instead of the elevator
- park farther away from the door to the grocery or other store
- walk over to see a friend
- walk to the store or the mailbox instead of driving
- take a nature walk with the kids
- find a friend to walk with
- walk around the block while talking on the phone
- get up and walk around the office
- get out of the office and take a walk at lunch

Purpose

The purpose of a pedometer is to provide information about how many steps and individual has taken. Pedometers that track distance walked or

---

---

calories burned can also be used to monitor this information. Many individuals who begin using a pedometer do so because they are curious about how many steps they are walking each day, or want to begin walking more steps each day.

Studies have shown that receiving feedback about performance helps lead to improved performance compared to receiving no feedback. Pedometers provide this feedback, and can be effective at encouraging increased daily activity. Pedometers that come with programs that allow for tracking performance over moths or weeks may be especially effective, although individuals can also track their own progress on a chart or graph each day.

Risks

There are no risks specific to wearing a pedometer. However, before starting a new **exercise** regimen it is important to consult a doctor. Beginning an exercise routine after a sedentary lifestyle can increase the risk of heart attack or stroke.

Most individuals who use pedometers use them to count the number of steps taken while walking, jogging, or running. There are risks associated with each of these activities. Running and jogging puts stress on the joints, especially the hip, knee, and ankle. These activities can also lead to strains, sprains, and **muscle pain**. Individuals who have balance problems or are pregnant are at an increased risk of falls and should be especially careful. To reduce the risk of sprains and falls walking, running, and jogging should be done on level ground in well-lit areas, such as on treadmills or tracks instead of on uneven pavement or trails.

Benefits

There are a wide variety of health benefits to being more active. Regular walking can increase overall fitness level, increasing muscle mass, stamina, agility, and flexibility. It can also improve balance, and reduce back pain and soreness. Walking is a good low impact fitness activity that can be enjoyed by people of all ages and fitness levels.

Increased daily activity can help an individual lose weight or maintain a healthy body weight. Maintaining a healthy body weight helps reduce the risk of **cardiovascular disease**, type 2 **diabetes**, and has been found to reduce the risk of some types of cancers. Regular physical activity such as walking can also help reduce **cholesterol**, and strengthen the heart. Lung function has also been shown to improve. Some studies have shown that exercising regularly into the senior years can even help to reduce the risk of dementia including **Alzheimer's disease**.

Preparation

There is no special preparation required to use a pedometer. Before using a new pedometer for the first time, the individual should read and follow any manufacturer's instructions for set up. Some pedometers have a set-up function that has the individual walk a specified number of steps. The pedometer then uses this to calculate a stride length to help with distance and other calculations.

Aftercare

There is no aftercare required for using a pedometer. After a brisk walk or run, the individual should stretch all of the major muscle groups to help prevent soreness.

Resources

BOOKS

Nottingham, Suzanne, and Jurasin, Alexandra. *Nordic Walking for Total Fitness*. Champaign, IL: Human Kinetics, 2010.

Tuminelly, Nancy. *Super Simple Walk and Run: Healthy and Fun Activities to Move Your Body*. Edina, MN: ABDO Publishing Company, 2012.

Williamson, Peggie. *Exercise for Special Populations*. Philadelphia: Wolters Kluwer Health/ Lippincott Williams and Wilkins, 2011.

PERIODICALS

Hartvigsen, Jan, et al. "Supervised and Non-Supervised Nordic Walking in the Treatment of Chronic Low Back Pain: A Single Blind Randomized Clinical Trial." *BMC Musculoskeletal Disorders* (2010) 1:30.

Wilson, Lee-Ann M. et al. "The Association Between Objectively Measured Neighborhood Features and Walking in Middle-Aged Adults." *American Journal of Health Promotion*. (March-April 2011) 25(4):E12–21.

WEBSITES

The Mayo Clinic. "Walking for Fitness? Make it Count with a Pedometer." http://www.mayoclinic.com/health/walking/SM00056_D/NSECTIONGROUP=2 (accessed July 28, 2011).

WebMD "Walking Faster May Lead to a Longer Life." http://www.webmd.com/healthy-aging/news/20110104/walking-faster-may-lead-to-a-longer-life (accessed July 28, 2011).

ORGANIZATIONS

Aerobics and Fitness Association of America, 15250 Ventura Boulevard, #200, Sherman Oaks, CA, 91403, (877) 968-7263, http://www.afaa.com.

American Council on Exercise, 4851 Paramount Drive, San Diego, CA, 92123, (888) 825-3636, http://www.acefitness.org.

American Nordic Walking Association, PO Box 491205, Los Angeles, CA, 90049, (323) 244-2519, Fax: (310) 459-8149, info@anwa.us, http://www.anwa.us.

International Nordic Walking Federation, Jollaksentie 27 A, Helsinki, Finland, FIN-00850, office@inwa-nordicwalking.com, http://www.inwa-nordicwalking.com.

Tish Davidson, AM

Performance-enhancing drugs

Definition

Performance-enhancing drugs include prescription and over-the-counter (OTC) medications, illegal "street drugs," and nutritional supplements that are believed to improve athletic performance. However the term "performance-enhancing drugs" most often refers to anabolic-androgenic steroids (AAS), a large family of compounds also called simply **anabolic steroids** or steroids. Nevertheless, various other compounds—including certain other hormones, stimulants, diuretics, and creatine—are considered to be performance-enhancing drugs.

Purpose

AAS are the most widely used—and abused—performance-enhancing drugs. AAS are growth inducers that were first developed in Europe in the 1930s to treat malnourishment and promote healing

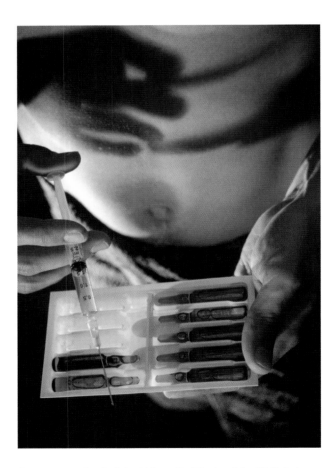

A man preparing to inject himself with steroids. (© Bob Jones Photography/Alamy)

following surgery. Their most common legitimate use today is for hormone-replacement therapy. Competitive weightlifters began using AAS in the 1950s and the drugs gradually spread to other sports, until their use became pervasive. At the high dosages used for performance enhancement, the anabolic effects of AAS rapidly build muscle, increasing both size and strength. They may also increase **energy** and reduce muscle damage or hasten repair, allowing athletes to train harder and more frequently, with faster recovery after workouts. The androgenic effects of AAS promote male sexual characteristics in both males and females. Some athletes report aggressive "rushes" from AAS that also may enhance performance.

Like AAS, human growth hormone (hGH), or somatropin, is an anabolic hormone. It may increase muscle mass and improve performance and endurance, although this has not been demonstrated conclusively.

Erythropoietin (EPO) is a hormone that increases red blood cell production and is used to treat anemia. Athletes have used EPO in attempts to increase the oxygen-carrying capacity of the blood to improve strength and endurance.

Beta-2 agonists, which are related to the hormone **epinephrine** (adrenaline), are bronchodilators that are widely used to treat conditions such as **asthma**. They may have performance-enhancing effects when consistently present at high levels in the blood.

Stimulants activate the central nervous system and increase heart rate and **blood pressure**. They can reduce **fatigue** and appetite and increase endurance, alertness, and aggressiveness.

Diuretics increase water loss and can decrease body weight, enabling some athletes to compete in lighter-weight classes that may give them a competitive advantage. Diuretics sometimes function as "masking" agents, diluting the urine so that prohibited performance-enhancing drugs cannot be detected.

Creatine is the most popular of the many nutritional supplements that are promoted as performance enhancers. Creatine phosphate is an important energy storage system in muscle and it is the first energy source utilized for activities such as sprinting and **weightlifting**. Creatine may also promote muscle growth and strength. Although creatine supplements may have small performance-enhancing effects for short bursts of muscle activity, there is no evidence that they enhance aerobic capacity or endurance.

Description

AAS

Anabolic-androgenic steroids include the male sex hormone testosterone and a large number of synthetic testosterone derivatives. AAS help metabolize proteins, increase the rate of skeletal muscle synthesis, and provide a "rush" that masks fatigue. AAS are taken orally as tablets or capsules, through the skin as ointments or transdermal patches, or injected into muscles. They are sometimes combined with creatine, **protein** powders, and/or various **antioxidants**.

More than 1,000 different AAS have been synthesized since the 1950s and there are many thousands of international brand names. Although AAS are illegal in the United States and prohibited by most athletic competitions, in some countries they are available over the counter. They are also widely available as veterinary and street drugs under a variety of names, as well as through physician prescriptions. The products of steroid **metabolism** can be detected in the urine for six months or longer after use and athletes are routinely screened for AAS. However the technology for detecting steroids in blood or urine—and distinguishing AAS use from the products of normal metabolism or legitimate medications—is often one step behind new "designer" steroid drugs.

Common AAS include:

- testosterone derivatives—methandrostenolone, fluoxymesterone, and methyltestosterone (rare)
- testosterone esters—testosterone propionate, cypionate, and enanthate
- dihydrotestosterone (DHT) derivatives—oxandrolone, stanozolol, and oxymetholone
- nandrolone derivatives—ethylestrenol, trenbolone, and nandrolone decanoate, one of the most widely abused injected AAS

Steroid precursors, such as dehydroepiandrosterone (DHEA) and androstenedione ("andro"), are marketed as performance-enhancing nutritional supplements. DHEA is converted to androstenedione in the adrenal glands, testes, and ovaries. Androstenedione is converted to the sex hormones testosterone and estradiol in both men and women. Scientific evidence indicates that these precursors are unlikely to be effective AAS, although their use as performance enhancers is illegal in the United States.

Other performance enhancers

The presence of abnormal concentrations of hormones—such as hGH, EPO, insulin, human chorionic gonadotropin (hCG), or adrenocorticotropin (ACTH), or their metabolites or markers—in blood or urine samples, or platelet-rich plasma (PRP) indicating treatment with platelets, are considered evidence of prohibited performance-enhancing drug use. Exceptions are made for demonstrated physiological or medical conditions.

Stimulants include caffeine, amphetamines, methamphetamine, and cocaine. Some prohibited stimulants, such as ephedrine and pseudoephedrine, are common in OTC nasal sprays, diet aids, and headache, cold, and flu remedies. Many medications that are commonly prescribed for asthma and other respiratory symptoms are also strong stimulants and some have anabolic properties.

Creatine supplements are commonly sold as powders, although other preparations are available. The liver produces about 0.07 oz (2 g) of creatine daily and it also is obtained from meat in the diet. Since muscles usually have adequate stores of creatine and any excess is removed by the kidneys, the value of creatine supplements for performance enhancement is questionable.

Recommended dosage

Since most performance-enhancing drugs are illegal or prohibited, there are no recommended dosages. Athletes may use AAS dosages that are 50–100 times higher than the dosages used for legitimate medical conditions, in which their anabolic effects may be unnoticeable. In one survey of AAS users, more than half reported taking 1,000 mg or more every week. AAS users also may practice stacking—taking two or more AAS in combination, using more than one route of administration, or mixing AAS with other drugs, such as stimulants or painkillers. Other AAS users practice cycling—alternating periods of steroid use with periods of abstinence—or pyramiding—increasing dosages over several weeks followed by decreasing dosages.

The loading dose of creatine monohydrate for adult athletic performance is generally 5 g, taken four times daily for one week. The adult maintenance dose is generally 2–5 g daily.

Precautions

The list of drugs prohibited by the World Anti-Doping Agency (WADA) is updated annually. All anabolic agents, peptide hormones, growth factors and related substances, hormone antagonists and modulators (that affect the activity of endogenous hormones in the body), beta-2 agonists (with certain exceptions), and diuretics and other masking agents are prohibited at all times. Stimulants, narcotics, cannabinoids, and glucocorticosteroids are prohibited in competitions. Certain sports also prohibit alcohol and beta-blockers. In general, a drug is prohibited if it meets two of the following three criteria: has the potential to enhance performance, poses a potential health risk, and violates the spirit of the sport.

Most performance-enhancing drugs pose serious potential health risks. Furthermore, side effects and potential complications from the drugs may lead to a deterioration of athletic performance. Some drugs, such as oxymetholone, a commonly abused AAS throughout the world, are considered carcinogens. People with medical conditions should never take performance-enhancing drugs.

Black market performance-enhancing drugs smuggled in from other countries or manufactured clandestinely are particularly dangerous, because they may be impure or mislabeled. Steroids that are designed to be undetectable by standard drug tests and have with no approved medical uses have never been tested for safety or effectiveness.

Performance-enhancing nutritional supplements are considered food by the U.S. Food and Drug Administration (FDA) and are not regulated to the same extent as drugs. They are sometimes contaminated with synthetic hormones or other harmful substances. Products that are advertised as alternatives to FDA-approved drugs or illegal AAS, or that warn that they may cause positive drug tests, should be viewed with suspicion.

Although creatine is sometimes used by athletes to increase their weight, its prolonged use is more likely to increase muscle water retention than muscle mass. There have also been reports of contaminated creatine supplements.

Interactions

Although interactions involving performance-enhancing drugs and dietary supplements have not been well-studied, AAS may interact with:

- anticoagulants, such as warfarin (Coumadin)
- carbamazepine
- insulin or oral diabetes medications
- corticosteroids
- eucaplyptus
- kava (*Piper methysticum*)

Creatine may have negative interactions with:

- caffeine
- non-steroidal anti-inflammatory drugs (NSAIDs), such as ibuprofen or naproxen
- diuretics

- cimetidine (Tagamet)
- probenecid

Complications

AAS

Although at typical medical dosages, AAS are considered relatively safe, with few side effects, at performance-enhancing dosages, they can cause a range of side effects, some that may be irreversible. Side effects of AAS and steroid precursors in men can include breast enlargement, shrunken testicles, impotence, enlarged prostate gland, and infertility. Women may develop a deeper voice, enlarged clitoris, and increased body hair. Side effects in both men and women can include:

- baldness
- severe acne
- feet and ankle swelling
- skin color changes
- insomnia
- excitability
- changes in sex drive
- diarrhea, nausea, and vomiting
- bladder irritation
- increased low-density lipoprotein (LDL) or "bad" cholesterol and decreased high-density lipoprotein (HDL) or "good" cholesterol
- suppression of normal hormonal pathways or harmful hormone imbalances

Unsafe injection of AAS can transmit HIV/AIDS and hepatitis B and C. One survey found that 13% AAS users acknowledged using such unsafe injection practices, such as sharing or reusing needles or sharing multi-dose vials of steroids.

It may be possible to become physically or psychologically addicted to AAS. Hormone supplementation may be required to restore normal hormonal function when AAS are withdrawn. Depression is the most serious symptom of AAS withdrawal. If untreated, can last for more than a year and lead to suicidal behaviors.

Other complications from performance-enhancing AAS can include:

- high blood pressure
- tendinitis and tendon rupture
- heart and circulatory problems, including early heart attacks and stroke
- kidney failure

Adrenal glands—The two glands located on top of the kidneys that secrete steroid hormones.

Anabolic—Causing muscle and bone growth and a shift from fat to muscle in the body.

Anabolic-androgenic steroids (AAS)—Anabolic steroids; illegal and prohibited testosterone derivatives that are synthesized as performance-enhancing and muscle-building drugs.

Androgenic—Testosterone-like, masculinizing effects.

Androstenedione—Andro; a steroid sex hormone that is secreted by the adrenal glands, testes, and ovaries, as a precursor of testosterone and estrogen, and marketed as a performance-enhancing drug.

Beta-2 agonists—Drug that bind to and activate beta-2 receptors, such as bronchodilators used to treat asthma and other lung diseases; sometimes used as performance-enhancing drugs.

Cholesterol—A steroid alcohol that is a precursor for hormones and other steroids.

Creatine—A nitrogen-containing organic acid that supplies muscles with energy.

Dehydroepiandrosterone (DHEA)—An androgenic steroid secreted by the adrenal cortex and an intermediate in the synthesis of testosterone; sometimes marketed as a performance-enhancing drug.

Diuretic—"Water pill;" a medication or other substance that increases urine excretion.

Erythropoietin (EPO)—A hormone made in the kidneys that stimulates red blood cell formation; a synthetic drug sometimes used as a performance enhancer.

Estradiol—The most physiologically active form of estrogen.

Estrogen—Any of several naturally occurring or synthetic steroid hormones that promote the growth and maintenance of the female reproductive system.

Hormones—Chemical messengers that are carried by the bloodstream to various organs where they affect functioning, often by stimulatory action.

Human growth hormone (hGH)—A growth-promoting human hormone; a recombinant version, often called somatropin, used by athletes to increase muscle mass.

Masking agent—A drug or other substance that renders another drug undetectable in the urine.

Over-the-counter (OTC)—A drug that can be purchased without a doctor's prescription.

Platelet—A clotting factor in the blood.

Steroids—A class of hormones and drugs that includes sex and stress hormones and growth-promoting substances.

Stimulant—A drug or other substance that produces a temporary increase in activity or efficiency.

Testosterone—The primary male sex hormone.

Tolerance—The requirement for higher doses of a substance to continue achieving the same effect.

Withdrawal—Unpleasant physiological and/or psychological changes that occur due to the discontinuation of a drug after prolonged regular use.

- severe liver problems, including jaundice, tumors, and cancer
- severe psychiatric disturbances, including depression
- aggressive behaviors, rage, or violence
- birth defects if used before or during pregnancy
- early puberty and premature cessation of bone growth in young people

Other performance enhancers

Side effects of hGH may include:

- joint pain
- muscle weakness
- fluid retention
- poor glucose regulation
- high fat levels in the blood
- carpal tunnel syndrome
- heart disease

EPO can increase the risk of heart attack, stroke, pulmonary edema, kidney disease, and cancer progression or recurrence. Its use by competitive cyclists during the 1990s is believed to have contributed to at least 18 deaths.

Possible side effects of beta-2 agonists include:

- nervousness
- rapid or irregular heart beat
- headaches

- sweating
- muscle cramps
- nausea

Side effects of stimulants can include:

- weight loss
- nervousness and irritability
- tremors
- insomnia
- mild high blood pressure
- dehydration
- heatstroke
- irregular or abnormal heartbeat
- tolerance, requiring higher dosages
- psychological addiction
- hallucinations
- convulsions
- stroke
- circulatory problems or heart attack

Diuretics at any dose affect the balance of fluids and salts in the body and cause **dehydration**. Use of diuretics by athletes increases the risk for:

- potassium deficiency
- muscle cramps
- dizziness
- exhaustion
- irregular heart beat
- drop in blood pressure
- heatstroke

Although creatine is generally considered safe for adults at recommended dosages, high doses have the potential to cause kidney or liver damage. Side effects may include weight gain, dehydration, muscle cramps

and strains, stomach pain, dizziness, nausea, diarrhea, and high blood pressure. Supplements may prevent the body from making its own natural stores of creatine.

Resources

BOOKS

Bjornlund, Lydia D. *How Dangerous Are Performance-Enhancing Drugs?* San Diego, CA: ReferencePoint, 2011.

May, Suellen, and D.J. Triggle. *Steroids and Other Performance-Enhancing Drugs.* New York: Chelsea House, 2011

Piehl, Norah, editor. *Performance-Enhancing Drugs.* Farmington Hills, MI: Greenhaven/Gale Cengage Learning, 2010.

Robinson, Tom, and Mikhail G. Epshteyn. *Performance-Enhancing Drugs.* Edina, MN: ABDO, 2009

Simon, Robert L. *Fair Play: The Ethics of Sport.* 3rd ed. Boulder, CO: Westview, 2010.

Sommers, Annie Leah. *College Athletes: Steroids and Supplement Abuse.* New York: Rosen, 2010.

Teitelbaum, Stanley H. *Athletes Who Indulge Their Dark Side: Sex, Drugs, and Cover-Ups.* Santa Barbara, CA: Praeger, 2010.

Thompson, Teri. *American Icon: The Fall of Roger Clemens and the Rise of Steroids in America's Pastime.* New York: Alfred A. Knopf, 2009.

Tilin, Andrew. *The Doper Next Door: My Strange and Scandalous Year on Performance-Enhancing Drugs.* Berkeley, CA: Counterpoint, 2011.

PERIODICALS

Gleaves, John. "No Harm, No Foul? Justifying Bans on Safe Performance-Enhancing Drugs." *Sports, Ethics and Philosophy* 4, no. 3 (December 2010): 269–83.

Handelsman, D.J. "Commentary: Androgens and "Anabolic Steroids": The One-Headed Janus." *Endocrinology* 152, no. 5 (May 2011): 1752–54.

Petersen, Thomas Søbirk. "Good Athlete—Bad Athlete? On the 'Role-Model Argument' for Banning Performance-Enhancing Drugs." *Sports, Ethics and Philosophy* 4, no. 3 (December 2010): 332–40.

Schmidt, Michael S. "Selig Says Steroid Era is Basically Over." *New York Times* (January 12, 2010): B14.

Wiesing, Urban. "Should Performance-Enhancing Drugs in Sport be Legalized Under Medical Supervision?" *Sports Medicine* 41, no. 2 (February 2011): 167–76.

WEBSITES

"Anabolic Steroid Abuse." National Institute on Drug Abuse. http://www.steroidabuse.org (accessed August 13, 2011).

"Anabolic Steroids." MedlinePlus. January 13, 2011. http://www.nlm.nih.gov/medlineplus/anabolicsteroids.html (accessed August 13, 2011).

"Athlete Handbook." U.S. Anti-Doping Agency. January 1, 2010. http://www.usada.org/files/active/athletes/AthleteHandbookFinal.pdf (accessed August 13, 2011).

Doheny, Kathleen. "FDA Targets Tainted Dietary Supplements." WebMD Health News. December 17, 2010. http://www.medscape.com/viewarticle/734487 (accessed August 13, 2011).

Kishner, Stephen. "Anabolic Steroid Use and Abuse." Medscape Reference. July 6, 2011. http://emedicine.medscape.com/article/128655-overview (accessed August 13, 2011).

Mayo Clinic Staff. "Performance-Enhancing Drugs: Know the Risks." Mayo Clinic Health Information. December 23, 2010. http://www.mayoclinic.com/health/performance-enhancing-drugs/HQ01105 (accessed August 13, 2011).

Mayo Clinic Staff. "Performance-Enhancing Drugs and Teen Athletes." Mayo Clinic Health Information. December 22, 2010. http://www.mayoclinic.com/health/performance-enhancing-drugs/SM00045 (accessed August 13, 2011).

"Mind Over Matter: Anabolic Steroids." NIDA for Teens. http://teens.drugabuse.gov/mom/mom_ster1.php (accessed August 13, 2011).

"NIDA InfoFacts: Steroids (Anabolic-Androgenic)." National Institute on Drug Abuse. July 2009. http://www.drugabuse.gov/infofacts/steroids.html (accessed August 13, 2011).

Werner, T.C., and Caroline K. Hatton. "Performance-Enhancing Drugs in Sports: How Chemists Catch Users." *Journal of Chemical Education* 88, no. 1 (January 1, 2011): 33–40. http://pubs.acs.org/doi/full/10.1021/ed100525f (accessed September 2, 2011).

ORGANIZATIONS

American College of Sports Medicine, P.O. Box 1440, Indianapolis, IN, 46206-1440, (317) 637-9200, Fax: (317) 634-7817, http://www.acsm.org.

National Institute on Drug Abuse, 6001 Executive Boulevard, Room 5213, Bethesda, MD, 20892-9561, (301) 443-1124, information@nida.nih.gov, http://www.drugabuse.gov.

United States Anti-Doping Agency, 5555 Tech Center Drive, Suite 200, Colorado Springs, CO, 80919-2372, (719) 785-2000, Fax: (719) 785-2001, (866) 601-2632, drugreference@usada.org, http://www.usada.org.

U.S. Food and Drug Administration, 10903 New Hampshire Avenue, Silver Spring, MD, 20993-0002, (888) INFO-FDA (463-6332), http://www.fda.gov.

Margaret Alic, PhD

Periodization

Definition

In general, the term periodization refers to the process of dividing an activity into blocks of time that repeat at regular intervals. In sports, athletics, and **exercise**, the term refers to a method of training in which a variety of training exercises are organized into a regular program that a person follows over extended periods of time, usually a year.

Purpose

Periodization training is used for a variety of reasons including to increase a person's muscle mass, to improve one's speed, to improve strength, and to build endurance strength. The program is devised to avoid **overtraining**.

Demographics

Proponents of periodization training claim that the program has beneficial effects on individuals of virtually any **age** or level of fitness, from "stay-at-home" moms to professional athletes. There appear to be no scientific data on the number of individuals who participate in periodization training programs. The program has, however, been adopted by and adapted to virtually every form of sporting activity from **bodybuilding** to **bicycling** to **rugby** to **fencing**.

Description

Periodization training usually consists of three distinct phases, known as the macrocycle, mesocycle, and microcycle. The term macrocycle (macro = "large") refers to a general plan designed to cover a single calendar year, about 12 months. It consists of three phases: preparation or pre-season, competition or in-season, and recovery or off-season (although alternative names are also used to describe these periods). The emphasis in the preparation period (typically lasting for eight to nine months of the year) is on improving one's general overall physical fitness. The schedule tends to emphasize a high volume of low intensity exercises. These exercises focus on both general physical skills and on sports-specific skills. Towards the end of the preparation period, the emphasis changes somewhat and greater stress is placed on a reduced volume of high intensity exercises.

The second phase of the macrocycle includes the actual time of competition, when one has supposedly reached his or her maximum level of general physical strength and specific sports skills. In most sports, this period of the macrocycle lasts for a relatively short period of time, normally only a few months out of the year, although that pattern differs significantly for various sports. The third phase of the macrocycle is the rest and restorative period, during which time the body is allowed to recuperate from the training and competition that has gone on for the greater part of the year. At the end of this period, the macrocycle begins once again with a new period of preparation.

Each macrocycle in a periodization training program is sub-divided into some number of mesocycles (meso = "mid-range") that, in turn, are further divided into a number of microcycles (micro = "very small"). Each microcycle typically lasts about a week in length, and each mesocycle consists of a small number (usually four to six) microcycles. Each microcycle is designed specifically to achieve some limited objective that fits into the overall scheme of the macrocycle program, promoting improvement in both general physical skills and skills associated with some specific sport. As an example, the schedule for the first microcycle in a mesocycle might consist of a variety of strength exercises, such as bicep curls, tricep push-downs, hamstring curls, dumbbell flat presses, and barbell squats, repeated a certain number of times at a given level of intensity in a certain pattern of repetitions. By contrast, the second week might employ some or all of the same exercises in a different pattern, with or without the addition of new exercises. The specific pattern of exercises selected for a microcycle is determined by a number of factors, including an individual's current physical condition, his or her short- and long-term goals, and the sport or activity for which one is training.

Origins

Athletes and trainers have been thinking about issues of periodization training for more than a century. As early as the 1910s, some coaches had observed that athletes that trained on the same exercises for extended periods of time actually became less skillful than those who had trained for shorter periods of time and/or in a greater variety of exercises. For a half century, however, these observations remained largely anecdotal in nature, with relatively little scientific research to see how various types of training programs affected skill level. Many (but not all) historians suggest that the modern era of periodization training originated with the studies of Russian **weightlifting** coach Lev Pavlovich Matveev, who first proposed the general outlines of macro-, meso-, and microcycles in his 1965 book, *Fundamentals of Sports Training*. The book contains a graph showing the progress of events in a

periodization macrocycle that has now become famous (although often much-altered) in the sport training world.

The training philosophy espoused by Matveev dominated much of athletic training in the Soviet Union and the Eastern Bloc during the 1950s and 1960s and is generally credited with the dominance of Soviet sports teams and individuals in international competitions such as the Olympic Games. That philosophy was popularized by Hungarian Olympic rower and trainer Tudor Bompa in his 1983 book *Theory and Methodology of Training*, which is still popular and currently in its fifth edition. Because of Bompa's impact on the program, he is often called the Father of Periodization. Bompa is currently emeritus professor at York University in Toronto, Canada.

Types

Many different variations in the basic periodization model have been developed over the past few decades. That model is now sometimes called linear periodization because changes in training volume and intensity occur gradually in a regular sequence over time. Another form of periodization training is called non-linear, or undulating, periodization because changes in training volume and intensity occur more frequently, sometimes on a daily basis with a given microcycle. Yet another form of periodization training is called conjugate training because it incorporates a variety of different skills during a single training session.

The concept of periodization has also been extended to nutritional planning. Nutrition periodization is simply a program for providing athletes with the nutritional elements they need for each phase of a periodization training program. As an example, one expert in the field, Bob Seebohar, has devised a nutritional program for each of the three stages of a periodization macrocycle. In that program, participants should aim for a diet that includes 3–7 grams/kilogram of body weight of **carbohydrates** per day, 1.2–2.5 grams/kilogram of body weight of **protein** per day, and 0.8–1.3 grams/kilogram of body weight of fat per day during the preparatory stage of the macrocycle. He then makes similar recommendations for the competition and recuperative parts of the macrocycle.

Duration and repetition

Selecting the duration and repetition patterns for specific exercises in all phases of the periodization training program are critical to the program's success. Literally hundreds of different combinations are possible, depending on the cycle involved, the needs of a specific individual, the level of competency of the individual, the sport involved, and a number of other factors.

Preparation

Anyone wanting to engaged in a program of periodization training has a very large supply of print and electronic sources to which to turn for further information. In addition, professional trainers are available to design and supervised individual periodization training programs. Finally, most amateur and professional sports teams now employ trainers who are familiar with the general principles and specific applications of periodization training for competitors in a wide variety of sports.

Risks

Relatively little research has been conducted on the potential risks of periodization training. Indeed, most proponents of periodization point to data that suggest that this form of training results in fewer injuries to athletes than do more traditional, non-periodized forms of training. The most important factor in that pattern appears to be the reduced number of injuries that occur as a result of overuse that occur in non-periodized, but not in periodized training programs.

Results

Most research on periodization training focuses on highly specific issues, such as the effects of various forms of periodization on selected skills among

QUESTIONS TO ASK YOUR DOCTOR

- Can you recommend an individual or a facility where I can learn more about periodization training?
- What information or opinions do you have about potential injuries that might result from periodization training?
- Whom can I consult to find out more about the concept of nutritional periodization to accompany a program of periodization training in which I might become involved?

participants in a particular sport. Reviews of research on the topic, however, tend to conclude thatperiodization training is more effective at improving strength, speed, and endurance compared to non-periodized training. Another topic of research has been the relative effectiveness of various types of periodization training, such as the comparison of undulating and linear periodization. The majority of that research appears to show that there is little difference in the effectiveness of any one kind of periodization compared to other types.

Resources

BOOKS

Bompa, Tudor O., and Greg Haff. *Periodization: Theory and Methodology of Training*, 5th ed. Leeds, UK: Human Kinetics, 2009.

Bompa, Tudor O., and Michael C. Carrera. *Periodization Training for Sports*, 2nd ed. Champaign, IL: Human Kinetics, 2005.

Kraemer, William J., and Steven J. Fleck. *Optimizing Strength Training: Designing Nonlinear Periodization Workouts*. Champaign, IL: Human Kinetics, 2007.

Seebohar, Bob. *Nutrition Periodization for Athletes: Taking Traditional Sports Nutrition to the Next Level*. Chicago: Bull Publications, 2011.

PERIODICALS

Cormie, Prue, Michael McGuigan, and Robert Newton. "Developing Maximal Neuromuscular Power: Part 2—Training Considerations for Improving Maximal Power Production." *Sports Medicine* 41, 2. (2011):125–46.

Fleck, S. J. "Periodized Strength Training: A Critical Review." *The Journal of Strength and Conditioning Research.* 1999 13(1): 82–89

Ford, Paul, et al. "The Long-Term Athlete Development Model: Physiological Evidence and Application." *Journal of Sports Sciences* 29, 4. (2011):389–402.

WEBSITES

Nutrition Periodization for Athletes. http://www.nsca-lift. org/HotTopic/download/Nutrition%20Periodization. pdf (accessed October 16, 2011).

Periodization: Latest Studies and Practical Applications. http://www.unm.edu/~lkravitz/Article%20folder/ periodization.html (accessed October 16, 2011).

The Periodization Bible. http://www.t-nation.com/ free_online_article/sports_body_training_perform- ance/the_periodization_bible;jsessionid= 1FF2E776D7CEC25D9BBCD5BE67D3FFB3- mcd01.hydra (accessed October 16, 2011).

"What Does 'Periodization' Mean and How Does It Work?" http://www.trifuel.com/training/triathlon-training/ what-does-periodization-mean-and-how-does-it-work (accessed October 16, 2011).

ORGANIZATIONS

National Athletic Trainers' Association, 2952 Stemmons Fwy, #200, Dallas, TX, 75247, (214) 637-6282, Fax: (214) 637-2206, http://www.nata.org/contact, http://www.nata.org/.

National Strength and Conditioning Association, 1885 Bob Johnson Drive, Colorado Springs, CO, 80906, (719) 632-6722, Fax: (719) 632-6367, (800) 815-6826, nsca@nsca-lift.org, http://www.nsca-lift.org/.

David E. Newton, AB, MA, EdD

Peripheral arterial disease

Definition

Peripheral arterial disease (PAD), also called peripheral vascular disease (PVD) or peripheral artery occlusive disease (PAOD), is a narrowing of blood vessels that restricts blood flow. It mostly occurs in the legs, but is sometimes seen in the arms. The disease can cause serious health problems and adversely affect the ability to walk. The best way to reduce one's risk from PAD is to regularly **exercise** and eat a healthy diet.

Description

PAD includes a group of diseases in which blood vessels become restricted or blocked. Typically, the patient has PAD from atherosclerosis. Atherosclerosis is a disease in which fatty plaques form in the inside walls of blood vessels. Other processes, such as blood clots, further restrict blood flow in the blood vessels. Both veins and arteries may be affected, but the disease is usually arterial.

All the symptoms and consequences of PAD are related to restricted blood flow. PAD is a progressive

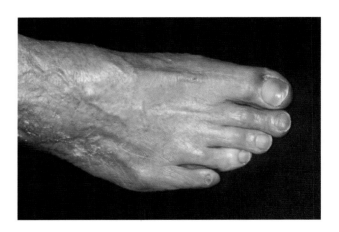

Signs of peripheral arterial disease are evident in this patient's foot. (© Dr. P. Marazzi/Photo Researchers, Inc.)

disease that can lead to gangrene of the affected area. It may also occur suddenly if an embolism occurs or when a blot clot rapidly develops in a blood vessel already restricted by an atherosclerotic plaque, and the blood flow is quickly cut off.

Demographics

About 12–14% of the general population has PAD. However, only one in four people have been diagnosed with it and are receiving treatment. As an individual ages, the risk of developing PAD increases. About 20% of people over age 70 have PAD. Generally, PAD affects about one in three diabetics over the age of 30.

Causes and symptoms

Causes

There are many causes of PAD. One major risk factor is smoking cigarettes; this includes both first hand and second hand smoking of tobacco products. Diseases that may predispose patients to develop PAD are diabetes (**diabetes mellitus**), dyslipidemia, **hypertension** (high **blood pressure**), Buerger's disease, hypertension, and Raynaud's disease.

The risk of developing PAD is two to four times greater for people with diabetes than the general population. Dyslipidemia occurs when a person has high low-density-lipoprotein (LDL, or "bad") **cholesterol** and low high-density-lipoprotein (HDL, or "good") cholesterol. These individuals have an increased chance of developing PAD as well. An elevated blood pressure, called hypertension, also causes an increased incidence of PAD. The risk for hypertension, tobacco smoking, high total cholesterol, and diabetes can be reduced by living a healthy lifestyle, including eating a diet low in fat and high in fruits and vegetables and exercising on a regular basis.

Symptoms

The main symptom of PAD is pain in the affected area. Early symptoms include an achy, tired sensation in the affected muscles, along with weakness or numbness. Together these feelings are called claudication. Since this disease is seen mainly in the legs, these sensations usually occur when **walking**. The symptoms may disappear when resting. As the disease becomes worse, symptoms occur even during light exertion and, eventually, occur all the time, even at rest. In the severe stages of the disease, the leg and foot may be cold to the touch and feel numb. The skin may become dry and scaly. If the leg is even slightly injured, ulcers, wounds, and sores may form because, without a good blood supply, proper healing cannot take place or take much longer than normal. The effected leg will also grow hair and the foot will grow nails much slower than normal.

At the most severe stage of the disease, when the blood flow is greatly restricted, gangrene can develop in those areas lacking blood supply. In some cases, PAD occurs suddenly. This happens when an embolism rapidly blocks blood flow to a blood vessel. The patient experiences a sharp pain, followed by a loss of sensation in the affected area. The limb becomes cold and numb, and loses color (pale) or turn bluish. If only one leg is affected, it is noticeably different in color from the other leg.

Diagnosis

PAD can be diagnosed by comparing blood pressures taken above and below the point of pain. The area below the pain (downstream from the obstruction) has a much lower or undetectable blood pressure reading. One such method is an ankle brachial pressure index (ABPI/ABI). Doppler ultrasonography and angiography are also used to diagnose and define this disease. Computed tomography (CT) scans are frequently performed to provide direct imaging of the arteries of the legs and feet.

Treatment

If the person is a smoker or user of tobacco products, they should stop immediately. Exercise is essential to treating this disease. The patient should walk until pain appears, rest until the pain disappears, and

---

then resume walking. The amount of walking a patient can do should increase gradually as the symptoms improve. Ideally, the patient should walk 30–60 minutes per day. Infections in the affected area should be treated promptly. Surgery may be required to attempt to treat clogged blood vessels. Limbs with gangrene must be amputated to prevent the death of the patient. A change of diet is also recommended. It should include plenty of foods such as fruits, vegetables, and grains and eliminate foods containing substantial amounts of **fats** and sugars.

Cholesterol should be managed with medication, such as statins (or HMG-CoA reductase inhibitors), that reduce the levels of cholesterol. If diabetes or hypertension is present, either one should be controlled to help with the treatment of PAD. For claudication, the drugs cilostazol (Pletal) or pentoxifylline (Trental) usually relieve associated symptoms.

Prognosis

The prognosis depends on the underlying disease and the stage at which PAD is diagnosed. Removal of risk factors, such as smoking, should be done immediately. In many cases, PAD can be treated successfully, but coexisting cardiovascular problems may ultimately prove to be fatal. Persons with PAD have an increased risk from cardiovascular problems, such as heart disease and heart attacks. Those with PAD and claudication have an increased risk of amputation of the effected limb.

Prevention

PAD can be prevented by getting help from a medical professional. If one smokes, quit as quickly as possible because tobacco use is the biggest risk factor for PAD. Several stop-smoking programs are available to help one to quit the habit. In addition, blood pressure and cholesterol should be checked and lowered to normal levels, if necessary. A healthy lifestyle that includes plenty of fruits, vegetables, and whole grains each day is very beneficial. When drinking milk products, make sure they are low-fat or no-fat. Foods containing saturated fats, trans-fat, cholesterol, sodium (salt), and added sugar should be avoided. If overweight, begin a program to lose weight. Include an exercise program to improve one's overall health, well being, and fitness level. The risk from PAD can be reduced when one's lifestyle is healthy.

Resources

BOOKS

Miller, Max. *The Quit Smoking Companion: The Daily Guide to Freedom from Cigarettes.* Charleston, SC: Book-Surge, 2009.

Mohler III, Emile R., and Alan T. Hirsch. *100 Questions & Answers About Peripheral Artery Disease.* Sudbury, MA: Jones and Bartlett, 2009.

Rokavec, Kathleen A. *The Hospital Book.* Raleigh, NC: Lulu.com, 2009.

Wallach, Jacques. *Interpretation of Diagnostic Tests,* 8th ed. Philadelphia: Lippincott Williams & Wilkins, 2006.

Zimring, Michael P. *Healthy Travel: Don't Travel Without It!* Laguna Beach, CA: Basic Health Publications, 2009.

WEBSITES

"Peripheral Artery Disease." Mayo Clinic. (April 21, 2010). http://www.mayoclinic.com/health/peripheral-arterial-disease/DS00537 (accessed November 9, 2011).

"Peripheral arterial disease." Texas Heart Institute. (August 2010). http://www.texasheartinstitute.org/hic/topics/cond/PAD.cfm (accessed November 9, 2011).

"Peripheral Artery Disease—Legs." *A.D.A.M. Medical Encyclopedia.* PubMed Health. (June 17, 2010). http://www.ncbi.nlm.nih.gov/pubmedhealth/PMH0001223/ (accessed November 9, 2011).

Stöppler, Melissa C. "Peripheral arterial disease." MedicineNet.com. (April 21, 2008). http://www.medicinenet.com/peripheral_vascular_disease/article.htm (accessed November 9, 2011).

ORGANIZATIONS

American College of Cardiology, Heart House, 2400 N St., NW, Washington, DC, 20037, (202) 375-6000, Fax: (202) 375-7000, (800) 253-4636, resource@acc.org, http://www.acc.org.

American Heart Association, 7272 Greenville Ave., Dallas, TX, 75231, (301) 223-2307, (800) 242-8721, http://www.heart.org.

Centers for Disease Control and Prevention, 1600 Clifton Rd., Atlanta, GA, 30333, (800) 232-4636, cdcinfo@cdc.gov, http://www.cdc.gov.

National Coalition for Promoting Physical Activity, 1100 H St., NW, Suite 510, Washington, DC, 20005, (202) 454-7521, Fax: (202) 454-7598, http://www.ncppa.org.

National Heart, Lung and Blood Institute, P.O. Box 30105, Bethesda, MD, 20824-0105, (240) 629-3255, Fax: (240) 629-3246, http://www.nhlbi.nih.gov.

John T. Lohr, PhD
Laura Jean Cataldo, RN, EdD
William A. Atkins, BB, BS, MBA

Personal training

Definition

Personal training is a service provided by fitness professionals to help clients reach their fitness goals. Clients hire trainers for their knowledge and experience, and trainers usually provide one-on-one training on a short-term or long-term basis at locations including the trainer's business, gyms, community centers, and clients' homes.

Purpose

The purpose of personal training is help a client achieve goals that are as varied as the people who hire personal trainers. Their clients include pregnant mothers who receive prenatal personal training, children and adults trying to lose weight, people seeking instruction in strength training or **muscle toning**, and older adults who want to improve their tennis skills.

A trainer at a gym or health club may give a session on instruction in how to use **exercise** equipment. This helps the client use the equipment correctly and gain the most benefit from it. People may also hire a trainer to provide this service in their homes.

Long-term personal training is also available at locations including the trainer's business, gyms, community centers, or the clients' home. The trainer is paid an hourly rate or a fee per session, and usually meets with the client one or more times per week. Trainers generally work with one client at a time, but some work with a small group of people who share the cost.

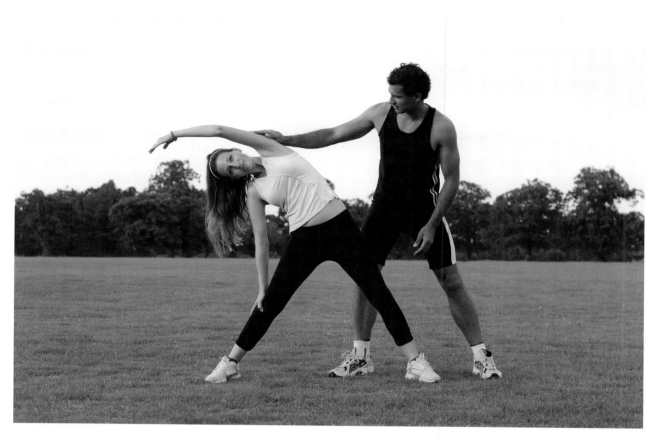

A trainer assists his client with stretches. *(© AISPIX/ShutterStock.com)*

The training service starts when the trainer designs a personalized program for a client or updates an existing program. The trainer develops the program and then supervises the clients' progress towards the goal. In addition to providing fitness knowledge, the trainer evaluates progress, and motivates the client to continue with the fitness plan. The trainer also updates the plan when as the client advances toward the goal.

Demographics

Personal trainers work with people of both genders, with clients ranging from young children to the elderly. **Weight loss** is often a goal, especially for children. According to the United States Centers for Disease Control and Prevention (CDC), about 17% of children between the ages of 2 and 19 were obese in 2007.

Contributing to the dramatic rise in childhood **obesity** is the lack of physical education programs in schools. Physical activity for children may be limited to those who play sports. As a result, some parents hire personal trainers to help their children lose weight.

Weight loss may also be the goal of adults who use personal trainers. In addition, fitness professionals help children and adults update a workout routine, learn or train for a sport, learn an activity such as weight training, prepare for an event like a triathlon or ski trip.

Furthermore, some trainers help older adults get into shape and stay fit as they **age**. Services for the aging population include weight-loss programs, weight training, and athletic training. A trainer could also help elderly clients maintain balance and coordination. This training helps to prevent falls and keep clients independent, allowing them to live in their homes.

Trainers may also work with people receiving from surgery and those diagnosed with conditions such as diabetes and **osteoporosis**.

Specialized trainers include fitness professionals certified by the American Council on Exercise (ACE) and referred to potential clients through an arrangement with AARP (formerly the American Association of Retired Persons).

History

Fitness training dates back to ancient times when a civilization's survival depended on the strength of its army. Spartans living in northern Greece began fitness training for boys at the age of 6, according to "The History of Fitness, " a 2002 article by Lance C. Dalleck and Len Kravitz.

The authors noted that the boys were turned over to the government and raised to be soldiers when they reached adulthood. The government also required that women were fit so that they produced strong children.

Fitness was also associated with fighting in ancient Greece. However, the Greeks also believed that there was a connection between a healthy mind and a healthy body. According to the article, young boys went to facilities for training in activities such as **gymnastics**, wrestling, **running**, and jumping. When boys reached the age of 14, they were trained through adulthood in gymnasiums. Boys and men received training from a gymnastic instructor and a *paidotribe*, an instructor regarded as the forerunner of the personal trainer and physical education instructor.

The *paidotribe* also trained males for competitions such as the Olympic games that were first held in Olympia in 776 BC. Some historians believe the games may be several centuries older, but they were not held on such an organized level.

Modern personal training

During the twentieth century, the public placed an emphasis on fitness training as a health issue. Among those credited with generating enthusiasm for this concept was Jack Lalanne, a fitness enthusiast described by *The New York Times* as the "Father of the Modern Fitness Movement." Born in 1914, Lalanne worked out with weights and opened a business in 1936 with a gym, juice bar, and spa in Oakland, California.

People were skeptical about his claims about the relationship between exercise and health. Lalanne said in an interview that people thought he was "a charlatan and a nut." Doctors warned that working out with weights would result in heart attacks and the loss of the sex drive.

Lalanne continued to advocate for exercise and a healthy diet. He advocated as a televised personal trainer, on "The Jack Lalanne Show," a daytime exercise program. The public attitude changed as the show went from a local offering in San Francisco in 1951 to a national program that aired from 1959 until the mid-1980s.

By that time, personal training had become an important part of the fitness scene. The National Academy of Sports Medicine (NASM) in 2009 gave Lalanne an honorary Certified Personal Training certification, an honor bestowed at his 95th birthday party. He died a year later.

Description

A personal trainer usually works with a client on a one-on-one basis, with training done in the clients' home or another location. Trainers usually charge from US$20–100 per hour, according to the American College of Sports Medicine (ACSM). There may be a discount for long-term packages or prepaid sessions.

Before training begins, the process starts with the client selecting a trainer. This process includes evaluating the trainer's experience and education, and establishing a training plan that covers details such as where and when training is held.

Establishing a plan

The issues to be decided include how often the client and trainer will meet. For some clients, meeting several times a week helps them meet fitness goals. Other clients may want periodic meetings where the trainer evaluates their progress through measures such as fitness testing.

The training process usually starts with an initial consultation and assessment, according to the ACE. This meeting for someone starting an exercise program could include tests to assess fitness in areas such as body-fat percentage, cardiorespiratory (aerobic) fitness, muscular strength, flexibility, posture, and balance.

The fitness evaluation will serve as the baseline for the program that the trainer creates. The personalized exercise program described by the ACE is based on the assessment and the client goals. The plan is structured around the FITT principle of training: frequency, intensity, type, and time.

FITT. Frequency is the number of times per week that an exercise is done. The ACSM recommends that healthy people do at least 30 minutes of moderate-intensity physical activity five days per week. During this aerobic activity, the person exercises enough to sweat but is able to talk to others. The ACSM recommendation for strength training is to do these resistance exercises at least two days per week. The workout should include from 8–12 repetitions of 10 exercises that target all of the major muscle groups.

Intensity refers to the amount of **energy** that the client exerts while training. Measurements for the amount of cardiorespiratory exercise include the **target heart rate**. This is the rate that the heart should pump during exercise achieve the maximum cardiovascular benefit. The rate is based on a percentage of the maximum heart rate, a figure based on factors including age and fitness level.

Intensity of resistance training could be measured by the amount of weight the client lifts or how many repetitions of an exercise that the client does.

The types of aerobic exercise include **walking**, running, dancing, **swimming**, and cycling. Types of resistance training include exercising with weights or resistance bands.

Time for **aerobic training** is based on the client's fitness level. The trainer may advise a client at a lower level to aim to stay within the target heart rate for 20 to 30 minutes. That amount could increase to up to an hour as the person becomes more fit. For resistance training, the person could exercise for 45 minutes to an hour, unless the training is intense. The trainer will then recommend a shorter exercise session.

Training sessions

During the sessions, the trainer will supervise exercise and provide motivational coaching, according to the ACE. The trainer could also relay information about the fitness topics such as the fundamentals of aerobic training and the safe use of equipment. The trainer will also advise the client about when to proceed to the next level of the fitness plan. At that time, the trainer will give additional instruction as needed.

Preparation

The individual hiring a trainer should begin by consulting a doctor to discuss what type of personal training is beneficial and whether any health conditions would place limits on this plan. Once the fitness goal is established, the next step is to locate a personal trainer.

Trainer expertise

Personal training covers many activities and sports. The scope of service depends upon the experience and education of the trainer. Although not all states regulate personal trainers in the United States,

certification is available from professional organizations and through continuing education programs.

In addition, some schools offer associate, bachelor, master, and doctoral degrees related to personal training.

A personal trainer should be certified and have at least an undergraduate degree and a strong background in anatomy and **kinesiology**, according to the ACSM. That background is needed because much of the training has to do with muscular strength and **endurance training**.

The ACSM is among the nationally recognized organizations that certify personal trainers. Certifying organizations accredited by the National Commission for Certifying Agencies in September 2011 included the American College of Sports Medicine, American Council on Exercise, National Academy of Sports Medicine, and National Strength and Conditioning Association. Certification is based on passing of an exam, and these organizations hold educational workshops to prepare candidates for the test and their careers.

Interviewing the trainer

The initial meeting with the trainer is similar to a job interview. In addition to verifying the trainer's expertise, the ACSM advises people to ask many questions before contracting with a trainer. These questions include how long the person has worked as a trainer, if the trainer has liability insurance, and if the person has first aid and CPR training. The client should also ask for references.

The client should also consider the trainer's personality, advises the ACSM. A trainer's overbearing manner could cause a client to end the relationship and stop exercising, while a patient trainer who communicates well may help a client reach his/her fitness goal.

Risks

As of September 2011, there were no national standards or minimum requirements for working as a personal trainer. As a result, there is a risk for the person who does not research the trainer's qualifications and education. An unqualified or underqualified trainer could put the client at risk through actions such as giving instructions that cause injury or urging the client to exercise more than is safe for that person.

Prescreening measures for clients recommended by the ACSM include asking many questions on topics ranging from the potential risks of certain exercises to how the trainer would handle an emergency situation.

Results

A qualified trainer will help a client define and reach fitness goals. The trainer provides knowledge and also motivates the client to implement goals that lead to a healthier life because the client will be aware of the importance of physical fitness.

Resources

WEBSITES

Dalleck, Lance. C, MS and Len Kravitz, Ph.D. " The History of Fitness. " University of New Mexico. UNM.edu. http://www.unm.edu/~lkravitz/Article%20folder/history. html (accessed September 17, 2011).

Goldstein, Richard. "Jack LaLanne, Founder of Modern Fitness Movement Dies at 96." *The New York Times.* (January 23, 2011). NYTimes.com. http://www.nytimes. com/2011/01/24/sports/24lalanne.html (accessed September 17, 2011).

"Selecting and Effectively Using A Personal Trainer." American College of Sports Medicine. ACSM.org. (accessed September 17, 2011).

ORGANIZATIONS

American College of Sports Medicine, 401 West Michigan Street, Indianapolis, IN, 46202-3233, (317) 637-9200, Fax: (317) 634-7817, http://www.acsm.org.

American Council on Exercise, 4851 Paramount Drive, San Diego, CA, 92123-1449, (858) 576-6500, Fax: (858) 576-6564, support@acefitness.org, http://www. acefitness.org/.

Liz Swain

Physical education in schools *see*
U.S. President's Council on Fitness, Sports, & Nutrition

Pilates

Definition

Pilates (pronounced pie-LAH-tes) or Physical Mind method, is a series of non-impact exercises designed by Joseph Pilates to develop strength, flexibility, balance, and inner awareness.

Purpose

Pilates promotes a feeling of physical and mental well-being and develops inner physical awareness. Since this method strengthens and lengthens the muscles without creating bulk, it is particularly beneficial for dancers and actors. Pilates is also helpful in preventing injuries and rehabilitating injuries, improving posture, and increasing flexibility, circulation, and balance.

Demographics

Pilates is a form of strength and flexibility training that can be done by someone at any level of fitness. The exercises can be adapted for people who have limited movement or who use wheelchairs.

Pregnant women who do Pilates exercises can develop body alignment, improve concentration, and develop body shape and tone after pregnancy. According to Joseph Pilates, "You will feel better in 10 sessions, look better in 20 sessions and have a completely new body in 30 sessions."

Although Pilates is often associated with dancers, athletes, and younger people who are interested in improving their physical strength and flexibility, a simplified version of some Pilates exercises is being used to lower the risk of hospital-related deconditioning in older adults. A Canadian study of hospitalized patients over age 70 found that those who were given a set of Pilates exercises that could be performed in bed recovered more rapidly than a control group given a set of passive range-of-motion exercises.

History

Joseph Pilates, the founder of the Pilates method (also simply referred to as "the method"), was born in Germany in 1880. As a frail child with rickets, **asthma**, and rheumatic fever, he was determined to become stronger. He dedicated himself to building both his body and his mind through practices that included **yoga**, zen, and ancient Roman and Greek exercises. His conditioning regime worked, and he

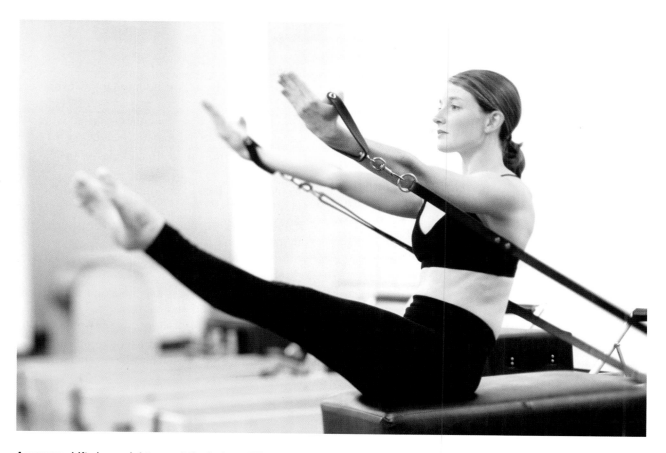

A woman shifts her weight gracefully during a Pilates routine. (© *Jim Cummins/Corbis*)

became an accomplished gymnast, skier, boxer, and diver.

While interned in England during World War I for being a German citizen, Pilates became a nurse. During this time, he designed a unique system of hooking springs and straps to a hospital bed in order to help his disabled and immobilized patients regain strength and movement. It was through these experiments that he recognized the importance of training the core abdominal and back muscles to stabilize the torso and allow the entire body to move freely. This experimentation provided the foundation for the style of conditioning and the specialized **exercise** equipment associated with the Pilates method.

Pilates emigrated from Germany to the United States in 1926. That same year he opened the first Pilates studio in New York City. Over the years, dancers, actors, and athletes came to his studio to heal, condition, and align their bodies.

Joseph Pilates died at age 87 in a fire at his studio. Although his strength enabled him to escape the flames by hanging from the rafters for over an hour, he died from smoke inhalation. He believed that ideal fitness is "the attainment and maintenance of a uniformly developed body with a sound mind fully capable of naturally, easily, and satisfactorily performing our many and varied daily tasks with spontaneous zest and pleasure."

Description

Over 500 exercises were developed by Joseph Pilates. "Classical" exercises, according to the Pilates Studio in New York, involve several principles: concentration, centering, flowing movement, and breath. Some instructors teach only the classical exercises originally taught by Joseph Pilates. Others design new exercises that are variations upon these classical forms in order to make the exercises more accessible for a specific person.

The appeal of the Pilates method to a wide population, coupled with a new interest in it on the part of rehabilitation therapists, suggests that further research studies may soon be underway. Dancers and actors originally embraced the Pilates method as a form of strength training that did not create muscle bulk. Professional and amateur athletes also use these exercises to prevent re-injury. Sedentary people find Pilates to be a gentle, non-impact approach to conditioning. Pilates equipment and classes can be found in hospitals, health clubs, spas, and gyms.

Preparation

During the initial meeting, an instructor will analyze the client's posture and movement and design a specific training program. Once the program has been created, the sessions usually follow a basic pattern. A session generally begins with mat work and passive and active **stretching**. In passive stretching, the instructor moves and presses the client's body to stretch and elongate the muscles. During the active stretching period, the client performs the stretches while the instructor watches their form and breathing. These exercises **warm up** the muscles in preparation for machine work. The machines help the client to maintain the correct positioning required for each exercise.

Two primary exercise machines are used for Pilates, the Universal Reformer and the Cadillac, along with several smaller pieces of equipment. The Reformer resembles a single bed frame and is equipped with a carriage that slides back and forth and adjustable springs that are used to regulate tension and resistance. Cables, bars, straps, and pulleys allow the exercises to be done from a variety of positions. Instructors usually work with their clients on the machines for 20–45 minutes. During this time, they are observing and giving feedback about alignment, breathing, and precision of movement. The exercises are done slowly and carefully so that the movements are smooth and flowing. This requires focused concentration and muscle control. The session ends with light stretching and a cool-down period.

Once the client has learned the basics from an instructor, either in one-on-one lessons or in a class, it is possible to train at home using videos. Exercise equipment for home use is available and many exercises can be preformed on a mat.

A private session costs between US$45–75 dollars, depending on location. Pilates is not specifically covered by insurance although it may be covered when the instructor is a licensed physical therapist.

Risks

The Pilates method is not a substitute for good physical therapy, although it has been increasingly used and recommended by physical therapists since the mid-1980s. People with chronic injuries are advised to see a physician.

Results

As of mid-2011, several studies have been done on the effectiveness of the Pilates method for a variety of patients. One study found that compared female breast cancer patients. A group that performed Pilates in addition to home exercises had improved outcomes on a variety of scores when compared to a group who only performed home exercises. Another study found that in elderly individuals Pilates significantly improved balance, general fitness, and quality of life factors.

Resources

BOOKS

Aikman, Louise. *Pilates Step-By-Step*. New York: Rosen Central, 2011.

Isacowitz, Rael. *Pilates Anatomy*. Champaign, IL: Human Kinetics, 2011.

Staugaard-Jones, Jo Ann. *The Anatomy of Exercise and Movement for the Study of Dance, Pilates, Sports, and Yoga*. Berkeley, CA: North Atlantic Books, 2011.

PERIODICALS

Dunleavy, Kim. "Pilates Fitness Continuum: Post-Rehabilitation and Prevention Pilates Fitness Programs." *Rehab Management* 23, no. 9 (October 2010): 10.

Lim, Edwin, et al. "Effects of Pilates-based Exercises on Pain and Disability in Individuals with Persistent Nonspecific Low Back Pain: A Systematic Review with Meta-Analysis." *Journal of Orthopaedic and Sports Physical Therapy* 14, no. 2 (February 2011): 70–80.

WEBSITES

"Pilates: A Low-Impact Way to Build Core Strength, Endurance, and Flexibility." MayoClinic.com. (June 8, 2009). http://www.mayoclinic.org/news2009-mchi/5346.html (accessed November 9, 2011).

Sarnataro, Barbara Russi. "The Benefits of Pilates." WebMD.com. (May 27, 2009). http://www.webmd.com/fitness-exercise/features/the-benefits-of-pilates (accessed November 9, 2011).

ORGANIZATIONS

Aerobics and Fitness Association of America, 15250 Ventura Blvd., #200, Sherman Oaks, CA, 91403, (877) 968-7263, http://www.afaa.com.

American Council on Exercise, 4851 Paramount Dr., San Diego, CA, 92123, (888) 825-3636, http//www.acefitness.org.

Rebecca J. Frey, PhD
Tish Davidson, AM

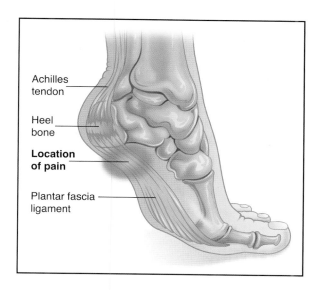

Pain or a burning sensation in the heel and bottom of the foot can be worsened most commonly in the first steps of the day, after sitting or standing for long periods of time, or after extreme activity. *(Electronic Illustrators Group. © 2012 Cengage Learning.)*

Plantar fasciitis

Definition

Plantar fasciitis is a condition in which the plantar facia—the arch tendon in the foot—becomes very painful, swollen, irritated, or inflamed when tiny tears occur on its surface. The condition is one of the most common orthopedic complaints relating to problems of the foot. Athletes are especially at risk from the condition due to excessive **running**, jumping, dancing, and other such activities that add stress to the foot, and the plantar facia.

Description

The plantar facia is a deep, wide band of fibrous connective tissue located on the bottom of the foot. It extends from the calcaneus (heel bone) to the sole of the foot and the proximal phalanges bones of the toes. This band that acts similar to a stretchy rubber band supports the muscles and arch of the foot. It continually contracts and lengthens as the foot moves, helping the foot absorb forces acting down upon it, such as the weight of the body.

When the plantar fascia is extremely over-stretched or repeatedly overused, such as from daily physical activities, exercising, and sporting events, it can develop the condition called plantar fasciitis. One result of the condition is pain caused by pointed, bony fragments that extend from the heel bone—known as heel spurs. The condition is frequently the cause of heel pain in humans—making for a painful foot, and even more so while **walking**.

Demographics

The Plantar Fasciitis Organization states that heel pain—the primary symptom of plantar fasciitis—affects almost two million Americans each year, causing mild discomfort to debilitating pain. The condition is common among athletes participating in high-impact sports and physical exercises in which excessive force is brought onto the heel and attached tissue. Such high-stress activities include ballet dancing, **dance** aerobics, **volleyball**, **basketball**, and long-distance running (especially running downhill or on uneven surfaces). Runners who roll their feet or flatten them (overpronate) are at high risk for plantar fasciitis because the action adds excess **stretching** to the plantar fascia. In addition, it is frequently found in non-athletes who are overweight or obese.

Plantar fasciitis is most commonly found in physically active people between the ages of 40 and 70 years of age. Women are more likely to get plantar fasciitis than are men. Pregnant women are more likely to get it than are women who are not pregnant or have not been pregnant. Obese people (or people who gain weight quickly) are more likely to get plantar fasciitis than normally weighted people because the excessive weight places more pressure on the feet.

Both men and women who wear shoes with inadequate foot support or soft soles are at increased risk from getting the condition. This includes shoes that are loose fitting (or are not tied, if containing laces), have thin soles, do not possess sufficient arch support, have little or no padding, and are high-heeled. For instance, high-heeled shoes cause the Achilles tendon to overly contract and shorten, causing strain on the tissue around the heel.

People with problems of the arches, such as those with flat feet, tight Achilles tendons, or high arches, are more prone to have the condition. An abnormal pattern of walking is also more likely to cause plantar fasciitis because body weight is not evenly distributed while walking. People who work at jobs that require long hours of standing or walking are especially prone to plantar fasciitis. Such occupations include teachers, factory workers, retail clerks and workers, postal carriers, and others.

Causes and symptoms

Causes

The plantar fascia absorbs the shock from impacts to the foot, such as in exercises, physical activities, and general walking around. The plantar fascia provides this support through the arch in the foot. However, if tension becomes too great, small tears can develop within the fascia. Excessive stretching and tearing of the fascia can cause it to become irritated or inflamed, leading to plantar fasciitis.

The most common cause of the condition is overly tight calf muscles. When the calf muscles are excessively tight for long periods, excessive pronation (abnormal rotational movement, also called overpronation) of the foot can occur. Foot overpronation leads to excessive stretching of the plantar fascia, eventually causing inflammation and pain, along with thickening of the tendon. As the tendon thickens, strength and flexibility are lost.

Increased risk of developing plantar fasciitis is caused by:

- advancing age
- being overweight or excessively overweight (obese); or sudden weight gain
- constantly stressing the feet through such activities as running
- medical conditions such as arthritis, diabetes, rheumatoid arthritis, or systemic lupus erythematosus (lupus); along with hormonal changes in pregnant women
- standing for long hours each day
- wearing high-heeled shoes frequently, or switching between flat- and high-heeled shoes on a regular basis
- wearing shoes that are not correctly fitted or those without proper arch support and cushioning
- having flat feet, or an exceptionally high arch in both feet
- having legs that are not equal in length or an abnormal walking style (gait) or unusual foot positioning while walking
- having tight Achilles tendons

Symptoms

Symptoms include pain on the underside of the heel that becomes worse and increases to stabbing pain after first getting out of bed after sleeping, or after **sitting** or standing for long periods during the day. Normally, the pain goes away after a few steps. Another symptom of plantar fasciitis is difficulty bending the affected foot. Athletes, such as runners, often develop plantar fasciitis when they have knee pain.

The most common complaint by people with plantar fasciitis is aching, burning, or stabbing pain on the bottom of the heel that is usually worse in the morning and may improve throughout the day. This pattern is due to the fascia ligament tightening during sleep, and becoming taut (and painful) when pressure is first placed on the foot when stepping out of bed. By the end of the day, the pain is usually replaced by a dull ache that improves with rest. Thus, the pain diminishes as the ligament relaxes (warms) throughout the day. However, the pain can easily return if during the day a person is forced to stand for long hours, or is conducting activities that involve lifting or carrying heavy items, any type of physical exertion, or suddenly standing after sitting for a long time. The stabbing pain is usually located in the heel of the foot, but may extend to the outside of the heel. The pain usually occurs in just one foot, although it can sometimes be felt in both feet at the same time.

Diagnosis

A medical professional diagnoses plantar fasciitis with a physical examination and a detailed medical history of the patient. Data about previous physical activities, foot problems, and other related information is gathered. The feet are examined, along with a visual observation of the patient walking and standing. Images may be taken of the feet, including computed tomography (CT) scans, magnetic resonance imaging (MRI) scans, and diagnostic sonography scans (also called ultrasonography). Other possible medical problems of the foot are eliminated before a diagnosis of plantar fasciitis can be made. Typical findings for plantar fasciitis from a medical examination includes redness and mild swelling and inflammation of the foot, along with tenderness on the bottom of the heel.

Treatment

Treatment for plantar fasciitis includes:

- massage therapy
- rest and application of ice or cold therapy on a regular basis
- stretching exercises (such as of the calf, Achilles tendon, and plantar fascia muscles)
- weight loss, if needed
- night splints to improve muscle flexibility, and prevent tightening of the plantar fascia
- orthotics such as foot supports; in more extreme cases, a walking boot or walking cast
- motion-control running shoes
- physical therapy
- taping across the plantar fascia to reduce the stress on the foot and increase healing time
- anti-inflammatory medications, such as nonsteroidal anti-inflammatory drugs (NSAIDs), including aspirin and ibuprofen
- local injections of corticosteroids

If symptoms from plantar fasciitis continues, it may be necessary to seek medical help from a doctor or podiatrist (a doctor specializing in problems of the feet). The widely held recommendation from the medical community is to seek help before the symptoms become excessive because by that time it is less likely that the pain will go away by itself. More advanced stages of the condition may necessitate surgery. When the treatment process is performed early on,

> ## KEY TERMS
>
> **Achilles tendon**—The tendon that connects the calf muscles to the heel bone.
>
> **Arthritis**—A condition of the joints that causes stiffness, swelling, or pain.
>
> **Calcaneus**—The heel bone.
>
> **Lupus**—Lupus erythematosus, a disease of the connective tissue.
>
> **Orthopedic**—Relating to disorders of the bones, ligaments, joints, and muscles.
>
> **Phalanges**—Bones forming the toes and fingers.
>
> **Plantar fascia**—Connective tissue that supports the arch in the foot.
>
> **Pronation**—Rotational movement of the foot at the subtalar and talocalcaneonavicular joints.
>
> **Rheumatoid arthritis**—An inflammatory condition that adversely affects the synovial joints of the body.

conservative (less invasive) treatment options usually solve the problem.

Surgery is an option when other possibilities have failed. One surgical technique is plantar fascia release that involves surgically cutting the plantar fascia ligament to relieve tension and reduce inflammation. Another technique, called coblation surgery, is a minimally invasive procedure that uses radio waves (a type of electromagnetic radiation) to remove the problem areas—what is called radio frequency ablation. Risks associated with surgery for plantar fasciitis include nerve damage, infection, rupture of the plantar fascia, and inability to reduce the pain and other symptoms.

Prognosis

If nothing is done to treat the problem, the pain is likely to become chronic. Other foot, knee, hip, or back problems may also result as the condition causes negative changes to occur in walking. If treated properly, the condition usually goes away without the need for surgery. Various outcomes are likely to result due to differences in the severity of the condition, along with other extraneous problems. Recovery times also widely vary.

Prevention

Preventing plantar fasciitis from occurring is very important. One way to prevent it is to maintain a

QUESTIONS TO ASK YOUR DOCTOR

- What specific exercises should I do to correct my problem?
- What activities should I avoid when pain occurs?
- What is likely causing my symptoms or condition?
- Will I need surgery?
- Will my health insurance pay for surgery or rehabilitation?
- Do I need other tests to confirm the diagnosis?
- What treatment do you recommend?
- How long after treatment do you expect my condition to improve?
- Is there anything else I can do to relieve my foot pain?
- If I do nothing, do I risk long-term complications?
- Should I see a specialist?
- Where can I learn more about plantar fasciitis?

healthy weight to height ratio, known as the **Body Mass Index** (BMI). The National Heart, Lung and Blood Institute maintains a BMI calculator at http://www.nhlbisupport.com/bmi/. A proper weight helps to reduce stress on the plantar fascia. Shoes that fit correctly and provide sufficient support to the heel, arch, and ball of the foot is also key to reducing the risk for plantar fasciitis.

Walking barefoot; wearing old, worn-out shoes; and wearing sandals and other types of footwear that provide little support for the foot increase the risk of having foot problems, including plantar fasciitis. Foot problems can also be avoided by gradually building up intensity when exercising and performing everyday physical activities. Warming up and stretching exercises are recommended before doing physical activities because it helps to prevent sudden stress on the feet, along with allowing the muscles to stretch in the foot before they must perform more strenuous exercises.

A gait analysis on a person's walking style is performed by a doctor to determine if overpronation is a problem. **Orthotics** or insoles can help to correct any problems with the feet. Taping the feet during **exercise** is sometimes done, especially for professional athletes and others involved in frequent high stress activities.

Resources

BOOKS

Berquist, Thomas, H., editor. *Imaging of the Foot and Ankle.* Philadelphia: Wolters Kluwer Health/Lippincott Williams & Wilkins, 2011.

Katch, Victor L., William D. McArdle, Frank I. Katch. *Essentials of Exercise Physiology.* Philadelphia: Wolters Kluwer/Lippincott Williams & Wilkins Health, 2011.

Miller, Mark D., Jennifer A. Hart, and John M. MacKnight, editors. *Essential Orthopaedics.* Philadelphia: Saunders/ Elsevier, 2010.

Noyes, Frank R, and Sue D. Barber-Westin, editors. *Noyes' Knee Disorders: Surgery, Rehabilitation, Clinical Outcomes.* New York: Thieme, 2006.

Yates, Ben, and Linda M. Merriman. *Merriman's Assessment of the Lower Limb.* Edinburgh: Churchill Livingstone/ Elsevier, 2009.

WEBSITES

"Plantar Fasciitis." Mayo Clinic. (March 15, 2011). http://www.mayoclinic.com/health/plantar-fasciitis/DS00508 (accessed November 12, 2011).

"Plantar Fasciitis, Heel Spurs, Heel Pain." Plantar Fasciitis Organization. (2010). http://www.plantar-fasciitis.org/ (accessed November 12, 2011).

"Understanding Plantar Fasciitis: The Basics." WebMD. (October 24, 2010). http://arthritis.webmd.com/understanding-plantar-fasciitis-basics (accessed November 12, 2011).

Vorvick, Linda J., and C. Benjamin Ma. "Plantar Fasciitis." MedlinePlus. (February 19, 2011). http://www.nlm.nih.gov/medlineplus/ency/article/007021.htm (accessed November 12, 2011).

ORGANIZATIONS

American Association of Orthopaedic Surgeons, 6300 N. River Rd., Rosemont, IL, 60018-4262, (847) 823-7186, Fax: (847) 823-8125, http://www.aaos.org.

American Pain Society, 4700 W. Lake Ave., Glenview, IL, 60025, (847) 375-4715, Fax: (847) 375-6479, info@ ampainsoc.org, http://www.ampainsoc.org.

Plantar Fasciitis Organization, http://www.plantar-fasciitis.org.

William A. Atkins, BB, BS, MBA

Play *see* **Recess and unstructured play**

Power yoga

Definition

Power **yoga** is an Americanized form of ashtanga yoga, also known as astanga, vinyasa, or classical yoga. Power yoga is designed to build strength, flexibility, and endurance through a fast-paced, physically demanding series of postures.

Purpose

Power yoga is pursued by experienced yoga practitioners who want a more strenuous workout and by athletes who want to balance their specialized training. Intensive training for a particular sport tends to cause tight muscles and uneven muscular development. Athletic training, even when it includes cross-training, can cause muscular and structural imbalances that may result in repeated injury. For example, although **running** develops strong leg muscles and increases cardiorespiratory capacity, it also disproportionately tightens and shortens the muscles of the backs of the legs, without working the other muscles of the body. Power yoga strengthens, loosens, and balances all of the muscles of the body. It can help to realign the muscles and restore range of motion to tight muscles. Thus, power yoga can help athletes avoid injury, while simultaneously building strength and endurance. Power yoga also emphasizes concentration, focus, and full attentiveness—attributes that are of particular importance to competitive athletes. Power yoga also incorporates practices that are designed to address specific types of sports injuries, as well as general pain that can result from **overtraining**.

Beryl Bender Birch, an originator of power yoga, formulated eight "axioms" to explain its purpose. To paraphrase:

- One must be hot to stretch—this is accomplished by performing strength work while stretching.

- Strength develops flexibility—strength work provides the heat that makes stretching both possible and safe and safe and that enables stretching to increase flexibility.

- Sports do not make a person physically fit; rather, sports create tight, shortened muscles and muscular imbalances due to repetitive training and the uneven use of muscle groups.

- Sports injuries are caused by structural and muscular imbalances that tend to develop over time, along with loss of range of motion and agility.

- Structural and muscular imbalances can be corrected with power yoga.

- Even iron bends when it is heated, and this applies to tight muscle tissue as well.

- Halting training does not correct structural and muscular imbalances.

- Regardless of one's physical fitness, one must ease into the practice of power yoga.

- Stretching is not a warm-up.

Demographics

Yoga's popularity has grown steadily in the United States and other Western countries since the 1960s. A 2008 survey sponsored by *Yoga Journal* found that 6.9% of American adults—15.8 million people—practiced yoga. Although the vast majority of yoga enthusiasts practice styles of **hatha yoga** other than power yoga, some components of power yoga, such as sun salutations for warming up, have been widely adopted by mainstream hatha yoga teachers and students. Power yoga has become increasingly popular among advanced hatha yoga students and teachers. Competitive athletes who incorporate power yoga into their workouts include swimmers, runners, climbers, cyclists, dancers, skiers, and amateur and professional golfers, tennis players, and **baseball**, **football**, and **basketball** players.

History

The practice of yoga dates back at least 5,000 years, to the Indus Valley of ancient India. The term yoga derives from a Sanskrit word meaning "union," the bringing together of the body and mind in perfect harmony. Passed down by oral tradition over the centuries, various branches of yoga evolved with different philosophies and practices. Ashtanga yoga was described by the Indian scholar Patanjali in his *Yoga Sutras* some 2,000 years ago. A branch of hatha yoga, Ashtanga yoga is an eight-fold or eight-limbed path to total physical, mental, and spiritual health. The eight limbs are restraints or moral commandments, observances or disciplined self-purification, postures or asanas, rhythmic controlled breathing or pranayama, withdrawal from the senses, concentration, meditation or dhyana, and absorption or super-consciousness.

Ashtanga yoga is based on an ancient Sanskrit text by Vamana Rishi called the *Yoga Korunta*. The text was passed down to Shri K. Pattabhi Jois (1915–2009) by his yoga guru Sri T. Krishnamacharya. Pattabhi Jois first began instructing Westerners in ashtanga yoga at his school in Mysore, India, in the 1970s. Two of those

KEY TERMS

Aerobic exercise—Activity that increases the body's requirement for oxygen, thereby increasing respiration and heart rate.

Asanas—Postures, stances, or poses of power yoga.

Ashtanga yoga—Astanga, classical, or power yoga; a physically strenuous form of hatha yoga.

Cross-training—Cross-conditioning; training in a sport that is complementary to the sport competed in; such as distance running and cross-country skiing or power yoga.

Drishti—"Gazing point;" the focus of the eyes in ashtanga and power yoga.

Hatha yoga—A broad category of yoga styles that are commonly practiced in the United States and other Western countries; power yoga is a strenuous form of hatha yoga.

Pranayama—Rhythmic breath control used in yoga.

Savasana—Relaxation in the corpse pose at the end of yoga practice.

Sun salutations—Surya namaskara; the warm-ups that begin every session of power yoga.

Tristhana—The three foci of attention in ashanga or power yoga—posture, breathing, and drishti.

Vinyasa—The connecting movement and breath between postures in ashanga and power yoga.

early students, Norman Allen and David Williams, passed the system on to their students, Beryl Bender Birch and Bryan Kest, respectively. Birch and Kest independently coined the term "power yoga," to make the practice more appealing to Western athletes and others interested in challenging workouts. Birch began adapting power yoga to the cross-training requirements of skiers, long-distance runners, and other traditional athletes. Birch's husband Thom Birch, a world-class runner who used power yoga successfully as physical therapy for injuries, helped popularize the workout. Over the past two decades, power yoga has come to refer to almost any strenuous yoga routine and aspects have been incorporated into gentler forms of hatha yoga.

Description

The three intrinsic principles of ashtanga yoga are vinyasa, tristhana, and internal purification. Vinyasa is the flowing movement from one posture to the next and the accompanying breath. In traditional ashtanga yoga, each asana is assigned a specific number of vinyasas. Vinyasas are said to heat the blood for internal cleansing and better circulation, eliminating toxins, disease, and pain from the internal organs. Sweating during practice then removes these impurities from the body and is therefore an important component of power yoga. Tristhana refers to the three foci of one's attention—posture, breathing, and the point of one's gaze or drishti. The postures purify, strengthen, and provide flexibility. Breathing is even, through the nose with the mouth

always closed, and with the length of the inhale matching that of the exhale. Gazing at one of the nine drishtis—such as the nose, hands, thumb, navel, or feet—stabilizes the mind. Internal purification is the removal of negative emotions—the six poisons of desire, anger, delusion, greed, envy, and laziness.

Power yoga emphasizes asanas—the third limb of the ashtanga path—with emphasis on strength, flow, and focus. Pranayama or breath control, the fourth limb, is essential for generating heat and **energy**. The fifth, sixth, and seventh limbs—withdrawal from outside distractions, concentration and focus, and meditation—are also important components of power yoga.

Power yoga routines vary greatly, from the prescribed order of traditional ashtanga yoga asanas to free-flowing routines that incorporate only certain postures, add postures from other yoga traditions, and/or vary the order of asanas. Asanas can be modified in various ways, depending on individual abilities and limitations. The pace of power yoga routines also varies, with some performed much faster than others. The common factor among power yoga workouts is that they are always strenuous. However power yoga is not aerobic **exercise**: one of its goals is to slow heart rate and respiration, rather than increase them. However people with low levels of fitness may approach aerobic levels of activity when first embarking on power yoga.

Sun salutations

Power yoga workouts begin with warm-ups called sun salutations, sometimes preceded by breathing exercises or simple postures. Sun salutations heat and loosen up the body, beginning with the spine, and simultaneously and sequentially contract and stretch opposing muscles. Sun salutations can constitute a complete workout on their own. There are two traditional series of sun salutations in ashtanga and power yoga. In general, three to five sun salutations are performed from each series. These can be modified to accommodate muscle tightness or injury. Sun salutations are usually the first asanas to be learned, along with simple finishing poses.

Surya namaskara A has nine vinyasas or positions:

- Beginning in mountain or attention pose, the arms and head reach up on an inhale.
- The upper body bends forward with the hands to the feet on an exhale.
- The chest lifts up on an inhale.
- The legs walk back to plank or push-up position on an exhale.
- The head and chest lift to upward-facing dog posture on an inhale.
- The body lifts into downward-facing dog posture on an exhale, possibly pausing for five breaths.
- The feet step forward to the third position on an inhale.
- The upper body returns to the forward bend on an exhale.
- The body returns to the first position on an inhale and exhales to mountain pose.

Surya namaskara B has 17 positions. It is similar to the A series, with the addition of warrior poses.

Primary series and closing

The postures of the primary power yoga series are learned one at a time, beginning with the primary standing postures. Standing postures include triangle and warrior poses, side stretches, and balancing poses for generating power and balance. Seated poses for strength and surrender include forward-bending, half-lotuses, spinal twisting, bridge poses, back-bending, and other hip-opening poses. Once the primary series has been mastered, the intermediate and then the advanced series are undertaken.

A power yoga closing sequence includes shoulder stands, legs-up-the-wall, the plow, fish, and embryo postures, headstands, and lotus poses. Power yoga practice always concludes with relaxation in the corpse pose or savasana.

QUESTIONS TO ASK YOUR DOCTOR

- Would you advise me to add power yoga to my exercise regimen?
- Do I risk injury from power yoga?
- Are there power yoga postures that I should avoid?
- Are there other precautions I should take when practicing power yoga?
- Can you recommend a power yoga teacher?

Preparation

Power yoga is learned gradually, over a period of time. Typical recommendations call for practicing in the morning or late afternoon, for at least 15–20 minutes, at least four or five days per week. Power yoga should be practiced on an empty stomach—usually at least three or four hours after eating. Practitioners should be clean and well-hydrated. The practice area should be free of distractions. Power yoga does not usually require any props or equipment, other than a non-stick yoga mat. Although books and DVDs are available, power yoga is best learned in a class that is appropriate for one's experience and ability level, with a qualified teacher. Classes that cater to beginners usually modify both the pace and the postures.

Risks

Beginners often find power yoga very difficult. This is especially true for athletes who are physically fit for their sport, but are very tight and out of balance. People sometimes have difficulty staying with power yoga long enough to experience its benefits. Power yoga can cause injuries, including torn muscles, tendons, and ligaments. For these reasons, it is very important to choose a power yoga teacher who encourages beginners, uses modifications and workarounds for difficult asanas, and strives to prevent injury.

Women should not perform inverted postures while menstruating and power yoga may not be appropriate for inexperienced women during pregnancy. Some postures, such as the upward-facing dog and back bends, should be modified or eliminated after the third or fourth month of pregnancy.

Results

People who learn power yoga and continue their practice on a regular basis often find it to be very beneficial. It can increase strength, range of motion, flexibility, and concentration. It can improve cardiovascular health and reduce tightness, tension, and stress. Power yoga can improve athletic performance, help prevent injury, and aid in rehabilitation from injury. Some athletes have found that by increasing their range of motion and reducing their fear of injury, power yoga enables them to train harder and longer.

Resources

BOOKS

Birch, Beryl Bender. *Boomer Yoga: Energizing the Years Ahead for Men & Women.* Portland, ME: Sellers, 2009.

Birch, Beryl Bender. *Power Yoga: The Total Strength and Flexibility Workout.* New York: Fireside, 1995.

Lark, Liz. *Astanga Yoga: Connect to the Core with Power Yoga.* London: Carlton, 2009.

Norberg, Ulrica. *Power Yoga: An Individualized Approach to Strength, Grace, and Inner Peace.* 2nd ed. New York: Skyhorse, 2011.

WEBSITES

"Ashtanga Yoga: The Practice." Shri K. Pattabhi Jois Ashtanga Yoga Institute. 2009. http://kpjayi.org/the-practice (accessed August 16, 2011).

"Ashtanga Yoga—Understanding the Method: Interview with Manju Pattabhi Jois." Ashtanga Yoga Germany. 2009. http://www.ashtanga-yoga-germany.com/Ashtanga%20-Yoga%20Germany%20Deutschland%20Ashtanga-Yoga-Germany.com%20Method%20Manju%20-Pattabhi%20Jois.html (accessed August 16, 2011).

Baptiste, Baron. "Power Warm-Ups." *Yoga Journal.* http://www.yogajournal.com/practice/1696 (accessed August 16, 2011).

"On the Mat—the Ashtanga Yoga Practice." AshtangaYoga.info. August 9, 2011. http://www.ashtangayoga.info/practice (accessed August 16, 2011).

"Yoga for Athletes." The Hard & the Soft Yoga Institute. http://www.power-yoga.com/AboutBeryl/Articles/YogaforAthletes/tabid/156/Default.aspx (accessed August 16, 2011).

ORGANIZATIONS

The Hard & the Soft Yoga Institute, P.O. Box 5009, East Hampton, NY, 11937, (631) 324-8409, info@ power-yoga.com, http://www.power-yoga.com.

Shri K. Pattabhi Jois Ashtanga Yoga Institute, #235 8th Cross, 3rd Stage, Gokulam, Mysore, India, Karnataka, 570002, +91 988 0185-500, shala@kpjayi.org, http://kpjayi.org.

Yoga Alliance, 1701 Clarendon Boulevard, Suite 110, Arlington, VA, 22209, (888) 921-YOGA (9642), http://yogaalliance.org.

Margaret Alic, PhD

Pre-participation screening

Definition

Participation in regular physical activity confers numerous health benefits. However, there are certain risks involved with physical activity. These hazards include risk of acute musculoskeletal injury, myocardial infarction, and sudden cardiac death. Given the public health goal of increasing the number of individuals participating in regular physical activity, there must be also be processes in place to identify those individuals at an increased risk of an exercise-related event. These processes should simultaneously be robust yet not in and of themselves should they provide a barrier to participation in physical activity. Pre-participation health screening involves various measures aimed at evaluating an individual's risk for adverse exercise-related events and formulating suitable recommendations in terms of starting, continuing, or progressing individual physical activity programs in a manner that prevents untoward events.

Purpose

There are several purposes to pre-participation screening, including the following:

- identify individuals who have contraindications for initiating an exercise program
- identify unique needs required of an individual for exercise testing and exercise prescription
- identify individuals with a diagnosed disease or condition who would benefit from exercising in a clinically/medically supervised program
- identify individuals at an increased risk for exercise-related events due to presence of cardiovascular disease risk factors, symptoms, or disease who should be referred for medical examination and physician-supervised exercise testing

Demographics

The extensiveness of pre-participation screening will depend on both the demographics of program participants and characteristics of the exercise/physical activity program. As the **age** range of program participants increases, it is expected that the degree of pre-participation screening will concomitantly increase. For example, the level of screening for college students looking to initiate an **exercise** program at the campus fitness center would likely be fairly brief and might only consist of a single step. Conversely, the pre-participation screening measures required for a **weight loss** program for type 2 diabetics would be expectedly more comprehensive. Along these same lines, if the physical activity program itself will only consist of moderate-intensity exercise, the extent of pre-participation screening once again will likely require a basic approach. On the other hand, if the physical demands of the program are higher (e.g., vigorous-intensity exercise or participation in a scholastic/collegiate sport), a more comprehensive process of pre-participation screening is warranted.

Current trends show that Americans are living longer while the number of U.S. citizens with chronic diseases continues to increase. In the past 100 years, life expectancy at birth in the United States increased from less than 50 years to more than 76 years. The United States Census Bureau has projected that by 2030, the number of adults 65 years of age and older will be approximately 70 million. Approximately 80% of individuals aged 65 years or older are living with at least one chronic health problem, and another 50% are living with two. Moreover, the presence of specific chronic conditions can lead to an even greater propensity of comorbidities. For instance, almost all individuals with type 2 diabetes have at least one other chronic condition and nearly half have three or more comorbidities. These factors make it increasingly likely that individuals entering a facility to initiate a physical activity/exercise program will be at an increased risk. Fitness and exercise professionals should be mindful of these facts when planning the pre-participation screening processes.

Description

Pre-participation screening procedures must provide valid and timely data to be considered appropriate; information on health and medical history, medications, **cardiovascular disease** risk factors, sign/symptoms of cardiovascular disease, and exercise/physical activity habits is commonly collected. Pre-participation screening processes can be generally split into either self-guided or professionally-guided categories.

Self-guided pre-participation screening

As its name implies, self-guided, pre-participation screening is steered by the individual seeking to start a physical activity/exercise program; and prior to beginning, wanting to know whether it is safe to do so or not. Screening tools used for these situations must be straightforward, simple to self-administer, and easy to interpret. Two such tools commonly used include the Physical Activity Readiness Questionnaire (PAR-Q) and the American Heart Association (AHA)/American College of Sports Medicine (ACSM) Health/Fitness Facility Pre-participation Screening Questionnaire. The purpose of using self-guided, pre-participation instruments, such as the PAR-Q, is to make individuals aware of any potential elevated risk they possess. In those instances where increased risk is indicated based on the screening tool, the individual is then encouraged to consult with their physician prior to initiating physical activity or exercise.

Professionally-guided pre-participation screening

Professionally-guided, pre-participation screening is performed by appropriately qualified (i.e., academically and certificated by a professional organization) fitness and exercise professionals. The processes in professionally-guided, pre-participation screening are more advanced and encompass identifying conditions, risk factors, signs, and symptoms that are linked with an increased risk of an adverse exercise-related event. In particular, risk stratification schema is beneficial in identifying those individuals who require further medical screening and exercise testing prior to engaging in vigorous-intensity exercise.

Preparation

In advance of the pre-participation screening process, fitness and exercise professionals should first familiarize themselves with those characteristics that are most likely to increase an individual's chances of an adverse exercise-related event; identification of these particular attributes during the screening process can help prevent future injuries. The characteristics associated with increased cardiovascular and other complications related to exercise can be placed into one of four different categories:

- Clinical status: Individuals who have a history of multiple myocardial infarctions, angina that is unstable or occurs at rest, abnormal heart rhythms at rest, or low serum potassium levels have an increased risk of an adverse exercise-related event.
- Exercise training habits: Individuals who disregard appropriate warm-up and cool down routines and consistently exceed their prescribed exercise training intensity (i.e., intensity violator) have an increased risk of an adverse exercise-related event.
- Exercise testing results: Individuals who are very low fit, have a drop in systolic blood pressure during increasing exercise intensity, experience myocardial ischemia with exertion, or experience serious abnormal heart rhythm with exertion are at an increased risk of an adverse exercise-related event.

KEY TERMS

Abnormal heart rhythm—Refers to an irregularity in the normal beating pattern of the heart.

Angina—Chest pain, discomfort, or tightness; stable angina is typically triggered by increased exertion or exercise. The symptoms of angina usually subside with reduced exertion and rest.

Cardiovascular disease risk factors—Physiological parameters whereby exceeding threshold values places one at an increased risk for developing cardiovascular disease; the specific risk factors used for risk stratification by the American College of Sports Medicine include age, family history for heart disease, high cholesterol, hypertension, obesity, physical inactivity, pre-diabetes, and smoking.

Co-morbidities—Refers to the presence of one or more disorders or diseases in addition to the primary disease; for instance an individual with cardiovascular disease and hypertension, obesity, and Parkinson's disease.

Intensity violator—An individual who consistently exercises at an intensity above their prescribed training intensity range.

Low serum potassium levels—Potassium is a normal electrolyte found in the body; lower than normal concentrations in the blood can cause numerous problems including abnormal heart beats and fatigue.

Myocardial infarction—In laymen's terms a heart attack; refers to changes to the heart tissue, with tissue death the principal one, due to sudden disruptions in oxygenated blood flow.

Sudden cardiac death—Abrupt and unexpected death due to cardiac causes; usually death occurs within one hour of the onset of symptoms.

Risk stratification—A pre-exercise screening process by which individuals at increased risk for an acute cardiac event are identified and subsequently referred for additional medical screening prior to starting an exercise program.

Unstable angina—Chest discomfort, pain, or tightness that occurs at rest and unpredictably; the severity and duration of the symptoms varies.

Untoward event—Refers to an adverse medical occurrence, for example a heart attack or bout of low blood sugar.

Warm-up— A 5 to 10 minute period of low-intensity activity preceding the conditioning phase.

• Other characteristics: Cigarette smokers and men have an increased risk of an adverse exercise-related event compared to non-smokers and women.

Risks

Overall, exercise is safe for most individuals, and exercise per se does not incite adverse cardiovascular events. The risk of an acute myocardial infarction or sudden death during exercise is higher in adults compared to their younger counterparts. The higher prevalence of cardiovascular disease in older adults is responsible for this elevated risk. The absolute risk of sudden death during vigorous-intensity, physical activity has been estimated to be one per year for every 15,000–18,000 people. Similarly, the risk of cardiac events associated with maximal exercise testing is related to the incidence of cardiovascular disease. Although, the overall risk remains relatively low; it has been reported that six cardiac events per 10,000 maximal exercise tests can be expected; the most elevated risk exists for those individuals with underlying or diagnosed cardiovascular disease. The key to minimizing untoward events is to identify those individuals who may be at an increased risk through appropriate pre-participation screening. Accordingly, the proper adjustments can be made to the physical activity/exercise program or exercise test protocol.

Results

The process of risk stratification assigns individuals into one of three risk categories (low, moderate, or high) based on the factors:

• presence or absence of known cardiovascular, pulmonary, and/or metabolic disease

• presence or absence of signs or symptoms suggestive of cardiovascular, pulmonary, and/or metabolic disease

• presence or absence of cardiovascular disease risk factors

Individuals categorized as low risk are those who have no signs or symptoms of nor have they been diagnosed with cardiovascular, pulmonary, and/or metabolic disease. These individuals also possess no more than one cardiovascular disease risk factor. Low risk-stratified individuals have minimal risk for an

QUESTIONS TO ASK YOUR DOCTOR

- Is it safe for me to begin a physical activity or exercise program?

- Are there any specific restrictions to my exercise program?

- Should I adjust my exercise program in any way to reduce the chances of injury or other exercise-related complications?

- Do I require a medical examination and exercise testing prior to beginning my exercise program?

- How much exercise should I do each week?

- Are there any local professionals or programs you can refer me to which can help me get started with my exercise?

acute cardiovascular event during exercise; this population can safely participate in either moderate-intensity or vigorous-intensity exercise.

Individuals categorized as moderate risk are those who have no signs or symptoms of nor have they been diagnosed with cardiovascular, pulmonary, and/or metabolic disease. However, these individuals possess two or more cardiovascular disease risk factors. As such, moderate risk-stratified individuals have an elevated risk for an acute cardiovascular event during exercise. Although it is appropriate for these individuals to begin a moderate-intensity exercise program, prior to engaging in vigorous-intensity exercise it is recommended that moderate risk-stratified individuals first undergo a medical examination and complete a physician supervised exercise test.

Individuals categorized as high risk are those who have one or more signs or symptoms of or have been diagnosed with cardiovascular, pulmonary, and/or metabolic disease. High risk-stratified individuals have a substantial risk for an acute cardiovascular event during exercise. Accordingly, it strongly recommended prior to engaging in either a moderate-intensity or vigorous-intensity exercise program that high risk-stratified individuals first undergo a medical examination and complete a physician supervised exercise test.

Resources

BOOKS

Ehrman, Jonathan K., editor. *ACSM's Resource Manual for Guidelines for Exercise Testing and Prescription*. Philadelphia: Lippincott Williams & Wilkins Health, 2010.

Heyward, Vivian, H., editor. *Advanced Fitness Assessment and Exercise Prescription*. Champaign: Human Kinetics; Wilkins, 2010.

Thompson, Walter R., editor. *ACSM's Guidelines for Exercise Testing and Prescription*. Philadelphia: Lippincott Williams & Wilkins Health, 2010.

PERIODICALS

Garber, C.E. et al. "Quantity and Quality of Exercise for Developing and Maintaining Cardiorespiratory, Musculoskeletal, and Neuromotor Fitness in Apparently Healthy Adults: Guidance for Prescribing Exercise." *Medicine and Science in Sports and Exercise*, (July 2011) 43(7):1334–59.

WEBSITES

"AHA/ACSM Health/Fitness Facility Preparticipation Screening Questionnaire." Doc.stoc.com. (July 21, 2011). http:// http://www.docstoc.com/docs/77953449/AHA-ACSM-Health-Fitness-Facility-Preparticipation-Screening (accessed August 22, 2011).

"Health screening guidelines." Mayoclinic.com. (August 18, 2011). http://www.mayoclinic.com/health/health-screening/WO00112 (accessed August 22, 2011).

"PAR-Q forms." Csep.ca. (August 20, 2011). http://www.csep.ca/english/view.asp?x = 698 (accessed August 22, 2011).

ORGANIZATIONS

American College of Sports Medicine, 401 West Michigan Street, Indianapolis, IN, U.S.A., 46206-1440, (317) 637-9200, Fax: (317) 634-7817, http://www.acsm.org/.

American Council on Exercise, 4851 Paramount Drive, San Diego, CA, U.S.A., 92123, (888) 825-3636, support@acefitness.org, http://www.acefitness.org/.

American Heart Association, 7272 Greenville Ave., Dallas, TX, 75231, 90245, (301) 223-2307, (800) 242-8721, http://www.americanheart.org.

Centers for Disease Control and Prevention, 1600 Clifton Road, Atlanta, GA, U.S.A., 30333, (800) 232-6348, cdcinfo@cdc.gov, http://www.cdc.gov/.

National Coalition for Promoting Physical Activity, 1100 H Street, N.W., Suite 510, Washington, D.C., U.S.A., 20005, (202) 454-7521, Fax: (202) 454-7598, http://www.ncppa.org/membership/organizations/.

Lance C. Dalleck, BA, MS, PhD

Pregnancy *see* **Prenatal exercise**

Prenatal exercise

Definition

Prenatal **exercise** is mild to moderate exercise done during pregnancy to increase muscle tone, improve flexibility, and increase positive self-image.

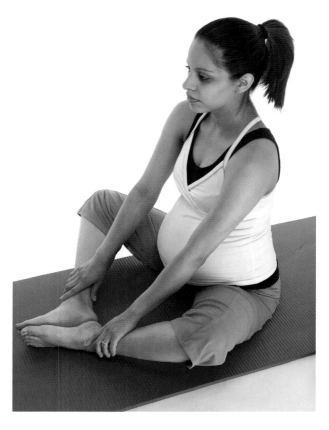

Pregnant woman holding butterfly pose during a prenatal yoga class. (© Ken Hurst/ShutterStock.com)

Purpose

Exercise during pregnancy can be beneficial for both the mother and the developing child. Mild to moderate exercise can reduce some of the negative side effects of pregnancy. It also is believed to help prevent some serious complications that can occur during pregnancy. To obtain the most benefits from exercise during pregnancy with the fewest risks of complications, the exercise should be low-impact and only mild to moderate in intensity. High-intensity workouts during pregnancy can lead to serious negative consequences for both the mother and developing child.

Demographics

A 1988 National Maternal and Infant Health Survey (NMIHS) of 9,953 randomly selected women found that 42% of all women reported exercising during their pregnancy. **Walking** was the most common form of exercise (43%). **Swimming** (12%) and aerobics (12%) were also exercises of choice.

As of 2011, there are no definitive statistics available as to how many pregnant women in North America have tried or presently practice prenatal exercise.

History

Exercise during pregnancy has long been thought to be a good idea to keep both the expectant mother and the developing baby healthy.

The American College of Obstetrics and Gynecology has recommended that pregnant women exercise 30 or more minutes per day on most days, as long as there are no conditions that could make exercise during pregnancy especially risky. Historically, exercise during pregnancy has been found to help the expectant mother feel better, gain less weight in the form of fat, decrease stress, and reduce muscle aches. In addition, exercise during pregnancy has been shown to help improve circulation, resulting in less leg cramps and swelling of ankles, and in the prevention of constipation and varicose veins. Some research has indicated that exercise during pregnancy reduces the risk of diabetes and high-blood pressure caused by pregnancy.

With the advent of personal trainers, many women have chosen to consult with these exercise professionals prior to embarking on prenatal exercise. In part, because working with a trainer or other certified professional throughout pregnancy can help ensure that the exercise routine is changed to continue to ensure safety as the pregnancy progresses. Personal trainers and other fitness professionals are certified by organizations such as the Aerobics and Fitness Association of American and other groups.

Description

Prenatal exercise is exercise undertaken during pregnancy. Common forms of prenatal exercise include most forms of low-impact, low intensity workouts. Walking is considered one of the best forms of prenatal exercise because it is unlikely to cause overheating, stress on the abdomen, or unnecessary bouncing. Swimming is also a recommended form of prenatal exercise because it has a low impact on the joints that are loosened and prone to injury because of the loosening during pregnancy. Caution should be exercised when swimming or working out in a heated pool because increased body temperature can harm the developing baby.

Light strength training, some forms of **yoga**, and exercise classes designed for pregnant women also are common forms of prenatal exercise. Exercising should be done wearing loose clothing and performed on an even surface where the risk of falling is reduced. Taking frequent breaks, resting, and **stretching** all help the expectant mother get the most of prenatal exercise

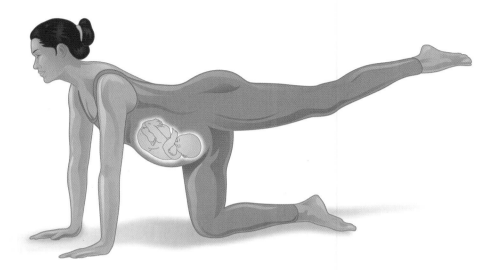

Prenatal exercise

Benefits of prenatal exercise

- Helps improve circulation
- Helps reduce back soreness and maintain mother's muscle tone
- May result in easier delivery, due to increases in muscle strength, endurance, and control of breath
- May reduce risk of gestational diabetes
- Helps keep weight gain within a healthy range

Potential risks of prenatal exercise

Hyperthermia
- An increase in the mother's body temperature can be passed on to the fetus, and therefore it is important for the mother to hydrate regularly and partake in low-impact activies.

Injury
- Falling may seriously harm the baby, and so great caution should be used in selecting exercise activities.

(Illustration by Electronic Illustrators Group. Reproduced by permission of Gale, a part of Cengage Learning.)

while reducing risks. Footwear that supports the arches of the feet helps reduce the strain on the lower back and can help improve balance.

Preparation

Drinking plenty of fluids before exercising can help to ensure proper **hydration**. Stretching for at least five minutes before beginning a workout may reduce the risk of injury.

After completing a workout another period of at least five minutes of stretching is recommended. Drinking additional fluids helps to replace those lost during exercise. It is especially important for pregnant women to **cool down** from exercise gradually.

If a pregnant woman chooses to exercise with a trained professional, she should ask what type of certifications he or she holds. Additionally, the exercise professional should have received special training in the exercise needs of pregnant women. Before beginning an exercise class she should check to ensure that the activity is appropriate for pregnant women. Classes specifically designed for pregnant women are often available at local gyms or community centers. Classes designed for individuals who are not pregnant may be too strenuous, require too much bouncing, or require non-recommended postures.

Risks

The main risks associated with exercising while pregnant are exercising too strenuously and falling because the center of gravity is changed as pregnancy progresses.

KEY TERMS

Aerobic exercise—Exercise that uses large numbers of muscle groups, such as brisk walking or jogging.

Cervix—The narrow, lower end of the uterus forming the opening to the vagina.

Chronic—A word used to describe a long-lasting condition. Chronic conditions often develop gradually and involve slow changes.

Diabetes mellitus—A disease in which insufficient insulin is made by the body to metabolize sugars.

Hypertension—Persistently high blood pressure.

Strength training—The use of resistance to increase the strength of specific muscles or muscle groups.

Women should consult their doctor before beginning any exercise program during pregnancy or before continuing their pre-pregnancy exercise routine. Although exercise during pregnancy is safe for most women, women with certain diseases, conditions, and complications may increase risk to themselves and their baby if they exercise. Women with diabetes, **asthma**, or high **blood pressure** may be told by their doctors to avoid exercise during pregnancy. What is safe depends on the specifics of the woman's general health, the pregnancy, and the seriousness of the condition. Women with a weak cervix, lowered placenta, or who have a history of miscarriages or premature births should not exercise while pregnant without a doctor's consent.

Women who are pregnant should not exercise strenuously. In general, the woman's heart rate should not exceed 140 beats per minute, she should not sweat excessively, and breathing should not be difficult. It should still be possible to talk normally while exercising.

Some exercises are not recommended for pregnant women. Contact sports, aerobics requiring bouncing, and any activity that may cause trauma or contact with the abdomen should be avoided. Exercising in hot weather or in a warm pool is not recommended because increased body temperature can have a negative impact on the baby. Women further along in pregnancy should not do exercises that require lying on the back, as this can decrease the amount of blood flowing to the developing baby. Exercises that put strain on the lower back, such as some types of **weightlifting**, should also be avoided.

As the pregnancy progresses, weight gain and an shifting center of gravity, along with loosening joints, make balancing more difficult. Therefore, exercises toward the end of pregnancy should be structured to reduce the risk of falling, tripping, and injury. Exercise routines should be reviewed and revised periodically throughout the pregnancy.

Results

There are many beneficial results associated with exercising during pregnancy. First and foremost, it can help expectant mothers look and feel better while reducing some of the stress that goes along with pregnancy. Exercising can reduce the occurrence of some of the negative side effects of pregnancy, such as sore back, constipation, and difficulty sleeping.

Exercising during pregnancy also can help reduce unwanted fat storage. Although it is healthy and usual to gain weight during pregnancy, exercise can help reduce the amount of excess fat accumulated during this time. Exercise can also help to keep muscle tone at pre-pregnancy levels for many women. Exercising during pregnancy may make delivering the baby easier through increased muscle strength, improved endurance, and improved breathing technique.

Some studies have shown that regular exercise during pregnancy can reduce the risk of preeclampsia, a serious condition in which blood pressure increases and **protein** is present in the urine. Preeclampsia can be very dangerous, even fatal, for both the mother and the developing baby. Exercise also has been found to reduce the risk of gestational diabetes. Gestational diabetes is diabetes that occurs during pregnancy, causing the body to change the way it uses sugar. Gestational diabetes can be extremely harmful to the developing baby.

Resources

BOOKS

Aberg, Anna. *The 30-Minute Pregnancy Workout Book: The Complete Light Weight Program For Fitness.* New York: St. Martin's Griffin, 2008.

American College of Obstetricians and Gynecologists, Women's, Health Care Physicians. *Your Pregnancy and Childbirth: Month to Month,* 5th ed. Washington, DC: American College of Obstetricians and Gynecologists, 2010.

Roizen, Michael F., and Mehmet C. Oz. *You Having a Baby: The Owner's Manual to a Happy and Healthy Pregnancy.* New York: Free Press, 2009.

Swank, Ann Marie, and Patrick Hagerman. *Resistance Training For Special Populations.* Clifton Park, NY: Delmar Cengage Learning, 2010.

QUESTIONS TO ASK YOUR DOCTOR

- Do I have any conditions that might mean I should not exercise while I am pregnant?
- Are my typical exercise activities still good choices for while I am pregnant?
- How soon after delivering the baby will I be able to exercise normally again?
- Can you recommend any local classes or centers that specialize in exercise during pregnancy?
- Do I have any conditions that might put me at high risk during certain types of exercise?
- What is a good way to contact your office if I experience any problems during exercise?

PERIODICALS

Duncombe, D., Wetheim, E. H., Skouteris, H., Paxton, S. K., and Kelly, L. "Factors Related to Exercise Over the Course of Pregnancy Including Women's Beliefs About the Safety of Exercise During Pregnancy." *Midwifery,* (August 2009), 25(4):430–8.

Fell, D. B., Joseph, K. S., Armson, B. A. and Dodds, L. "The Impact of Pregnancy on Physical Activity Level." *Maternal and Child Health Journal,* (September 2009), 13(5): 597–603.

Kalisiak, B., and Spitznagle, T. "What Effect Does an Exercise Program for Healthy Pregnant Women Have on the Mother, Fetus, and Child?" *Physical Medicine and Rehabilitation,* (March 2009), 1(3): 261–6.

ORGANIZATIONS

American Pregnancy Association, 1431 Greenway Drive, Suite 800, Irving, TX, 75038, (972)550-0140, Fax: (972)550-0800, questions@americanpregnancy.org, www.americanpregnancy.org.

National Health &Exercise Science Association, 3701 Flintridge Court, Brookeville, MD, 20833, (301)576-0611, 1-866-481-5957, Fax: (301)685-1819, info@nhesa.org, www.nhesa.org.

Tish Davidson, AM
Laura Jean Cataldo, RN, EdD

President's Challenge

Definition

The President's Challenge is America's primary physical activity and fitness initiative and a cornerstone of the **U.S. President's Council on Fitness, Sports, & Nutrition**.

Purpose

The purpose of the President's Challenge is to motivate all Americans to increase their physical activity, fitness, and health. Scientific evidence conclusively demonstrates that as little as 150 minutes of moderate-intensity physical activity—such as brisk walking—every week has significant health benefits for adults. Children require a minimum of 60 minutes of daily physical activity. The President's Challenge is aimed at youth and adults of all ages. It can be utilized by individuals, groups of friends, schools, and organizations. The President's Challenge provides research-based information, easy-to-use tools, fun motivators, and awards.

Demographics

An estimated 34 million adult Americans are obese and many more are overweight. Only 35% of adults aged 18 and older engage in regular leisure-time physical activity and 33% engage in no leisure-time physical activity. Almost one-third of American children are overweight or obese, including almost 40% of black and Hispanic children. Only one-third of high-school students get the recommended amount of physical activity. The President's Challenge is aimed at Americans of all ages and abilities, including those with disabilities. It hopes to reach individuals, educators, schools, homeschoolers, workplaces, and community groups and organizations.

Description

Participation in all President's Challenge programs is free. Its website provides program descriptions, entry forms, information about the benefits of fitness, and advice on setting activity and fitness goals. It also has suggestions for increasing and maintaining activity specific levels, specific activities, and encouraging students and employees to become physically active. The website includes a **body mass index** (BMI) calculator.

Origins

The President's Challenge was founded in the early 1960s by President John F. Kennedy as a youth fitness test. It has promoted physical activity and **exercise** through its school-based youth fitness testing program for more than half a century. The President's Challenge is administered through a co-sponsorship agreement between the President's Council on Fitness, Sports, & Nutrition and the Amateur Athletic Union (AAU). Over the years it has expanded to include four separate challenges: the youth physical fitness test, the adult fitness test, the Presidential Activity Lifestyle Award (PALA), and the Presidential Champions Award.

Youth physical fitness test

The youth physical fitness test is designed to measure the physical fitness of children and teens and to be used as a tool by educators for improving fitness. It measures fitness levels on five activities:

- Abdominal strength and endurance is measured by the number of curl-ups performed correctly in one minute, with a partner holding down the student's feet, or by performing a target number of three-second partial curl-ups with a partner cupping the student's head.
- Speed and agility are measured by timing a shuttle run.
- Heart/lung endurance is assessed by the time on a 0.25–1-mi (0.4–1.6-km) run/walk.
- Upper-body strength and endurance is measured by the number of properly performed pull-ups or right-angle three-second push-ups, or by length of time for a flexed-arm hang.
- Flexibility of the lower back and hamstrings are assessed by a V-sit reach test—the arm distance held for three seconds while sitting upright with the legs apart—or by a sit-and-reach test that requires a specially constructed box.

There is no limit to the number of attempts a student can make at each activity. Awards are offered for all students who complete the activities, based on their fitness level scores. The Participant Physical Fitness Award is for students who participate in all five activities, but score below the 50th percentile on one or more. The National Physical Fitness Award is for students who score above the 50th percentile on all five activities. The Presidential Physical Fitness Award is for students who score at or above the 85th percentile on all activities.

After creating an online account, educators can use the free Fitness File software to enter student scores, track tests, compare their students' scores with national percentiles, and generate reports. It is recommended that students be tested twice a year, in the fall and spring, to measure their progress over the year. The percentile standards for each award are based on the 1985 National School Population Fitness Survey. The standards were validated in 1998 through comparison with a large 1994 nationwide sample.

Adult fitness test

The adult fitness test is for those aged 18 and older who are in good health. It estimates health-related fitness components that can lower the risk for medical complications such as high **blood pressure**, diabetes, or **low back pain**. The adult fitness test assesses:

- aerobic fitness—the ability of the heart and lungs to supply the muscles with oxygen—as determined by heart rate after a 1-mi (1.6-km) walk or by time on a 1.5-mi (2.4-km) run
- muscular strength and endurance—the ability to easily perform normal activities while protecting the lower back from injury—as measured by the number of half sit-ups performed in one minute and the number of correctly performed standard or modified push-ups
- flexibility—the ability to move joints through their proper range of motion—as measured by the farthest distance in a sit-and-reach test
- waist circumference and BMI or the proportion of body fat, as determined using a table or online calculator (weight in pounds, divided by height in inches squared, multiplied by 703; weight in kilograms divided by height in meters squared)

After completing the activities, participants enter their results online and receive evaluations. Participants retake the test to measure their progress as they increase their physical activity. Eventually they may choose to enroll in the PALA or Presidential Champions challenges.

PALA

The PALA challenge is for everyone—from young children to seniors—who want to incorporate physical activity into their everyday lives. The PALA is also an important component of the Let's Move! initiative, a program developed by First Lady Michelle Obama to combat childhood **obesity**. Obama's goal was to double the number of youth earning the PALA by the end of the 2010–2011 school year. The President's Council on Fitness, Sports, & Nutrition expanded upon that goal with the Million PALA Challenge, a call for one million Americans to enroll in and earn the PALA by September 2011.

The PALA challenge is designed to jumpstart a regular fitness routine through a six-week commitment to daily physical activity. For children and teens between the ages of six and 17, the goal is to be active for 60 minutes daily, at least five days per week, for six out of eight weeks. Alternatively, daily activity steps can be counted with a **pedometer**, with a goal of 11,000 daily steps for girls and 13,000 steps for boys. The goal for adults aged 18 and older is to be active for 30 minutes daily, at least five days per week, for six out of eight weeks. Alternatively, daily activity steps can be counted using a pedometer, with a goal of 8,500 daily steps.

Body Mass Index (BMI)—A measure of body fat; the ratio of weight in kilograms to the square of height in meters.

Hamstrings—The three muscles at the back of the thigh.

Let's Move—First Lady Michelle Obama's initiative for combating childhood obesity that incorporates aspects of the President's Challenge.

Obesity—Excessive weight due to accumulation of fat, usually defined as a body mass index of 30 or above or body weight greater than 30% above normal on standard height-weight tables.

Overweight—A body mass index between 25 and 30.

Pedometer—Step counter; a device that counts each step by detecting hip motion.

Percentile—A rank in a population that has been divided into 100 equal groups; thus, test results in

the 50th percentile indicate that half of those who took the test scored higher and half scored lower.

Presidential Activity Lifestyle Award (PALA)—A component of the President's Challenge, the PALA is a six-week commitment to daily physical activity, designed for everyone from young children to seniors.

Pull-up—An exercise or test of upper-body strength in which the suspended body is pulled up by the arms.

Push-up—Press-up; a test or exercise in which the body is lowered and pushed up with the arms.

Sit-up—A common test or exercise for strength and endurance of the abdominal muscles.

Validation—The extent to which a test measures the trait that it is designed to assess.

After creating an individual online account, progress can be tracked online with a free personal activity log. A paper log is also available. Times can be logged in intervals as short as five minutes, although activity periods of ten minutes or longer are preferred. Pedometer steps or distances for some activities, such as biking, can also be logged. There are more than 100 activities to choose from, including **walking**, **running**, playing tag, **basketball**, tennis, **yoga**, gardening, or mopping the floor. Any physical activity that uses large muscle groups and burns **energy** counts toward the PALA. The activity tracker notifies participants when their goals have been reached and they can order their awards. Participants can earn the PALA in less than two months and then work toward additional PALA awards or move on to the Presidential Champions challenge.

The PALA has been adopted by schools, workplaces, community groups, and teams of friends, as well as individuals and families. Schools have incorporated it into their existing fitness programs or implemented special six-week programs culminating in an awards celebration. The General Mills Foundation, a President's Challenge partner, sponsors PALA Family Fitness Nights through its Box Tops for Education (BTFE) program. Other President's Challenge partners promoting the PALA include the National Recreation and Park Association, Boys and Girls Clubs of America, and the YMCA.

Presidential Champions

The Presidential Champions challenge is for physically active children and adults who have completed the PALA and want to increase the intensity and frequency of their activities. It is a point-based program available only online. Points, based on the amount of energy burned with each activity, are logged into the free online activity tracker. A bronze award requires 40,000 points, a silver 90,000 points, a gold 160,000 points, and a platinum award requires one million points. There is no time limit and there are a wide variety of activities to choose from—from running or playing **golf** to learning karate or walking the dog. Running five miles every day will earn a bronze award in about six weeks. Moderate exercise will take somewhat longer. As with the PALA, activities can be logged in increments as short as five minutes, although at least 10-minute increments are preferable. Pedometer steps or distances for activities such as biking can also be logged. The activity tracker notifies participants when they have reached their goals and can order awards.

The Presidential Champions challenge is open to individuals and groups. It encourages competitions between classrooms, co-workers, and friends, as well as yearly challenges.

School recognition programs

The President's Challenge selects elementary and secondary schools as Demonstration Centers for renewable three-year terms. To become a Demonstration Center, schools must:

- encourage health appraisals for all students
- provide regular physical education
- promote their physical education programs; for example, through take-home materials or local newspaper articles
- develop programs for helping sedentary students increase their daily physical activities
- provide students with motivational tools
- monitor annual student progress
- offer students opportunities for participating in the President's Challenge
- arrange for others to observe their programs in action

Advocates

Educational institutions, corporations, government agencies, and medical, scientific, and nonprofit organizations can partner with the President's Challenge as advocates. There are a wide range of advocate activities, including subsidizing youth awards, sponsoring employee health and wellness programs, and incorporating the President's Challenge into special promotions and initiatives. Advocates and other partners receive special access and recognition.

Preparation

Before embarking on the President's Challenge, educators should review the medical status of each student to identify any medical, orthopedic, or other health issues. Students should be taught correct techniques for all activities, including running style and pacing.

Adults should complete the Preparticipation Screening Questionnaire, provided by the American Heart Association and American College of Sports Medicine, before performing the adult fitness test, to assess their risk for cardiovascular events. Some people may need to take additional steps prior to exercise testing. The one-mile walk of the adult aerobic fitness test should only be attempted by those who routinely walk for 15–20 minutes, or the equivalent, several times per week. The 1.5-mi (2.4 km) run should only be attempted by those who routinely run continuously for at least 20 minutes three or more times per week.

The Mayo Clinic has designed a simple four-step assessment, based on the President's Challenge, for embarking on a fitness program. It is available at http://

> ## QUESTIONS TO ASK YOUR DOCTOR
>
> - Am I healthy enough to take the adult fitness test?
> - What is my body mass index (BMI)?
> - Am I healthy enough for the Presidential Activity Lifestyle Award (PALA) challenge?
> - How much physical activity do you recommend?
> - What physical activities do you recommend for me?

www.mayoclinic.com/health/fitness/SM00086. The assessment is repeated six weeks after beginning an exercise program and periodically thereafter, with goals adjusted as fitness improves. A physician or personal trainer can offer additional guidance based on the results of the assessment.

Risks

Although any physical activity carries a risk of injury, healthy adults are at low risk for cardiovascular events—dizziness, fainting, irregular heartbeat, or rarely, a heart attack—from exercise testing. However some risk factors or diseases can increase one's risk. Overall, there are about six abnormal cardiovascular events per 10,000 adults who undergo exercise testing.

Results

More than 50 million children and teens have been recognized by the President's Challenge for their fitness achievements. More than one million Americans aged six and older have earned a PALA or Presidential Champions Award. In addition to awards at every level of the President's Challenge, T-shirts are available for the PALA and Presidential Champions challenges. Schools with excellent physical education programs are eligible for State Champions and Demonstration Center awards.

Resources

BOOKS

Bakewell, Lisa. *Fitness Information for Teens.* 2nd ed. Detroit: Omnigraphics, 2009.

PERIODICALS

"The President's Challenge: Physical Activity & Fitness Awards Program." *Strategies: A Journal for Physical and Sport Educators* 24, no. 2 (November-December 2010): S19–22.

WEBSITES

"Am I Healthy Enough to Take the Test?" The President's Challenge Adult Fitness Test. http://www.adultfitnesstest. org/riskQuestionaire.aspx (accessed July 25, 2011).

"Exercise and Physical Activity." Eunice Kennedy Shriver National Institute of Child Health & Human Development. February 2, 2011.http://www.nichd.nih.gov/health/topics/Exercise_and_Physical_Activity.cfm (accessed July 22, 2011).

Let's Move! America's Move to Raise a Healthier Generation of Kids. http://www.letsmove.gov (accessed July 24, 2011).

Mayo Clinic Staff. "How Fit Are You? See How You Measure Up." Mayo Clinic. February 19, 2011. http://www.mayoclinic.com/health/fitness/SM00086 (accessed September 1, 2011).

"Physical Activity Guidelines for Americans." Office of Disease Prevention & Health Promotion, U.S. Department of Health and Human Services. November 4, 2009. http://www.health.gov/paguidelines (accessed July 24, 2011).

The President's Challenge Adult Fitness Test. http://www.adultfitnesstest.org/ (accessed July 22, 2011).

ORGANIZATIONS

Amateur Athletic Union, P.O. Box 22409, Lake Buena Vista, FL, 32830, (407) 934-7200, Fax: (407) 934-7242, (800) AAU-4USA, http://aausports.org.

American College of Sports Medicine, P.O. Box 1440, Indianapolis, IN, 46206-1440, (317) 637-9200, Fax: (317) 634-7817, http://www.acsm.org.

American Heart Association, National Center, 7272 Greenville Avenue, Dallas, TX, 75231, (800) AHA-USA-1 (242-8721), http://www.heart.org.

Office of Disease Prevention and Health Promotion, U.S. Department of Health and Human Services, 1101 Wootton Parkway, Suite LL100, Rockville, MD, 20852, (240) 453-8280, Fax: (240) 453-8282, http://odphp.osophs.dhhs.gov.

President's Challenge, 501 North Morton Street, Suite 203, Bloomington, IN, 47404, Fax: (812) 855-8999, (800) 258-8146, preschal@indiana.edu, http://www.presidentschallenge.org.

President's Council on Fitness, Sports, & Nutrition, 1101 Wootton Parkway, Suite 560, Rockville, MD, 20852, (240) 276-9567, Fax: (240) 276-9860, fitness@hhs.gov, http://www.fitness.gov.

Margaret Alic, PhD

Protein

Definition

Proteins are compounds composed of carbon, hydrogen, oxygen, and nitrogen that are arranged as strands of amino acid. They play an essential role in the cellular maintenance, growth, and functioning of the human body. Serving as the basic structural molecule of all the tissues in the body, protein makes up nearly 17% of the total body weight. To understand protein's role and function in the human body, it is important to understand its basic structure and composition.

Description

Proteins are all around us. Much of the body's dry weight is protein; even bones are about one-quarter protein. The animals humans eat and the microbes that attack an individual's body are likewise largely protein. Leather, wool, and silk clothing are nearly pure protein. The insulin that keeps a patient with diabetes alive and the clot-busting enzymes that may save heart attack patients are also proteins. Proteins can even be found working at industrial sites—protein enzymes produce not only the high-fructose corn syrup that sweetens most soft drinks, but also fuel-grade ethanol (alcohol) and other gasoline additives.

Function

Within human bodies and those of other living things, proteins serve many functions. They digest foods and turn them into **energy**; they move the body and move molecules about within cells; they let some substances pass through cell membranes while keeping others out; they turn light into chemical energy, making both vision and photosynthesis possible; they allow cells to detect and react to hormones and toxins in their surroundings; and, as antibodies, they protect the body against foreign invaders. There are numerous types of proteins—possibly more than 100,000.

Amino acids

Amino acids are the fundamental building blocks of protein. Long chains of amino acids, called polypeptides, make up the multicomponent, large complexes of protein. The arrangement of amino acids along the chain determines the structure and chemical properties of the protein. Amino acids consist of the following elements: carbon, hydrogen, oxygen, nitrogen, and, sometimes, sulfur. The general structure of amino acids consists of a carbon center and its four substituents that consist of an amino group (NH_2), an organic acid (carboxyl) group (COOH), a hydrogen atom (H), and a fourth group known as the R-group. These four groups determine the structural identity and chemical properties of the amino acid. The first three groups are common to all amino acids. The basic amino acid structure is $R-CH(NH_2)-COOH$.

The human body uses twenty different forms of amino acids. These forms are distinguished by the fourth variable substituent, the R-group, that can be a chain of different lengths or a carbon-ring structure. For example, if hydrogen represents the R-group, the amino acid is known as glycine, a polar but uncharged amino acid; while the methyl (CH_3) group is known as alanine, a nonpolar amino acid. The chemical components of the R-group essentially determine the identity, structure, and function of the amino acid.

The structural and chemical relatedness of the R-groups allows classification of the twenty amino acids into chemical groups. Amino acids can be classified according to optical activity (the ability to polarize light), acidity and basicity, polarity and nonpolarity, or hydrophilicity (water-loving) and hydrophobicity (water-fearing). These categories offer clues to the function and reactivity of the amino acids in proteins. The biochemical properties of amino acids determine the role and function of protein in the human body.

Of the twenty amino acids, eleven are considered nonessential (or dispensable), meaning that the body is able to adequately synthesize them, and nine are essential (or indispensable), meaning that the body is unable to adequately synthesize them to meet the needs of the cell. They must be supplied through the diet. Foods that have protein contain both nonessential and essential amino acids, the latter of which the body can use to synthesize some of the nonessential amino acids. A healthful diet should consist of a sufficient and balanced supply of both essential and nonessential amino acids in order to ensure high levels of protein production.

Protein quality: nutritive value

Meat, milk, eggs, poultry, and seafood and soya are considered high-quality, "complete" proteins because they have all the essential amino adds (protein's building blocks) in adequate amounts. Those sources are considered more complete than vegetable protein, such as beans, peas, and grains, also considered a good—even if not complete—source of amino acids. Except for soy, plant sources—nuts, beans, seeds, and grains—are deficient in or contain low levels of one or more of the essential amino acids. But plant foods contain other vital nutrients (such as phytochemicals and fiber) not found in animal foods. Dietitians recommend that a healthy diet consist of foods from a variety of sources and include 10–20% of daily **calories** from protein (poultry, fish, dairy, soy protein, nuts, legumes, eggs, peanut butter, and vegetable sources). Incomplete proteins can be combined to provide all the essential amino acids, though combinations of incomplete proteins must be consumed at the same time, or within a short period of time (within four hours), to obtain the maximum nutritive value from the amino acids. Such combination diets generally yield a high-quality protein meal, providing sufficient amounts and proper balance of the essential amino acids needed by the body to function.

Protein processing: digestion, absorption, and metabolism

Protein digestion begins when the food reaches the stomach and stimulates the release of hydrochloric acid (HCl) by the parietal cells located in the gastric mucosa of the GI (gastrointestinal) tract. Hydrochloric acid provides for a very acidic environment that helps the protein digestion process in two ways: (1) through an acid-catalyzed hydrolysis reaction of breaking peptide bonds (the chemical process of breaking peptide bonds is referred to as a hydrolysis reaction because water is used to break the bonds); and (2) through conversion of the gastric enzyme pepsinogen (an inactive precursor) to pepsin (the active form). Pepsinogen is stored and secreted by the chief cells that line the stomach wall. Once converted into the active form, pepsin attacks the peptide bonds that link amino acids together, breaking the long polypeptide chain into shorter segments of amino acids known as dipeptides and tripeptides. These protein fragments are then further broken down in the duodenum of the small intestines. The brush border enzymes that work on the surface of epithelial cells of the small intestines hydrolyze the protein fragments into amino acids.

The cells of the small intestine actively absorb the amino acids through a process that requires energy. The amino acids travel through the hepatic portal vein to the liver, where the nutrients are processed into glucose or fat (or released into the bloodstream). The tissues in the body take up the amino acids rapidly for glucose production, growth and maintenance, and other vital cellular functioning. For the most part, the body does not store protein, as the **metabolism** of amino acids occurs within a few hours.

Amino acids are metabolized in the liver into useful forms that are used as building blocks of protein in tissues. The body may utilize the amino acids for either anabolic or catabolic reactions. Anabolism refers to the chemical process through which digested and absorbed products are used to effectively build or repair bodily tissues, or to restore vital substances broken down through metabolism. Catabolism, on the other hand, is the process that results in the release of energy through the breakdown of nutrients, stored materials, and cellular substances. Anabolic and catabolic reactions work hand-in-hand, and the energy produced in catabolic processes is used to fuel essential anabolic processes. The vital biochemical reaction of glycolysis (in which glucose is oxidized to produce carbon dioxide, water, and cellular energy) in the form of adenosine triphosphate, or ATP, is a prime example of a catabolic reaction. The energy released, as ATP, from such a reaction is used to fuel important anabolic processes, such as protein synthesis.

The metabolism of amino acids can be understood from the dynamic catabolic and anabolic processes. In the process referred to as deamination, the nitrogen-containing amino group (NH_2) is cleaved from the amino acid unit. In this reaction that requires vitamin B_6 as a cofactor, the amino group is transferred to an acceptor keto-acid that can form a new amino acid. Through this process, the body is able to make the nonessential amino acids not provided by a patient's diet. The keto-acid intermediate can also be used to synthesize glucose to ultimately yield energy for the body, and the cleaved nitrogen-containing group is transformed into urea, a waste product, and excreted as urine.

Vital protein functions

Proteins are vital to basic cellular and body functions, including cellular regeneration and repair, tissue maintenance and regulation, hormone and enzyme production, fluid balance, and the provision of energy.

CELLULAR AND TISSUE PROVISIONING. Protein is an essential component for every type of cell in the body, including muscles, bones, organs, tendons, and ligaments. Protein is also needed in the formation of enzymes, antibody, hormones, blood-clotting factors, and blood-transport proteins. The body is constantly undergoing renewal and repair of tissues. The amount of protein needed to build new tissue or maintain structure and function depends on the rate of renewal or the stage of growth and development. For example, the intestinal tract is renewed every couple of days, whereas blood cells have a life span of 60 to 120 days. Furthermore, an infant uses as much as one-third of the dietary protein for building new connective and muscle tissues.

HORMONE AND ENZYME PRODUCTION. Amino acids are the basic components of hormones, which are essential chemical signaling messengers of the body. Hormones are secreted into the bloodstream by endocrine glands, such as the thyroid gland, adrenal glands, pancreas, and other ductless glands, and regulate bodily functions and processes. For example, the hormone insulin is secreted by the pancreas and works to lower the blood glucose level after meals. Insulin is made up of 48 amino acids.

Enzymes play an essential kinetic role in biological reactions and are composed of large protein molecule. Enzymes facilitate the rate of reactions by acting as catalysts and lowering the activation energy barrier between the reactants and the products of the reactions. All chemical reactions that occur during the digestion of food and the metabolic processes in tissues require enzymes. Enzymes are vital to the overall function of the body, and indicate the fundamental and significant role of proteins.

FLUID BALANCE. The presence of blood protein molecules, such as albumins and globulins, are critical factors in maintaining the proper fluid balance between cells and extracellular space. Proteins are present in the capillary beds—one-cell-thick vessels that connect the arterial and venous beds. They cannot flow outside the capillary beds into the tissue because of their large size. Blood fluid is pulled into the capillary beds from the tissue through the mechanics of oncotic pressure, in which the pressure exerted by the protein molecules counteracts the **blood pressure**. Therefore, blood proteins are essential in maintaining and regulating fluid balance between the blood and tissue. The lack of blood proteins results in clinical edema, or tissue swelling, because there is insufficient pressure to pull fluid back into the blood from the tissues. The condition of edema is serious and can lead to many medical problems.

ENERGY PROVISION. Protein is not a significant source of energy for the body when there are sufficient amounts of carbohydrate and **fats** available, nor is protein a storable energy, as in the case of fats and **carbohydrates**. However, if insufficient amounts of carbohydrates and fats are ingested, protein is used for energy needs of the body. The use of protein for energy is not necessarily economical for the body, because tissue maintenance, growth, and repair are compromised to meet energy needs. If taken in excess, protein can be converted into body fat. Protein yields slightly more usable energy (4 kcal/g) than carbohydrates (3.75 kcal/g). Although not the main source of usable energy, protein provides the essential amino acids needed for adenine, the nitrogenous base of ATP, as well as other nitrogenous substances, such as creatine phosphate (nitrogen is an essential element for important compounds in the body).

Role in human health

On a per kilogram basis, protein requirements in humans are highest in infancy and gradually decline throughout life, except in circumstances such as pregnancy, lactation, and illness. The Recommended Daily Intake (RDI) suggests protein requirements based on age incrementally. The amount of protein needed also depends on body weight, but it is not a linear relationship. A person who weighs 400 lb (181 kg) does not need four times as much protein as a person weighing 100 lb (45 kg). From birth to three months, protein needs are at their highest (2.2 g/kg of body weight). The requirement for adult males and females is 0.8 g/kg. This amount is equal to about 63 g of dietary protein for a male aged 25–50 years who weighs 174 lb (79 kg), and 50 g for a female aged 25–50 years who weighs 139 lb (63 kg). The average Western diet contains ample amounts of protein.

Special needs of athletes

Most people in the United States have sufficient amounts of protein in their diet. The RDI values of protein are generally considered enough protein for individuals who engage in recreational sports and fitness activities. Professional athletes, such as runners, triathletes, dancers, and individuals who play sports professionally may have increased protein needs. These needs may be increased during times of intense physical training when new muscle is being built.

Athletes should be careful about where their protein comes from. Specialty protein bars and shakes may contain incomplete proteins and may contain high levels of fat and calories. It is recommended that proteins come from natural animal and plant sources and be only minimally processed. Athletes who are vegetarian or vegan should pay special attention to mix different incomplete proteins in each meal to ensure that their bodies can produce all of the amino acids needed for good health.

Certain athletes such as dancers, gymnasts, and wrestlers who are especially weight conscious may be at an increased risk for protein deficiency if they do not eat enough to ingest all of the protein necessary each day. The nitrogen balance index (NBI) is used to evaluate the amount of protein used by the body in comparison with the amount of protein supplied from daily food intake. The body is in the state of nitrogen (or protein) equilibrium when the intake and usage of protein is equal. The body has a positive nitrogen balance when the intake of protein is greater than that expended by the body. In this case, the body can build and develop new tissue. Since the body does not store protein, the overconsumption of protein can result in the excess amount being converted into fat and stored as adipose tissue. The body has a negative nitrogen balance when the intake of protein is less than

that expended by the body. In this case, protein intake is less than required, and the body cannot maintain or build new tissues.

Common diseases and disorders

Most people in industrialized countries eat more protein than they need. In the United States, true protein deficiency is rare except when excess protein is lost and protein requirements are increased, as in cases of:

- burns
- fever
- fractures
- surgery
- wasting and/or cachexia associated with cancer (approximately half of all cancer patients experience cachexia, a wasting syndrome that induces metabolic changes leading to a loss of muscle and fat)
- chronic renal failure, when the patient is undergoing hemodialysis or peritoneal dialysis

Protein-modified diets

High-protein diets are designed to provide about 1.5 g of protein for each kilogram of body weight. Complex proteins, such as milk and meats, should make up one-half to two-thirds of the daily protein requirement. High-protein diets are recommended for people who have:

- an increased need for protein due to protein-calorie malnutrition; severe stress; or conditions such as AIDS, cancer, or burns with high metabolic rates that lead to the loss of large amounts of protein

- malabsorption syndromes, celiac disease, or other disorders characterized by poor food absorption

A low-protein diet excludes dairy products and meats, and requires that about three-fourths of the daily allowance of protein come from high-value protein sources. Supplements may be prescribed to prevent amino-acid deficiencies. Low-protein diets are used in treatment of conditions such as liver cirrhosis and kidney disease (excluding chronic renal failure patients who have increased protein needs because of losses that occur during dialysis).

Protein deficiency

A negative nitrogen balance represents a state of protein deficiency, in which the body is breaking down tissues faster than they are being replaced. The ingestion of insufficient amounts of protein, or food with poor protein quality, can result in serious medical conditions in which an individual's overall health is compromised. The **immune system** is severely affected; the amount of blood plasma decreases, leading to medical conditions such as anemia or edema; and the body becomes vulnerable to infectious diseases and other serious conditions. Treatment or prevention of this condition lies in adequate consumption of protein-rich foods.

Resources

BOOKS

Bean, Anita. *The Complete Guide to Sports Nutrition*, 6th ed. London: A. and C. Black, 2009.

Kruskall, Laura J. *Fitness Professionals' Guide to Sports Nutrition and Weight Management*. Monterey, CA: Healthy Learning, 2010.

Shryer, Donna, and Jodi Forschmiedt. *Peak Performance: Sports Nutrition*. New York: Cavendish Benchmark, 2010.

Smolin, Lori A., and Mary B. Grosvenor. *Nutrition for Sports and Exercise*, 2nd ed. New York: Chelsea House, 2010.

PERIODICALS

Fuhrman, Joel, and Deana K. Ferreri. "Fueling the Vegetarian (Vegan) Athlete." *Current Sports Medicine Reports* 9, no. 4 (July-August 2010): 233–241.

Tipton, Kevin D. "Nutrition for the Acute Exercise-Induced Injuries." *Annals of Nutrition and Metabolism* 57, Supplement 2 (2010):43–53.

WEBSITES

Osterweil, Neil. "The Benefits of Protein." WebMD. (2004). http://www.webmd.com/fitness-exercise/guide/benefits-protein (accessed November 9, 2011).

"Protein". National Center for Chronic Disease Prevention and Health Promotion. (October 19, 2011). http://www.cdc.gov/nutrition/everyone/basics/protein.html (accessed November 9, 2011).

ORGANIZATIONS

American Dietetic Association, 120 S. Riverside Plaza, Suite 2000, Chicago, IL, 60606, (800) 877-1600, http://www.eatright.org.

American Society for Nutrition, 9650 Rockville Pike, Bethesda, MD, 20814, (301) 634-7050, Fax: (301) 634-7892, http://www.nutrition.org.

National Association of Sports Nutrition, 7710 Balboa Ave., Suite 311, San Diego, CA, 92111, (888) 694-0317, http://nasnurtition.com.

Office of Dietary Supplements, National Institutes of Health, 6100 Executive Blvd., Room 3B01, MSC 7517, Bethesda, MD, 20892-7517, (301) 435-2920, Fax: (301) 480-1845, ods@nih.gov, http://ods.od.nih.gov.

Tish Davidson, AM

Protein drinks *see* **Energy drinks**

Protein metabolism and exercise

Definition

Up to 40% of the **protein** found in the body exists as muscle tissue. The turnover and replacement of this protein mass is called protein **metabolism**. Protein metabolism in muscle accounts for about one-half to one-third of the total protein turnover in the body.

KEY TERMS

Amino acids—Small organic molecules that are the building blocks of proteins. There are 20 essential amino acids that must be present in the diet.

Insulin—A pancreatic hormone involved in systemic control of energy storage (glucose and fat reserves) in response to food intake.

Protein—A polymer of amino acids comprised of peptide linkages (amide bonds). Proteins are the major structural elements of muscle.

Description

The basic building block of muscle is protein. The balance between protein production versus protein breakdown determines whether muscles grow or shrink. Physical activity or **exercise**, particularly in the form of resistance exercise, results in net synthesis of protein, and muscle growth. However, the ability of exercise to change protein metabolism involves a complex interplay between the type of physical activity (intensity, frequency, duration), dietary considerations, and hormonal input.

Function

Muscle mass is governed by a use-disuse principle. With increased physical activity, muscles adapt by growing larger (**muscle hypertrophy**), whereas in sedentary states the loss of mechanical activity leads to muscle breakdown (atrophy).

The acute metabolic response of muscle is actually a net increase in protein breakdown. This increase in protein breakdown serves several positive physiological functions. Proteins are built from small organic molecules called amino acids. The degradation of protein in response to exercise enables muscle to produce a steady supply of amino acids that are required as key intermediates in aerobic metabolism via the Krebs cycle. Second, protein degradation mobilizes amino acids, particularly alanine, into the bloodstream for use by the liver to regenerate glucose (alanine-glucose cycle). Third, mechanical stresses can damage the specialized cellular structures that are important for muscle contraction, and increased protein turnover ensures that any such structural defects are removed and repaired in an efficient manner. However, to offset this protein degradation, protein synthesis rates are rapidly increased in the post-exercise recovery phase.

A key determinant of the protein synthesis rate in muscle is the availability of free amino acids. This availability is controlled by the levels of amino acids in the bloodstream that, in turn, is dependent on diet. Dietary consumption of protein in the post-recovery period is critical for the ability of muscle to increase its mass in response to exercise. In fact, fasting after exercise leads to muscle atrophy. Diet also modulates the anabolic (growth) response of muscle to exercise by changing the level of the hormone, insulin. Insulin and insulin-like growth-factor are known to decrease the rate of protein degradation in muscle, and can help tilt the balance of protein metabolism in favor of protein synthesis.

Due to the adaptive nature of protein metabolism in muscle, increased protein synthesis rate in the exercise recovery period may lead simply to homeostasis (maintenance of existing tissue) rather than muscle growth. The anabolic response of muscle to exercise follows a threshold rule, wherein future growth often requires the mechanical stress on the muscles to exceed the levels previously experienced. Hence, body builders must continually lift heavier loads to grow larger muscles. Moreover, this explains why dynamic or low-impact exercise regimes, while beneficial to overall (especially cardiovascular) health, do not promote robust muscle growth. Research studies on the anabolic effects of dynamic exercise often produce conflicting conclusions depending on whether they study trained subjects (whose muscles may have already maximized their responses) or untrained subjects. While the details of how muscles establish the threshold for this anabolic response are incompletely understood, it appears to be due in part to the fact that trained muscles also show decreased protein degradation during the acute phases of exercise.

Role in human health

Because of the pivotal role of protein metabolism in maintaining and building muscle mass, there is great interest in trying to use nutritional supplements to enhance muscle production in athletes. Evidence suggests that protein types can affect muscle anabolism through increased protein synthesis. Milk protein in particular has shown some beneficial effects for athletes. Diets that meet the energetic demands of the individual and derive 12–15% of their total **calories** from protein are considered sufficient to support the metabolic needs of muscle. The timing and quantity of protein consumption are important in influencing protein synthesis. Approximately 20 g of protein should be consumed after exercise and at subsequent meals following training.

QUESTIONS TO ASK YOUR DOCTOR

- Is my exercise routine safe and appropriate?
- Does my diet contain adequate sources of protein?
- Are there any potential side effects from the supplements I am taking?

Resources

BOOKS

Mougios, Vassilis. *Exercise Biochemistry*. Champaign, IL: Human Kinetics, 2006.

Silbernagl, Stefan, and Agamemmnon Despopoulos. *Color Atlas of Physiology*. New York: Thieme, 2009.

PERIODICALS

Rennie, Michael J. "Protein and Amino Acid Metabolism During and After Exercise and the Effects of Nutrition." *Annual Review of Nutrition* 20 (2000): 457–83.

WEBSITES

Quinn, Elizabeth. "High Protein Diets and Sports Performance." About.com—Sports Medicine. (September 10, 2010). http://sportsmedicine.about.com/od/sportsnutrition/a/HighProteinDiet.htm (accessed November 22, 2011).

Daniel M. Cohen, PhD

Q

Qigong

Definition

Qigong (pronounced "chee-gung," also spelled *chi kung*) is translated from the Chinese to mean "energy cultivation" or "working with the life energy."

Purpose

Qigong is an ancient Chinese system of postures, exercises, breathing techniques, and meditations. Its techniques are designed to improve and enhance the body's *qi*. According to traditional Chinese philosophy, qi is the fundamental life **energy** responsible for health and vitality.

Demographics

In China, qigong exercises are practiced on a daily basis by an estimated 100 million people. Western population data is not well known, however, a 2009 article in *The Journal of Alternative and Complementary Medicine* states that in 2002 there were over 500,000 individuals practicing qigong in the United States, with most purporting to practice for the benefit of maintaining health.

Qigong has been subject to much government regulation in China, from banning to increased requirements for teachers. It has not yet been regulated in the United States. Different schools may provide teacher training, but there are no generally accepted training standards. Western medicine generally does not endorse any of the traditional Chinese healing systems that utilize the concept of energy flow in the body, largely because this energy has yet to be isolated and measured scientifically. New research is being conducted using sophisticated equipment that may verify the existence of energy channels as defined by the Chinese system. Despite the lack of scientific validation, the results of energy techniques, including qigong and acupuncture, have gained widespread interest and respect. One California group of qigong practitioners now conducts twice-yearly retreats to improve their skills and energy level. Qigong masters have demonstrated to Western observers astounding control over many physical functions, and some have even shown the ability to increase electrical voltage measured on their skin's surface. Most of the research and documentation of qigong's effectiveness for medical conditions has been conducted in China, and is slowly becoming more available to English readers.

History

Qigong originated before recorded history. Scholars estimate qigong to be as old as 5,000–7,000 years. Tracing the exact historical development of qigong is difficult, because it was passed down in secrecy among monks and teachers for many generations. Qigong survived through many years before paper was invented, and it also survived the Cultural Revolution in China of the 1960s and 1970s that banned many traditional practices.

Qigong has influenced and been influenced by many of the major strands of Chinese philosophy. The Taoist philosophy states that the universe operates within laws of balance and harmony, and that people must live within the rhythms of nature—ideas that pervade qigong. When Buddhism was brought from India to China around the seventh century A.D., **yoga** techniques and concepts of mental and spiritual awareness were introduced to qigong masters. The Confucian school was concerned with how people should live their daily lives, a concern of qigong as well. The **martial arts** were highly influenced by qigong, and many of them, such as **t'ai chi** and kung fu, developed directly from it. Traditional Chinese medicine also shares many of the central concepts of qigong, such as the patterns of energy flow in the body. Acupuncture and acupressure use the same points on the body that qigong seeks to stimulate. In China, qigong masters have been renowned physicians and healers. Qigong is often prescribed by Chinese physicians as part of treatment.

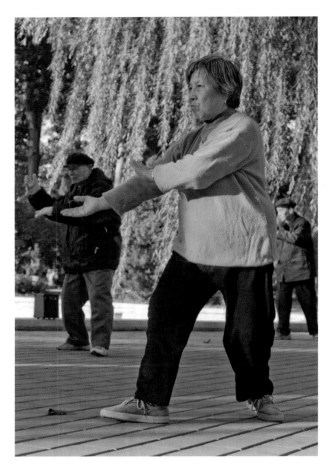

Woman in Ritan park, Beijing, using Qigong breathing exercise. *(© diyiming / Alamy)*

Due to the political isolation of China, many Chinese concepts have been shrouded from the Western world. Acupuncture was only "discovered" by American doctors in the 1970s, although it had been in use for thousands of years. With an increased exchange of information, more Americans have gained access to the once-secret teachings of qigong. In 1988, the First World Conference for Academic Exchange of Medical Qigong was held in Beijing, China, where many studies were presented to attendees from around the world. In 1990, Berkeley, California hosted the First International Congress of Qigong. In the past decade, more Americans have begun to discover the beneficial effects of qigong that motivate an estimated 60 million Chinese to practice it every day.

Description

Basic concepts

In Chinese thought, qi, or chi, is the fundamental life energy of the universe. It is invisible, but present in the air, water, food, and sunlight. In the body, qi is the unseen vital force that sustains life. We are all born with inherited amounts of qi, and we also get acquired qi from the food we eat and the air we breathe. In qigong, the breath is believed to account for the largest quantity of acquired qi, because the body uses air more than any other substance. The balance of our physical, mental, and emotional levels also affect qi levels in the body.

Qi travels through the body along channels called meridians. There are 12 main meridians, corresponding to the 12 principal organs as defined by the traditional Chinese system: the lung, large intestines, stomach, spleen, heart, small intestine, urinary bladder, kidney, liver, gallbladder, pericardium, and the "triple warmer" that represents the entire torso region. Each organ has qi associated with it, and each organ interacts with particular emotions on the mental level. Qigong techniques are designed to improve the balance and flow of energy throughout the meridians, and to increase the overall quantity and volume of qi. In qigong philosophy, mind and body are not separated as they often are in Western medicine. In qigong, the mind is present in all parts of the body, and the mind can be used to move qi throughout the body.

Yin and yang are also important concepts in qigong. The universe and the body can be described by these two separate but complementary principles that are always interacting, opposing, and influencing each other. One goal of qigong is to balance yin and yang within the body. Strong movements or techniques are balanced by soft ones, leftward movements by rightward, internal techniques by external ones, and so on.

Practicing qigong

There are thousands of qigong exercises. The specific ones used may vary depending on the teacher, school, and objective of the practitioner. Qigong is used for physical fitness, as a martial art, and most frequently for health and healing. Internal qigong is performed by those wishing to increase their own energy and health. Some qigong masters are renowned for being able to perform external qigong, by which the energy from one person is passed on to another for healing. This transfer may sound suspect to Western logic, but in the world of qigong there are some amazing accounts of healing and extraordinary capabilities demonstrated by qigong masters. Qigong masters generally have deep knowledge of the concepts of Chinese medicine and healing. In China, there are hospitals that use medical qigong to heal patients, along with herbs, acupuncture, and other techniques. In these hospitals, qigong healers use external qigong and design specific internal qigong exercises for patients' problems.

There are basic components of internal qigong sessions. All sessions require **warm-up** and concluding exercises. Qigong consists of postures, movements, breathing techniques, and mental exercises. Postures may involve standing, **sitting**, or lying down. Movements include stretches, slow motions, quick thrusts, jumping, and bending. Postures and movements are designed to strengthen, stretch, and tone the body to improve the flow of energy. One sequence of postures and movements is known as the "Eight Figures for Every Day." This sequence is designed to quickly and effectively work the entire body, and is commonly performed daily by millions in China.

Breathing techniques include deep abdominal breathing, chest breathing, relaxed breathing, and holding breaths. One breathing technique is called the "Six Healing Sounds." This technique uses particular breathing sounds for each of six major organs. These sounds are believed to stimulate and heal the organs.

Meditations and mind exercises are used to enhance the mind and move qi throughout the body. These exercises are often visualizations that focus on different body parts, words, ideas, objects, or energy flowing along the meridians. One mental **exercise** is called the "Inner Smile," during which the practitioner visualizes joyful, healing energy being sent sequentially to each organ in the body. Another mental exercise is called the "Microscopic Orbit Meditation," in which the practitioner intently meditates on increasing and connecting the flow of qi throughout major channels.

Discipline is an important dimension of qigong. Exercises are meant to be performed every morning and evening. Sessions can take from 15 minutes to hours. Beginners are recommended to practice between 15–30 minutes twice a day. Beginners may take classes once or twice per week, with practice outside of class. Classes generally cost US$10–20 per session.

Preparation

Qigong should be practiced in a clean, pleasant environment, preferably outdoors in fresh air. Loose and comfortable clothing is recommended. Jewelry should be removed. Practitioners can prepare for success at qigong by practicing at regular hours each day to promote discipline. Qigong teachers also recommend that students prepare by adopting lifestyles that promote balance, moderation, proper rest, and healthy diets, all of which are facets of qigong practice.

KEY TERMS

Martial arts—Group of diverse activities originating from the ancient fighting techniques of the Orient.

Meridians—Channels or conduits through which qi travels in the body.

Qi—Basic life energy, according to traditional Chinese medicine.

Yin/yang—Universal characteristics used to describe aspects of the natural world.

Risks

Side effects may occur during or after qigong exercises for beginners, or for those performing exercises incorrectly. Side effects may include dizziness, dry mouth, **fatigue**, headaches, insomnia, rapid heartbeat, shortness of breath, heaviness or numbness in areas of the body, emotional instability, anxiety, or decreased concentration. Side effects generally clear up with rest and instruction from a knowledgeable teacher.

Beginners should learn from an experienced teacher, as performing qigong exercises in the wrong manner may cause harm. Practitioners should not perform qigong on either full or completely empty stomachs. Qigong should not be performed during extreme weather, which may have negative effects on the body's energy systems. Menstruating and pregnant women should perform only certain exercises.

Results

Qigong may be used as a daily routine to increase overall health and well-being, as well as for **disease prevention** and longevity. It can be used to increase energy and reduce stress. In China, qigong is used in conjunction with other medical therapies for many chronic conditions, including **asthma**, allergies, AIDS, cancer, headaches, **hypertension**, depression, mental illness, strokes, heart disease, and **obesity**.

A long-term study of qigong began in 1999 at the Center for Alternative and Complementary Medicine Research in Heart Disease at the University of Michigan; it focuses on the speed of healing of graft wounds in patients undergoing coronary bypass surgery. The National Center for Complementary and Alternative Medicine (NCCAM) has been funding studies of qigong since 2000. The breathing techniques of qigong are being studied intensively by Western physicians as a form of therapy for anxiety-related problems and for disorders involving the vocal cords. Qigong is also

QUESTIONS TO ASK YOUR
DOCTOR

- How will qigong benefit me?

- Do I have any physical limitations that would prohibit my undertaking qigong?

- What tests or evaluation techniques will you perform to see if qigong has been beneficial for me?

- Will qigong interfere with my current medications?

- What tests or evaluation techniques can you perform to see if my fitness and nutritional choices promote a healthy condition in conjunction with qigong?

- What symptoms are important enough that I should seek immediate treatment?

being used in the rehabilitation of patients with severe asthma or **chronic obstructive pulmonary disease** (COPD). As studies of qigong continue in Western medicine in United States, additional beneficial results may emerge.

Resources

BOOKS

Barea, Christina. *QiGong Illustrated.* Champaign, IL: Human Kinetics, 2010.

Hoffman, Ronald L. *How to Talk with Your Doctor: The Guide for Patients and Their Physicians Who Want to Reconcile and Use the Best of Conventional and Alternative Medicine,* 2nd ed. Laguna Beach, CA: Basic Health Publications, 2011.

Mayor, David F., and Marc S. Micozzi. *Energy Medicine East and West: A Natural History of QI.* Philadelphia: Churchill Livingstone, 2011.

Micozzi, Marc., S. *Fundamentals of Complementary and Alternative Medicine.* New York: Saunders, 2010.

Pelletier, Kenneth R. *The Best Alternative Medicine,* Kindle ed. New York: Simon & Schuster, 2010.

Ting, Tienko. *Natural Chi Movement: Accessing the World of the Miraculous.* Berkeley, CA: North Atlantic Books, 2011.

PERIODICALS

Baker, S. E., C. M. Sapienza, and S. Collins. "Inspiratory Pressure Threshold Training in a Case of Congenital Bilateral Abductor Vocal Fold Paralysis." *International Journal of Pediatric Otorhinolaryngology* 67 (April 2003): 413–416.

Biggs, Q. M., K. S. Kelly, and J. D. Toney. "The Effects of Deep Diaphragmatic Breathing and Focused Attention on Dental Anxiety in a Private Practice Setting." *Dental Hygiene* 77 (Spring 2003): 105–113.

Birdee, Gurjeet S., et al. "T'ai Chi and Qigong for Health: Patterns of Use in the United States." *The Journal of Alternative and Complementary Medicine* 15 (September 2009): 969–973.

Emerich, K. A. "Nontraditional Tools Helpful in the Treatment of Certain Types of Voice Disturbances." *Current Opinion in Otolaryngology and Head and Neck Surgery* 11 (June 2003): 149–153.

Golden, Jane. "Qigong and Tai Chi as Energy Medicine." *Share Guide* (November-December 2001): 37.

Johnson, Jerry Alan. "Medical Qigong for Breast Disease." *Share Guide* (November-December 2001): 109.

Ram, F. S., E. A. Holloway, and P. W. Jones. "Breathing Retraining for Asthma." *Respiratory Medicine* 97 (May 2003): 501–507.

Tsang, H. W., C. K. Mok, Y. T. Au Yeung, and S. Y. Chan. "The Effect of Qigong on General and Psychosocial Health of Elderly with Chronic Physical Illnesses: A Randomized Clinical Trial." *International Journal of Geriatric Psychiatry* 18 (May 2003): 441–449.

ORGANIZATIONS

International Chi Kung/Qi Gong Directory, 2730 29th St., Boulder, CO, 80301, (303) 442-3131.

National Center for Complementary and Alternative Medicine (NCCAM), 9000 Rockville Pike, Bethesda, MD, 20892, (888) 644-6226, http://nccam.nih.gov.

Qi: The Journal of Traditional Eastern Health and Fitness, P.O. Box 221343, Chantilly, VA, 22022, (202) 378 3859

Qigong Human Life Research Foundation, P.O. Box 5327, Cleveland, OH, 44101, (216) 475-4712

Qigong Magazine, P.O. Box 31578, San Francisco, CA, 94131, (800) 824-2433

Douglas Dupler, MA
Rebecca J. Frey, PhD
Laura Jean Cataldo, RN, EdD

Quadraplegic athletes *see* **Paraplegic and quadraplegic athletes**

Quadricep exercises

Definition

The quadriceps femoris, also called the quadriceps or simply quads, is a large muscle group that consists of four muscles located on the front of the thigh. (Quadriceps is used both in the singular and plural sense.) The four muscles of the quads are the rectus femoris, vastus medialis, vastus intermedius, and vastus lateralis. As the strongest muscle in the human

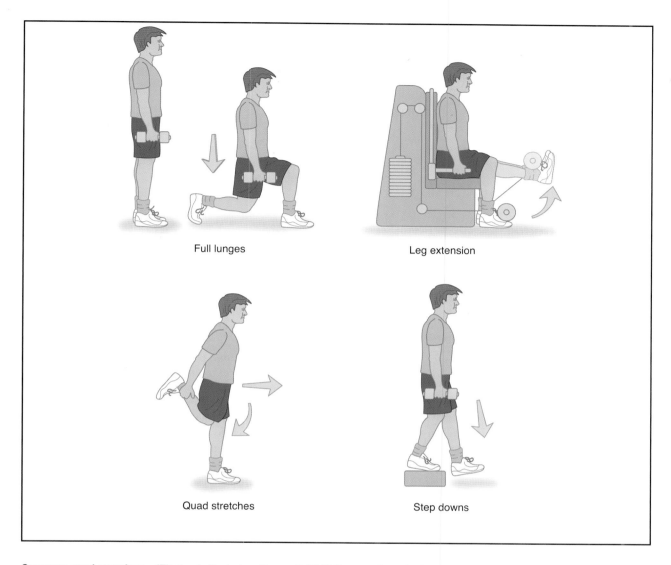

Full lunges

Leg extension

Quad stretches

Step downs

Common quad exercises. *(Electronic Illustrators Group. © 2012 Cengage Learning.)*

body, it is important to **exercise** the quadriceps on a regular basis to maintain a healthy and fit body.

Purpose

The quadriceps, all four of the muscles, are used as extensor muscles for the knee joint. They are necessary for humans to be able to walk, run, jump, squat, and perform other such actions. In addition, the rectus femoris, one of the four muscles, is used as a flexor of the hip because it is attached to the ilium (the uppermost, and largest, bone of the pelvis). The vastus medialis, another quad muscle, also helps to stabilize the patella (kneecap) and the knee joint during the gait process.

The quadriceps absorb much of the stress that is placed on the knees while doing such activities as

walking, jumping, and **running**. They are also responsible for straightening the knees and stabilizing the kneecaps. Exercise of the quadriceps is very important for overall physical health, and is crucial for good health of the knees.

Demographics

Whether young or old, physically fit or not, the regular exercising of the quads is very important for maintaining (or re-gaining) a healthy body. To keep the body in shape, the quadriceps should be strong so the lower body, especially the knees, can move the upper body around in its daily activities. Such exercises are especially important when performing athletic competitions and physical fitness events such as

KEY TERMS

Compression—The state of having been reduced in volume or mass by the application of pressure.

Condyle—A rounded part at the end of a bone that forms a moving joint with a cup-shaped cavity in another bone.

Gait—The manner by which one moves such as walking, jogging, or running.

Femur—The main bone in the thigh.

Flexor—A muscle that bends a joint or limb when it is contracted.

Patella—Another name for the kneecap.

Trochanter—Either of two knobs on the upper femur, to which the muscles between the thigh and the pelvis are attached.

playing **football**, **baseball**, **basketball**, **tennis**, ice and field **hockey**, **soccer**, and bowling, and performing such activities as riding a bicycle, mowing the grass, climbing the stairs, hiking in a forest, and skiing down a hill.

Description

The quadriceps is the extensor muscle for the knee. Located on the front and sides of the femur, these four muscles—rectus femoris, vastus medialis (internus), vastus intermedius, and vastus lateralis (externus)—are located on the front of the thigh and attached to the kneecap through the quadriceps tendon.

The rectus femoris is positioned on the middle of the thigh. Originating at the ilium (the largest and uppermost bone of the pelvis), the rectus femoris covers a majority of the other three muscles of the quads. Also beginning at the femur, the rectus femoris covers the area from the trochanters (part of the thighbone) to the condyles (the round prominence at the end of the femur). The vastus lateralis is on the lateral side of the femur (outer side of the thigh), while the vastus medialis is on the medial side of the femur (inner side of the thigh). The vastus intermedius—located between the vastus lateralis and the vastus medialis—is on the front of the femur (top of the thigh).

Common exercises that benefit the quadriceps include:

- All four quad stretch: While on the hands and knees, lift the right leg off the floor and hold its foot with the right hand. While keeping the knee fully flexed, stretch the quadriceps and extend the hips by thrusting them towards the floor. Hold the position for ten to 20 seconds. Repeat with the left leg and hand.
- Full lunges: With palms positioned inward while holding weights at the sides, step forward with one leg and bend that knees to 90°. (The exercise can also be done without weights.) The other (rear) knee should almost touch the floor. Then, push back to the original standing position. Repeat with the other side.

- Leg extension: Using a knee extension exercise machine, place the front of the ankles under the pads. Slowly straighten the knees. Then, return to the starting position. Repeat as necessary.
- Leg presses: A leg press machine is used in which a person pushes a weight away from the body with the use of their legs. Sometimes resistance replaces the use of a weight. In one method, a vertical or diagonal leg press machine is used with weights attached directly to the machine on a rail system. The user sits below the rail system and pushes the weights upward with their feet so the weights climb the rails. With the other method, the person sits upright and pushes forward with the feet onto a plate that is attached to a weight stack with the use of cables.
- Step downs: Hold weights (such as dumbbells) in the hands with the arms straight down at the sides. Stand on a step with both feet. Slowly step down with one leg and then step back up with the same leg. Repeat with the other leg.
- Squats: While holding a barbell on the shoulders behind the neck, lower the torso similar to sitting into a chair by bending the legs. (The exercise can also be done without any weights.) The distance lowered can be several inches. Slowly return to the original position by raising the torso to a standing position. Without weights, stand with the back up against a wall and lower the body a few inches by bending the legs. Return to the standing position. A squat machine can also be used. It uses a set of weights connected to a platform. Sit or lie with the feet against the platform. Then push against the platform to lift the weights. Repeat such exercise eight to 12 times, or until the feet become fatigued. They benefit the quadriceps, along with the buttocks and upper thighs.

These and similar exercises are important to keep the quadriceps in good shape. Weak quad muscles can lead to knee-related injuries and worst of all, loss of leg mobility due to a breakdown of the quadriceps mucles.

Preparation

The quadriceps should be stretched before and after exercising. **Stretching** these muscles keeps them long and flexible, allowing them to work more efficiently. Quadriceps that are well exercised are less at risk to be injured. When stretching the quadriceps, hold a stretch for about 30 seconds. Remain stationary—do not introduce any bouncing motions into the stretching exercise because such action can lead to damage of these muscles.

There are various stretching exercises for the quadriceps. One of them is the standing quadriceps stretch. With both feet positioned side-by-side, raise the left foot toward the buttocks, so the thigh is about parallel to the floor. When the muscle begins to stretch a burning sensation is felt at the front of the thigh. Hold this stretch for about 30 seconds and then lower the leg back to its original position. Repeat the stretch with the other leg.

Another quadriceps exercise is one performed lying down. While lying on the floor on the stomach, hold the right ankle and pull it toward the buttocks. Continue the motion until the quads begin to burn. Hold the position for about 30 seconds. Then, lower the leg. Repeat with the left leg.

Risks

Various quadriceps injuries can occur, especially in activities involving jumping, kicking, or sprinting. The rectus femoris is frequently at the center of the injury because it crosses both the hip joint and knee joint—the only quad muscle so positioned. Located at these two critical positions, the rectus femoris is more susceptible to injury. A common site of injury is at or around the musculotendinous junction, the location where the muscle meets the tendon just above the knee.

All of the quad muscles can be injured due to being compressed against the femur bone (what is called a compression injury). This type of injury is usually quite painful and can be temporarily disabling if serious enough. However, it rarely becomes a permanent disability. Other injuries to the quadriceps range from simple strains to more disabling muscle ruptures. The most common injury to the quads is a contusion. It is frequently caused by a direct impact to the anterior thigh from an object, such as another person's helmet while playing football.

Injuries while exercising the quadriceps is also possible. A common injury during exercise is what is called jumper's knee (patellar tendinopathy), a strain at a muscle of the quadriceps that occurs at the conjoined muscle tendon junction. Risks from quadriceps exercises can be minimized by first seeking medical advice from a trusted medical professional. Make sure the body is ready for quad exercises by gradually

---

QUESTIONS TO ASK YOUR DOCTOR

- Should I attempt quadriceps exercises? If so, what type of exercises should I do?
- What are some good quadriceps exercises for me to do?
- How often should I exercise my quad muscles?
- What quadriceps exercises should I avoid?
- Should I see a medical or fitness expert before trying exercises?
- What types of lifestyle changes will help with my exercises?

---

building up an exercise routine. If the exercise feels comfortable for the quad muscles, then it is appropriate for one's level. Never do too much and risk injuring the muscles. Never perform exercises if pain is present. Mild discomfort is natural when doing exercises, especially then the muscle is being stretched.

To avoid injuries and to minimize the chance of more serious injuries when they occur:

- always warm-up and stretch before doing exercises; and stretch afterwards
- make sure to gradually add weights to an exercise routine (if using weights)
- stop exercising when feeling pain
- rest if an injury occurs; get medical attention if needed

Results

Health benefits are obtained when performing a moderate amount of physical exercise daily, such as exercises for the quads. Regular physical activity plays a beneficial role in preventing disease and improving overall health status. Specifically, strong quadriceps are essential for good performance in any athletic endeavour or physical activity. Well-toned and developed quads provide the necessary power to swim the length of a pool, run up and down a basketball court, or run a **marathon** race. Strong quads are also important for living an independent and healthy life.

Resources

BOOKS

Hall, John E. *Guyton and Hall Textbook of Medical Physiology*. Philadelphia: Saunders/Elsevier, 2011.

Katch, Victor L., William D. McArdle, and Frank I. Katch. *Essentials of Exercise Physiology*. Philadelphia: Wolters Kluwer/Lippincott Williams & Wilkins Health, 2011.

Micheli, Lyle J., editor. *Encyclopedia of Sports Medicine*. Thousand Oaks, CA: SAGE, 2011.

Moorman III, Claude T., and Donald T. Kirkendall, editors. *Praeger Handbook of Sports Medicine and Athlete Health*. Santa Barbara, CA: Praeger, 2011.

Plowman, Sharon A., and Denise L. Smith. *Exercise Physiology for Health, Fitness, and Performance*. Philadelphia: Wolters Kluwer Health/Lippincott Williams & Wilkins, 2011.

Stone, Robert J., and Judith A. Stone. *Atlas of Skeletal Muscles*. New York: McGraw-Hill, 2012.

WEBSITES

DeBerardino, Thomas M. *Quadriceps Injury*. WebMD. (January 19, 2010). http://emedicine.medscape.com/article/91473-overview (accessed November 9, 2011).

Exercise. Texas Heart Institute. (December 2010). http://www.texasheartinstitute.org/hic/topics/hsmart/exercis1.cfm (accessed November 9, 2011).

Godman, Heidi. *Description of a Quadricep Stretch*. LiveStrong.com. (June 3, 2011). http://www.livestrong.com/article/462306-description-of-a-quadricep-stretch/ (accessed November 9, 2011).

"Quadriceps Stretch." *A Guide to 10 Basic Stretches*. Mayo Clinic. (February 23, 2011). http://www.mayoclinic.com/health/stretching/SM00043&slide = 4 (accessed November 9, 2011).

Thigh: Quadriceps. ExRx.net. http://exrx.net/Lists/ExList/ThighWt.html#anchor172012 (accessed November 9, 2011).

Wheeless III, Clifford R. "Quadriceps Muscle." *Wheeless' Textbook of Orthoaedics*. (May 12, 2011). http://www.wheelessonline.com/ortho/quadriceps_muscle (accessed November 9, 2011).

Weir, Jen. *The Quadriceps and Muscle Atrophy*. LiveStrong.com. (March 28, 2011). http://www.livestrong.com/article/366527-the-quadriceps-muscle-atrophy/ (accessed November 9, 2011).

ORGANIZATIONS

American Alliance for Health, Physical Education, Recreation and Dance, 1900 Association Dr., Reston, VA, 20191-1598, (703) 476-3400, (800) 213-7193, http://www.aahperd.org.

American College of Sports Medicine, 401 W. Michigan St., Indianapolis, IN, 46202-3233, (317) 637-9200, Fax: (317) 634-7817, http://www.acsm.org.

American Council on Exercise, 4851 Paramount Dr., San Diego, CA, 92123, (888) 825-3636, support@acefitness.org, http://www.acefitness.org.

National Coalition for Promoting Physical Activity, 1100 H St., NW, Suite 510, Washington, DC, 20005, (202) 454-7521, Fax: (202) 454-7598, http://www.ncppa.org.

President's Council on Fitness, Sports and Nutrition, 1101 Wootton Parkway, Suite 560, Rockville, MD, 20852, (240) 276-9567, Fax: (240) 276-9860, http://www.fitness.gov.

William A. Atkins, BB, BS, MBA

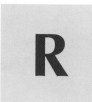

R

Racquetball

Definition

Racquetball is a sport played on a court with four walls, usually indoors, that requires a racquet and a small blue ball that is hollow and made of rubber. It can be played by two, three, or four players.

Purpose

In racquetball, the object of the game is to score points, which a player can only do when serving, similar to the game of tennis. To do so, the player must win a serve or rally (back-and-forth hitting of the ball). If the returning player wins the rally, it is called a "side out" and the returner now becomes the server. If the serving player (or team) wins a rally, he or she scores the point and the opportunity to serve again. The rally ends when one of the players is unable to reach the ball for their shot before it touches the floor twice or is unable to hit the ball so that it touches the front wall of the court before it touches the floor. A player also loses a rally if he or she is called for hindering another player.

Demographics

According to the International Racquetball Federation (IRF), 5.6 million Americans play racquetball each year, and the game is enjoyed in 90 countries by 14 million players. The U.S. Racquetball Association has at least 3 million members. Most are in the 25 to 44 year-old **age** group; the average age of an association member is about 30 years old. About 60% are men and 40% are women. The IRF holds junior and senior world championships each year for its member countries around the world. Junior championships are for girls and boys ages 10 to 18. Senior championship events are held for women and men ages 35 through 85 and over.

History

According to historical accounts, racquetball began in the 1800s when British men who could not pay their debts had to go to special prisons. Most of these men came from well-to-do backgrounds and had played tennis in their younger years. They began hitting balls against the prison walls with their tennis racquets and called the game "rackets." In no time, the game also was being played by schoolchildren against brick walls of school buildings.

Soon the game traveled to Canada with British Army soldiers, then to the United States. It onces was an Olympic event. A man named Joe Sobek, who was a tennis pro, played **handball** but found that it hurt his hands. Handball is similar to racquetball in purpose, but not in equipment. In handball, the ball is slightly smaller and harder, and the players use no racquets. Sobek combined rules from **squash** and handball to create a new game and designed racquets that were smaller than tennis racquets, introducing about 25 samples in 1950 at his local Young Mens Christian Association (YMCA). It turns out that the YMCA had just added thousands of handball courts in their gyms all around the country. He worked with a company to design the perfect ball to work with his racquets and the American sport of racquetball was born. Sobek now is referred to as "The Father of Racquetball."

Sobek began promoting his sport and eventually worked with Robert Kendler, head of the U.S. Handball Association, to start the International Racquetball Association in the late 1960s. The first tournament was held in Connecticut in 1963. Gut string was added to the rackets and throughout the 1970s, the racquet changed designs and materials. Aluminum alloy frames were introduced in 1971, and fiberglass frames the following year. By 1979, graphite frames were made, and the biggest change came in 1984, when large, oversized racquets became standard for most players. The handles still were shorter than those of tennis racquets, but the heads were much larger.

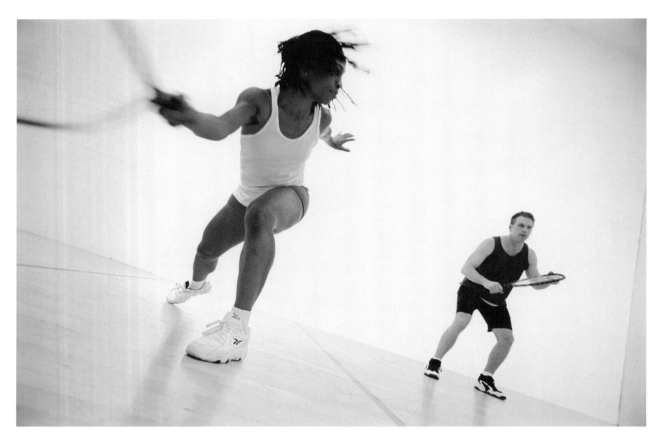

Adults participate in a racquetball match. (© Dennis O'Clair/Corbis)

Some amateur and professional players have grown in popularity and helped better position the sport for growth. By the mid-1980s, popularity of the sport declined and many sports clubs closed some of their courts. The IRF says that the decline leveled off and the game is more popular again. There have been world championships in racquetball held twice a year since 1981 and the game was accepted as a sport in the Pan American Games in 1995. A U.S. Open championship is held yearly; it offers prize money for professional players. Supporters and players are trying to position racquetball as an Olympic Sport in the future.

Description

Racquetball is a competitive sport that involves returning a rubber ball with a strung racquet. When two players play, it is called a singles game (one player against the other). Doubles play involves two teams, with two players each; doubles can be men's, women's, or mixed (a player of each sex on each team). Another version of the game that can be played for fun but not in official competitions involves three players. It is called cutthroat. The serving side scores points when the server hits a serve that can't be returned at all (an ace), or wins a rally. There are four walls on a racquetball court. The ball can touch any of these walls in a rally, as long as it does not touch the floor twice before the player returns it, or touch the floor before it touches the front wall. A serve must hit the front wall before touching the floor or another wall or it is deemed a sideout for the server. If the players are in a doubles match, loss of serve is called "handout" and the other player on the team serves.

Rules

There are many rules regarding serves, but in general, the serve must hit the front wall first and be longer than a line marked as the service line, but shorter than the back wall. It also cannot hit the ceiling without first touching a side wall or hit three walls before touching the floor. In every division except the most advanced (open division), players get two chances to serve the ball correctly. In the open division, they get only one chance. The receiver cannot hit the ball before it passes a plane marked by a line on the court, but can hit a ball in the air as soon as it passes

KEY TERMS

Anaerobic—Exercising at a level that the body must work to replace oxygen.

Corneal abrasions—A scratch on the surface of the cornea. The cornea is the eye's clear outer layer.

Retinal detachment—Retinal detachment is when the retina separates from the tissues under it. The retina is the transparent tissue on the back wall of the eye.

that point. He or she must hit the ball before it touches the floor a second time. The returned ball can hit any wall first, but must hit the front wall before touching the floor. Failing to return the serve or any ball in a rally is a point for the server. Players also must observe rules about making sure the opponent is ready and that each do not block the other or hinder play.

These rallies continue, with the player who wins the rally either scoring a point if he or she is server, or switching to the serving side if he or she is a receiver. The match is not over until one player or team wins two games. The first two games are played to 15 points. If each side wins a game, they play a tiebreaker to 11 points.

Doubles play offers other rules about where players stand during serves and how the players exchange serving. Racquetball played for recreation usually does not have referees. Players should become familiar with all rules and etiquette of the game, such as definitions of technical fouls, hinders, and equipment requirements. Tournament play may involve referees, but players must closely follow rules set forth by the IRF and USAR. Tournament play is based on skill levels; a doubles team plays at the level of the more highly skilled player.

Preparation

Learning the official rules of racquetball is part of preparation for the sport. Another way to prepare is to watch a match in action. Many clubs have competition courts with clear glass walls for spectators, and others can be viewed from above. Referees call matches from above the court, and there are walkways that spectators also can view matches from. Once hooked, a future racquetball player only needs to purchase or borrow the appropriate equipment and be sure he or she is in condition to play this high-intensity sport.

Equipment

Racquets vary widely in price, but new players can purchase starter racquets for as little as US$20. Some clubs also loan racquets when players reserve courts. Advanced players spend up to US$200 on their racquets.

Balls usually come in cans of two; they're typically blue, but can be other colors, and only cost a few dollars. A special glove is important to help maintain grip on the racquet handle, especially when sweating. It's not required, but is a good idea. Any type of court shoe (tennis shoe) helps players move around the wooden floor of the racquetball court quickly and safely. Finally, eyewear is essential. Tournament play requires special goggles that help protect the eyes from injury if a racquet or ball hits the player. The racquetball court generally is located at a private gym, but may be found at community college or recreational facilities. It has four walls, a ceiling that opens at the back, and a door in the back wall where players enter. Lines mark the service box and service line. Standard court size is about 20 feet wide and 40 feet deep.

Conditioning and training

Racquetball is a highly aerobic sport, equivalent to about **running** three 10-minute miles or 30 minutes of **martial arts** training. Preparing for competitive play means good anaerobic conditioning, healthy muscles and joints, and good reflexes. Strength training, **stretching**, and programs that help condition athletes for quick, short bursts of activity can help prepare them for racquetball. The muscles used most include the forearms, rotator cuffs, upper back, shoulders, quadriceps, triceps, hamstrings, chest, and calf muscles.

Risks

There is risk of injury in racquetball, as with any high-intensity, high-impact sport. Players could twist knees or ankles, fall, or damage shoulders or wrists from repetitive strains. Probably the most common and risky injury particular to racquetball, however, is eye damage. Retinal detachment or corneal abrasion are the two injuries that can occur when hit in the eye with the fast-moving rubber ball. Symptoms of corneal abrasion include redness, tearing, and feeling like there is something in the eye. Retinal detachment causes bright flashes or areas of grayness in vision. The chance of these injuries is a reason why rules require use of safety goggles. Players also can be hit with racquets or balls, but should be able to pay attention and get out of the way in most instances. Any competitive sport carries some risk of injury.

Results

According to the California State Racquetball Association, players can burn more than 600 **calories** an hour. That's also the average time it takes to play a three-game match. Playing the game increases coordination and flexibility. A study from the Netherlands that lasted two years showed that regular intensive **exercise** from sports such as racquetball helped improve joints in people who had rheumatoid **arthritis**. The study also found psychological benefits; people felt more optimistic and better able to cope with their conditions.

Resources

PERIODICALS

"Bouncing Off the Walls. Chasing After a Racquet Ball Will Burn UP Calories and Get Your Heart Racing." *Daily Herald (Arlington Heights, IL)*. (April 21, 2008):2.

Chang, Huang J. "Retinal Detachment." *Journal of the American Medical Association*. 302 (November 25, 2009,):2274.

"Corneal Abrasions." *Clinical Reference Systems*. (February 1, 2010).

"Long-term, High-intensity, Weight-bearing Exercise Benefits Patients." *Obesity, Fitness, and Wellness Week*. (September 27, 2003):8.

WEBSITES

California State Racquetball Association. "New to Racquetball?" CaliforniaStateRacquetball.org. http://www.californiaracquetball.org/new_to_racquetball.htm (accessed September 10, 2011).

Scwartz, Shannon. "The History of Racquetball. From Prisong to Country Clubs." TheHistoryof.net. http://www.thehistoryof.net/history-of-racquetball.html (accessed September 11, 2011).

USA Racquetball. "Rules and Regulations." USRA.org. http://usra.org/Rules.aspx (accessed September 10, 2011).

ORGANIZATIONS

International Racquetball Federation, Colorado Springs, CO, U.S., http://www.internationalracquetball.com.

USA Racquetball, 1685 West Uintah Street, Suite 103, Colorado Springs, CO, U.S., 80904, (719) 635-5396, Fax: (719) 635-0685, http://usra.org.

Teresa G. Odle, B.A., ELS

Recess and unstructured play

Definition

Recess is a break in the school day, during which children can engage in unstructured play. Unstructured play is child-initiated play without formal rules or guidelines.

Purpose

The purpose of recess and unstructured play is to allow children to control their own activities in a way that leads to improved social, verbal, and other skills. Recess allows the child to take a break from the rigorous structure of the classroom setting, move around and **exercise**, leading to improved classroom performance overall.

Recess and unstructured play are also important for the child's fitness and physical well being. Many activities children choose to participate in during recess or unstructured play are very active. Made up ball games, tag, and **running** during made up games of pretend, are good ways for children to get exercise. Childhood **obesity** has been increasing in the United States, and some experts believe this can be traced in part to the reduction in unstructured play seen in recent decades. The exercise during unstructured play not only aids in the **energy expenditure** necessary for maintaing a healthy weight, but also benefits heart and **bone health**.

Demographics

Recess and unstructured play is an activity available for both genders, all socioeconomic backgrounds, and all ethnicities. The primary target is toddlers and preschoolers, but time for unstructured play should continue into elementary school or even junior high school.

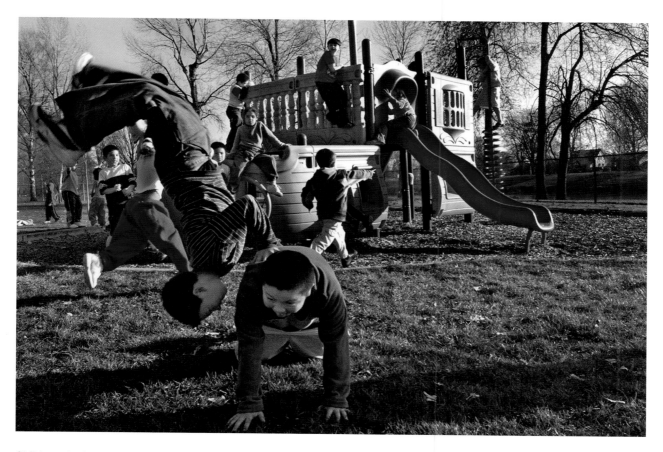

Children playing on a playground. (© AP Images/Greg Ebersole)

History

In the United States the time spent in recess and unstructured play has been decreasing since the mid 1980s. Children spend more time engaged in structured activities such as sports, academic classes, music lessons, and other achievement-oriented and adult-directed activities. Children also spend more time in front of the computer, television, and video games than ever before, further reducing the amount of time spent in unstructured play.

Description

Unstructured play is any play in which there is no specific set of rules previously defined, and in which the activity is not adult directed. Children typically engage in unstructured play when left to their own devices without specific instructions. For example, children told to play in the backyard without any other directions will quickly invent a game of tag, play a game of let's pretend, or make up a new ball game.

Not all unstructured play is imaginative play, but imaginative play is a core type of unstructured play, believed to have special benefits for the child. During games of let's pretend, children frequently invent complex universes with many characters each with their own back story and personality.

It is often difficult for achievement-oriented parents to allow long periods of unstructured play, as it does not appear to have any direct or measurable benefits. However, unstructured play is extremely important to the child's normal and healthy growth and development. Parents should examine their child's schedule to ensure that he or she is engaging in enough unstructured play each week. Some ways to encourage unstructured play are:

• Turn off the television. Even having it on in the background may reduce unstructured play.

• Show the child a new activity, such as using a paper bag as a puppet or making mud pies, then let them use their own imagination to extend the activity without adult direction.

- Do not provide instant entertainment. Boredom can quickly produce imaginative and unstructured play.
- Let children run around. It is sometimes difficult to do, but unstructured play is often loud and rambunctious. Allowing safe chaos can encourage unstructured play.
- Choose a preschool that stresses unstructured play, or an elementary school that provides two daily recesses for the lower grades.

Play therapy is a type of therapy used with young children to help with a variety of problems. During play therapy, the child is given a set of materials to choose from and allowed to play in an unstructured way while the therapist watches and sometimes asks questions. Play therapy should only be done by therapists who have been specially trained in its correct use. Such therapists generally receive a master's degree or doctorate in clinical psychology, with additional training specifically in play therapy. The Association for Play Therapy provides continuing education and maintains a list of approved education centers for the teaching of play therapy.

Preparation

There is no preparation required for unstructured play. Left to their own devices without a structured activity, most children initiate unstructured play by themselves. Although unstructured play does not require anything more than a child and an imagination, props and toys can add to the fun. Dress-up clothes, play cooking equipment, balls and other sports equipment, puppets, or almost anything else can be used as a prop during unstructured play. Adults can provide the props, or suggest a direction for the child (e.g., showing a child how a sock on the hand can be used as a puppet), but the play should be child-driven and child-directed.

Risks

There are no risks to unstructured play. Although there may always be some risks to allowing children to run, climb, and play, these risks are small and are far outweighed by the benefits of unstructured play. Playing on playgrounds can result in falls and cuts, scrapes, and bruises. Climbing equipment is a source of many recess and play accidents, the vast majority of which are not serious.

Results

There are numerous benefits to recess and unstructured play, many of which are just beginning to be rigorously demonstrated through scientific studies.

KEY TERMS

Obesity—Excessive weight, defined as a Body Mass Index (BMI) of 25 or above.

Play therapy—A type of therapy in which a child engages in unstructured play that provides the therapist insight into the child's mind and allows the child to work through problems.

Recess allows children to take a break from the focused attention required during classroom activities. It also allows them to participate in physical activities that can help increase attention back in the classroom, relieve stress, and improve mood.

Unstructured play has been found to be an integral part of a child's healthy development, both intellectually and socially. One study found that children who were in a preschool that emphasized structured activities were more likely to have committed a felony by the time they were 23 than their peers who were in a preschool that emphasized unstructured play.

Many stressful things happen in a child's daily life. The challenges of going to a new school, interacting with peers, and family life can lead to stress and anxiety. Unstructured play, both alone and with other children, has been found to reduce stress. One study looked at children who were stressed by the first day at a new preschool. Children who were allowed to play for 15 minutes were less stressed at the end of that time than children who were read a story by the teacher for 15 minutes. Psychologists hypothesize that unstructured play allows children to control their environment and work through the problems that are stressing them in a way that is **age** appropriate and makes sense to the child.

During unstructured play, children can imagine new worlds and make up games in any way they choose. This helps foster the creativity that is a cornerstone of academic and intellectual achievement later in life. Children can practice new skills they have learned during unstructured play, such as kicking a ball (a gross motor skill) or making mud pies (a fine motor skill). This type of play helps improve **hand-eye coordination**, balance, and manual dexterity.

Unstructured play also helps a child's social and intellectual development. During unstructured group play, children work through problems, learn to compromise, learn to work together to reach mutual goals, and learn to make up and follow rules together. This helps develop understanding of other people's points of view, and helps the child learn social skills that are the basis for healthy social interactions later in life.

Resources

BOOKS

Beresin, Anna R. *Recess Battles: Playing, Fighting, and Story-telling*. Jackson, MS: University Press of Mississippi, 2010.

Bullard, Julie. *Creating Environments for Learning: Birth to Age Eight*. Upper Saddle River, NJ: Merrill, 2010.

Smith, Peter K. *Children and Play*. Malden, MA: Wiley-Blackwell, 2010.

PERIODICALS

Haug, Ellen, et al. "The Characteristics of the Outdoor School Environment Associated with Physical Activity." *Health Education Research* 25, no. 2 (April 2010): 248–156.

Kalish, Meredith, et al. "Outdoor Play: A Survey of Parent's Perceptions of their Child's Safety." *Journal of Trauma-Injury, Infection, and Critical Care* 69, Supplement 4 (October, 2010): S218–22.

O'Connor, Chloe, and Karen Stagnitti. "Play, Behavior, Language and Social Skills: The Comparison of a Play and a Non-Play Intervention Within a Specialist School Setting." *Research in Developmental Disabilities* 32, no. 3 (May-June, 2011): 1205–2011.

WEBSITES

Francis, Meagan. *How to Get Kids to Play Outdoors*. WebMD. (July 1, 2008). http://www.webmd.com/parenting/features/kids-play-outdoors (accessed November 9, 2011).

Playground Injuries: Fact Sheet. Centers for Disease Control and Prevention. (January 19, 2009). http://www.cdc.gov/HomeandRecreationalSafety/Playground-Injuries/playgroundinjuries-factsheet.htm (accessed November 9, 2011).

ORGANIZATIONS

Aerobics and Fitness Association of America, 15250 Ventura Blvd., Suite 200, Sherman Oaks, CA, 91403, (877) 968-7263, http://www.afaa.com.

American Council on Exercise, 4851 Paramount Dr., San Diego, CA, 92123, (888) 825-3636, http://www.acefitness.org.

International Association for the Child's Right to Play, http://www.ipausa.org.

Tish Davidson, AM

Rehydration and recovery after exercise

Definition

Hydration is the act of supplying the body with adequate levels of water. Water must be continually replaced due to moisture lost during evaporation from respiration and sweating and from fluid loss due to urination. Approximately 60–70% of the body is comprised of water (70% represents water content in lean body mass), and up to 70% of the brain consists of water, so it is important that water balance is safely maintained within the body with proper hydration.

Purpose

Adequate hydration before, during, and after **exercise** is essential to the performance and health of athletes and non-athletes alike. Exercise generally induces higher levels of evaporative sweating that occurs as a bodily function to help reduce the rise in body temperature created during aerobic activity. An increase in sweating creates a greater loss of water and puts the body at risk for **dehydration**. Dehydration can inhibit athletic performance, and can jeopardize health in crucial ways. If the loss of water due to dehydration is significant, performance may suffer dramatically, and the health of the athlete may be compromised. However, overdrinking, or hyperhydration, can also create health concerns. Being knowledgeable about best hydration practices, and aware of what liquids are best to consume during times of exercise, is key to better performance, better health, and proper recovery.

Description

Body water is lost usually through increased sweating. Sweating occurs in order to cool the body down, because as the muscles work faster and harder during exercise, they continually generate more heat, increasing core body temperature. As water is lost through the process of sweating, it is being removed both at the intra-and extracellular level, which alters electrolyte levels and increases heart rate. This begins

ROBERT CADE (1927–2007)

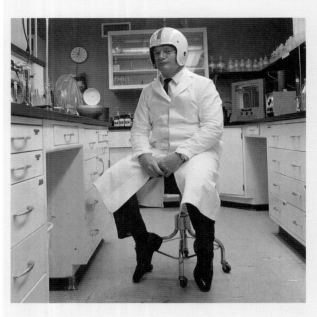

(© Lynn Pelham/Sports Illustrated/Getty Image)

Robert Cade earned his Bachelor of Science degree at the University of Texas, and then taught at the University of Florida College of Medicine.

In 1965, the Florida Gators football coach was concerned about the extreme dehydration of his players in the Florida heat. In need of a solution, he consulted with Cade. Cade worked with a team of doctors to develop a drink fortified with glucose and electrolytes. The initial formula tasted horrible, but after several iterations, the product was patented. Gatorade gained national attention during the 1967 Orange Bowl. The Gators defeated Georgia Tech, and the Georgia Tech coach said, "We didn't have Gatorade; that made the difference."

Gatorade is now a billion dollar product, available in many flavors and sold worldwide. Cade was inducted into the University of Florida Athletic Hall of Fame in April 2007. In November of 2007, Cade died as a result of kidney failure.

to limit the ability of the body to transfer heat from the muscles to the skin where it can then be released into the environment in order to help cool the body back to core temperature. If this does not occur properly, heat injury may result.

When dehydration during exercise occurs, the body is affected in a systemic way. When one system is impacted due to dehydration, others are affected. For example, the **cardiovascular system** begins to work harder (heart rate increases), impacting the thermoregulatory system that, in turn, impacts the **muscular system**. This makes continual hydration very important; multiple systems are compromised, and bringing those systems back into balance after they're impacted takes **energy** the body needs for repair and recovery in the normal course of exercise.

Precautions

Dehydration of greater than 2%of body weight negatively affects endurance performance. However, losses of up to 7% can be tolerated in strength and power sports without affecting performance. Hydration takes place with the intake of fluids as well as during the digestion of meals. Certain fluids assist with hydration better than others such as isotonic drinks whish have the fastest absorption rate; and the intake of some fluids can actually induce dehydration, such as strongalcoholic beverages that act as diuretics.

The American College of Sports Medicine recommendation is for athletes preparing to exercise to consume around 4-7ml/kg body weight of fluid 4 hours before exercise starts. They should then be sure to allow enough time between ingestion and exercise in order for their bodies to eliminate any excess water. The recommendations go further to urge athletes to consume fluids throughout exercise, beginning early and replenishing consistently to compete with the loss of fluids through sweating. Fluids consumed are best when cooler than ambient temperature (between 59°F and 72°F [15–22°C]) since this assists the body in its effort to regulate its core temperature which is rising in the course of exertion, and because cooler liquids are more palatable to most people, thus inspiring the urge to continue hydrating.

During exercise lasting longer than one hour, or in conditions of high heat or humidity, flavored sports drinks are recommended over water alone when they contain electrolytes, sodium, and any flavor that encourages drinking. (By the time an individual feels thirsty, dehydration has already begun.) Electrolytes are essential because they help with the transmission of nerve impulses and the contraction of muscles. Electrolytes are ionized particles—sodium, calcium, potassium, and chloride—that support the transfer of nutrients into cells, and assist with the elimination of wastes from the cell. It is important to offset electrolyte loss during times of excessive sweating in order to help the body maintain a homeostatic state, and to assist the body in muscle repair, and cellular nutrient exchange.

Sodium is added to sports drinks for two reasons: it helps to generate greater thirst, therefore ensuring that the urge to hydrate continues, but most importantly, because fluids with the right sodium content mimic the salinity of the blood causing them to be more quickly absorbed into the blood than water alone, which has no salt content. For athletes or individuals preparing to exercise for less than one hour, hydrating with water may be best, but for high endurance exercise lasting one or more hours, high quality sports drinks with sodium, electrolytes, carbohydrate, and some **protein** content may be preferred. **Carbohydrates** are added to sports drinks because for intense workouts and **endurance training**, muscle **fatigue** can set in. Carbohydrates are metabolized into glucose that is fuel for muscles, and can be readily used by the body during intensive workouts. This allows the body to continue working, and may even help in the recovery process after exercise.

When temperatures take a sudden rise, or when athletes are going to be performing in climates warmer than what they are accustomed to, hydration becomes a greater concern due to higher losses of sweat. Body temperature is also likely to rise more dramatically, impacting performance in important ways. A process known as acclimatization—where an athlete gradually prepares his or her body for the new conditions—is recommended. When temperatures are warmer, and where humidity percentages are higher, sweat rate generally increases for the same duration of exercise. This will require greater fluid intake before, during, and after exercise. It is strongly advised that hydration practices be well monitored especially during the first week of exercise in a new climate.

Aftercare

After exercise, training, or a competition event, rehydration should take place to make up for any fluids lost during the workout. It is suggested that rehydration occur during the two hours immediately following exercise, and that fluids used to rehydrate contain proper electrolyte and carbohydrate levels. The aim here should be to restore 25-50% of sweat losses from during the exercise event in order to reestablish balance

within the body and to be prepared to acquire best levels of fitness for the next event. Compensation for urine losses during the rehydration process should be made if the rehydration process must be rapid. It is further recommended that cooler fluids (between 50-59°F) are best, as are sports drinks incorporating electrolytes, sodium, and carbohydrates.

Certain athletes, such as wrestlers, boxers, rowers, those competing in judo, and body builders, typically do not hydrate before or during training because they train hard to fit into a lower weight class before competition. This is by design, as it improves their ability to compete, however it is especially critical for these athletes to hydrate post-match or competition. Stressing muscles in a dehydrated state weakens them, and puts stress on the body as a whole. It is strongly advised that taking measures such as using diuretics, exercising in saunas, or wearing rubber suits in order to advance dehydration so that one may fit into a lower weight class is not done. These measures can result in dangerous levels of dehydration that may be injurious to athletes.

The recovery process after exercise is just as important for individuals seeking to maintain fitness, achieve healthy immunity, control weight, and ward off chronic and other disease, as it is for competitive athletes. Research indicates that building gradually into an exercise routine is best, rather than stressing muscles and endurance immediately and too consistently. Muscles need time to repair and recover. Working out two days in a row and then allowing a day of rest is advised.

It is advisable to incorporate an appropriate warm up and **cool down** routine into any workout. Warm up prepares the muscles for more strenuous activity and may help prevent injury such as muscle pulls and tears. Lactic acid builds up during the course of exercise and slowing muscle movement before stopping altogether helps to ensure that lactic acid won't create undue muscle stiffness post exercise. Gentle **stretching** after exercise is also advisable. This is another way to help with the release of lactic acid build up in order to reduce the possibility of muscle stiffness after exercise or competition, and will help to increase flexibility that is beneficial to overall health and fitness.

Research indicates that it may be beneficial to consume complex carbohydrates, high quality proteins, and possibly branch chain amino-acid rich foods within 60 minutes after exercise in order to expedite recovery. Leucine is an amino acid that has been observed to positively affect skeletal muscle, helping in its repair by stimulating protein synthesis,

KEY TERMS

Acclimatize—The process of adapting to a new climate, altitude, or temperature.

Amino acid—An organic compound containing an amino group NH_2.

Creatine kinase—An enzyme present in the muscle, brain, and other tissues of vertebrates. Creatine kinase catalyzes the transfer of a phosphate group from adenosine triphosphate to creatine, producing adenosine diphosphate and phosphocreatine that reacts to store energy in the muscles and brain tissue.

Cortisol—A corticosteroid produced by the adrenal cortex that mediates metabolic responses in the body. It has anti-inflammatory and immunosuppressive properties, but may rise in response to physical or psychological stress.

Diuretic—Increases urination.

Electrolyte—Ionized salts that appear in the blood and urine and that play an important metabolic role, assisting in the delivery of nutrients into—and waste products out of—cells.

Glycogen—A carbohydrate molecule essential to the way glucose is stored in muscle and liver tissues.

Hydration—The act of supplying the body with adequate water.

Hyperhydration—Accelerated hydration.

Leucine—A white chrystalline essential amino acid.

Salinity—Consisting of salt.

Testosterone—A male hormone produced by the testes and responsible for producing male secondary sex characteristics.

---

providing fuel to the muscle, and maintaining blood glucose. Leucine is observed to have its most valuable impact on muscles during the recovery phase after exercise, rather than before or during. Leucine can be found in meats and some dairy products, and it is often added to protein bars and some sports drinks. The recommendation for BCAA is 0.03–0.05g/kgBW per hour or 2–4g/hour during exercise and recovery

Carbohydrates are a necessary part of the recovery phase because the body breaks them down into glucose that is metabolized into fuel for every cell. A body that is properly fueled and has rested after exercise is more prepared for the next round of exercise or competition. Researchers state that facing exercise without proper hydration or fuel for muscles and cells is counterproductive to fitness and to goals in competition, and may lead to accelerated health concerns.

Complications

Weighing oneself before and after exercise and hard training is very important. Experiencing a 3% loss in body weight in water can result in performance losses of 20–30%. Reaching a % loss in body weight in water is likely to create a medical emergency.

When dehydration becomes too severe, or if external conditions are such that body temperature rises too high, heat injury or exhaustion may become a complication. If the body's temperature rises to between 101–104°F (38–40°C), muscle weakness and fatigue sets in. At 104–105°F (40–40.5°C), a person becomes confused, and begins to experience extreme muscle weakness and imbalance. Above 105°F (40.5°C), the body ceases to sweat, and loss of consciousness sets in.

Continued thirst, irritability, persistent discomfort, nausea, vomiting, sensations of heat around the neck and/or head, and diminished performance are all signs of extreme dehydration. An athlete experiencing these conditions with no mental distress or diarrhea should immediately begin to rehydrate. Any athlete suffering these conditions along with confusion and gastrointestinal complaints should be seen immediately by emergency medical personnel.

There has been some research done on the subject of hyperhydration which some athletes attempt before exercise. Hyperhydration, however, has proven to cause side effects such as headaches and gastrointestinal distress that may inhibit athletic performance markedly.

On the subject of recovery, where it is lacking and can pose a danger to the athlete or individual, there is the subject of over-training. Exercise physiologists discuss a condition known as *over-reaching*, wherein someone who exercises frequently at maximum levels, and especially competitive athletes in long term training, find themselves experiencing symptoms in which their bodies no longer permit them to exercise or perform at the levels they are attempting to push them toward. Over-reaching begins as severe muscle soreness and stiffness, becoming severe muscle fatigue. The condition can present with mood changes such

QUESTIONS TO ASK YOUR DOCTOR

- How can I best defend against dehydration when exercising if I'm unable to hydrate during exercise?
- Given our local climate, my body weight, and my usual course of exercise, do you recommend that I hydrate with water or with a sports drink?
- Given my training and recovery routine, is it likely that I'm putting my body at risk for over-reach or over-training syndrome?
- Are there further recovery techniques you would suggest I add to my current post exercise routine?

as tension, depression, anger, and confusion. Resting heart rate becomes elevated, muscle glycogen stores deplete, and there is an increase in creatine kinase. Cortisol and testosterone levels may also increase. When over-reaching becomes more severe, it may be referred to as *overtraining syndrome*. An individual suffering this may need to cease exercising for many weeks, sometimes months.

Results

Hydration is responsible for maintaining intra-and-extracellular water balance in the body, and for continuing function of body systems—cardiovascular, muscular, thermoregulatory, et al. Dehydration induced by increase sweating in exercise can result in compromised performance, and may pose serious health risks to athletes and non-athletes. Some symptoms of dehydration are extreme thirst, fatigue, confusion, irritability, nausea, vomiting, gastrointestinal disturbance, cessation of sweating, and even loss of consciousness.

Electrolyte replacement is critical during and after exercise because of the important role electrolytes play in body chemistry. Electrolytes play an key function in muscle contraction and the delivery of nerve impulses, and they are further critical because they help in delivering nutrients into cells, and in eliminating waste material out of cells.

Both hydration and electrolyte replacement are an important part of overall recovery in exercise. The muscles need time after training to repair and strengthen. Incorporating steps such as warming up and cooling down may help to prevent injury and accelerate the recovery period after exercise. Over-exercising or training too hard for too long without

rests can pose damaging results to an athlete or individual. Severe muscle and other fatigue, diminished capacity to perform, mood changes like tension, irritability, depression, or, anger, and elevated levels of cortisol may result. These symptoms are known as over-reaching or **overtraining** syndrome, and may take many weeks or months of rest for recovery.

Resources

BOOKS
Armstrong, Lawrence E. "Heat Acclimatization." *Encyclopedia of Sport Medicine and Science* (1998).

Ronald J. Maughan, John B. Leiper, and Susan M. Shirreffs. "Hydration and Perforance: Rehydration and Recovery After Exercise." *Journal of Sports Nutrition*5 (1995).

Douglas J. Casa, Lawrence E. Armstrong, Susan K. Hillman, et al. "National Athletic Trainers' Association Position Statement: Fluid Replacement for Athletes." *Journal of Athletic Training* 35, 2 (2000): 212-224.

Victor A. Convertino, Lawrence E. Armstrong, Edward F. Coyle, Gary W. Mack, et al. "Position Statement: Exercise and Fluid Replacement." *American College of Sports Medicine*. 28, 1 (1996).

Peterson, Angela. "Overtraining." *Proposition for Debate*. Curtin University: 1999.

WEBSITES
Horowitz, Stephen M. "Recovery and Exercise." (accessed September 21, 2011).

"Eating Proper Foods at Right Time After Exercise Can Speed Recovery." ScienceDaily.com, Last modified, July, 13, 1999. (accessed September 18, 2011).

ORGANIZATIONS
American College of Sports Medicine, P.O. Box 1440, Indianapolis, IN, 46206-1440, (317) 637-9200, Fax: (317) 637-7817, (888) 463-6332, http://www.acsm. org/.

National Association for Health and Fitness, 65 Niagara Square, Room 607, Buffalo, NY, 14202, (716) 851-4052, wellness@city-buffalo.org, http://www.physicalfitness. org/contact-us.php.

Julie Jordan Avritt

Reproductive system, female

Definition

The female reproductive system is composed of organs that produce female eggs (called female gametes or ova), provide an environment for fertilization of the egg by a male sperm (male gamete), and support the development and expulsion of a fetus in pregnancy and childbirth.

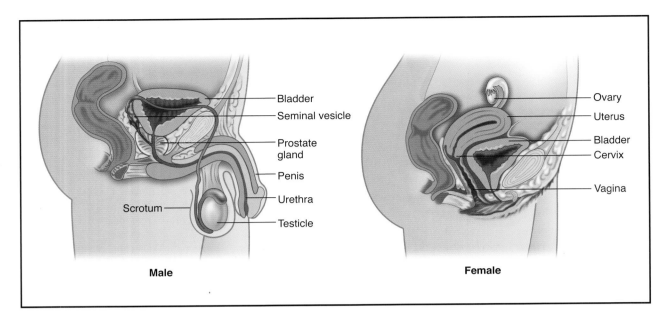

The male and female reproductive systems. *(Electronic Illustrators Group. © 2012 Cengage Learning.)*

Description

The normal female reproductive system is composed of external and internal genitals (genitalia).

External genitals

The external genitals (together, they are called the vulva) are composed of the genital structures visible from outside the body: the greater lips (labia majora), the lesser lips (labia minora), the clitoris, and the opening of the vagina to the outside (the other end of the vagina opens inside the body to the uterus). The labia majora are two large lips that protect the other external genitals. The outer surface of these lips is covered with oil-secreting (sebaceous) glands; their inner surface has hair. The lesser lips (labia minora) are found just inside the greater lips and protect the immediate opening to the vagina (this opening is called the "introitus," Latin for "entrance") and the opening to the urethra (that carries urine from the bladder out of the body). The clitoris is a small structure found at the top of the lesser lips; it is very sensitive to stimulation and may become erect. The perineum is the area between the vagina and the anus in the female (in the male, the perineum is the area between the scrotum and the anus). Two glands, one located on either side of the introitus, are called Bartholin's glands. They secrete a mucus that provides lubrication during sexual intercourse.

Internal genitals

The internal genitals are the vagina, the uterus (womb), the fallopian tubes, and the ovaries. The vagina extends approximately 3 to 4 inches (7 to 10 cm) from the outside of the body to the opening of the uterus. The lower third of the vagina (closest to the outside) is encircled by muscles that control its opening and closing. The uterus is the organ found at the top of the vagina and consists of two main parts: the neck (cervix) and the body (corpus). The neck is the opening of the uterus to the vagina that allows sperm to enter the uterus and allows menstrual fluid to exit. The neck is an important means of protecting the body of the uterus from disease-causing germs; a thick mucus normally covers the neck of the uterus but changes in consistency during ovulation to allow sperm to penetrate. The body of the uterus is the main part of the uterus. It can enlarge to hold a developing fetus during pregnancy. The inner lining of the body of the uterus is called the endometrium, which thickens and then sheds menstrual fluid during each menstrual period if fertilization does not occur.

The fallopian tubes (also called the oviducts or uterine tubes) are muscular structures that extend from the upper edges of the uterus to the ovaries. The fallopian tubes facilitate the transfer of a mature egg from one of the two ovaries to the body of the uterus. A fallopian tube is the site of normal fertilization. The ovaries are a pair of small oval-shaped structures and are suspended near the fallopian tubes by ligaments. A human female will not produce any new developing eggs (oocytes) after she is born. Although she is born with approximately two million eggs, only about 300,000 to 400,000 remain at onset of puberty, and only about 300 of these will develop fully and enter a fallopian tube for possible fertilization. The eggs start as oocytes and develop in what are called ovarian or Graafian follicles, small spherical sacs that burst when the mature egg (called an ovum) is ready to be released into a fallopian tube for possible fertilization, or for discharge in the menstrual fluid if fertilization does not take place.

The human egg is a round cell that, when mature, is surrounded by a number of protective layers (the oolemma, zona pellucida, and zona radiata). It contains half the number of chromosomes of a human cell that is not egg or sperm (that is, 23 instead of 46 chromosomes) and is therefore called a haploid (one-fold) cell. When the egg is fertilized by sperm, the resulting cell will have the full number of 46 chromosomes and will be considered a diploid (two-fold) cell.

Function

Menstruation

The menstrual cycle ranges from 21 to 40 days in most women, with an average cycle lasting 28 days. The first time a girl has a period (the onset of menstruation) is called "menarche"; the permanent cessation of menstruation some decades later is called "menopause" and marks the traditional end of a woman's ability to reproduce. In the 1990s, women past menopause have been impregnated with another woman's egg after it has been fertilized by artificial insemination, and these older women have successfully given birth to healthy babies.

Menstruation occurs when the lining of the uterus begins to shed menstrual fluid; the first day of bleeding is the first day of the menstrual cycle. The menstrual cycle has two phases. The follicular phase extends from the first day of the cycle until immediately before a mature egg gets released from the ovary.

In the second phase of the menstrual (ovulatory) cycle, called the "luteal" phase, the mature follicle bursts and releases an egg, a process called ovulation. The second phase of the menstrual cycle lasts approximately fourteen days until the first day of the next period (using as an example the average 28 day menstrual cycle). The ruptured empty follicle collapses to form the corpus luteum.

Fertilization

During the ovulatory phase of the menstrual cycle, the mature egg is released from the ovary and swept into the fallopian tube. If sperm cells are present in the fallopian tube, fertilization may occur. Pregnancy begins at the moment of fertilization (also called conception), when the sperm penetrates the egg. The fertilized egg, also called a zygote, then begins to move down the fallopian tube into the uterus, where it implants itself in the thick tissue of the lining of the uterus. In the uterus, this replicating cluster of cells is called a blastocyst; after two weeks of development, it is called an embryo; eight weeks after conception, it is called a fetus.

Hormones

A complex balance of hormones is required for reproduction. There are two main groups of hormones that are necessary for normal functioning of the female reproductive system.

The first group contains hormones of the central nervous system (CNS). A part of the brain called the hypothalamus is the main area of hormonal control; it secretes so-called releasing hormones that travel to the pituitary gland located at the base of the brain. Gonadotropin-releasing hormone (GnRH) secreted by the hypothalamus triggers the release of gonadotropic hormones from the anterior pituitary gland. Gonadotropin refers to any hormone that stimulates the gonads (the structures capable of producing eggs or sperm, that is, the ovaries or the testicles), regulates their development and their hormone-secreting functions, and contributes to the production of eggs or sperm.

There are two gonadotropic hormones secreted by the anterior pituitary gland: the follicle-stimulating hormone (FSH) and the luteinizing hormone (LH). The development of the ovarian follicles is dependent upon these hormones. FSH (as its name suggests) stimulates the development of several follicles in each cycle. During the first half of the follicular phase, increasing levels of FSH cause maturation of ovarian follicles (only one follicle will mature completely). It is the LH that begins the second phase of the menstrual cycle, when a surge of LH causes the mature follicle to burst and release an egg. FSH and LH also control the production of ovarian hormones (the second group of hormones regulating the female reproductive system).

The ovarian hormones in turn are divided into two groups: ovarian peptide hormones and ovarian steroid hormones.

There are two ovarian peptide hormones, inhibin and relaxin. Inhibin is secreted by the granulosa cells of the follicles. It inhibits the releasing of FSH from the anterior pituitary gland and also inhibits the release of GnRH from the hypothalamus. Thus inhibin has a role in controlling further follicular development. Relaxin is produced near the end of pregnancy by the corpus luteum and promotes relaxation of the birth channel.

There are two biologically extremely active ovarian steroid hormones: estrogen and progesterone. Estrogen is produced by the granulosa cells of developing follicles and by the corpus luteum following ovulation. This production of estrogen is dependent upon luteinizing hormone (LH). The most potent estrogenic hormone in human beings is estradiol. It is synthesized and secreted by ovarian follicles, specifically by the theca interna cells (these cells synthesize androstenedione, which is then converted into estradiol and estrone). Estradiol can also be synthesized by the fetoplacental unit and, perhaps, by the adrenal cortex. It has the following biological functions: to promote the growth and maturation of the female secondary sex characters, to induce estrus in conjunction with progesterone to prepare the endometrium for implantation of a fertilized ovum, and to support pregnancy.

Progesterone is a hormone produced by the corpus luteum. (It can also be secreted by the placenta and by the adrenal cortex.) Together with estrogen, it prepares the endometrium for implantation of the fertilized ovum, it maintains the uteroplacentofetal unit, and it promotes the development of the fetus.

Another important endocrine organ secreting the steroid hormones (estrogen and progesterone) is the placenta. It helps maintain the uterine mucosa during pregnancy. The placenta also produces and secretes chorionic gonadotropic hormone. The actions of human chorionic gonadotropin (hCG) resemble those of LH. The presence of hCG in urine in early pregnancy is the basis of most pregnancy tests. Human chorionic gonadotropic hormone maintains the secretory integrity of the corpus luteum.

Common diseases and conditions

Infertility

Infertility is diagnosed when a sexually active couple is unable to get the woman pregnant (or she is unable to carry a pregnancy to a successful childbirth) after one year of attempts. There are numerous reasons why infertility may occur:

• low number or lack of sperm cells produced by the male

• lack of ovulation (no eggs released from ovaries)

• abnormal fallopian tubes

• occurrence of what would normally be the lining of the uterus somewhere else than in the uterus (endometriosis), such as in the fallopian tubes

• problems with thick mucus in the neck of the uterus (Hence, sperm are not able to enter the uterus.)

A number of techniques may be used to assist a couple in getting the woman pregnant. These include fertilization in a dish (in vitro fertilization, IVF; *in vitro* is Latin for "in glass"). Eggs are removed from the woman, placed in a culture dish, and fertilized by sperm, then inserted into the uterus for implantation. An alternate technique is gamete intrafallopian transfer, or GIFT. Male and female reproductive cells are removed from the man and woman and then transferred to the fallopian tube where fertilization may take place naturally.

Cancer

Cancer (uncontrolled and abnormal new growth of cells) may occur in any of the structures of the reproductive system, male or female. Common types of cancer in women include the following:

• Cancer of the uterus (uterine carcinoma). It is the most common cancer of the female reproductive system.

• Cancer of the neck of the uterus (cervical carcinoma). It may be caused by the sexually-transmitted human papillomavirus or HPV.

• Cancer of the ovaries (ovarian carcinoma). It has the highest death rate of all cancers of the female reproductive system.

• Cancer of the external genitals (vulvar carcinoma). It is usually a type of skin cancer.

• Cancer of the vagina (vaginal carcinoma). It may be caused by the sexually-transmitted human papillomavirus (HPV).

• Cancer of the fallopian tubes. It is the rarest cancer of the female reproductive system.

• Tumors that form in the uterus during or after pregnancy (hydatidiform moles).

Other

Amenorrhea is the absence or abnormal stopping of menstrual periods. A number of factors may abnormally stop menstruation. They include abnormal production of LH and FSH, excessive exercise, extreme stress, and near starvation.

Painful menstruation, that is, menstruation with severe cramps or aches is called dysmenorrhea. It may be caused by excessive production of prostaglandins (the hormones that cause the uterus to contract forcefully at childbirth, thus squeezing the fetus into the vagina) or by diseased genitals.

Premenstrual syndrome (PMS) occurs during the luteal phase of the menstrual cycle and is characterized by numerous symptoms. These include changes in mood and behavior, cramps, headaches, fluid retention, and fatigue. Approximately 40% of menstruating women complain of some sort of PMS.

Toxic shock syndrome (TSS) is a rare but devastating disease associated with tampon use. Although the exact cause of the disease is not known, it has been linked to infection by *Staphylococcus aureus*. If *S. aureus* enters the vagina, it is possible that tampon use could promote the growth of these deadly bacteria. *S. aureus* may then secrete poisons (toxins) that enter the bloodstream and lead to TSS. Symptoms start with fever, vomiting, diarrhea, and low blood pressure, but may eventually involve multiple organ systems and result in death.

Effect of fitness and nutrition

The Centers for Disease Control and Prevention note that risk factors such as high cholesterol, high blood pressure and obesity, are predominately linked to heart disease and stroke. In fact, heart disease is the number one cause of death in women, according to the American Heart Association. Lifestyle changes such as a maintaining a healthy diet and routine exercise regimen can have a significant impact on lowering these risks and other health complications.

Fitness for women can often be a priority low on the "to do" list. Demands such as work, family needs, meal preparation, etc. can all work to relegate time for exercise to the back burner. Maintaining a regular fitness routine however, is more than just something to fit in on occasion to feel good, it is important for maintaining a healthy body inside and out, as well as in the prevention of illnesses associated with a sedentary lifestyle such as diabetes and hypertension.

With time being at a premium, some women find taking three, brisk 10 minute walks in the morning, afternoon and evening is best for them. Going to a step–aerobic class is great, but not always feasible if classes are not at an opportune time. Some women enjoy alternating slow paced and fast paced activities (called interval training), such as alternating between a walk mode and a run mode. No matter what exercise routine, you should always do a warm up and cool down period. This will help muscles warm up, and aid in the prevention of muscle injury. Remember that you will build stamina, exercise intensity, and endurance over time, such as progressing from walking, to brisk walking, to jogging. Start with 10 minutes of exercise 3 times a day and work up from there. It is a good idea to alternate aerobic activity one day, with strength training the other day.

Keep your bones strong. Due to the reduction in estrogen levels, older women and menopausal women are especially at risk for osteoporosis so they should include strength training exercises in their fitness routine.

Remember, it's not all about aerobics. Lifting weights, doing yoga and Pilates, working with resistance bands, and even floor exercises such as push ups, are all good, and varied forms of exercise, all of which are good in the long run.

Making time to participate in a fitness routine is important for a variety of reasons. Exercise helps to:

- Stimulate movement in the gastrointestinal tract to prevent constipation.
- Expand and oxygenate your lungs.
- Move blood throughout the circulatory system.
- Stimulate the lymphatic system.
- Relax and contract muscles throughout the entire body, increasing muscle tone and skin turgor.
- Promote and maintain good range of motion of the limbs.
- Accelerate a release of endorphins, improving mood, energy, and libido.
- Burn calories and aids in the reduction of body fat which in turn, helps in weight control.
- Enhance heart health (especially aerobic exercise), aiding in the prevention of high cholesterol and high blood pressure. While cholesterol levels can be lowered by reducing weight and eating less saturated fatty foods, a key ingredient in a cholesterol lowering program is a regular and systematic physical training program.
- Maintain a healthy weight, avoiding propensity toward insulin resistance, diabetes, and resulting complications of diabetes.
- Give you more energy. Although you may feel tired after a good workout, you will have more energy in the long run.
- Make you feel good about yourself by taking charge of your weight, health, and well being.
- Reduce stress and aid in achieving a more restful night of sleep.
- Strengthen bones to help prevent osteoporosis.

- Stimulate white blood cell movement (especially brisk physical activity), making the immune system strong.
- Make you more aware of the food you eat— especially after having done a robust workout. After all, there is a minimal sense of accomplishment in taking part in a vigorous workout, then "blowing it" by choosing less than healthy food choices.
- Make you feel satisfied and rewarded about being disciplined in your choice to take time and take action, to be good to yourself, especially when achieving predetermined fitness goals along the way.

The American Heart Association recommends 30 minutes of exercise five times a week in conjunction with a heart healthy diet regimen. Pregnant or post-partum women should first check with their doctor before beginning an exercise program.

Give yourself time to make small, incremental and beneficial changes in the look and feel of your body as you continue on your exercise journey. Results will not be overnight, so pay attention to your level of energy and the way your clothes fit to spur you on, rather than just looking at numbers on a scale. Other rewards may be seen in better blood pressure readings and blood lab values during your next visit to the doctor.

A good exercise program should start off slowly and progress moderately and at a safe degree of intensity, keeping in mind how your fitness level will change over time. Pay attention to your level of energy before, during, and after exercising, to help you decide when and how, to progress to the next level of intensity and duration, and type of exercise. Women naturally have and store, more fat on their bodies than men do, so an exercise regimen must take these differences into account. A professional trainer may be of help when putting together an exercise schedule and routine.

Exercise can be done at your local gym and can be very enjoyable when done with other women of the same age group. Some women prefer to work out at home using resistance bands, exercise balls, dumb-bells, and exercise videos. Still others, enjoy participating in a trainer–led yoga, stretching, or Pilates class. All are fine forms of exercise to help get in shape and maintain a healthy physique. Varying routines and a change in exercise locations helps avoid boredom or sagging motivation.

When working out, remember that women need to pay special attention to strength training, as well as aerobic exercise. Light weights will help add lean muscle (not bulk) to keep bones strong, reducing the

KEY TERMS

Amenorrhea—Abnormal absence or stopping of menstrual cycles.

Dysmenorrhea—Painful menstruation.

Endometrium—The inner lining of the uterus.

External genitals—The greater lips (labia majora), the lesser lips (labia minora), the clitoris, and the opening of the vagina.

Follicle—A small spherical sac located in an ovary in which an oocyte develops and matures; when the follicle bursts, the mature egg (ovum) is released into the fallopian tube. Only about 300 follicles burst during a woman's lifetime.

Gamete—A one-fold (haploid, that is, having 23 instead of 46 chromosomes) cell involved in sexual reproduction; the male gamete is the sperm; the female gamete is the egg.

Internal genitals—The vagina, uterus, fallopian tubes, and ovaries.

Menarche—The first menstrual cycle in a girl's life.

Menopause—The permanent stopping of menstrual cycles, traditionally marking the end of a woman's ability to reproduce.

Menstruation—The discharge of the lining of the uterus (endometrium) as it sheds during the menstrual cycle when pregnancy does not take place.

Zygote—A two-fold (diploid, that is having 46 chromosomes) cell resulting from fertilization of the female egg by a sperm.

chance for osteoporosis. Exercises that target core muscles of the abdomen and back, are important to keep muscles both strong, and limber. These muscles help maintain posture and balance, as well as keep the pelvic floor muscles strong—which help in prevention of bladder "leaks" and also enhance the sexual experience by keeping vaginal muscles strong.

Women over the age of 50, should pay special attention to maintaining proper balance and form when exercising, as so avoid falls and other injury to the body. Muscle and bone takes longer to heal in populations over age 50, so take care to maintain safety. Putting together a good routine with an exercise professional may be beneficial.

Healthy pregnant and postpartum woman should also be physically active. In fact, pregnant women who are in good physical shape, have been shown to have an easier delivery and more comfortable, shorter period of recovery after giving birth. Moderate activity such as brisk walking is good to keep the lungs clear and the heart strong. Moderate activity also helps maintain good blood circulation in the legs and aids in the prevention of swelling of the ankles. Most doctors advise women to wait six weeks (longer if you've had a caesarean section) before exercising. If you've had a caesarean section be careful not do any heavy lifting so as to avoid straining abdominal muscles. If you are pregnant or have recently given birth, check with your doctor before beginning a fitness program.

Adhering to a healthy nutrition program in conjunction with a good fitness program has multiple benefits for women. A healthy, well balanced diet augments the benefits of fitness by helping women attain or maintain a body that is lean, strong, and within a healthy weight range. Looking good also boosts self confidence and often increases a women's desire to be more active and engage in social activities. This is especially important for new mothers needing energy to care for their newborns and other young children or school age siblings in the family.

For pregnant women, a healthy diet is important to healthy fetal development. Mothers who are breast-feeding may need to increase their caloric intake. Check with your doctor. Typically women do not need to eat a lot of additional food to stay healthy when pregnant, usually an additional 300 calories per day, when added to an already healthy–calorie diet, is sufficient.

After giving birth, women will lose about 10 pounds. Some weight loss may occur for a few weeks following birth due loosing excess water weight. Gradual changes in diet and exercise will allow for a continued reduction in weight and an increase in tone. Remember to focus on healthy eating to keep up your energy level.

Researchers at the Mayo Clinic note that obesity as well as malnutrition, contributes to infertility in women. This may be due in part, to improper pituitary gland function (which is necessary for hormone production) as a result of deficient minerals, vitamins, and other important nutrients in the diet. Studies have also shown that a diet high in trans fat (such as that found in fast food) may also be linked to infertility in women although the reason for this is unclear.

There's no news that women's bodies look different from men's but there is a need to keep in mind that women have different vitamin, mineral and caloric needs than men, as well. The American Heart

QUESTIONS TO ASK YOUR DOCTOR

- What are the indications that I may have a problem with my reproductive system?
- What diagnostic tests are needed for a thorough assessment?
- Why do I have painful periods?
- Can you give me information about what to expect during pregnancy?
- What tests or evaluation techniques can you perform to see if my fitness and nutritional choices promote a healthy condition?
- What treatment options do you recommend for me?
- What physical or health limitations do you foresee?
- What symptoms are important enough that I should seek immediate treatment?

Association reports that diets rich in fruits and vegetables, lean protein, whole grains and fiber, and low in saturated fat, help women lower their risk for heart disease, stroke, high blood pressure, and high cholesterol. Women should keep in mind that their nutritional needs may vary with age and the amount of daily activity they engage in on a regular basis. Talk to your doctor about increasing your calcium, vitamin D, and other vitamins and minerals, as these daily requirements may increase with age. Women should talk to their obstetrician about increasing certain vitamins and minerals such as folate, and taking prenatal vitamins while they are pregnant.

The American Cancer Society notes that the risk for breast cancer increases in women who are obese, sedentary, and who eat a diet high in saturated fats. There is some evidence that ovarian, colon, and cervical cancer may also be associated with these risk factors. A women's risk for cancer can be lowered by reducing weight, exercising, and eating a healthy diet low in saturated fats.

Remember to read food labels to examine not only calorie, fat, carbohydrate, and protein content, but also to determine serving size in relation to these numbers. Dieticians may be of assistance in understanding these food labels. A well balanced fitness and nutrition regimen can improve not only the way you look and feel, but also have a positive impact on the health and quality of your life.

Resources

BOOKS

Goldberg, Nieca., MD. *Dr. Nieca Goldberg's Complete Guide to Women's Health.* New York, NY: Ballantine Books, 2009.

Heffner, Linda J., and Danny J. Schust. *The Reproductive System at a Glance,* 3rd ed. New York, NY: Wiley–Blackwell, 2010.

Kandeel, Fouad., ed. *Female Reproductive and Sexual Medicine.* Totowa, NJ: Humana Press, 2011.

McDowell, Julie., ed. *Encyclopedia of Human Body Systems.* Santa Barbara, CA: Greenwood, 2010.

Ogle, Amy, MS., RD., and Lisa Mazzullo, MD. *Before Your Pregnancy: A 90-Day Guide for Couples on How to Prepare for a Healthy Conception.* New York, NY: Ballantine Books, 2011.

Redwine, David B., MD.*100 Q&A About Endometriosis.* New York, NY: Jones-Bartlett, 2008.

Rizzo, Donald C. *Introduction to Anatomy and Physiology.* Clifton Park, NY: Delmar, 2011.

Schuiling, Kerri D., and Frances E. Likis. *Women's Gynecologic Health,*2nd ed. New York, NY: Jones–Bartlett, 2011.

ORGANIZATIONS

American College of Obstetricians and Gynecologists, 409 12th St. SW, P.O. Box 96920, Washington, DC, 20090-6920, (202) 638-5577, http://www. acog.org.

National Institutes of Health (NIH), 9000 Rockville Pike, Bethesda, MD, 20892, (301)496-4000, http://www.nih.gov/index.html.

National Women's Health Resource Center. Healthy-Women, 157 Broad St., Suite 106, Red Bank, NJ, 07701, (877) 986-9472, http://www. healthy women.org.

U.S. National Library of Medicine, 8600 Rockville Pike, Bethesda, MD, 20894, http://www.nlm.nih.gov/medlineplus/medlineplus.html.

Stéphanie Islane Dionne
Laura Jean Cataldo, RN, Ed.D.

Reproductive system, male

Definition

The male reproductive system is composed of organs that work together to produce sperm and deliver them to the female reproductive tract for fertilization of the ovum.

Description

The normal male reproductive system is composed of numerous anatomical structures, including the testis, the excretory ducts, the auxiliary glands, the penis, and the various hormones that control reproductive functions.

Testis

The testis is responsible for the production and maturation of sperm in a process called spermatogenesis. It is also the site of synthesis and secretion of androgens (male sex hormones). The testes (plural) develop in the abdomen and descend into the scrotum in the normal male. The scrotum is a muscular sac in which the testes hang from the spermatic cord.

The testis is subdivided into the tubular compartment and the interstitial compartment. The tubular compartment is composed of up to 900 seminiferous tubules, which are populated by three main types of cells: germ cells, peritubular cells, and Sertoli cells. Germ cells become mature sperm in the spermatogenic process. Peritubular cells produce various factors that aid in the transportation of mature sperm to the epididymis. Sertoli cells secrete various factors that determine the sperm production and testis size of an adult male.

Androgens are produced in the interstitial compartment of the testis. Leydig cells are responsible for the production and secretion of testosterone. Immune cells such as macrophages and lymphocytes are also found in the interstitial compartment, and aid in the proliferation and hormone production of Leydig cells.

Sperm cells are composed of a head (containing the nucleus and acrosome), the body (containing the mitochondria, or energy-producing organelles), and the tail. The nucleus contains the cell's genetic material (chromatin) while the acrosome contains enzymes that are capable of penetrating the protective layers around the egg. The mitochondria provide energy for tail motility; this is essential for movement of the sperm through the female reproductive tract.

Excretory ducts

The excretory ducts are responsible for the transfer of sperm from the seminiferous tubules of the testis to the urethra and include the epididymis, the vas deferens, and intratesticular ducts. The epididymis is a tubular structure through which sperm exiting the seminiferous tubules pass. Testicular sperm are not fully mature and would not be able to fertilize an ovum (egg). Complete maturation occurs in the epididymis in the two to twelve days that sperm are typically stored before being passed to the vas deferens. The vas deferens functions to carry mature sperm from the epididymis to the urethra; it is also called the ductus deferens. Secretions from the auxiliary glands are mixed with sperm in the vas deferens to form semen.

Auxiliary glands

The auxiliary glands include two bulbourethral glands, one prostate, and two seminal vesicles. These glands contribute the secretions that compose semen. The bulbourethral glands (also called the glands of Cowper) secrete a fluid that lubricates the urethra prior to ejaculation. The prostate secretes a fluid rich in zinc, citric acid, choline, and various proteins. The secretions of the seminal vesicle are high in fructose (an energy source for sperm) and prostaglandins (fatty acid derivatives).

Penis

The penis is the male organ of sexual reproduction and consists of three elongated bodies that cause erection, the two corpora cavernosa and the corpus spongiosum. These tissues become engorged with blood when stimulated by the nervous system during arousal. Blood is supplied by the superficial and deep arterial systems (which carry blood to the penile skin and erectile tissue, respectively). The urethra runs through the corpus spongiosum to the glans penis (distal end of the penis). The organ is covered with loose skin that forms the prepuce (foreskin) over the glans penis.

Function

Endocrine control

Normal reproductive function is dependent on complex interactions between various hormones. A portion of the brain called the hypothalamus secretes releasing hormones that travel to the pituitary gland, located at the base of the brain. The secretion of gonadotropin-releasing hormone (GnRH) from the hypothalamus triggers the release of luteinizing hormone (LH) and follicle-stimulating hormone (FSH) from the pituitary gland. LH stimulates testosterone production by Leydig cells in the testis, and FSH promotes spermatogenesis.

Male sexual act

The male sexual act can be divided into three main steps: erection, emission, and ejaculation. Erection is the result of increased blood flow to the erectile tissues of the penis; stimulation of the nervous system during arousal causes a release of acetylcholine (a neurotransmitter) that in turn causes vasodilation (increase in the diameter of blood vessels). Emission is the passage of sperm and secretions into the urethra mediated by release of the hormone adrenaline. Ejaculation occurs when the sperm are forced from the urethra by contraction of the bulbocavernous muscles. A release of noradrenaline causes the blood vessels in the penis to contract, decreasing blood flow and resulting in detumescence (loss of erection).

Fertilization

In order to fertilize the ovum, ejaculated sperm must move into the vaginal tract, pass through the cervix, survive in the uterus, and enter the fallopian tubes. Usually only healthy, motile sperm will reach the ovum and have the opportunity to fertilize it. Numerous protective layers (including the oolemma, the zona pellucida, and the zona radiata) surround the ovum, and sperm cells must penetrate each of these layers for fertilization to occur. Binding of a sperm cell to the zona pellucida induces the acrosome reaction, which permits the sperm to penetrate the zona pellucida and reach the egg membrane. The sperm and egg membranes fuse to form a zygote, and subsequent reactions prevent the binding of additional sperm cells to the egg membrane.

Common diseases and conditions

Diseases of the male reproductive system are classified based on the localization (e.g., testis, pituitary gland, etc.) and cause (e.g., congenital malformation, cancerous tumor, etc.) of the disorder.

Some common examples of andrological disorders include:

- Infertility: Male infertility may be the symptom of multiple disorders. A blockage in both of the vas deferentia or a testicular disorder may result in the complete absence of sperm (azoospermia). Low sperm counts might result from a prolonged increase in scrotal temperature—as in the case of a varicocele, a disturbance in testicular blood circulation. Retrograde ejaculation is another cause of male infertility; semen travels in the wrong direction, up the urethra to the bladder instead of down toward the penis.

- Hypogonadism: This describes a condition in which there is decreased sexual development and growth of the testes. Hypogonadism may result from tumors, hormone imbalances, or chromosomal abnormalities. Its symptoms (after puberty) include voice alteration, decreased size of testes, gynecomastia (enlargement of mammary glands), an infantile penis, or osteoporosis.

- Erectile dysfunction: It is estimated that the incidence of erectile dysfunction (ED) is twice as high as that of coronary heart disease. ED may result from reduced penile blood flow, low serum levels of testosterone, use of psychotropic drugs, alcohol abuse, metabolic disorders such as diabetes mellitus, or muscle cell impairment.

- Prostate cancer: The prostate surrounds the urethra and secretes seminal fluids. Prostate cancer is the second most common cause of cancer death of men in the United States, and the second most commonly diagnosed form of cancer (after skin cancer).

Effect of fitness and nutrition

Regular exercise is important for the physical, mental, and emotional health of men. Exercise promotes:

- weight maintenance or weight loss
- cardiovascular efficiency
- musculoskeletal strength and flexibility
- improved functioning of the metabolic, endocrine, and immune systems
- bone density
- lower cholesterol levels
- recovery from illness, injury, or surgery
- mental and emotional wellbeing

Men most often stick with an exercise program when they enjoy the activity, whether as an individual, with a partner, or with a group or team. Exercise can take place at home, outdoors, at a health club or fitness center, or as part of an after–work group activity. Working out with a friend, utilizing a personal trainer, competing, or setting personal goals can help maintain motivation.

The most efficient cardiovascular exercises for improving physical fitness include:

- brisk walking
- jogging
- running
- bicycling
- stair climbing
- elliptical cross-training on exercise machines
- aerobics
- swimming
- rowing

Many men enjoy exercise benefits while engaging in a sports activity. These activities may include:

- basketball
- soccer
- softball
- racquetball
- squash
- tennis

- volleyball
- golfing

Making time to participate in a fitness routine is important for a variety of reasons. Exercise helps to:

- Stimulate movement in the gastrointestinal tract to prevent constipation.
- Expand and oxygenate your lungs.
- Move blood throughout the circulatory system.
- Stimulate the lymphatic system.
- Relax and contract muscles throughout the entire body, increasing muscle tone and skin turgor.
- Promote and maintain good range of motion of the limbs.
- Accelerate a release of endorphins, improving mood, energy, and libido.
- Burn calories and aids in the reduction of body fat which in turn, helps in weight control.
- Enhance heart health (especially aerobic exercise), aiding in the prevention of high cholesterol and

high blood pressure. While cholesterol levels can be lowered by reducing weight and eating less saturated fatty foods, a key ingredient in a cholesterol lowering program is a regular and systematic physical training program.

- Maintain a healthy weight, avoiding propensity toward insulin resistance, diabetes, and resulting complications of diabetes.
- Give you more energy. Although you may feel tired after a good workout, you will have more energy in the long run.
- Make you feel good about yourself by taking charge of your weight, health, and well being.
- Reduce stress and aid in achieving a more restful night of sleep.
- Strengthen bones to help prevent osteoporosis.
- Stimulate white blood cell movement (especially brisk physical activity), making the immune system strong.
- Make you more aware of the food you eat—especially after having done a robust workout, so you generally make healthier food choices.
- Make you feel satisfied and rewarded about being disciplined in your choice to take time and take action, to be good to yourself, especially when achieving predetermined fitness goals along the way.

The American Heart Association recommends 30 minutes of exercise five times a week in conjunction with a heart healthy diet regimen. A regular exercise routine and nutritious diet will also help in weight management.

Men should be sure to include not only weight training, but aerobic, strength, and flexibility training, as well. Incorporating a variety of different types of training helps boost muscle mass, tone, metabolism, endurance, and overall well being. Loss of muscle mass generally occurs around age 40 and strength training in particular. will help generate and maintain muscle function and physique for men in this age group or older.

Many men enjoy circuit training as an exercise program. Circuit training combines cardiovascular exercise, endurance, and strength training exercise, as individuals move between various machines at set intervals.

Men should pay attention to their nutritional needs before, during, and after exercising. Many foods enhance a good exercise regimen, and help muscles recover well after a good workout so paying particular attention to vitamin, mineral, and fluid replenishment is important. Balanced nutrition should

include lean protein, unsaturated fats, complex carbohydrates, and plenty of water.

Vitamin B6 in particular, as well as eating garlic, onions, scallions leeks and chives (allium vegetables), may help reduce the risk of benign prostatic hypertrophy (BPH) and prevent the loss of testosterone. Eating fish high in omega-3 fatty acids can also help protect from prostate disease and infection. A blood test measuring prostate-specific antigen (PSA) can be performed by your physician to help determine prostate health. The American Cancer Society recommends yearly testing for all men aged 50 or older, and earlier testing for men with known cancer risks.

A good exercise program should start off slowly and progress moderately and at a safe degree of intensity, keeping in mind how your fitness level will change over time. Pay attention to your level of energy before, during, and after exercising, to help you decide when and how, to progress to the next level of intensity, duration, and type of exercise. A professional trainer may be of help when putting together a fitness schedule and routine.

Give yourself time to make small, incremental and beneficial changes in the look and feel of your body as you continue on your exercise journey. Results will not be overnight, so pay attention to your level of energy, changes in your physique, and the way your clothes fit to spur you on, rather than just looking at numbers on a scale. Other rewards may be seen in better blood pressure readings and blood lab values during your next visit to the doctor.

Remember to read food labels to examine not only calorie, fat, carbohydrate, and protein content, but also to determine serving size in relation to these numbers. Dieticians may be of assistance in understanding these food labels. A well balanced fitness and nutrition regimen can improve not only the way you look and feel, but also have a positive impact on the health and quality of your life.

Resources

BOOKS

Heffner, Linda J., and Danny J. Schust. *The Reproductive System at a Glance,* 3rd ed. New York, NY: Wiley–Blackwell, 2010.

Katz, Aaron E., MD. *The Definitive Guide to Prostate Cancer: Everything You Need to Know about Conventional and Integrative Therapies.* Emmaus, PA: Rodale Books, 2011.

McDowell, Julie., ed. *Encyclopedia of Human Body Systems.* Santa Barbara, CA: Greenwood, 2010.

Nieschlag, Eberhard., Hermann. M. Behre., and Susan Nieschlag, eds. *Andrology: Male Reproductive Health and Dysfunction,* 3rd ed. New York, NY: Springer, 2009.

Rizzo, Donald C. *Introduction to Anatomy and Physiology.* Clifton Park, NY: Delmar, 2011.

PERIODICALS

Lue, Tom F. "Erectile Dysfunction." *New England Journal of Medicine* (June 2000): 1802–1813.

ORGANIZATIONS

American Society of Andrology, 74 New Montgomery, Suite 230, San Francisco, CA 94105, (415) 764-4823, http://www.andrologysociety.com.

National Institutes of Health (NIH), 9000 Rockville Pike, Bethesda, MD, 20892, 301-496-4000, http://www.nih.gov/index.html.

U.S. National Library of Medicine, 8600 Rockville Pike, Bethesda, MD, 20894, http://www.nlm.nih.gov/U.S. National Library of Medicine, 8600 Rockville Pike, Bethesda, MD, 20894, http://www.nlm.nih.gov/medlineplus/medlineplus.html.

Stéphanie Islane Dionne
Laura Jean Cataldo, RN, Ed.D.

Respiratory system

Definition

The respiratory system consists of organs that deliver oxygen to the circulatory system for transport to all the cells of the body. The respiratory system also assists in the removal of carbon dioxide (CO_2), thus preventing a deadly buildup of this waste product in the body.

Description

The respiratory system consists of the upper and lower respiratory tracts, extending from the nose to the lungs.

The upper respiratory tract encompasses the:

• nose
• pharynx, more commonly called the throat

The lower respiratory tract includes the:

• larynx, also called the voice box
• the trachea or windpipe, which splits into two main branches called bronchi
• tiny branches of the bronchi called bronchioles
• the lungs

These organs all work together to provide air to and from the lungs. The lungs then operate in conjunction with the circulatory system to deliver oxygen and remove carbon dioxide.

Breathing is an unconscious process carried out on a constant basis and is necessary for survival. Under normal conditions, a person takes 12–20 breaths per minute, although newborns breathe at a faster rate, at approximately 30–50 breaths per minute. The breathing rate set by the respiratory center can be altered by conscious control, for example, by holding the breath. This alteration occurs when the part of the brain involved in thinking, the cerebral cortex, sends signals to the diaphragm and rib muscles to momentarily ignore the signals from the respiratory center. If a person holds his or her breath too long, carbon dioxide accumulates in the blood, which then causes the blood to become more acidic. The increased acidity interferes with the action of enzymes, which are specialized proteins that coordinate all biochemical reactions in the body. To prevent too much acid from building up in the blood, special receptors located in the brainstem and in the blood vessels of the neck called chemoreceptors monitor the acid level in the blood. These chemoreceptors send nervous signals to the respiratory center when acid levels are too high, which overrides the signals from the cerebral cortex, forcing a person to exhale and then resume breathing. The blood acid level is brought back to normal levels by exhalation, which expels the carbon dioxide. Irreversible damage to tissues occurs, followed by the failure of all body systems, and ultimately, death if the respiratory system's tasks are interrupted for more than a few minutes.

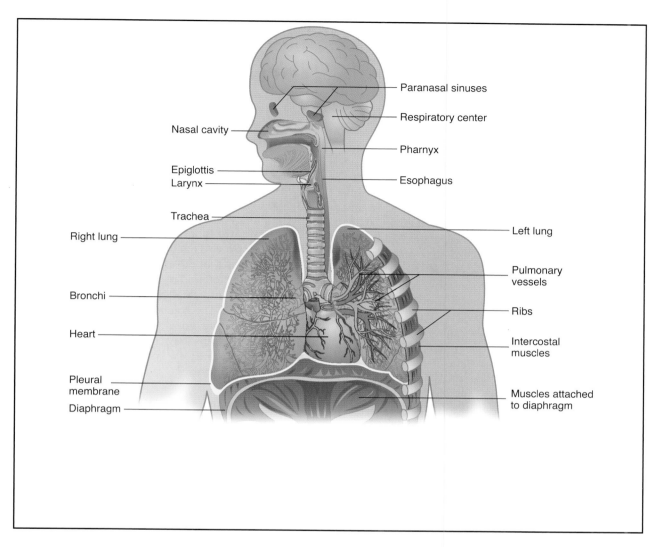

Labels: Nasal cavity, Epiglottis, Larynx, Trachea, Right lung, Bronchi, Heart, Pleural membrane, Diaphragm, Paranasal sinuses, Respiratory center, Pharynx, Esophagus, Left lung, Pulmonary vessels, Ribs, Intercostal muscles, Muscles attached to diaphragm

The respiratory system. *(Electronic Illustrators Group. © 2012 Cengage Learning.)*

Nasal passages

The flow of air begins in the nose, which is divided into the left and right nasal passages and ends in the lungs. The nasal passages are lined with epithelial cells, a mucous membrane composed mostly of a layer of flat, closely packed cells. Each epithelial cell is fringed with thousands of tiny fingerlike extensions of the cells called cilia. Goblet cells are specialized cells that produce mucus, and are among the epithelial cells. Mucus is a thick, moist fluid that coats epithelial cells and cilia. Beneath the mucous membrane, near the surface of the nasal passages, are many tiny blood vessels called capillaries. The nasal passages play two critical roles in transporting air to the pharynx. First, the nasal passages filter air to remove potentially disease-causing particles. Secondly, they moisten and warm the air to protect the respiratory system.

Filtering air through the nasal passage prevents airborne bacteria, viruses, smog, dust particles, and other potentially disease-causing substances from entering the lungs or the bronchioles. Just inside the nostrils are coarse hairs that assist in trapping airborne particles as they are inhaled. The particles then drop down onto the mucous membranes in the lining of the nasal passages. The particles are then propelled out of the nose or downward to the pharynx by the wave of mucus created by the cilia in the mucous membranes. From the pharynx, mucus is swallowed and travels to the stomach where subsequently the particles are destroyed by stomach acid. If there are more particles in the nasal passages than the cilia can cope with, a reflex will be triggered producing a sneeze. The sneeze, designed to flush out the polluted air, is due to particles building up on the mucus and irritating the membrane below it.

Pharynx

As air leaves the nasal passages, it flows to the pharynx, which is a short, funnel-shaped tube about 13 cm (5 inches) long. The pharynx is also lined with a mucous membrane and ciliated cells that filter air from the nasal passages. The pharynx also includes the tonsils, which are lymphatic tissues that contain white blood cells. If any impurities escape the hairs, cilia, and mucus of the nasal passages and pharynx, the white blood cells attack the disease-causing organisms. To prevent these organisms from moving further into the body, the tonsils are strategically located. One pair of growths of lymphoid tissue, referred to as the adenoids, is located high in the rear wall of the pharynx. Two tonsils called the palatine tonsils are positioned on either side of the tongue at the back of the pharynx. Another pair called the lingual tonsils is found deep in the pharynx at the base of the tongue. The tonsils may become swollen with infection during their fight against disease-causing organisms.

Larynx

Air passes from the pharynx to the larynx, which is approximately 2 inches (5 cm) long and situated near the middle of the neck. The larynx is comprised of several layers of cartilage, a tough and flexible tissue.

In addition to transporting air to the trachea, the larynx serves other functions such as:

- It prevents food and fluid from entering the air passage which would cause choking.
- Its mucous membranes and cilia-bearing cells help filter air.
- It plays a primary role in producing sound.
- The cilia in the larynx move airborne particles up toward the pharynx to be swallowed.

A thin, leaf-like flap of tissue called the epiglottis prevents food and fluids from entering the larynx from the pharynx. The epiglottis is held in a vertical position, like an open trap door when a person is breathing. When swallowing, a reflex forces the larynx and the epiglottis to move toward each other. This reflex diverts food and fluids to the esophagus. The swallowing reflex may not work if one eats or drinks too rapidly, or laughs while swallowing. Food or fluid enters the larynx and a coughing reflex is initiated to clear the obstruction. This situation may cause life-threatening choking if coughing does not clear the larynx of the obstruction.

Trachea, bronchi, and bronchioles

Air is passed from the larynx into the trachea, the largest airway in the respiratory system. The trachea is a tube located just below the larynx, approximately 5 to 6 inches (12 to 15 cm) long. Fifteen to 20 C-shaped rings of cartilage form the trachea. Air passes freely at all times because the trachea is held open by the rings of sturdy cartilage. The open part of the C-shaped cartilage rings is situated at the back of the trachea with the ends connected by muscle tissue. The trachea branches into two tubes at its base, located just below where the neck meets the trunk of the body. These two tubes are called the left and right bronchi and they deliver air to the left and right lungs, respectively. The bronchi branch into smaller tubes called bronchioles within the lungs. The trachea, bronchi, and the first few bronchioles are lined with mucous membranes and ciliated cells; thus they contribute to the cleansing action of the respiratory system by moving mucus upward to the pharynx.

Alveoli and lungs

The bronchioles divide many more times in the lungs into an upside-down tree-like structure with progressively smaller branches. Tiny air sacs called alveoli are at the end of the branches. Some of the bronchioles are no larger than 0.5 mm (0.02 inches) in diameter. The alveoli comprise most of the lung tissue, with about 150 million alveoli per lung, and resemble bunches of grapes. The alveoli send oxygen to the circulatory system while removing carbon dioxide. Alveoli have thin elastic walls, thus allowing air to flow into them when they expand; they collapse when the air is exhaled. Alveoli are arranged in clusters, and each cluster is surrounded by a dense network of capillaries. The walls of the capillaries are very thin; thus the air in the wall of the alveoli is very near to the blood in the capillaries (only about 0.1 to 0.2 microns). Carbon dioxide is a waste product that is dumped into the bloodstream from the cells. It flows throughout the body in the bloodstream to the heart, and then to the alveolar capillaries. The oxygen diffuses from the alveoli to the capillaries since the concentration of oxygen is much higher in the alveoli than in the capillaries. From the capillaries, the oxygen flows into larger vessels and is then carried to the heart where it is pumped to the rest of the body. The forces of exhalation cause the carbon dioxide to go back up through the respiratory passages and out of the body. Numerous macrophages are interspersed among the alveoli.

Macrophages are large white blood cells that remove foreign substances from the alveoli that have not been previously filtered out. The presence of the macrophages ensures that the alveoli are protected from infection; they are the last line of defense of the respiratory system.

The lungs are the largest organ in the respiratory system and resemble large pink sponges. The left lung is slightly smaller than the right lung since it shares space with the heart, which is also located in the left side of the chest. Each lung is divided into lobes, with two in the left lung and three in the right. A slippery membrane called the pleura covers the lungs and lines the inside of the chest wall. It helps the lungs move smoothly during each breath. Normally, the two lubricated layers of the pleura have very little space between them. They glide smoothly over each other when the lungs expand and contract.

The diaphragm is the most important muscle involved in respiration. It lies just under the lungs and is a muscle shaped like a large dome. The sternum (or breastbone), ribs, and spine protect the lungs and the other organs in the chest. Twelve pairs of ribs curve around the chest and are joined to the vertebrae of the spine. The intercostal muscles are also important for respiration. They lie between the ribs and assist in breathing by helping to move the rib cage.

Function

The main function of the respiratory system is the delivery of oxygen and removal of carbon dioxide. To achieve this purpose, the nervous system controls the flow of air in and out of the lungs while maintaining a regular rate and pattern of breathing. Regulation is controlled by the respiratory center, a cluster of nerve cells in the brain stem. These cells simultaneously send signals to the muscles involved in inhalation: the diaphragm and rib muscles. The diaphragm flattens out when stimulated by a nervous impulse. The thoracic or chest cavity contains the lungs. The volume of the cavity expands with the downward movement of the diaphragm, thus expanding the lungs. The rib muscles also contract when stimulated, which pulls the rib cage up and out, at the same time expanding the thoracic cavity. This movement reduces pressure in the chest. When the volume is increased in the thoracic cavity, air rushes into the lungs to equalize the pressure. This nervous stimulation is quick, and when it is over, the diaphragm and rib muscles relax and a person exhales.

Working in conjunction with the circulatory system, the oxygen-rich blood travels from the lungs through the pulmonary veins into the left side of the heart. From there, blood is pumped to the rest of the body. Blood that is oxygen-depleted, but carbon dioxide-rich, returns to the right side of the heart through two large veins called the superior and inferior venae cavae. This blood is then pumped through the pulmonary artery to the lungs, where oxygen is picked up and carbon dioxide is released. This process is repeated continually under normal circumstances.

Other functions the respiratory system assist in just by normal respiration are the regulation of acid–base balance in the body, a critical process for normal cellular function. It also protects the body against toxic substances inhaled as well as against disease-causing organisms in the air. The respiratory system also assists in detecting smell using the olfactory receptors located in the nasal passages. Furthermore, it aids in producing sounds for speech.

Common diseases and conditions

The diseases and disorders of the respiratory system can affect any part of the respiratory tract and may range from mild to life-threatening conditions such as:

- Colds—A virus that targets the nasal passages and pharynx. Symptoms include a stuffy and runny nose.
- Hay fever and asthma—Allergic reactions that may occur when the immune system is stimulated by pollen, dust, or other irritants. A runny nose, watery eyes, and sneezing characterizes hay fever. In asthma, because the bronchi and bronchioles are temporarily constricted and inflamed, a person has difficulty breathing.
- Bronchitis—Characterized by inflamed bronchi or bronchiole membranes, resulting from viral or bacterial infection or from chemical irritants.
- Emphysema—A non-contagious disease that results from multiple factors including: smog, cigarette smoke, infection, and a genetic predisposition to the condition. Emphysema partially destroys the alveolar tissue and leaves the remaining alveoli weakened and enlarged. When a person exhales, the bronchioles collapse, trapping air in the alveoli. This process eventually impedes the ability to exchange oxygen and carbon dioxide, leading to breathing difficulties.
- Pneumonia—Infections caused by bacteria or viruses can lead to this potentially serious condition. The alveoli become inflamed and fill with fluid, impairing the flow of oxygen and carbon dioxide between the capillaries and the alveoli.
- Tuberculosis—A condition caused by a bacterium that attacks the lungs and occasionally other body

tissues. Left untreated, the disease destroys lung tissue.

- Laryngitis—An inflammation of the larynx caused by irritants such as cigarette smoke, overuse of the voice, or a viral infection. People with laryngitis may become hoarse, or they may only be able to whisper until the inflammation is reduced.

- Lung cancer—Occurs in those individuals who are exposed to cancer-causing agents, such as tobacco smoke, asbestos, or uranium; or who have a genetic predisposition to the disease. Treatments are very effective if the cancer is detected before the cancer has spread to other parts of the body. About 85% of cases are diagnosed after the cancer has spread; thus the prognosis is very poor.

- Respiratory distress syndrome (RDS)—Refers to a group of symptoms that indicate severe malfunctioning of the lungs affecting adults and infants. Adult respiratory distress syndrome (ARDS) is a life-threatening condition that results when the lungs are severely injured, for example, by poisonous gases, in an automobile accident, or as a response to inflammation in the lungs.

- Wheezing—A high-pitched whistling sound produced due to air flowing through narrowed breathing tubes. It may have many causes such as asthma, emphysema, pneumonia, bronchitis, etc.

- Shortness of breath or dyspnea—This condition may have multiple causes such as asthma, emphysema, hyperventilation, obesity, cigarette smoking, lung disease, excessive exercise, etc.

- Chronic respiratory insufficiency (or chronic obstructive pulmonary disease; COPD)—A prolonged or persistent condition characterized by breathing or respiratory dysfunction resulting in reduced rates of oxygenation or the ability to eliminate carbon dioxide. These rates are insufficient to meet the requirements of the body and may be severe enough to impair or threaten the function of vital organs (respiratory failure).

Some of the most common symptoms of respiratory disorders are a cough, shortness of breath, chest pain, wheezing, cyanosis (bluish discoloration), finger clubbing, stridor (a crowing sound when breathing), hemoptysis (coughing up of blood), and respiratory failure. These symptoms do not necessarily signify a respiratory problem, but can be a sign of another problem. For example, chest pain may be due to a heart or a gastrointestinal problem.

Cystic fibrosis is a genetic disease that causes excessive mucus production and clogs the airways.

Acidosis is a condition resulting from higher than normal acid levels in the body fluids. It is not a disease but may be an indicator of disease. Respiratory acidosis is due to a failure by the lungs to remove carbon dioxide, therefore reducing the pH in the body. Several conditions such as chest injury, blockage of the upper air passages, and severe lung disease may result in respiratory acidosis. Blockage of the air passages may be due to bronchitis, asthma, or airway obstruction resulting in mild or severe acidosis. Regular, consistent retention of carbon dioxide in the lungs is referred to as chronic respiratory acidosis. This disorder results in only mild acidosis because of an increased bicarbonate (alkali) production by the kidneys.

Alkalosis is a condition resulting from a higher than normal level of base or alkali in the body fluids. Respiratory alkalosis results from decreased carbon dioxide levels caused by conditions such as hyperventilation (a faster breathing rate), anxiety, and fever. The pH becomes elevated in the body. Hyperventilation causes the body to lose excess carbon dioxide in expired air and can be triggered by altitude or a disease that reduces the amount of oxygen in the blood. Symptoms of respiratory alkalosis may include dizziness, lightheadedness, and numbing of the hands and feet. Treatments include breathing into a paper bag or a mask that induces rebreathing of carbon dioxide.

Effect of fitness and nutrition

Most people who exercise know firsthand, the effect that exercise has on their respiratory rate. Exercise activity necessitates interchange with the respiratory system and many beneficial physiological responses, as a result.

As we take part in calisthenics, aerobics, or other exercise activities our metabolism increases with movement of the body, that is, the muscular, respiratory, and the circulatory system. When we work harder and increase motion, our respiratory rate increases both in rate and depth, and our pattern of breathing may change as well. Increasing our respiratory rate expands the lungs as we inhale and exhale oxygen and carbon dioxide. This lung expansion necessitates active movement of the muscles of the diaphragm (expansion and contraction) as we increase our lung capacity (tidal volume). As we increase body movement and breathing we clear the respiratory tract and stimulate the lungs while the cardiovascular and circulatory system circulate oxygen-rich blood throughout the body. In addition the body temperature increases, further necessitating good respiratory function to help keep body temperature in balance.

KEY TERMS

Acidosis—A dangerous condition in which the blood and body tissues are less alkaline (or more acidic) than normal.

Alkalosis—Excessive alkalinity of the blood and body tissue.

Bronchi—The trachea branches into two tubes at the base of the trachea called the left and right bronchi, which extend from the trachea to deliver air to the left and right lungs, respectively. The bronchi branch into smaller tubes called bronchioles within the lungs.

Bronchioles—The bronchioles are no larger than 0.5mm (0.02 inches) in diameter and divide many times in the lungs to form a tree-like structure; they have progressively smaller branches and tiny air sacs called alveoli at the end.

Capillaries—Tiny blood vessels that lie beneath the mucous membrane, near the surface of the nasal passages.

Carbon dioxide (CO_2)—A gaseous waste product that is dumped into the bloodstream from the cells;

a byproduct of respiration, it is released upon exhalation of air from the body.

Cilia—Each epithelial cell is fringed with thousands of these tiny fingerlike extensions of the cells.

Diaphragm—The diaphragm is involved in inhalation. It lies just under the lungs and is a muscle shaped like a large dome.

Epiglottis—A thin, leaflike flap of tissue that prevents food and fluids from entering the larynx from the pharynx.

Mucus—A thick, moist fluid that coats epithelial cells and cilia.

pH—the negative logarithm of H+ (hydrogen) concentration. Acid-base balance can be defined as homeostatis (equilibrium) of the body fluids at a normal arterial blood pH ranging between 7.37 and 7.43.

Thoracic cavity—Also called the chest cavity, it is the portion of the ventral body cavity located between the neck and the diaphragm. It is enclosed by the ribs, the vertebral column, and the sternum. It is separated from the abdominal cavity by the diaphragm.

Some exercises and physical activities that enhance the respiratory system include:

- aerobics
- bicycling
- circuit or cross-training on exercise machines
- cross-country skiing
- jogging
- jumping rope
- moderate or brisk walking
- rowing
- running
- stair climbing
- swimming
- water exercise

All of these exercises promote cardiovascular fitness, including improved heart function and increased heart, lung, and muscle endurance.

Yoga is also a popular activity that enhances the respiratory system, as participants pay particular attention to their breathing during yoga sessions. **Bikram yoga** is a style of **hatha yoga** developed by Bikram Choudhury and includes a specific series of 26 breathing exercises and asanas (body postures)

designed to help move oxygenated blood throughout the entire body. **Iyengar yoga** also utilizes specific breathing exercises and patterns. Individuals with diminished lung function due to age–related changes, smoking, or other factors, generally find the breathing activity associated with yoga to be beneficial.

Pilates is a low–impact form of exercise that requires deep breathing exercises while progressing from one movement to the next. Many individuals find the controlled, balanced, rhythmic flow of this exercise very appealing.

When weightlifting, individuals should inhale prior to moving the weight, and exhale when exerting force with movement of the weight. Take care to avoid breath–holding, as doing so prevents lung expansion and much needed oxygen from getting to muscle groups. Breath–holding may also cause an unsafe increase in **blood pressure**.

As always, consult with your doctor before beginning an exercise program.

A good exercise routine should start off slowly and progress moderately and at a safe degree of intensity, keeping in mind how your fitness level will change over time. Pay attention to your breathing rate and level of exertion before, during, and after exercising, to help you decide when and how, to progress to the next level of intensity, duration, and type of exercise. The American Heart Association maintains that the "talk test" is useful to consider when exercising. That is, if you can talk and hold a moderate conversation while exercising, you are working at a safe and sustainable level of activity. If however, you cannot hold a conversation or are having breathing difficulty, you are working too hard. A professional trainer may be of help when putting together a fitness schedule and activity routine.

The American Heart Association recommends 30 minutes of exercise five times a week in conjunction with a heart healthy diet regimen. A regular exercise routine and nutritious diet will also help in weight management. Remember to read food labels to examine not only calorie, fat, carbohydrate, and **protein** content, but also to determine serving size in relation to these numbers. Dieticians may be of assistance in understanding these food labels.

A balanced, systematic, and routine workout offers individuals numerous fitness benefits including:

• weight control
• good circulation
• promotion of good heart health
• strength
• tone
• overall well-being

As noted previously, respiratory conditions such as allergies, asthma, and bronchitis, increase mucus and inflammation in the respiratory tract. Certain foods have been found to help reduce symptoms caused by these breathing ailments. Foods high in **antioxidants** such as many fruits and vegetables, minimize free radicals in the body. Free radicals cause internal "rust" and inflammation to the cells and foods high in free radicals such as green leafy vegetables, citrus fruits, and berries help decrease lung inflammation. Warm (not hot) fluids such as light soups and teas may help loosen mucus and soothe the respiratory tract, as well. Avoid milk or cream–based products as they thicken mucus, making the respiratory tract more difficult to clear.

Making good nutritional choices and developing a healthy exercise regimen is beneficial to the respiratory system and the entire body as a whole. Give yourself time to make small, incremental changes in the look and feel of your body as you continue on your journey. Results will not be overnight, so pay attention to your level of **energy**, changes in your physique,

QUESTIONS TO ASK YOUR DOCTOR

• What are the indications that I may have a problem with my respiratory system?
• What diagnostic tests are needed for a thorough assessment?
• What kind of fitness program should I follow?
• What tests or evaluation techniques can you perform to see if my fitness and nutritional choices promote a healthy condition?
• What treatment options do you recommend for me?
• What physical or health limitations do you foresee?
• What measures can be taken to prevent respiratory system problems?
• How can my quality of life be improved?
• What symptoms are important enough that I should seek immediate treatment?

and the way your clothes fit to spur you on, rather than just looking at numbers on a scale. Other rewards may be seen in better blood pressure readings and blood lab values during your next visit to the doctor. A strong, effective respiratory system will support your wellness efforts. A well balanced fitness and nutrition regimen can improve not only the way you look and feel, but also have a positive impact on the health and quality of your life.

Resources

BOOKS

Harper, Bob. *Are You Ready! Take Charge, Lose Weight, Get in Shape, and Change Your Life Forever*. New York: Broadway Books, 2009.

Kohlstadt, Ingrid. *Food and Nutrients in Disease Management*. Boca Raton, FL: CRC Press, 2009.

Lechner, Andrew. *Respiratory: An Integrated Approach to Disease*. New York, NY: McGraw–Hill Professional, 2011.

Manocchia, Pat. *Anatomy of Exercise: A Trainer's Inside Guide to Your Workout*. Richmond Hill, ONT: Firefly Books, 2009.

McConnell, Alison. *Breathe Strong, Perform Better*. Champaign, IL: Human Kinetics, 2011.

McDowell, Julie., ed. *Encyclopedia of Human Body Systems*. Santa Barbara, CA: Greenwood, 2010.

Plant, Jane., and Gill Tidey. *Eating for Better Health*. New York, NY: Virgin Books, 2010.

Rizzo, Donald C. *Introduction to Anatomy and Physiology.* Clifton Park, NY: Delmar, 2011.

Shils, Maurice E. *Modern Nutrition in Health and Disease,* 11th ed. New York, NY: Lippincott Williams & Wilkins, 2012.

West, John B., MD., PhD. *Respiratory Physiology: The Essentials,* 9th ed. New York, NY: Lippincott Williams & Wilkins, 2011.

PERIODICALS

Baker, Frank, et al. "Health risks associated with cigar smoking." *Journal of the American Medical Association* 284, no. 6 (2000):735–740.

Beckett, W. S. "Current concepts: occupational respiratory diseases." *New England Journal of Medicine* 342 (2000):406–413.

Napoli, Maryann. "Alleviating cold symptoms: what works, what doesn't." *Healthfacts* (January 2001). http://www.findarticles.com/cf_0/m0815/2001_Jan/68277444/p1/article.jhtml.

ORGANIZATIONS

American Heart Association, 7272 Greenville Avenue, Dallas, TX, 75231, (800) 242-8721, http://www.americanheart.org.

American Lung Association, 1301 Pennsylvania Ave. NW, Suite 800, Washington, DC, 20004, (202) 785-3355. http://www.lungusa.org.

American Medical Association, 515 N. State St., Chicago, IL, 60654, (800) 621-8335, http://www.ma-assn.org.

National Heart Lung and Blood Institute (NHLBI), P. O. Box 30105, Bethesda, MD, 20824-0105, (301) 592-8573, TTY: (240) 629-3255, http://www.nhlbi.nih.gov.

National Institutes of Health (NIH), 9000 Rockville Pike, Bethesda, MD, 20892, 301-496-4000, http://www.nih.gov/index.html.

U.S. National Library of Medicine, 8600 Rockville Pike, Bethesda, MD, 20894, http://www.nlm.nih.gov/medlineplus/medlineplus.html.

Crystal Heather Kaczkowski, MSc
Laura Jean Cataldo, RN, EdD

Risk stratification *see* Pre-participation screening

Rock climbing

Definition

Rock climbing is a recreational and competitive sport in which a person attempts to ascend a natural or artificial rock face carrying gear that may range from purely safety devices to more complex equipment that provides both safety and mechanisms for making the climb possible.

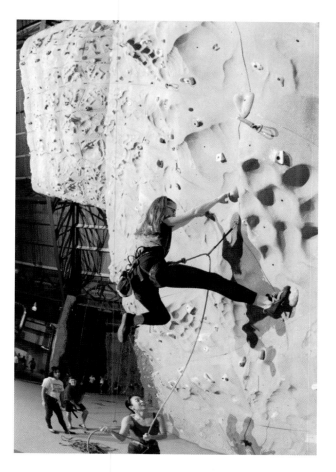

A woman ascends a rock climbing wall. *(© AP Images)*

Purpose

Many rock climbers enjoy the sport for the pure pleasure that it brings, both in terms of accomplishing a physical task that challenges one's body to the utmost and in terms of the interface with nature that it provides. Competitive rock climbers have, in addition to this goal, the objective of triumphing over opponents in completing a given course in the least amount of time, or covering the largest part of a predesignated course in a given period of time.

Demographics

The most complete data on participation in rock climbing in the United States comes from annual surveys conducted by the Outdoor Foundation. The most recent survey (2011) was based on interviews with 38,742 Americans aged six and over; results of that survey were extrapolated to the total U.S. population. The survey estimated that 2,198,000 Americans participated in traditional, ice, and mountaineering climbing in 2010, and another 4,770,000 participated in indoor rock climbing.

These numbers were relatively constant for the latter category over the period from 2006 to 2010, although they represented an increase of 38.6% for indoor climbing over the same period. For purposes of comparison, other outdoor sports included **adventure racing** (1,339,000 participants), birdwatching (13,320,000), canoeing (10,553,000), **skateboarding** (6,808,000), surfing (2,767,000), and trail **running** (5,136,000).

Another good source of demographic data on rock climbing is the British Mountaineering Club, which keeps regular records of the numbers and characteristics of rock climbers in Great Britain. In a 2003 survey, the club found that the majority of rock climbers surveyed were between the ages of 19 and 30 (37%) and 31 and 45 (44%), with only 1% under the age of 18 or over the age of 65. In all age groups, men were in the majority by far, making up 84% of all those in the 19 to 30 and 89% of those in the 31 to 45 age group. Some anecdotal evidence seems to suggest that, at least in the United States, the proportion of women rock climbers has begun to increase significantly over the last decade.

History

Rock climbing appears to be as old as human history in at least mountainous parts of the world. For residents of the Andes, the Rockies, the Alps, and other mountain ranges, people have probably always had to travel at least occasionally over difficult terrain to obtain food, launch attacks on enemies, explore new territories, or other basic human activities. Rock climbing may also have been enjoyed as a form of recreation.

Some historians date the origin of modern mountain climbing to 1492, when a captain in the French army, Antoine de Ville, ascended to the summit of Mont Aiguille (Mount Inaccessible). Other discrete episodes of rock climbing were recorded over the next four centuries, but most experts agree that the sport cannot be said to have originated until the 1880s, when it became popular in three disparate geographical areas at almost the same time, the Lake District and Wales in Great Britain, near Dresden in Saxony, and the Dolomites in northeastern Italy. The leading figure during this time was a member of the British aristocracy, Walter Parry Haskett Smith. Although trained in the law, Smith spent much of his time pursuing athletic adventures, one of which involved the ascent of the 70-ft (21-m) Napes Needle in the English Lake District. Word of Smith's accomplishment spread throughout the country and inspired a new interest in the sport of rock climbing. The sport was just developing in the United States at almost the same

time. In 1869 John Muir had made apparently the first free solo ascent of Cathedral Peak in what is now Yosemite National Park, and six years later, 28 year-old George Anderson made the first ascent (in his bare feet) of Half Dome, also in Yosemite. He used a variety of climbing implements, including a climbing rope and fixed eye bolts for holds in the rock.

Competitive rock climbing dates to post-World War II Soviet Union, when the first speed events were introduced. These events at the time, and for some time afterwards, were limited to citizens of the USSR only. The first international event occurred in 1985 at Bardonecchia, Italy, not far from Torino. That event, the Sportroccia, was held on a mountain in Valle Stretta and was won by German climber Stefan Glowacz. The event was repeated the following year and an indoor competition at a gymnasium in the Lyon suburb of Vaulx-en-Velin was added to the competition. By the late 1980s, rock climbers were provided with a number of competitive events in which to participate, culminating in the first World Cup in 1989.

The governing body for rock climbing was originally the Union Internationale des Association d'Alpinisme (International Mountaineering and Climbing Federation; UIAA), established in 1932 for the "study and solution of all problems regarding mountaineering." The UIAA assumed responsibility for all aspects of rock climbing until 2006 when it decided to create a separate organization to deal with climbing competition exclusively, the International Federation of Sport Climbing (IFSC), which continues to be a separate, self-governing part of UIAA.

Description

A variety of rock climbing styles are used:

• Bouldering is a style of rock climbing that takes place on relatively short routes at heights from which it is relatively safe to fall. The climber uses no special equipment except for the possibility of a bouldering pad to break a person's fall from the rock and a spotter who watches the climb from below and gives advice to the climber and tries to direct her or him away from dangerous parts of the climbing rock.

• Free climbing is a form of rock climbing in which the climber relies entirely on his or her hands and feet to make an ascent. Any equipment is used solely for safety purposes, and not to aid in the ascent itself. For example, a climber may be attached to a top rope belay system or on safety anchors installed in the rock along the route. But essentially the climber's success depends entirely on his or her own physical strength, endurance, and skill.

- Traditional, or trad, climbing is a variation of free climbing in which the climber installs a safety device during the ascent and removes them as soon as they are no longer needed. As in free climbing, the devices installed are used only for safety purposes, and not to assist in the ascent.

- Sport climbing is another version of free climbing except that the safety devices needed for the climb are permanently installed (or at least not installed by the climber during the climb). Again, the devices are not used to aid in the ascent, but just to provide additional safety for the climber.

- Aid climbing involves the use of devices installed into the face of the rock by the climber to help with the ascent. At one time, the usual procedure was to drive some type of object, such as a piton (a metal spike), into the rock to serve as an anchor in climbing. Climbers ascend in pairs, the leader (who goes first) and the belayer (who remains at some distance behind the leader). The two are connected by a rope that is also connected to one of the anchors in the rock. If the leader should fall, the belayer controls the rope in such a way as to keep the leader from falling to the ground. Ascent takes place as leader and belayer move upward from one anchor point to the next. A variety of devices are used in aid climbing to make the ascent possible. In recent years, the most popular (because it is the least damaging to the rock) has been a camming device, which provides a tight attachment to the rock.

- Free soloing might be regarded as the purest form of rock climbing in that the climber relies on her or his own body only, with no gear of any kind, either for the purpose of protection or to aid in the ascent. Free soloing is probably the riskiest form of rock climbing in that a climber who falls during this type of ascent faces a high likelihood of severe injury or death.

- Deep water soloing is a version of free soloing in that the climber selects a rock that lies above deep water, which provides the sole means of protection should the climber fall from the rock.

- Top-roping is perhaps the safest method of rock climbing because the climber is attached to a rope that travels over a support system at the top of the rock. A belayer holds the other end of the rope and can control the motion of the climber in case of an emergency.

- Indoor climbing is the most popular version of rock climbing; in fact, it is twice as popular in the United States as the traditional outdoor version of the sport. The sport is usually practiced on non-rocky material, such as tough plastic, in a gymnasium-like setting. Many people learn indoor climbing on a rock fitted with a top rope system and proceed to bouldering and other versions of the sport.

Competitive rope climbing falls into one of four major categories. In all forms of competition, climbers ascend by means of a number of fixed anchors over which they traverse during their ascent. Climbers must focus not on the placement of the anchors, but on the most efficient way of moving from one anchor to the next. The first category of competitive climbing is a speed climb. The winner is the person that covers a designated route in the shortest possible time. The other three types of climbing focus on difficulty and speed, rather than speed alone. In red point climbing, a variety of climbing routes are available to the climber, each of different difficulty and with a different point value. The climber must select the most difficult route he or she can follow in the fastest time to achieve a maximum score. Competitions may also involve on-sight or flash events. In the former case, competitors are allowed to have one preview examination of the wall to be climbed and then one attempt to climb the wall. The person who ascends the farthest on the wall in a given time period is the winner. In flash events, competitors are allowed to watch each other attempt their ascent and to comment among themselves before, but not during, the ascent.

Preparation

Rock climbing is a very demanding sport that requires superior strength, endurance, flexibility, and balance. The sport also requires mental and emotional qualities, such as the willingness to face unknown and potentially very dangerous situations and the ability to deal with sudden, potentially life-threatening conditions on the face of a wall.

Equipment

The minimum personal apparel required for rock climbing is as simple as that required for **swimming**. Some climbers attempt a climb in nothing more than shorts or a skimpy bathing suit. For all but the very best climbers, other equipment is appropriate, such as shorts or long pants, a sleeveless or sleeved shirt, socks and shoes, a helmet, and gloves. The choice of personal apparel depends to a significant degree on the climber's self-confidence, the extent to which he or she needs or wants to be in contact with the rock, the protection one needs, along with other factors.

Many forms of rock climbing require a variety of equipment needed for safety purposes or to be used in the ascent. This equipment may include:

- Climbing holds: Rubber or plastic grips that come in a variety of shapes. They are attached to a wall by means of bolts or t-nuts to provide climbers with objects to grip or stand on during their ascent.
- Climbing harness: A device worn by a climber to which a rope or other safety device can be attached.
- Belays and rappels: Closeable or closed devices, respectively, to which ropes can be attached.
- Climbing ropes: Ropes used for the ascent in a climb or as a safety system for preventing a person from falling during a climb.
- Carabiners: Spring-loaded loops used for attaching various parts of a climbing system to each other. They snap on to other components of a system quickly and securely.
- Quickdraws: A short piece of rope or strap with loops at each end used to attach a rope to a carabiner.
- Climbing shoes: Specialized designed shoes with soles adapted to hold tightly to rock surfaces, flexible enough to fit into tight places in the rock, and otherwise adapted to the special demands placed on feet by climbing.
- Fingerboards: Strips of wood or plastic with depressions into which the fingers can be placed to provide a training tool for finger strength and placement.
- Bouldering pad or crash pad: Used to provide protection for climbers who fall during bouldering or other short-distance climbs.
- Powdered chalk: An essential element of the rock climber's kit; it is used to increase friction and improve the grip on a rocky surface.

Training and conditioning

A training program for rock climbers should focus on the body parts that are especially important in the sport, namely the arms, fingers, shoulders, legs, and feet. The **exercise** program should take into consideration any particular weakness the individual may have. For example, pull-ups are very helpful for increasing upper body strength. Forearm curls develop forearm strength, which is essential in maintaining one's grip strength. Rock climbers, like all athletes, should be aware of the importance of **stretching** and **warm-up** exercises in preparing the body for a climb and in general training and conditioning exercises. One should also remember the necessity of allowing one's body to rest between exercises and avoiding the risks associated with overuse.

Trainers also recommend a variety of sport-specific exercises in preparation for climbing. For example, an exercise in which a climber uses both hands to ascend

and wall and then repeats the exercise using one hand only. Preparation for climbing involves a number of mental factors, such as scoping out the course before hand, looking for potential hand and foot holds and watching for potential rest stops along the way.

Risks

One of the most comprehensive studies of rock climbing injuries was reported in 2009 by two researchers at Nationwide Children's Hospital in Columbus, Ohio, Nicolas G. Nelson and Lara B. McKenzie. The researchers reviewed the records of 40,282 patients who had been treated in emergency departments between 1990 and 2007 for rock climbing injuries. They found that patients between the ages of 20 and 39 accounted for more than half of all injuries with males accounting for more than twice as many injuries as females. The most common injuries were those to the lower extremities involving sprains, strains, and fractures. In particular, the body part most frequently involved in injury was the ankle (19.2% of all injuries), with sprains and strains being the most common type of injury. Less common than fractures, strains, and sprains were lacerations (17.1% of all injuries), soft tissue injuries (16.9%), and dislocations (4.3%). By far the most common cause of injury during rock climbing was a fall (77.5% of all injuries), compared by hitting an object (7.1%) or being hit by an object (6.4%). Overall, just over 11% of all those who were injured required hospitalization, a high fraction for sports-related injuries.

A similar study was reported in the *British Journal of Sports Medicine* in 2008 of 201 active rock climbers, 163 male and 38 female climbers. About half of all respondents reported at least one injury in the preceding year, for a total of 275 distinct injuries. The most common type of injury was a chronic injury caused by overuse (33% of all injuries), followed by acute injuries caused by stressful moves required as part of a climb (28%), and acute injuries resulting from a fall (10%). The principal location of injuries were fingers and shoulders.

Results

Specialists in sports medicine note that rock climbers can reduce their risk for injury by following a few common-sense guidelines, such as being certain that one stretches and warms up before taking part in the sport, by understanding the demands of the sport and one's own physical limitations, ,and by remembering the risks of **overtraining** and including adequate rest periods within and between training periods.

Resources

BOOKS

Brown, Katie. *Girl on the Rocks: A Woman's Guide to Climbing with Strength, Grace, and Courage.* Guilford, CT: Falcon Guides, 2008.

Hörst, Eric J. *Learning to Climb Indoors.* Guilford, CT: Falcon Guides, 2006.

Hörst, Eric J. *Training for Climbing: The Definitive Guide to Improving Your Climbing Performance.* Guilford, CT: Falcon Guides, 2003.

Luebben, Craig. *Rock Climbing: Mastering Basic Skills.* Seattle: Mountaineers Books, 2004.

WEBSITES

Allred, Trevor. *Start Climbing.* rockclimbing.com. (April 1, 2010). http://www.rockclimbing.com/Articles/ Introduction_to_Climbing/Start_Climbing_Part_1_ Introduction_Overview_1.html (accessed November 9, 2011).

Rock Climbing Glossary. REI. http://www.rei.com/ expertadvice/articles/rock%20climbing%20glossary. html (accessed November 9, 2011).

Types and Formats of Rock Climbing Competitions. indoorclimbing.com. http://www.indoorclimbing.com/ comp_types.html (accessed November 9, 2011).

ORGANIZATIONS

International Federation of Sport Climbing, Corso Ferrucci 122, Torino, Italy, 10141, 39011 385 39 95, Fax: 39011 412 17 73, office@ifsc-climbing.org, http://www.ifsc-climbing.org.

Union Internationale des Associations d'Alpinisme (International Mountaineering and Climbing Federation), Monbijoustrasse 61 Postfach, CH-3000 Bern 23, Switzerland, 41(0) 31 370 1828, Fax: 41(0) 31 370 1838, http://www.theuiaa.org/contact.html, http://www.theuiaa.org.

David E. Newton, AB, MA, EdD

Rotator cuff injury

Definition

A rotator cuff injury is a tear, sprain, strain, or inflammation of the rotator cuff muscles or tendons in the shoulder. They connect the upper arm bone with the shoulder blade.

Description

Rotator cuff injury is known by several names, including pitcher's shoulder, swimmer's shoulder, and tennis shoulder. As these names imply, the injury occurs most frequently in athletes in sports requiring the arm be moved over the head repeatedly, such as weight lifting. Rotator cuff **tendinitis** is an inflammation of the shoulder tendons while a rotator cuff tear is a ripping of one or more of the tendons.

Tendons of four muscles make up the rotator cuff. The muscles are the supraspinatus, infraspinatus, teres minor, and subscapularis. The tendons attach the muscles to four shoulder bones: the shoulder blade (scapula), upper arm bone (humerus), and the

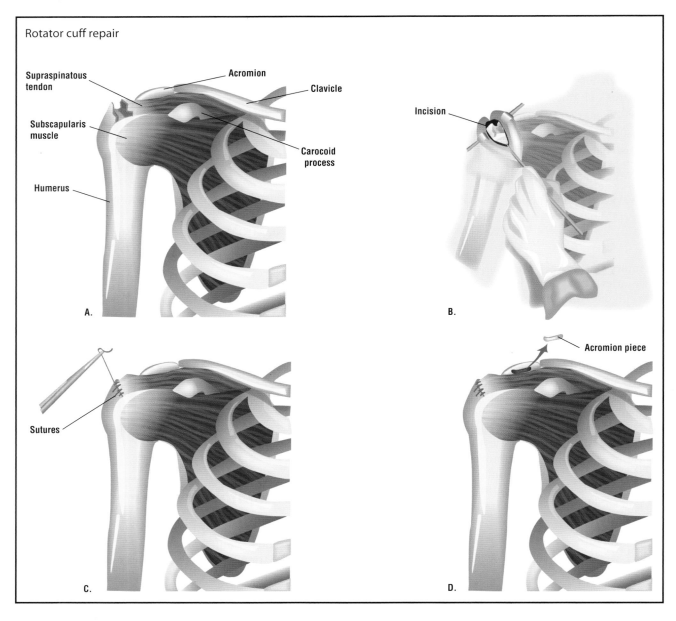

Rotator cuff repair

Supraspinatous tendon

Acromion

Clavicle

Subscapularis muscle

Carocoid process

Humerus

A.

Incision

B.

Sutures

C.

Acromion piece

D.

The process of repairing the rotator cuff. *(Diagram by PreMediaGlobal. Reproduced by permission of Gale, a part of Cengage Learning.)*

collarbone (clavicle.) The rotator cuff tendons can also degenerate due to **age**, usually starting around age 40.

A rotator cuff injury includes any type of irritation, inflammation, or damage to the rotator cuff muscles or tendons. Types of injuries and conditions include:

• Tendinitis: Inflammation of the rotator cuff due to overuse or overload, fairly common in sports such as baseball, tennis, and racquetball. It can also be caused by stress to the shoulders while doing weight-bearing exercisesperforming certain activities, such as

weightlifting. Tendinitis, if not treated, can weaken tendons and cause chronic degeneration or a tear.

• Bursitis: Irritation or inflammation of the fluid sac (bursa) between the shoulder joint and rotator cuff tendons.

• Strain or tear: A rotator cuff strain can occur when the arm cannot move freely in a wide range of motion without feeling pain because one or more of the tendons is strained. Treatments for mild to moderate strains include stretching and strengthening exercises to prevent stiffness and weakness of the muscles. Stress from overuse of the muscle or tendon can cause it to tear.

- Sprain: Rotator cuff sprains are stretched or torn ligaments caused by an extreme bend or twist of the upper arm or the shoulder. The common treatment for a sprained rotator cuff is rest, placing ice on the sore area, compression, and keeping the shoulder elevated.

Demographics

Rotator cuff injuries are fairly common in athletes, including **baseball** pitchers, and people whose shoulder muscles and tendons are subjected to repetitive motion, such as javelin and shot putt throwers. They occur mostly in males, especially those over age 40. Younger males can also injure the rotator cuff; injuries in high school and college baseball players is not uncommon.

Causes and symptoms

There are areas of the rotator cuff tendons that have poor blood supply, causing the tissue to heal and maintain itself from normal use. These regions in particular are slow to heal following a strain or tear. Tearing and inflammation in athletes is usually due to hard and repetitive use, especially in baseball pitchers. In non-athletes over age 40, the injuries usually occur during improper lifting of heavy objects.

Normal wear and tear, poor posture, and falling are common causes of rotator cuff injuries. Fitness-related causes include:

- Lifting an object that is too heavy or lifting it improperly, especially overhead, such as a barbell or dumbbell.
- Pulling an object, such as an archery bow.
- Repetitive stress that injures shoulder tendons and muscles, caused by activities such as baseball pitching and throwing, archery, tennis, and racquetball.

The two primary symptoms of a rotator cuff injury are pain and weakness in the shoulder or arm. A partial tear may cause pain but still allow normal arm movement. A complete tear usually leaves the injured person unable to raise the arm away from the side.

Symptoms of a rotator cuff injury include:

- pain or soreness in the shoulder, especially when reaching overhead, reaching behind the back, and lifting, pulling, or sleeping on the injured side
- weakness or loss of strength in the shoulder or upper arm

KEY TERMS

Arthrogram—A test done by injecting dye into the shoulder joint and then taking x rays. Areas where the dye leaks out indicate a tear in the tendons.

Arthroscopy— A procedure that uses a small fiber optic scope inserted through a small incision in the skin to see inside the shoulder.

Cortisone—A hormone produced naturally by the adrenal glands or made synthetically.

Magnetic resonance imaging (MRI) scan—A special radiological test that uses magnetic waves to create pictures of an area, including bones, muscles, and tendons.

Tendinitis—Inflammation of the tendons.

- a loss or decrease in the range of motion of the shoulder
- a tendency to keep the affected shoulder inactive

Diagnosis

Diagnosis is usually made after a physical examination, often by a sports medicine physician or an orthopedic surgeon. X rays are sometimes used in diagnosis but the most effective test is an arthrogram. A magnetic resonance imaging (MRI) scan or ultrasound scan is sometimes used to determine muscle and tendon tears.

Treatment

The primary treatment is resting the shoulder and, for minor tears and inflammation, applying ice packs to reduce inflammation and pain. Over-the-counter non-steroidal anti-inflammation medications can be used for pain. These drugs include aspirin, ibuprofen (Advil and Motrin), naproxen (Aleve), and acetaminophen (Tylenol). Anti-inflammatory medications may also be prescribed by a physician. As soon as pain decreases, physical therapy is usually begun to help regain normal range of motion. If pain persists after several weeks, the physician may inject cortisone into the affected area.

Serious tears to the rotator cuff tendons usually require surgery to repair. Sometimes during surgery, bone spurs or calcium deposits are removed. The surgery is performed either as an open incision or arthroscopy. Arthroscopy uses a small fiber optic scope inserted through a small incision in the skin to see inside the shoulder. It allows surgeons to view joint problems without major surgery. Depending on the

QUESTIONS TO ASK YOUR DOCTOR

- What exercises will strengthen my rotator cuff?
- Can my injury be treated without surgery?
- What pain and anti-inflammatory medication will help relieve my pain or soreness?
- How can I prevent future rotator cuff injuries?
- Is physical therapy a treatment option for me?
- What are the risks associated with rotator cuff injury treatment, including surgery?

problem that is found, surgeons may use small tools inserted through additional incisions to repair the damage, such as a torn tendon that fails to heal naturally. Using arthroscopy, for example, a surgeon may reattach the torn ends of a ligament or reconstruct the ligament using a piece (graft) of healthy ligament from the patient. Because arthroscopy uses tiny incisions, it results in less trauma, swelling, and scar tissue than conventional surgery, which in turn decreases hospitalization and rehabilitation times. Problems can be diagnosed earlier and treated without serious health risks or more invasive procedures. Furthermore, since injuries are often addressed at an earlier stage, operations are more likely to be successful. Other surgical options include partial or total shoulder replacement.

There are no effective alternative medicine treatments for rotator cuff injuries.

Prognosis

The prognosis for recovery from minor rotator cuff injuries is excellent. For serious injuries, the prognosis is usually good, but requires up to six weeks of physical therapy following surgery. Full recovery may take several months. In rare cases, the injury is so severe it requires tendon grafts and muscle transfers. If a tendon has been torn for too long, the injury may not be repairable.

Prevention

The best prevention is to avoid repetitive overhead movements and to develop shoulder strength in opposing muscle groups. Other preventative measures include doing regular shoulder exercises, taking frequent breaks from activities that use repetitive arm and shoulder motions, sufficiently resting the shoulders during sports that require repetitive arm motion, and apply application of heat or cold at the first indication of shoulder pain or soreness.

Resources

BOOKS

Andrews, James R., et al. *The Athlete's Shoulder.* Burlington, MA: Churchill Livingstone, 2008.

Hamil, Douglas P. *Effectiveness of Nonoperative and Operative Treatments for Rotator Cuff Tears.* Hauppauge, NY: Nova Science Publishers, 2011.

Kirsch, John M. *Shoulder Pain? The Solution & Prevention, Second Edition.* Gilroy, CA: Bookstand Publishing, 2010.

PERIODICALS

Condor, Bob. "Shouldering the Load." *Tennis* (November-December 2009): 52.

Degon, Ryan, and Dennis Wilkenfeld. "Keeping the Shoulder Safe." *Coach and Athletic Director* (November 2009): 10.

Palacios, Enrique, and Karen Palacios-Jansen. "Retooling Your Swing After Rotator Cuff Injury." *Golf Fitness Magazine* (March-April 2008): 12.

Sohn, Emily. "Shrug Off Shoulder Pain." *Prevention* (April 2009): 161.

Stoppani, Jim. "Rear Deltoids." *Flex* (September 2010): 98.

WEBSITES

Rotator Cuff Injuries. Shoulder-Pain-Management.com. http://www.shoulder-pain-management.com/rotatorcuffinjuries.html (accessed October 30, 2011).

Rotator Cuff Injury. Mayo Clinic. (August 21, 2010). http://www.mayoclinic.com/health/rotator-cuff-injury/DS00192 (accessed October 30, 2011).

ORGANIZATIONS

American Physical Therapy Association, 1111 N. Fairfax St., Alexandria, VA, 22314-1488, (703) 684-2782, Fax: (703) 684-7343, (800) 999-2782, memberservices@apta.org, http://www.apta.org.

American Shoulder and Elbow Surgeons, 6300 N. River Rd., Suite 727, Rosemont, IL, 60018, (847) 698-1629, Fax: (847) 823-0536, ases@aaos.org, http://www.ases-assn.org.

National Institute of Arthritis and Musculoskeletal and Skin Diseases, 1 AMS Circle, Bethesda, MD, 20892-3675, (301) 495-4484, Fax: (301) 718-6366, (877) 226-4267, NIAMSinfo@mail.nih.gov, http://www.niams.nih.gov.

Ken R. Wells

Rowing

Definition

Rowing is a sporting activity in which one or more individuals propel a boat across water by means of one or two oars. The term usually does not include purely recreational activities, such as canoeing and kayaking, but is limited to boats of relatively similar structure used primarily for racing competitions.

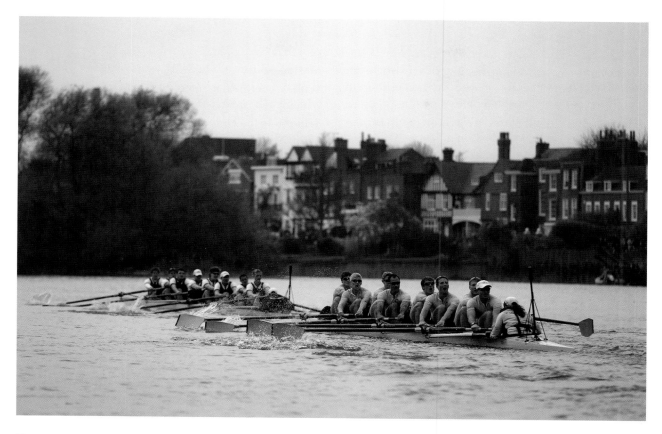

The teams row during the 157th Oxford and Cambridge University Boat Race on the River Thames on March 26, 2011 in London, England. (© Richard Heathcote/Getty Images Sport/Getty Images)

Purpose

In a rowing competition, the purpose of a rower or rowing team is to complete a prescribed course in the lowest time of all competitors.

Demographics

A number of surveys have been conducted to determine who it is that participates in rowing. Those surveys tend to show that rowers are generally well educated, with more than 90 percent having earned college degrees, more than half of whom also have graduate degrees. They also tend to be financially well to do, with just under half (about 45 percent in one survey) having annual incomes of more than US$100,000 and about a quarter (25 percent) with incomes of less than US$50,000 annually. Participants are approximately equally divided between males (55 percent) and females (45 percent), with the largest category of participants belonging to the Masters category (**age** 21 and over) and the next largest, to the high school (30 percent) and college (20 percent) categories. Many rowing organizations and facilities have developed special programs

that reach out to individuals of all ages, both genders, and all skill levels, offering instruction and events for children, senior citizens, and individuals with disabilities.

History

As with many other sports, such a **swimming, running**, and **rock climbing**, rowing has a very old history that dates back millennia, to the time when people engaged in these activities for both personal and commercial use, as adjuncts to military activities, and as a source of recreation. History is replete with descriptions of contests between oared boats, such as the regattas held in Venice from the late thirteenth century onwards. One of the first such races held in the United States was a contest between a Cape Cod whaler and a Dutch boat called a pettiauger held in New York in 1756. Some historians date the first modern-day-style rowing competition to a race held on the Thames River in England between two eight-oared cutters in 1788. During the nineteenth century, rowing became more popular in Great Britain, Canada, and Australia with contested events becoming increasingly popular, along with

KEY TERMS

Coxswain—A non-rowing member of a rowing team who sets the pace for rowers and keeps them informed of their status in a race.

Elite—In the United States, a rower who has been a member of a US Rowing National Team.

Intermediate—In the United States, a rower who has not yet advanced to the role of Senior or Elite rower.

Junior—A rower who has not attained the age of 19.

Master—A rower who is 21 years of age or older.

Scull—A term that refers to a rowing situation in which each rower uses two oars.

Senior—In the United States, a rower who has won a certified race over 2000 meters in the United States or Canada.

Shell—The boat used in a rowing competition.

Sweep—A term that refers to a rowing situation in which each rower uses a single oar.

organizations to promote and oversee the sport. The first college boat club to be organized was apparently founded at Oxford University in 1815, to be followed by the first boat club in the United States in 1823, the Knickerbocker Club in New York City. In 1829, probably the most famous of all continuing boat races was held at Henley-on-Thames between Oxford and Cambridge in a contest that has been repeated almost every year since. The U.S. counterpart of that race, between Harvard and Yale, was first held in 1852 on Lake Winnepesaukee, a race that has also been repeated almost every year since, although now on the Thames River in New London, Connecticut.

Rowing was scheduled to be a part of the first modern **Olympics** Games, held in Greece in 1896, but the event was cancelled when bad weather at the port of Piraeus made competition impossible. The sport was included in the second Olympic Games four years later, and has been included in every Olympiad since then. The 2008 Olympic Games in Beijing included 14 separate rowing events, with the singles sculls being won by Olaf Tufte for men, of Norway, and Rumyana Neykova for women, of Bulgaria. The winning eights were the teams from Canada, for men, and the United States, for women.

The Federation Internationale des Societes d'Aviron (International Federation of Rowing Associations, or FISA) was organized in 1892 in response to the rapidly growing popularity of the sport. At the time, betting was an integral part of the sport, and it became obvious to afficionados that some type of governing body was essential to avoid the most corrupt aspects of the sport. FISA continues to be the international governing body for the sport. It sponsors a number of championships, including the World Rowing Cup, determined by a series of three races each summer since 1997; the World Rowing Junior Championship and the World Rowing Under 23 Championship, both held annually since 1967; and the World Rowing Masters Regatta, held annually since 1973. The FISA continues to be the international sponsoring body for the participation of rowing in the quadrennial Olympic Games.

Description

Rowing events are categorized on the basis of four characteristics: the number of oars used by a rower; the number of rowers in a boat; the presence or absence of a coxswain; and the weight of rowers in the boat:

- Sculling is a form of rowing in which the rower(s) uses two oars. Sweeping refers to the situation in which the rower(s) uses only one oar. Boats used for sculling and sweeping are essentially identical in construction (except for the number of oars), and are sometimes referred to simply as shells. The terms "scull" and "sweep" refer only to the number of oars used in the event.

- A rowing event can include boats that carry one, two, three (rare), four, or eight rowers, either male or female. A boat with one rower is called a single scull (1x-). The shorthand representation indicates that there is one rower ("1") in a sculling boat ("x") without a coxswain ("-"). A boat with two rowers is called a double (2x-), a coxed pair (2+), or a coxless pair (2-); with four rowers, a quadruple (or quad) with a coxswain (4x+) or without a coxswain (4x-) or a coxed four (4+) or coxless four (4-); and with eight rowers, an octuple (8x+) or an eight, which always has a coxswain (8 or 8+).

- Competitors may also be classified according to weight, with the "lightweight" category reserved for rowers of some maximum weight, or for boats with some maximum average weight per rower. For men, the maximum weight per individual is 160 pounds with a limited average weight for the boat of 155 pounds. For women, the comparable weights are 130 pounds and 125 pounds.

The length of all world championship and Olympic races is 2,000 meters, divided by markers at each 500 meter point. The course typically consists of six lanes, out of which boats may stray provided that they do not impede the passage of another boat. Each boat is permitted one false start at the beginning of the race, but is disqualified in the case of two false starts. The coxswain does not participate in the actual rowing, but is an essential member of the team in steering the shell and directing the rest of the crew as to the speed of strokes they are to use and their position in the race.

Preparation

An observer might get the impression that rowing is a sport that emphasizes upper body muscle strength in particular. While that observation is partly true, it is also incomplete in the regard that rowers use their whole body in their sport. Indeed, many rowing trainers argue that matches are won or lost on the basis of participants' lower body strength, especially leg strength, and endurance.

Equipment

Rowers require minimum clothing for participation in the sport: usually a sleeveless shirt, shorts, and suitable sox and shoes. Sunglasses may also be necessary, depending on weather conditions.

Essential equipment for rowing includes, of course, the shells themselves and the oars used to propel them. Shells range in length from about 27–58 ft (8.2–17.6 m), with a width of (0.28–0.590 m). Historically, shells were made out of wood, but today they are usually made of some lightweight composite material, such as honeycombed carbon fiber. Oars range in length from about 2.5 meters to about 3.6 meters with a blade at one end about 50 centimeters long and 25 centimeters wide. The blade is traditionally painted in some distinctive color associated with the individual rower(s) or team.

Training and conditioning

As with most sports today, rowing training programs consist of a complete set of exercises designed to improve a person's strength, flexibility, endurance, speed, and balance. These programs usually include a wide range of aerobic, strength, power, and other training regimes. An example of the training program recommended for rowers is one provided by the International Federation of Rowing Associations, found at http://www.rathburn.net/rowing/training.html That program outlines a year-round agenda that includes frequent **stretching** and **warm-up** exercises, **interval training**, Fartlek training, speed exercises, body weight **circuit training**, endurance strength. training, and maximal strength training.

A device of special value for indoor training is the ergometer rowing machine, which mimics (but not perfectly) in many respects the behavior of a shell on water. Athletes row for periods of 20 to 40 minutes at a time on the machine, with times required to complete certain interludes (like the five minutes required for the best times in an actual race) recorded by the device. The ergometer has become so popular among rowers that there now exists a world indoor racing championship similar to water rowing using the machine. The winner of that event, the 2011 C.R.A.S.H.-B men's championship, was Conlin McCabe of the University of Washington, and the women's champion was Kaisa Pajusalu, of Estonia.

Risks

One of the most comprehensive studies of rowing injuries is now more than ten years old. It studied a cohort of elite rowers over a ten-year period, and was reported in 1997. According to that study, chronic overuse injuries were by far the most common source of injury among participants in the study. Among males, the most common sites of injury were the lumbar spine, the forearm and wrist and the knee. Among females, the most common locations were the chest, lumbar spine, and forearm and wrist. Researchers observed that these injuries were very often the consequence of repetitive motions unrelieved by breaks between practices and between practice and participation in an event.

A more recent study, reported in 2005, noted that demographic studies since 1997 had been rare or absent, and most of what sports physicians know about rowing injuries comes from anecdotal evidence. The 2005 researchers concluded that the primary injuries observed for rowers appear to be nonspecific **low back pain**, specific low back injuries (spondylolysis, sacroiliac joint dysfunction, and disc herniation), rib stress fractures, costochondritis, costovertebral joint subluxation, intercostal **muscle strain**, and nonspecific shoulder pain. **Blisters** and abrasions were also seen commonly among rowers, a category of less severe conditions than strains, sprains, muscle tears, and other more serious problems.

Results

Virtually all studies on the risks and injuries associated with rowing emphasize the importance of adequate training and conditioning exercises in preparation for a competition. Rowers who have developed strength, endurance, balance, flexibility, and other characteristics are less likely to be injured than are those who have not worked on those fitness components. Perhaps the single most important way of avoiding injuries is to know and remember the role of repetitive motion in the sport and to train in such a way as to avoid overuse injuries by following appropriate **periodization** training programs and occasionally taking breaks from training.

Resources

BOOKS

Churbuck, D. C. *The Book of Rowing*. New York: Overlook, 2008.

McArthur, John. *High Performance Rowing*. Ramsbury, UK: Crowood Press, 2005.

Nolte, Volker. *Rowing Faster*, 2nd ed. Champaign, IL: Human Kinetics, 2011.

Roberts, M. B. *Crew: The Rower's Handbook*. New York: Sterling, 2007.

Sayer, Bill. *Rowing and Sculling: The Complete Manual*, new and expanded edition. London: Robert Hale, 2006.

WEBSITES

Dudhia, Anu *Physics of Rowing*. http://www.atm.ox.ac.uk/rowing/physics/index.html (accessed August 31, 2011).

Rowing 101 USRowing.org. http://www.usrowing.org/About/Rowing101.aspx (accessed August 31, 2011).

Rowing News Rowing News. http://rowingnews.com/ (accessed Accessed on August 31, 2011).

ORGANIZATIONS

Fédération Internationale des Sociétés d'Aviron (International Federation of Rowing Associations), Avenue de Cour 135; Case Postale 18, 1000 Lausanne 3, Switzerland, 4121 617 8373, Fax: 4121 617 8375, info@fisa.org, http://www.fisa.org/home/default.sps.

United States Rowing Association, 201 S. Capitol Ave., Suite 400, Indianapolis, IN, 46225-1068, (317) 237-5656, Fax: (317) 237-5646, (800) 314-4769, members@usrowing.org, http://www.usrowing.org/.

David E. Newton, A.B., M.A., Ed.D

Rugby

Definition

Rugby, also called rugby **football**, is a type of football that first started in the United Kingdom. Specifically, it originated from the Rugby School, an independent, public boarding school located in Rugby, Warwickshire, England. In modern society, rugby is organized within two primary sports: Rugby League and Rugby Union. Both are characterized by kicking and dribbling of the ball with the feet, along with passing of the ball with the hands. However, they differ somewhat in the rules (laws) applied to each.

Purpose

The purpose of rugby is to have players from two opposing teams working together for the ultimate goal of grounding the ball past their opponent's goal line and score the greater number of points during two periods of play. The hoped for result at the end of the game is score more points than the opponent, which ultimately makes that team victorious over the other team.

Demographics

Rugby can be played by people of all ages and abilities. Because rugby is a contact sport, children are introduced to the sport gradually. They learn the game through modified rules and activities that make it less dangerous, such as through play involving no contact.

Rugby is played in over 40 countries of the world. The countries where rugby is most popular is Australia, France, Jamaica, New Zealand, South Africa, the United Kingdom, and Wales.

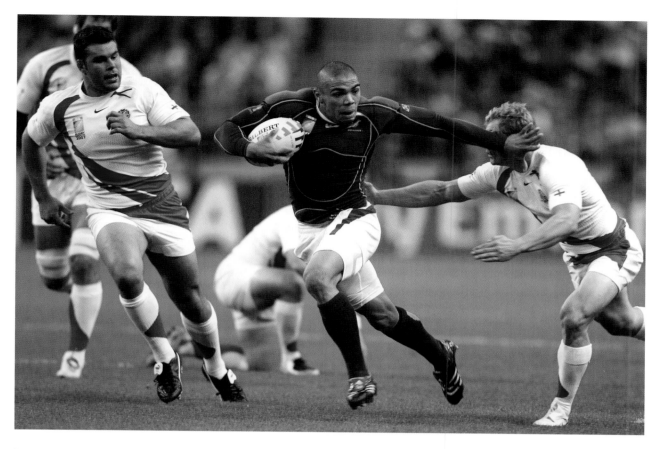

International Rugby Board World Cup Match in 2007, England vs. South Africa. *(© Christian Liewig/Corbis)*

The Rugby League International Federation, headquartered in Sydney, Australia, coordinates professional rugby in about 30 nations, where 12 of the countries have full international member status. The top countries within the Rugby League include Australia, New Zealand, and England. Two major professional competitions are held regularly: the Australasian National Rugby League and the European Super League. The Rugby League World Cup, its top international competition, is held every four years on average. Held in Australia, it was last won in 2008 by New Zealand. The next World Cup will be held in 2013 by England.

The Rugby Union has teams in over 100 countries around the world—being considered the most popular form of rugby in the world. As of the end of 2010, 118 unions (countries) were members of the International Rugby Board (IRB, with headquarters in Dublin, Ireland), the governing body of the Rugby Union. The first-tier countries include Argentina, Australia, England, France, Ireland, Italy, New Zealand, Scotland, South Africa, and Wales. Other countries include Brazil, Canada, Chile, Columbia, Fiji, Georgia, Japan, Namibia, Portugal, Romania, Samoa, Spain, Tonga, the United States, and Uruguay. In 1995, the IRB removed the rules that prevented players at the highest level of its organization from accepting money for playing rugby. The IRB conducts its Rugby World Cup every four years. The winner of the competition receives the Webb Ellis Cup. The cup was won last by South Africa in the 2007 competition held in Paris, France. The next competition is scheduled to take place in 2011 in New Zealand, with Japan hosting the 2015 event and England, the 2019 competition.

History

Various football-type games were played from the fifth to sixteenth centuries in England. They were played between neighboring towns. Few rules were made and huge numbers of players often opposed each other in these unruly games. The simple goal of each game was to move an inflated "pig's bladder" to markers located on opposite ends of a town.

NEW ZEALAND ALL BLACKS HAKA

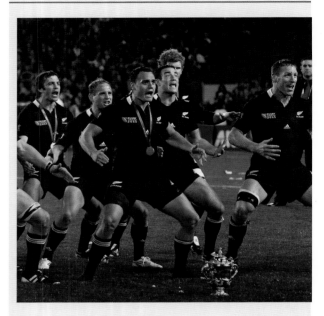

(© Paul Thomas/CSM/Landov)

The New Zealand national rugby team (All Blacks) adopted a traditional war dance—the Haka—to perform before every match. This started in 1884, when the first New Zealand global team performed this dance before the match. Initially the war dance was performed while the team wore their native costumes, but this practice quickly went by the wayside.

The All Blacks rugby spectators enjoy this Haka pregame tradition. The Haka has been termed "The greatest ritual in world sport." However, the opponents' reaction varies greatly, with some ignoring the celebration and others treating the tradition with respect. Sometimes there has been resulting controversy based on the opponents' reactions. For instance, during the 2011 World Cup, the French team approached the All Blacks team as they performed the Haka. The French players stood within ten feet of the celebratory war dance, and were fined as a result.

Frequently, authorities tried to make the games illegal because of their very violent nature.

From this beginning, the modern game of rugby was developed and organized at the Rugby School, located about 80 mi. (130 km) northwest of London, during the mid-eighteenth century. During its first one hundred years, players were allowed to handle the ball but no one could run toward their goal with the ball in their hands. **Running** with the ball was introduced sometime in the middle of the nineteenth century. At that time, the Rugby School created the first recognized written rugby rules, and it became a widely played game around the world. Soon, two distinct types of rugby developed: handling and non-handling.

The Football Association formed using the non-handling form of rugby, with the Rugby Football Union (Rugby Union) later forming in 1871.. Near the end of the nineteenth century, amateur players began to play for money. The Northern Rugby Union was formed in 1895. In the twentieth century, specifically in 1922, the Rugby Football League (Rugby League) formed. Rugby is very popular throughout most of the world.

Description

The professional form of rugby is called the Rugby League, with 13 players on each team during the start of each match. The amateur game (now professional at its highest level, as of 1995), called the Rugby Union or the Rugby Football Union, is played with 15 men on each team during the start of play. Players for the Rugby Union include eight forwards, seven backs (which include one full back, two half-backs, and four three-quarter backs).

The Rugby League, sometimes also called Rugby League Football, has positions that are divided between forwards and backs. The forwards are further divided into: hooker, prop, second-row forward, and loose forward. The backs are divided into: full back, right wing threequarter, right center threequarter, left center threequarter, left wing threequarter, stand-off half (or five-eighth), and scrum half (or half-back).

Forwards are generally larger and stronger than backs. They primarily run with the ball, make openings for the backs, and tackle their opponents. Backs are usually smaller in size and faster in speed.

The ball and uniform

Rugby is played with an oval-shaped inflated ball made from leather. It is 11 to 12 in. (28 to 30 cm) long, along with being 23 to 24 in. (58 to 62 cm) in (long-axis) circumference and weighing 14 to 15 oz. (400 to 440 gm). Rugby players wear jerseys, shorts, and shoes, but do not wear any type of protective equipment or padding.

The field and periods

The game is played on a field that extends approximately 109.4 yd. (100 m) in its longer length, with a goal line on each end. At the center of each goal line is positioned a goal post. An "in goal" area is located beyond the goal line, being approximately 24.1 yd. (22 m) in depth. The shorter length (of the field is approximately 75.5 yd. (69 m) wide. Each side line is bounded by "touch lines," which are approximately 10.9 yd. (10 m) apart. Halfway down the field, dividing the field into half, is the "halfway" line.

Professional rugby is played within two 40-minute periods, with a half-time rest period of no more than five minutes. The two teams reverse sides at the beginning of the second period. Games, usually called matches, can be delayed by no more than two minutes for any specific reason per delay. Substitutions (interchanges) are allowed in rugby, with substitutes permitted to stand on the sidelines (called the "bench") at the start of the game.

Officials

A referee officiates the match. The referee is the only one that applies the laws of rugby, along with being the timekeeper for the game. In addition, two "touch" judges officiate at rugby matches. The touch judges guide rugby play from the touch zones and signal with a flag when the ball or a player crosses the touch line on either side of the playing field.

The game

A rugby match starts with a kickoff from the center of the halfway line. The ball must be kicked past the ten-yard line of the opponent. The players on the opposing can then kick, dribble, pass, or run with the ball if they are on the "onside"; that is, they are behind the ball in the direction it is being advanced. If an opponent gets the ball, they can also tackle the player. When a tackle occurs, the tackled player must immediately release the ball so that it can be picked up or kicked by a player on the opposing team.

Rugby is scored when the ball is grounded in the opponent's in goal area. The score is called a "try." When a try is scored, four points are awarded to a team in Rugby Union and three points in Rugby League. After a try, the scoring team can also score by place-kicking the ball. A successful place-kick is awarded an additional two points. A team can also score with a penalty kick for a goal. The Rugby Union awards three points for a successful penalty kick, while the Rugby League awards two points. Scoring can also be made by drop-kicking the ball for a goal for three points, for both the Rugby Union and Rugby League.

In all forms of play, the ball cannot be passed forward toward a team's goal. Passes can only be made laterally (to the side) or backward with respect

to the motion toward the team's goal. In addition, players on the same team as the player carrying the ball cannot be ahead of this person.

During the matches, players cannot contact ("charge") each other except with their shoulders. Contacting players, or obstructing a player's motion, who are not holding the ball is illegal. The referee will call a penalty for the following willful actions: striking, tripping, and holding. When penalized, the opposing team receives a penalty kick at the site where the penalty was made.

Matches continue without a break except for time taken for penalty plays, out-of-bounds ("in touch") plays, and after a score occurs. A score will cause a kickoff to occur at the center of the halfway line. After a referee-issued penalty is completed, play re-starts with a "set scrummage," also called a tight scrummage. This involves a player awarded the penalty to roll the ball into a tunnel formed by opposing team members; specifically, groups of forwards in three rows with the goal to push their opponents away from the ball so they can kick ("heel") the ball toward their teammates who are located behind the line.

A "loose scrummage" occurs when players from each side close around the ball without any referee action. The group of players forming the loose scrummage push against their opponents in the attempt to kick the ball behind them as other players wait to receive the ball from them.

When the ball goes out of bounds, play is restarted with a "line-out," in which both groups of forwards line up at the point where the ball goes out of bounds, either at a right angle or straight out from their opponents. The referee than throws the ball down the middle of the opposing teams and over their heads so the teams can fight for control.

Preparation

Warming up is important, as it is with any type of **exercise** or physical activity, because it helps to prepare the muscles before they are asked to do more strenuous work. Such a **warm-up** period may consist of about five minutes of light exercise or **walking**. Doing stretches are also recommended during the warm-up routine.

Once finished playing rugby, it is a good idea to spend about five minutes cooling down. Light exercise, such as walking, along with **stretching**, helps the body to settle back down to its normal routine.

Risks

Rugby is a fast-paced, highly intense sport to play. Because it is a heavy contact sport, injuries will occur. Injuries in rugby are more frequent than they are in American football or **soccer**. Adolescents and teenagers from the ages of ten to 18 years experience the most injuries. Boys are at higher risk from injuries than are girls.

Most injuries occur while involved with tackling, either being tackled or doing the tackling. Common injuries occur to the fingers and thumbs, along with those to the legs, arms, and hands. Many injuries are muscular strains or contusions (bruising), sprains, dislocations, fractures, lacerations, and overuse injuries. Nearly one out of seven injuries occurs as the result of sprains or strains to the ankles. Head injuries, including **concussion**, are also a big concern to rugby players.

Injuries can be minimized by preparing for games with adequate conditioning and stretching exercises. Pre-season conditioning is especially important because injuries are likely when one first begins

playing. Such conditioning should include a gradual increase in the intensity and duration of the game. Proper techniques and tactics should also be learned to help minimize injuries. Correct tackling, offensive and defensive skills, and other such methods are highly important for avoiding serious injuries.

Results

Playing of rugby helps to improve the strength in the upper and lower parts of the body. It also improved cardiovascular fitness and endurance. One's speed and agility also benefits from the playing of rugby.

Resources

BOOKS

Biscombe, Tony, and Peter Drewett. *Rugby: Steps to Success*. Champaign, IL: Human Kinetics, 2010.

De Klerk, Andrew. *International Rugby Encyclopedia*. Johannesburg: 30 Degrees South, 2009.

Harris, John. *Rugby Union and Globalization: An Odd-shaped World*. Houndmills, Basingstoke, Hampshire, U.K.: Palgrave Macmillan, 2010.

Lipscombe, Trevor Davis. *The Physics of Rugby*. Nottingham: Nottingham University Press, 2009.

WEBSITES

A Beginner's Guide to Rugby. International Rugby Board. (March 25, 2009). http://www.irb.com/newsmedia/news/newsid = 2030335.html (accessed August 18, 2011).

Rivera, Larry. *Rugby World Cup*. About.com. http://goaustralia.about.com/cs/eventsfestivals/a/rugbyhistory.htm (accessed August 18, 2011).

Rockwood, Dan. *A Brief History of Rugby*. Guardian.co.uk. (October 6, 2003). http://www.guardian.co.uk/sport/2003/oct/06/rugbyworldcup2003.rugbyunion6 (accessed August 23, 2011).

Rugby. OMBAC. (July 16, 2010). http://ombac.org/ombac_rugby/rulesofrugby.htm (accessed August 23, 2011).

Rugby Injuries. BC Injury Research and Prevention Unit. http://www.injuryresearch.bc.ca/Publications/Fact%20Sheets/rugby%20fact%20sheet.pdf (accessed August 23, 2011).

ORGANIZATIONS

International Rugby Board, Huguenot House; 35-38 St. Stephen's Green, Dublin, Ireland, 00353 (1) 240-9200, Fax: 00353 (1) 240-9201, irb@irb.com, http://www.irb.com/.

National Rugby League, Australia, http://www.nrl.com/.

Rugby Football League, 4851 Paramount Drive, San Diego, CA, 92123, (888) 825-3636, http://www. therfl.co.uk/.

Rugby League International Federation, Sydney, Australia, http://www.irb.com/.

William A. Atkins, B.B., B.S., M.B.A.

Running

Definition

Running is a means of locomotion used by many species of animals, including humans, whereby they travel across an area by propelling themselves with rapid movements of their legs and feet.

Purpose

Running has many functions for an animal, including the pursuit of food, escape from a predator, and, in many cases, the pure joy of a recreational activity. Among humans, the first two of these objectives has become, over time, a less common motivation for running than the last. Humans now run primarily for the pleasure it provides, to improve one's general overall health, or to win a competition with other humans.

Demographics

Data and statistics on running in the United States are compiled and published annually by the non-profit organization Running USA (the "National Runner Survey"). Its most recent survey (2011) provided the following information about "core runners," defined as individuals who tend to enter running competitions of one kind or another and tend to train year around. (This information was obtained from the responses of 11,264 runners nationwide. These data correspond rather closely with surveys conducted by two running magazines, *Runner's World*, and *Running Times*.)

- Overall, core runners are serious about their sport, reporting that they practice or compete an average of 224 days out of the year for an average total distance per runner of 1,357 miles per year. These numbers contrast significantly with data for more casual fitness runners and joggers who, according to surveys by the Sporting Goods Manufacturing Association, run an average of 85 days per year.

- The average female runner is 38.6 years of age, married (61.9 percent of respondents), college educated (78.7 percent), and financially well off (69.0 percent with a household income of more than US$75,000). She has been running for an average of 11 years and has competed in seven competitive events in the preceding 12 months. She tends to run or jog four or more hours a week for an average distance of about 23 miles. Her favorite race is the half marathon (38.1 percent of respondents), followed by the 5K race and marathon.

- The average male runner is 44.8 years of age, married (73.5 percent of respondents), college educated (78.8 percent), and financially well off (76.4 percent with a household income of more than US$75,000). He has been running for an average of 16 years and has competed in nine competitive events in the preceding 12 months. He tends to run or jog four or more hours a week for an average distance of about 29.5 miles. His favorite race is the half marathon (38.1 percent of respondents), followed by the 5K race, the 10K race, and marathon.

- The primary motivation for running for both men and women is exercise. The second most important motivating factor for women is weight control, but for men, it is inertia, in the sense that they started running in school and just continued to do so ever since.

- Core runners report that they purchase an average of 3.2 pairs of running shoes per year (3.0 pairs for women and 3.4 pairs for men), with a total estimated expenditure for shoes of US$2.31 billion annually.

- Nearly 84 percent of respondents to the survey chose half marathon, 5K, 10K, and marathon as their races of choice. Other races in which individuals compete are the 12K, 15K, 10 mile, 8K, 4 mile, 5 mile, ultramarathon, and 1 or 3 mile (in order of preference).

- Different sources report slightly different divisions between male and female runners, ranging from 46.2 percent male/53.8 percent female in the National Runner Survey to 56.5 percent male/43.5 percent female in the Running Times survey, with the Runner's World reporting a 49.8 percent male/50.2 percent female split.

- In all surveys runners are by far members of the Caucasian race, with numbers ranging from 88.4 percent in the Runner's World survey to 91.9 percent in the Running Times survey.

- The National Sporting Goods Association (NSGA) provides somewhat more limited data on running patterns, the most important of which may be changes in participation over time. In its most recent survey (2011), NSGA reported that 35.5 million Americans reported taking part in some type of running or jogging activity at least once in the previous 12 months, an increase of 10.3 percent over the preceding year, and an increase of 55.7 percent over 2000 results.

History

Running for the pursuit of food or to escape predators was almost certainly a part of the daily life of early humans dating back more than four million years ago. Running as a recreational and/or competitive activity is much more recent, but still an ancient

KEY TERMS

Elite runner—A runner who runs professionally or who has attained some level of distinction in her or his field of running.

Iliotibial band syndrome (ITB)—A type of hip injury.

Jogging—A moderate form of running in which the primary goal is recreational rather than winning a competition.

Medial tibial stress syndrome (MTSS)—The technical name for shin splits.

tradition. Perhaps the earliest competitive races were those held in Egypt about 3800 years before the birth of Christ. Competitors ran back and forth between two pillars about 800 meters apart for four laps. Among the earliest written records of running races were those held in connection with the Tailteann Games in Ireland between 632 bce and 1171 ce. Perhaps most famously running races were an integral part of the Olympic Games held in Greece, the first games dating to 776 bce.

The excitement of betting on a running race probably first developed in England in the seventeenth century, when nobles placed wagers on which of their servants would prevail in various types of foot races. The first use of scientific training principles of the sport of race running is sometimes traced to the work of Finnish distance runner Paavo Nurmi and his associate Lauri Pihkala. Today, many kinds of competitive racing events exist, ranging from short-distance races (sprints) of 100 and 200 meters to medium-distance races of 800 metes and a mile to long-distance races of half marathons and marathons.

Description

Foot racing can be divided, in general, into two major categories: events in which participants compete with each other for some type of recognition, such as a cash award or a trophy or some kind, and recreational running, in which a person runs simply for the **exercise**, to improve one's overall fitness, to lose weight, or just for the joy of running. One form of recreational running is called jogging. Jogging is simply a form of running at a slower pace than in most other forms of running. It has the advantage of placing less stress on the runner and, therefore, reducing the risk of physical damage as a result of participating in the sport.

Preparation

The type of preparation required for running depends on the purpose of the running activity. Individuals who run for the purpose of recreation generally do not engage in a detailed program of preparation (such as, for example, weight training), although they should always perform some simple **warm-up** exercises, such as **stretching** and jogging in place to prepare the body for the forthcoming exercise. Recreational runners also benefit from a simple program of preparation that consists of **walking** exercises first, followed by jogging exercises, followed by progressively more challenging runs, until one has reached the level of performance with which she or he is comfortable. Selecting the proper running gear, especially good running shoes, is also part of the amateur runner's program of preparation.

Elite runners, those who participate in the sport for more than just recreational reasons, often develop more rigorous programs of preparation that may include strength, speed, and **endurance training**. They also focus more closely on nutritional programs that prepare their bodies for the demands placed by frequent practice and competition and, especially, long distance runs characteristic of **marathon** and ultra marathon competitions.

Equipment

Running requires relatively little specialized equipment, usually just a shirt and shorts. The most important piece of equipment is running shoes. A great variety of running shoes is available, each designed for a specific type of running. A novice runner should seek the advice of a qualified shoe expert to decide precisely the type of shoe needed by that individual.

Risks

Running might appear to be a rather benign sport in terms of the risk it poses to the participant. After all, there is little or no contact with another person, as there is in most sports. Yet, the stress placed on the body by slamming the feet and legs onto the ground in a continuous pattern can have a number of serious effects on the body. In a 2009 survey by the running magazine Runner's World, for example, two-thirds of respondents reported that they had suffered some type

QUESTIONS TO ASK YOUR DOCTOR

- What type of preparatory exercises do you recommend prior to recreational running?
- What is the most common running-related injury that you see, and how can I best avoid this type of injury?
- What suggestions do you have for the type of running shoe I should purchase?
- Is there a specific type of running activity that you recommend for a person of my age and experience

of injury in the preceding year that prevented them from running for at least some minimal period of time. The most common types of injuries reported in the 2011 Running USA's "State of the Sport" survey were **blisters** (30.9 percent of respondents); knee injuries (22.7 percent); iliotibial band syndrome (ITB; a hip injury; 15.6 percent); **plantar fasciitis** (an inflammation of the foot pad; 14.0 percent); shin splints [also known as medial tibial stress syndrome (MTSS); 12.7 percent]; hamstring pulls (12.3 percent); and miscellaneous foot (12.0 percent), hip (11.9 percent), and low back (10.4 percent) injuries

Prevention

Sports medicine specialists suggest that most running injuries can be prevented by proper preparation for the sport. The best way of avoiding running injuries, according to the American Orthopaedic Society for Sports Medicine is to stretch and warm up before beginning to run. Other preparatory steps should include making sure that one has the best available running shoes, to take sufficient rest periods between training and running, to run on the best possible surface, to make sure one drinks adequate amounts of

water during a run, and to avoid large changes in one's running regime (such as the length of the run or the elevation over which one runs) in a short period of time.

Resources

BOOKS

Burfoot, Amby. Runner's World Complete Book of Running: Everything You Need to Know to Run for Fun, Fitness and Competition, revised edition. Emmaus, PA: Rodale, 2010.

Maharam, Lewis G. *The Running Doc's Guide to Healthy Running: How to Fix Injuries, Stay Active, and Run Pain-Free.* Boulder, CO: Velo Press, 2011.

Noakes, Timothy. *Lore of Running,* 4th ed. Champaign, IL: Human Kinetics, 2003.

Puleo, Joe, and Patrick Milroy. *Running Anatomy.* Champaign, IL: Human Kinetics, 2010.

Tucker, Ross, and Jonathan Dugas. *Runner's World, the Runner's Body: How the Latest Exercise Science Can Help You Run Stronger, Longer, and Faster.* New York: Rodale, 2009.

WEBSITES

2011 Marathon, Half-Marathon and State of the Sport Reports. Running USA. http://www.runningusa.org/node/76115#76664 (accessed October 18, 2011).

Cool Running http://www.coolrunning.com/ (accessed October 18, 2011).

Running and Jogging Injuries. American Orthopaedic Society for Sports Medicine. http://www.sportsmed.org/uploadedFiles/Content/Patient/Sports_Tips/ST%20Running%20and%20Jogging%2008.pdf (accessed October 17, 2011).

Running Tips and Training Programs for Beginners to Marathon Runners. Tips4Running. http://www.tips4running.com/ (accessed October 18, 2011).

ORGANIZATIONS

American Running Association, 4405 East-West Hwy., Suite 405, Bethesda, MD, 20814, Fax: (301) 913-9520, (800) 776-2732, http://www.americanrunning.org/m/contact/, http://www.americanrunning.org/.

David E. Newton, A.B., M.A., Ed.D

S

Scubadiving *see* **Ocean sports**

Senior fitness

Definition

Older adults can be defined as men and women 65 years and older and adults aged 50-64 years with clinically significant chronic conditions and/or functional limitations that impact movement ability, fitness, or physical activity. Senior fitness refers to good health in all categories of physical fitness, including cardiorespiratory, muscle-strengthening, flexibility, and balance.

Purpose

Poor fitness leads to functional limitations, and ultimately loss of functional capacity and decreased independence in seniors. Importantly though, it should not be assumed that chronological **age** is equivalent to physiological or functional age. Individuals of similar ages can differ remarkably in functional capacity, which in turn affects how they respond to **exercise**. Although it is inevitable that physiological function will decline with age, the rate and magnitude of change in fitness parameters are dependent on a complex mixture of genetics, individual health, presence of disease/injury, and exercise history. In particular, regular exercise plays a critical role in preserving fitness; this confers several important benefits including prevention of various chronic diseases (e.g., type 2 diabetes, **cardiovascular disease**), maintaining cardiorespiratory fitness, and the prevention of functional limitations and disabilities.

Demographics

There is a strong association between physical fitness and function; for example, high levels of cardiorespiratory and muscular fitness permit an individual to more easily perform functions such as stair climbing and lifting. In turn, sufficient execution of these functions allows individuals to successfully complete personal hygiene tasks, housework, and other activities of daily living. By comparison, poor muscle fitness or flexibility can lead to impairments in function; for instance, bending and kneeling may be more challenging or restricted. These functional limitations can inhibit tasks such as dressing, gardening, and other related activities of daily living. Research has highlighted the important link between fitness and functional limitations; it has been shown that for both men and women, individuals with the lowest level of cardiorespiratory fitness have four-to-five fold increased prevalence of functional limitations compared to those individuals with the highest levels of cardiorespiratory fitness.

Description

Cardiorespiratory fitness is arguably the most important goal of an exercise program for older adults because low cardiorespiratory fitness may contribute to premature mortality in middle-aged and older adults. The literature suggests a 15% reduction in mortality for a 10% improvement in cardiorespiratory fitness. Seniors should strive to fulfill the population-wide recommendation of moderate-intensity aerobic activity for a minimum of 30 minutes, five days a week (or 150 minutes) or vigorous-intensity aerobic activity for a minimum of 25 minutes, three days a week (or 75 minutes) or an equivalent combination of both. If older adults cannot fulfill these guidelines due to debilitating chronic conditions, it is important that they are still encouraged to be as physically active as their condition permits. It is also imperative that seniors are counseled to avoid physical inactivity.

Aging is associated with a reduction in muscle mass that contributes to decreased muscle strength and a decline in functional capacity. Undeterred, the process

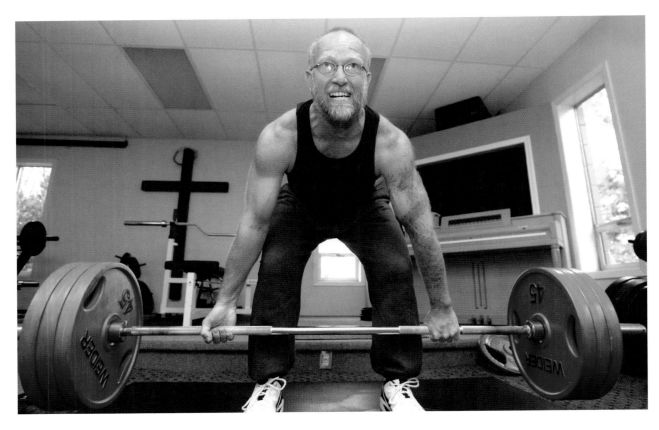

An older gentleman improves his physique by lifting weights. *(© AP Images/Matthew Putney)*

can ultimately result in balance impairments, mobility problems, and lack of independence for seniors. Furthermore, decreased muscle mass plays a role in the development of glucose intolerance and type 2 diabetes. For these reasons, seniors should be encouraged to participate in a resistance training program to attenuate the loss of muscle mass and muscular fitness. It is recommended that seniors perform a single set of eight to 10 exercises using the major muscle groups on two to three nonconsecutive days of the week. The level of effort for resistance training activities should be moderate to high; on a 10-point scale, where no movement equates to 0, and maximal effort equates to 10, moderate-intensity effort equals 5 or 6, and high-intensity effort equals 7 or 8. This amount of effort should permit seniors to perform 10 to 15 repetitions. Various dynamic muscle strengthening activities are recommended for seniors, including machine and free weights, weight-bearing **calisthenics**, and resistance bands.

Flexibility is an essential component of fitness and decreases with age and physical inactivity. Poor flexibility, coupled with decreased musculoskeletal strength, has been associated with a diminished ability to perform activities of daily living. Consequently, the beneficial effect of static **stretching** on the achievement and maintenance of flexibility should not be overlooked. The last decade has seen much scientific inquiry on the topic of stretching and performance/ risk of injury. Present research findings suggest that there are no ergogenic benefits, and potentially detrimental effects (decreased muscle strength and endurance, impaired balance, and diminished reaction time), to the incorporation of static stretching exercises into the **warm-up** routine. These findings are consistent among different populations and research designs, including untrained and trained individuals, recreational and competitive athletes, men and women, and with or without an aerobic warm-up. Those fitness and exercise professionals that work with seniors should be mindful of this evidence when designing programs and consider sequencing the workout so that flexibility follows the aerobic and resistance training components. For flexibility training it is recommended that static stretching exercises of the major muscle groups be performed a minimum of two days per week, although up to daily is not inappropriate, at a moderate intensity (i.e., 5 or 6 on a 0 to 10 scale).

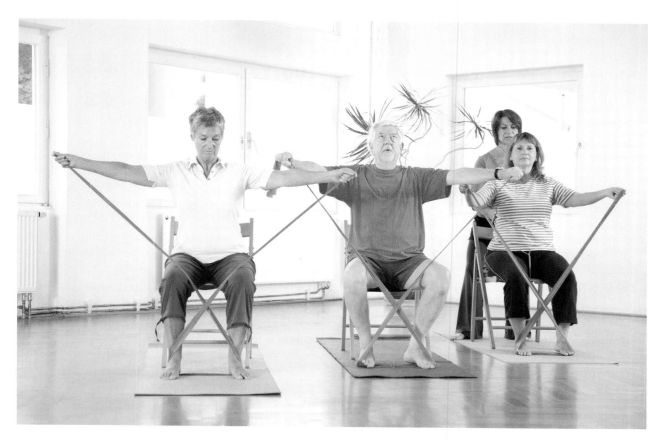

Some seniors using resistance bands to enhance their workout. *(© iStockPhoto. com/Christopher Pattberg)*

Fall incidence rates pose a serious health problem for seniors. In addition to an increased risk of falls, diminished balance and mobility may limit activities of daily living or participation in leisure-time activities. Accordingly, balance exercises should be included in all senior's exercise programs. It has been recommended that **balance training** be performed three days per week for 10 to 15 minutes each session. Balance training can be integrated into various phases of the exercise session, including warm up, main component, or cool-down.

Preparation

Seniors preparing to begin a fitness program can benefit from completion of baseline exercise testing. Those whom are at high risk (e.g., individuals with cardiovascular, metabolic, and/or pulmonary disease) will be assured it is appropriate to initiate exercise. Results from exercise tests also are useful with establishing a safe and effective fitness program, identifying fitness goals, and for interpreting the successfulness of the program at a later point in time. Depending on the individual, adjustments to the exercise testing protocol may be warranted. For example, a cycle ergometer exercise testing protocol may suit some seniors limited by poor balance, weight-bearing limitations, or vision problems more so compared to a **treadmill** exercise testing protocol. Additionally, it is likely that seniors will require a lower starting exercise testing workload, and subsequently progress with smaller workload increments throughout the test, relative to their younger adult counterparts.

Researchers have developed a battery of fitness tests specifically for seniors that can be employed by fitness and exercise professionals to quantify function in different areas of physical fitness, including cardiorespiratory, muscular fitness, flexibility, and balance. These tests include the following:

- Six-minute walk test: assessment of cardiorespiratory fitness

- Chair stand test: assessment of cardiorespiratory and leg muscle fitness

- Arm curl test: assessment of arm muscle fitness

KEY TERMS

Arteriovenous oxygen difference—The difference in blood oxygen content between arterial and venous blood.

Balance—Ability to remain upright and steady.

Cardiorespiratory fitness—The ability of the cardiovascular and pulmonary systems to supply oxygenated blood to the skeletal muscles during exercise and/or physical activity.

Comorbidities—The presence of one or more disorders or diseases in addition to the primary disease; for instance an individual with cardiovascular disease and hypertension, obesity, and Parkinson's disease.

Ejection fraction—The fraction of blood pumped by the left ventricle each beat; technically it is stroke volume divided by end-diastolic volume.

Flexibility—The ability to move joints through the full range of motion.

Functional capacity—The ability to carry out activities of daily living; for example, getting dressed, household chores, and running errands.

Functional limitations—Compromised ability to carry out activities of daily living; for instance, requiring assistance with personal hygiene or

needing to take an elevator rather than being able to walk up stairs.

Maximal cardiac output—Total volume of blood capable of being pumped by the left ventricle per minute during intense exercise.

Maximal heart rate—Refers to the maximal heart rate that can be elicited in an individual during intense exercise or exertion; this value can either be estimated (most commonly using 220-age) or directly measured from a maximal exercise test.

Maximal oxygen uptake—The highest rate at which oxygen can be taken up and consumed by the body during intense exercise.

Maximal stroke volume—Maximal difference between end-diastolic volume and end-systolic volume during intense exercise.

Muscular fitness—An overarching term characterizing the health of an individual's skeletal muscle; can be reflected in the capacity to generate sufficient muscle strength and endurance for various tasks.

Static stretching—Type of stretching in which muscle is gradually lengthened to the point of mild discomfort and then subsequently held for a short period of time (e.g., 30 seconds).

- Chair sit and reach test: assessment of flexibility
- Eight-foot up and go test: assessment of balance
- Scratch test: assessment of flexibility

For seniors who have difficulty adjusting to exercise or fitness testing protocols, the test may need to be either restarted or repeated on a separate day.

Risks

Current trends show that Americans are living longer while the number of U.S. citizens with chronic diseases continues to increase. In the past 100 years, life expectancy at birth in the United States increased from less than 50 years to more than 76 years. The U.S. Census Bureau has projected that by 2030, the number of adults 65 years of age and older will be approximately 70 million. Approximately 80% of individuals aged 65 years or older are living with at least one chronic health problem, and another 50% are living with two. The presence of specific chronic conditions can lead to an even greater propensity of comorbidities. For instance, almost all clients with type 2 diabetes have

at least one other chronic condition and nearly half have three or more comorbidities. These factors make it increasingly likely that fitness and exercise professionals will be interacting with many individuals other than apparently healthy adults.

Prior to initiating a fitness program, a medical examination and physician supervised exercise test is warranted for those seniors planning to participate in vigorous-intensity activities. Conversely, if seniors are only planning to engage in moderate-intensity activities a medical examination and physician supervised exercise test is not essential; however, it would not be deemed inappropriate either.

Results

An awareness of the physiological aspects of aging assist fitness and exercise professionals in establishing realistic and safe exercise tests and exercise programs for seniors. The following reductions in physiological capacities have been reported between the ages of 20 and 80: maximal oxygen uptake (50%), maximal cardiac output (25%), maximal heart rate (25%), maximal stroke volume (15%), ejection fraction (15%), and arteriovenous oxygen difference (25%). There are also expected declines, at a rate per decade past the age of 50, in muscle mass (6%), muscle strength (12-14%), and bone mass (10-15%) associated with the aging process. It is important to understand that while previously sedentary seniors initiating an exercise program can expect improvements in each of the physical fitness components, because of the natural decline in function associated with aging, fitness and exercise professionals should interpret maintenance of function as a successful outcome. For example, research suggests an average 1% decrease in cardiorespiratory fitness per year. A 65 year old senior who engages in a fitness program for five years and experiences no change in their cardiorespiratory fitness level over that time has had a successful outcome; the inevitable decline in physiological function, in this case cardiorespiratory fitness, has been delayed.

Resources

BOOKS

Ehrman, Jonathan K., editor. *ACSM's Resource Manual for Guidelines for Exercise Testing and Prescription.* Philadelphia: Lippincott Williams & Wilkins Health, 2010.

Heyward, Vivian, H., editor. *Advanced Fitness Assessment and Exercise Prescription.* Champaign: Human Kinetics; Wilkins, 2010.

Rikli, Roberta E., and C. Jessie Jones. *Senior Fitness Test Manual.* Champaign, IL: Human Kinetics, 2001.

Rose, Debra J. *Fall Proof! A Comprehensive Balance and Mobility Training Program.* Champaign, IL: Human Kinetics, 2010.

Thompson, Walter R., editor. *ACSM's Guidelines for Exercise Testing and Prescription.* Philadelphia: Lippincott Williams & Wilkins Health, 2010.

PERIODICALS

Garber, C.E., et al. "Quantity and Quality of Exercise for Developing and Maintaining Cardiorespiratory, Musculoskeletal, and Neuromotor Fitness in Apparently Healthy Adults: Guidance for Prescribing Exercise." *Medicine and Science in Sports and Exercise* 43, no. 7 (July 2011):1334–59.

Nelson, M.E., et al. "Physical Activity and Public Health in Older Adults: Recommendation from the American College of Sports Medicine and the American Heart Association." *Medicine and Science in Sports and Exercise* 39, no. 8 (August 2007): 1435–45.

WEBSITES

Fitness. Mayo Clinic. (March 19, 2011). http:// http:// www.mayoclinic.com/health/fitness/MY00396 (accessed October 1, 2011).

Rikli, Roberta, and Jessie Jones. *Five Senior Fitness Tests.* Sitandbefit.org. http://www.sitandbefit.org/senior_fitness_tests (accessed October 1, 2011).

Healthy Aging. National Center for Chronic Disease Prevention and Health Promotion. (2011). http:// www.cdc.gov/aging/ (accessed October 1, 2011).

ORGANIZATIONS

American College of Sports Medicine, 401 West Michigan St., Indianapolis, IN, 46206-1440, (317) 637-9200, Fax: (317) 634-7817, http://www.acsm.org.

American Council on Exercise, 4851 Paramount Dr., San Diego, CA, 92123, (888) 825-3636, support@ acefitness.org, http://www.acefitness.org.

The American Geriatrics Society, 40 Fulton St., 18th Floor, New York, NY, 10038, (212) 308-1414, Fax: (212) 832-8646, info.amger@americangeriatrics.org, http:// www.americangeriatrics.com.

American Society on Aging, 71 Stevenson St., San Francisco, CA, 94105-2938, (415) 974-9600, Fax: (415) 974-0300, (800) 537-9728, http://www.asaging.org.

Centers for Disease Control and Prevention, 1600 Clifton Rd., Atlanta, GA, 30333, (800) 232-6348, cdcinfo@ cdc.gov, http://www.cdc.gov.

Lance C. Dalleck, BA, MS, PhD

Senior fitness testing

Definition

Senior fitness testing assesses aerobic fitness, muscular strength and endurance, and flexibility in older people, as well as in others with physical limitations that make standard fitness testing inappropriate, dangerous, or impossible. Senior fitness testing may include standard fitness tests that are appropriate for seniors or are easily adapted to their special needs or limitations. Other tests are designed specifically for seniors and may include assessments of manual dexterity, fine- and gross-motor coordination, and agility. In particular, senior fitness testing aims to assess functional fitness—the ability to carry out daily tasks safely and effectively. Therefore the tests involve everyday activities, such as **walking**, standing up from a chair, bending, lifting, and **stretching**.

Purpose

Older adults require aerobic capacity or cardiorespiratory fitness, muscular strength and endurance, and flexibility, not just to enjoy their "golden years," but to be able to accomplish daily tasks and continue to live independently. Furthermore, more adults than ever are continuing to work long past traditional retirement **age**. Although physical abilities tend to decline with age, much of this decline is preventable, and possibly even reversible, with appropriate physical activity and fitness. Senior fitness testing can detect and address physical weaknesses at an early stage, before serious functional limitations develop. Test results can be used to develop individualized strength and conditioning routines for use at home or in physical therapy.

Description

Most senior fitness tests are simple to conduct and do not require specialized equipment. They usually include components of three similar test batteries:

- the American Alliance for Health, Physical Education, Recreation, & Dance (AAHPERD) Functional Fitness Test, for adults over age 60 with poor fitness but who are not frail
- the Groningen Fitness Test for the Elderly (GFE), developed by Human Movement Sciences at the University of Groningen in the Netherlands
- the Senior Fitness Test or Fullerton Functional Test, developed by Roberta Rikli and Jessie Jones as part of the LifeSpan Wellness program at Fullerton University

Aerobic fitness

Walking tests are commonly used to measure the aerobic fitness of seniors. Since walking tests may not require maximal aerobic capacity, they may not be appropriate for younger or more physically fit seniors.

The Groningen walk test is a variation of the standard beep test without sharp turns. It is performed on a flat, rectangular course of 54.69 ft. (16.67 m) by 27.33 ft. (8.33 m), for a perimeter of 164 ft. (50 m), with six alternating yellow and orange marker cones placed every 27.33 ft. (8.33 m). The course is walked counterclockwise around the cones to the pace of beeps on a recording, beginning at 2.5 mph (4 kph). Every three minutes, the pace increases by 0.62 mph (1 kph), to a maximum of 4.35 mph (7 kph). The test continues until the subject quits, fails to keep pace, or completes the last stage. Failing to keep pace is defined as being more than 9.8 ft. (3 m) from the next cone for two consecutive beeps. The score is the number of 54.69-ft. (16.67-m) stages completed, with 66 as the highest possible score.

The 0.5-mile (880-yd., 0.8-km, 805-m) walk tests aerobic endurance. It can be performed on a track or field with marked distances. Participants walk at their own pace, but as quickly as possible. Rest stops are permitted. The time is recorded in minutes and seconds.

The six-minute timed walking test is an adaptation of the Cooper 12-minute run. The rectangular course is 45 yd. (41 m) by 5 yd. (4.6 m) with cones at regular intervals. Subjects walk as quickly as possible at their own pace and can rest in chairs placed at intervals. The distance covered in six minutes is measured.

The two-minute step-in-place test is appropriate for people who use orthopedic devices or have trouble balancing. The subject stands straight against a wall and a tape is placed halfway between the knee cap and the top of the hipbone. The subject marches in place, lifting the knees to the height of the tape. Holding onto the wall or a stable chair and resting are permitted. The score is the number of times the right knee is lifted to the tape in two minutes.

Strength and endurance

The arm-curl test is a seated biceps curl that measures upper-body muscular strength and endurance. Seated in a chair without armrests, the subject grasps a weight in a suitcase grip (palm facing the body), using the stronger or dominant arm and seated near that side of the chair. Women use 4–5-lb. (1.8–2.3-kg) weights and men use 8-lb. (3.6-kg) weights. The arm is held straight down beside the chair and the upper arm is held against the body or held steady by a partner, so that only the lower arm moves. The forearm is curled up through the elbow's full range of motion and the palm is gradually turned upward. The arm is returned to the starting position through its full range of motion. The arm curl is repeated as many times as possible in 30 seconds.

The handgrip-strength test assesses upper-body strength by measuring the isometric strength of the hand and forearm with an instrument called a dynamometer. The handgrip test is often used to test overall strength. The dynamometer is gripped with the hand hanging by the side and squeezed as tightly as possible. The best of three attempts is scored, with a 30-second rest between attempts.

The chair-stand test for the lower body assesses leg strength and endurance. A straight-backed or folding chair, with a seat 17 in. (44 cm) high and without armrests, is placed against a wall. The subject sits in the center of the seat, with feet shoulder-width apart and flat on the floor. One foot may be slightly in front of the other. The arms are crossed at the wrists and held close to the chest. The subject stands completely up and sits completely down as many times as possible in 30 seconds. The arms can be used for assistance or safety.

Flexibility

The back-scratch test measures upper-body flexibility, especially shoulder range of motion. With the subject standing, one hand reaches over the shoulder as far as possible down the middle of the back, with the

KEY TERMS

Aerobic fitness—Aerobic capacity; cardiorespiratory fitness; the maximum amount of oxygen that can be transported by the heart, lungs, and blood to the muscles and utilized by the muscles during exercise.

Biceps—The large flexor muscle of the front of the upper arm.

Body mass index (BMI)—A measure of body fat; the ratio of body weight in kilograms to the square of height in meters.

Circumduction—Movement of a limb or extremity such that the end closest to the body remains fixed while the other end describes a circle; such as circling the arm from the shoulder.

Dynamometer—A device for measuring force, such as the strength of the arms, grip, back, or legs.

Fine-motor skills—Control of the smaller muscles of the body, especially in the hands, feet, and head, for activities such as writing and crafts.

Functional fitness—The physical ability to safely and effectively carry out tasks of daily life.

Gross-motor skills—Control of the large muscles of the body, including the arms, legs, back, abdomen, and torso, for activities such as sitting and walking.

Isometric—Muscular contraction against resistance without significant change in muscle-fiber length.

Normative—Test performance assessment based on results previously achieved by a selected sample of subjects, rather than by independent or absolute standards.

palm touching the back and the fingers downward. The other arm is placed around the back, palm out, and reaches as far up as possible, trying to touch or overlap the middle fingers of the upper hand. An assistant aligns the fingers of the two hands, measures the distance to the nearest 0.5 in. (1.3 cm), and records the best of two attempts.

The shoulder-circumduction test also assesses shoulder flexibility. A cord with one fixed handle and one sliding handle is adjusted to the subject's shoulder width. Holding a handle in each hand, the subject passes the cord from the front of the body, overhead, and as far back as possible with the arms extended. The score is the fanning-out angle recorded with an instrument.

The chair sit-and-reach test measures lower-body (trunk and leg) flexibility. It is a variation of the standard sit-and-reach flexibility test. The subject sits in a straight-back or folding chair about 17 in. (44 cm) high, placed against a wall. With one foot flat on the floor, the other leg is extended with the knee straight, the heel on the floor, and the ankle bent at 90°. With one hand on top of the other and the tips of the middle fingers even, the subject inhales and then exhales and, bending at the hips, reaches toward the toes of the extended foot. The back should be straight and the head up. The farthest reach is held for two seconds. The distance from the fingertips to the toes is measured to the nearest inch.

Manual dexterity, coordination, balance, and agility

The block-transfer test assesses fine-motor skills by measuring the speed at which blocks can be moved in a specific sequence. In a typical test, 40 blocks are moved from holes in one board to holes in a board farther away, in a given sequence, as quickly as possible.

The reaction-time test of fine-motor skills requires a special hand-held module. When the red light in the middle of the module comes on, the subject responds as quickly as possible by pushing a button at the top. The light comes on at intervals of four–nine seconds. The module displays the reaction times in milliseconds. After three practice trials, 15 trials are recorded.

The soda-pop test measures arm and hand coordination. The subject is seated at a table with an elbow bent about 100–120° and the thumb up. In one version of the test, a soda can in a drawn circle is grasped, inverted into an adjacent empty circle, and then returned to its original position in the first circle as quickly as possible. The process is repeated with two more cans. In another version, six soda cans are turned over in a specified order as fast as possible.

Seniors with poor balance are at risk for falls and injury. The balance board or platform test measures balance and agility. The wooden balance platform is about 20 in. (51 cm) square, with a 0.8-in.-wide (2-cm-wide) beam down the middle of the bottom. Stoppers at the corners prevent the board from tilting more than 18°. The subject stands on the platform with the toes pointed outward 15° and the heels 6 in. (15 cm) apart and tries to keep the platform balanced for 30 seconds. The best time of three trials is recorded.

The eight-foot-up-and-go test measures coordination, balance, agility, and speed. A straight-back or folding chair about 17 in. (44 cm) high is placed against a wall. A cone or other marker is set 8 ft. (2.4 m) away. Starting from a fully seated position with hands on the knees and feet flat on the floor, the subject stands and walks as quickly as possible around the cone and sits back in the chair, and the process is timed. A cane or walker may be used.

Precautions

Seniors, as well as anyone who is overweight or has a history of high **blood pressure** or heart disease, should consult a physician before undergoing fitness testing. Medical screening questionnaires are commonly used before testing. Medical assistance, first-aid supplies, and resuscitation equipment should be available in the testing area. Examiners should be trained in recognizing dangerous symptoms and have an emergency action plan in place.

All safety precautions should be followed. Chairs should be placed against a wall or otherwise stabilized. Tests should never involve **running**, bouncing, quick movements, or stretching to the point of pain. A test should be terminated immediately if the subject reports pain, dizziness, nausea, excessive **fatigue**, or other symptoms. Patients with severe **osteoporosis** should not perform the chair sit-and-reach test.

Preparation

The purpose and procedures of each test should be carefully explained. Most senior fitness tests involve one or more practice trials, but these should not cause fatigue. A trial to practice pacing is helpful for the 0.5-mile and six-minute walks.

Aftercare

Test results are clearly explained and may be compared with standardized norms for the subject's gender and age. Specific suggestions for improving fitness should be included. A report may be forwarded to the subject's physician.

Complications

Senior fitness tests are designed to be safe for the elderly and those with physical limitations. Therefore they seldom involve complications.

Results

Tests are scored and interpreted in various ways. The Senior Fitness Test uses normative data based on nationwide performance scores of more than 7,000 men and women between the ages of 60 and 94 who

---

WHAT TO ASK YOUR DOCTOR

- Should I undergo senior fitness testing?
- What tests or test battery do you recommend?
- Who should administer the tests?
- Are there any precautions I should take during the tests?
- What information will the tests give me?

---

were living independently. Calculators and software are available. Some test results, such as for the six-minute walk, are calculated taking into account gender, age, height, and for women, **body mass index** (BMI). However results are often interpreted in functional terms. For example, fewer than 11 arm curls in 30 seconds indicates risk for the inability to perform activities requiring arm strength. Fewer than eight chair stands in 30 seconds indicates risk for the inability to perform activities requiring leg strength. Taking more than nine seconds on the 8-foot-up-and-go test is considered a risk for being unable to move safely from one place to another.

If the fingertips touch on a scratch test, the score is zero. If they overlap, the score is the positive distance; otherwise the score is the negative distance. Scores are age-dependent, but in general, men whose fingertips are more than 8 in. (20 cm) apart and women whose fingertips are more than 5 in. (13 cm) apart are at risk for poor performance in activities that require upper-body flexibility.

Resources

BOOKS

Lemmink, K.A.P.M., et al. "The Groningen Fitness Test for the Elderly: Composition and Application in Large-Scale Fitness Events." In *Physical Activity, Aging and Sports: Toward Healthy Aging—International Perspectives. Part 2*, edited by S. Harris, E. Heikkinen, and W.S. Harris, 221–230. Albany, NY: Center for the Study of Aging of Albany, 1995.

Osness, W.H., et al. *Functional Fitness Assessment for Adults Over 60 Years (a Field Based Assessment)*. Reston, VA: American Alliance for Health, Physical Education, Recreation, and Dance, 1990.

Rikli, Roberta E., and C. Jessie Jones. *Senior Fitness Test Manual*. Champaign, IL: Human Kinetics, 2001.

PERIODICALS

Wiacek, Magdalena, et al. "Deterioration of Basic Coordinative Parameters Defines Life Quality of Elderly." *Archives of Gerontology and Geriatrics* 49, no. 2 (September-October, 2009): 212–14.

WEBSITES

Rikli, Roberta, and Jessie Jones. "Five Senior Fitness Tests." Sit and Be Fit. http://www.sitandbefit.org/senior_fitness_tests (accessed August 10, 2011).

"The Senior Fitness Test." Topend Sports. January 13, 2011. http://www.topendsports.com/testing/senior-fitness-test.htm (accessed August 9, 2011).

ORGANIZATIONS

American Alliance for Health, Physical Education, Recreation, & Dance, 1900 Association Drive, Reston, VA, 20191-1598, (703) 476-3400, (800) 213-7193, http://www.aahperd.org.

The AAHPERD is a consortium of five national organizations—the American Association for Health Education, American Association for Physical Activity and Recreation, National Association for Girls and Women in Sport, National Association for Sport and Physical Education, and National Dance Association. The AHPERD is organized into six district associations with more than 22,000 members who are interested in promoting healthy, active, and creative lifestyles. The AAHPERD has developed a senior fitness testing protocol.

Cooper Institute, 12330 Preston Road, Dallas, TX, 75230, (972) 341-3200, Fax: (972) 341-3227, (800) 635-7050, fitnessgram@cooperinst.org, http://www.cooperinstitute.org.

The Cooper Institute is a nonprofit research and education organization founded in 1970 by Dr. Kenneth H. Cooper, the "Father of Aerobics." It is dedicated to global preventive heath care for children and adults through science and education, with an emphasis on the role of exercise.

Sit and Be Fit, P.O. Box 8033, Spokane, WA, 99203-0033, (509) 448-9438, Fax: (509) 448-5078, sitandbefit @sitandbefit.org, http://www.sitandbefit.org/.

Sit and Be Fit is a nonprofit organization that has produced the award-winning public television series, *Sit and Be Fit*, since 1987.

Margaret Alic, PhD

Shoulder stability

Definition

Shoulder stability is the normal condition of the shoulder, one that bring about a full range of movement to the shoulder's ball-and-socket joint, including being able to lift up and rotate the arms over the head. This ability to have the maximum range of motions in

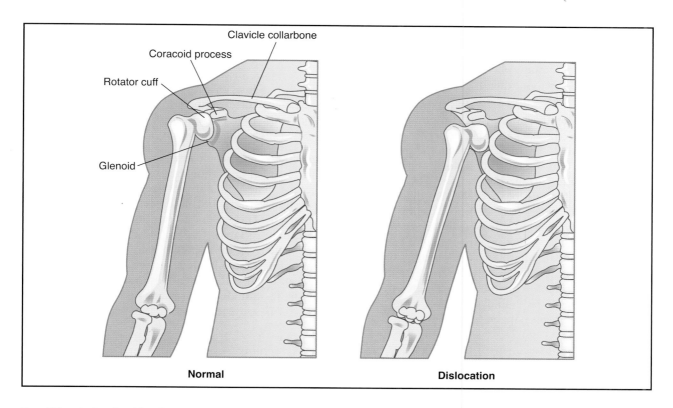

Repetitive strain, shoulder dislocation, and multidirectional instability are three common ways a shoulder's full range of motion can be affected. (Electronic Illustrators Group. © 2012 Cengage Learning.)

various directions allows the shoulder to be used in many different ways for daily tasks and for physical activities such as **exercise** and sporting events.

However, because of this large range of motions that the shoulder can perform, injuries to this area are more likely possible, which can lead to instability. Shoulder instability occurs when the head of the upper arm bone is forced out of the shoulder socket. This action can result from overuse over many years; a sudden, unexpected injury; or from genetics (heredity). In its more serious form, it is called chronic shoulder instability.

Description

The shoulder consists of three bones: the clavicle (collarbone), the humerus (bone in upper arm), and the scapula (shoulder blade). A shallow socket, called the glenoid socket, is contained in the shoulder blade where the ball (head) of the upper arm bone resides. The ball remains centered in the glenoid socket with strong connective tissue—what is called the shoulder capsule. This bone and connective tissue, along with muscles and ligaments keep the shoulder stable.

However, the head of the upper arm bone can be forced out of the shoulder socket from a sudden injury, such as from a sporting activity. It can also be forced out from long-term overuse, such as repeated use as a swimmer, tennis player, or other such athlete. It can also be forced out due to genetics; that is, from being born with loose ligaments around the shoulder.

The head of the upper arm can come out only partially from the socket. This condition is called shoulder subluxation. In other cases, the dislocation can be a total one. A complete dislocation means the ball comes all the way out of the socket. This condition is called shoulder dislocation. When this happens repeatedly, the ligaments, tendons, and/or muscles around the shoulder have become loose or torn. This causes the shoulder to become loose, and it can easily slip out of place—what is called chronic shoulder instability. Once chronic shoulder instability is present, it is difficult to maintain the centered position of the arm bone in the shoulder socket. Consequently, shoulder dislocations happen frequently.

Demographics

Shoulder instability is found most often in cases of trauma. Sporting events, such as contact type events found in **football**, see the most cases of shoulder instability. It is often diagnosed in young athletes. However, it also occurs commonly in all **age** groups in such everyday accidents as falling down the stairs, falling off a bicycle, or slipping on the ice or another slippery surface. Some people are prone to shoulder instability because they are genetically predisposed to it (that is, they were born with increased risk to it). In addition, repetitive activities that one performs adds to the risk of getting shoulder instability, such as throwing sports, **swimming**, impact/contact sports, and even certain types of working jobs.

Causes and symptoms

Causes

There are three frequent situations that cause the shoulder to become unstable. These are:

- serious prior shoulder injury (dislocation): an injury to the head of the upper arm bone can cause the socket bone and the ligaments at the front of the shoulder to become injured. After the ligament has been injured on one or more occasions, it may heal looser than it was before the injury. This can lead to shoulder instability and eventually to chronic shoulder instability. When this happens the shoulder may be at increased risk for repeated dislocations.

- repetitive strain: repetitive over-the-head motions of the arms, such as that in tennis, swimming, baseball (especially pitchers), and volleyball in sports, or in some jobs, can cause the shoulder capsule and ligaments in the shoulder to stretch (become looser than normal). This can cause repeated stress, or what is medically called cumulative microtrauma. When the ligaments stretch they become looser, making it more likely for shoulder instability.

- genetics: some people are born with naturally looser ligaments in their shoulders when compared to most people. They do not have a history of injury or repetitive strain, but still have instability in their shoulder. These people often have multidirectional instability; that is, the ball of the upper arm may dislocate from the socket in many directions. People that are double-jointed (a condition called joint laxity) usually also have loose joints. They may be prone to shoulder dislocations just because they are born with loose joints.

Symptoms

Common symptoms of chronic shoulder instability include:

- pain, sometimes severe
- swelling of the area around the shoulder

KEY TERMS

Cardiovascular—Relating to the heart and blood vessels of the body.

Clavicle—The long, curved bone that connects the upper breastbone to the shoulder blade in humans.

Humerus—The long bone in the upper arm of humans.

Magnetic resonance imaging—An imaging method that uses electromagnetic radiation to obtain images of soft tissues.

Scapula—Either of two large flat bones that form the back of the shoulder in humans.

Subluxation—Partial dislocation.

- clicking noises from the shoulder area, especially during exercise or while engaging in sports activities that require shoulder
- deformity of the shoulder
- sense of partial paralysis of the arm
- repeated dislocations of the shoulder
- numerous cases of the shoulder not being able to perform one or more of its normal functions
- persistent abnormal sensation in or around the shoulder that feels like the joint is loose or not stable; that the shoulder is about to come out of place or has repositioned itself back into its socket

Diagnosis

If having problems with a shoulder that is unstable, visit the family doctor or other such medical professional. This trained medical person will analyze past medical history and the current symptoms involving the shoulder. Certain movements may be asked by the doctor to determine if looseness is present in the shoulder.

The doctor is likely to order imaging test to help confirm the diagnosis. Such tests as x-ray scans and magnetic resonance imaging (MRI) scans may be used to show any injuries to the bones and tissues around the shoulder, along with any problems with the ligaments and tendons in that area.

Treatment

Instability in the shoulder is usually first treated with non-surgical methods. These include modifications in lifestyle, activities that directly cause shoulder problems. A non-steroidal anti-inflammatory medication, such as aspirin and ibuprofen, will help to reduce the pain and swelling. The application of ice immediately after the injury will help, too.

If warranted, physical therapy and/or rehabilitation may help to strengthen the shoulder muscles. Specific exercises may help to bring increased stability to the shoulder. The exercises build strength within the muscles that perform internal and external rotation of the joint. If weights are used, they should be less than five pounds. At this time, the patient will usually be required by the doctor to wear a sling to support the injured shoulder.

If patients continue to be bothered by shoulder instability, then additional exercises may be recommended by the doctor to strengthen the muscles around the shoulder. These exercises will frequently include flexion (bending) and extension (extending) movements with weights ranging from five to ten pounds, with the amount of weight depending on the injury's severity. **Stretching** exercises are also recommended to regain the full range of motion within the joint. In some case, cortisone injections may be recommended. At this point, a sling may or may not be necessary.

As the injured area recovers, the patient should eventually regain full range of motion within the shoulder. Therapy usually concludes at this point. At the end of therapy, regular movements should be possible, such as those that initially caused the shoulder instability. However, while therapy is nearly finished, the patient should at home continue to perform exercises that increase muscle strengthening and mobility. Exercises should consist of weights with a minimum of 15 pounds.

In more serious cases, such as chronic shoulder instability, the doctor may recommend surgery to repair torn or stretched ligaments in the shoulder. Arthroscopic surgery is one surgical method. Small instruments and incisions are used to look inside the shoulder to pinpoint the problem. For instance, if the capsule of the shoulder has been injured an arthroscopic procedure is performed called thermal capsular shrinkage. In the procedure, a heated probe is inserted to shrink the capsule so it secures more tightly into the tissue. In simple surgical cases, this minimally invasive surgery may be the better option to choose.

However, when the surgery involves complex procedures, then open surgery is most likely the better answer. Open surgery involves making a large incision over the shoulder and repairing the injured parts while the patient is unconscious. Sometimes a procedure called Bankart repair is performed to fix ligament tears around the shoulder. After the surgery, the shoulder will in most cases be entirely immobile so the healing process can proceed as fast as possible. Once the doctor recommends the shoulder can be moved, a rehabilitation program may be set up to help strengthen the shoulder ligaments. This will also help to improve the shoulder's range of motion.

Prognosis

The prognosis of further joint dislocation in young people is usually quite high, but the chance of such continuing dislocation becomes lower as one ages. At any age, the risk of further dislocations is quite possible. In addition, risks of further bleeding and injuries to the blood vessels, incorrect healing, infection, and nerve damage are always possible.

Prevention

The prevention of shoulder instability includes maintaining strength within the rotator cuff and the shoulder blade. Exercises that build and maintain muscle strength in those areas helps to keep the shoulder stable. In addition, learning the correct techniques when performing repetitive tasks or actions, such as throwing, helps to minimize the chances of shoulder instability.

Resources

BOOKS

Beers, Mark H. *The Merck Manual of Diagnosis and Therapy.* Pahway, Merck, 2006.

Micheli, Lyle J., editor. *Encyclopedia of Sports Medicine.* Thousand Oaks, CA: SAGE, 2011.

Moorman III, Claude T., and Donald T. Kirkendall, editors. *Praeger Handbook of Sports Medicine and Athlete Health.* Santa Barbara, CA: Praeger, 2011.

Plowman, Sharon A., and Denise L. Smith. *Exercise Physiology for Health, Fitness, and Performance.* Philadelphia: Wolters Kluwer Health/Lippincott Williams & Wilkins, 2011.

Rich, Brent E., and Mitchell K. Pratte. *Tarascon Sports Medicine Pocketbook.* Sudbury, MA: Jones and Bartlett Publishers, 2010.

Sutton, Amy L, editor. *Fitness and Exercise Sourcebook.* Detroit: Omnigraphics, 2007.

WEBSITES

Chronic Shoulder Instability. American Academy of Orthopaedic Surgeons. http://orthoinfo.aaos.org/topic.cfm?topic = A00529 (accessed September 27, 2011).

Physical Therapy for Chronic Shoulder Instability. eHow. com. http://www.ehow.com/way_5586085_physical-therapy-chronic-shoulder-instability.html (accessed September 28, 2011).

Shoulder Instability. Cleveland Clinic. http://my.cleveland clinic.org/disorders/shoulder_instability/or_overview. aspx (accessed September 28, 2011).

ORGANIZATIONS

American Alliance for Health, Physical Education, Recreation and Dance, 1900 Association Drive, Reston, VA, 20191-1598, (703) 476-3400, (800) 213-7193, http://www.aahperd.org/.

American Association of Orthopaedic Surgeons, 6300 North River Road, Rosemont, IL, 60018-4262, (847) 823-7186, Fax: (847) 823-8125, http://www.aaos.org/.

American Council on Exercise, 4851 Paramount Drive, San Diego, CA, 92123, (888) 825-3636, support@acefitness.org, http://www.fitness.gov/.

American College of Sports Medicine, P.O. Box 1440, Indianapolis, IN, 46206-1440, (317) 634-9200, Fax: (317) 634-7817, http://www.acsm.org/.

National Coalition for Promoting Physical Activity, 1100 H Street, N.W., Suite 510, Washington, DC, 20005, 1 (202) 454-7521, Fax: 1 (202) 454-7598, http://www.ncppa.org/membership/organizations/.

National Strength and Conditioning Association, 1885 Bob Johnson Drive, Colorado Springs, CO, 80906, (719) 632-6722, Fax: (719) 632-6367, (800) 815-6826, http://www.nsca-lift.org/.

President's Council on Fitness, Sports and Nutrition, 1101 Wootton Parkway, Suite 560, Rockville, MD, 20852, (240) 276-9567, Fax: (240) 276-9860, http://www.fitness.gov/.

William A. Atkins, BB, BS, MBA

Sitting

Definition

Sitting is a period of relative inactivity or rest in which is person is seated with the buttocks and thighs supporting the upper torso, which is basically in an upright position. Although sitting is a normal everyday activity, excessive sitting can be detrimental to maintaining a healthy and fit body, and can be a contributing factor to various medical problems.

Purpose

Sitting is used daily by humans as a way to rest or to maintain a sedate position while performing various types of work. There are various positions, postures, and general ways used in sitting—such as with parallel aligned legs or cross-legged; on a chair or floor; or sitting with legs down below the waist or raised above—but in each case the result is the same: a person is in a seated position while engaged in rest or some sedentary activity such as reading, watching TV, or listening to music.

Demographics

All humans sit periodically throughout their daily lives. Some sit more than others. Recently, medical studies have noted the negative impacts to excessively long periods of sitting, increasing the risk of such medical problems as **cardiovascular disease**, diabetes, **hypertension** (high **blood pressure**), high **cholesterol**, increased blood sugar triglyceride levels, **obesity**, and even some forms of cancer.

Long periods of sitting are becoming more common in today's society as increasing numbers of people have jobs that require more mental activities than physical ones. In addition, much leisure time activities are centered around recreational sitting, such as watching television or playing video games.

Description

Sitting is commonly performed on the floor with the knees either bended or unbent. An object such as a wall is sometimes used to support the back or the arms can be positioned so the upper body leans upon them. There are various ways to sit, but in each the buttocks and thighs are supporting the upper half of the body (torso).

American epidemiologist Steven Balir, from the Department of Public Health at the University of South Carolina (Columbia), puts sitting in perspective when he states, "Let's say you do 30 minutes of **walking** five days a week (as recommended by federal health officials), and let's say you sleep for eight hours. Well, that still leaves 15.5 hours" in the day."

The issue of excessive sitting has been recently raised in the medical community because of the distinct possibility that it increases the risk of cardio-vascular (heart) disease, obesity, type 2 diabetes, and other medical conditions. It has even been associated with increased risk of premature death.

Research

An Australian study that was published online in the *European Heart Journal* on January 11, 2011, found that long periods of sitting were associated with "worse indicators of cardio-metabolic function and inflammation, such as larger waist circumferences, lower levels of HDL ("good") cholesterol, and higher levels of C-reactive **protein** (an important marker of inflammation) and triglyerides (blood fats)."

The study, which was conducted on American participants, went on to state that these problems were even found in people who exercised on a regular basis but still sat long hours. They concluded that regular respites from sitting, even standing for a little as a minute, were better than sitting continuously for long times. Dr. Genevieve Healy, from the University of Queensland (Brisbane, Australia), commented on the problem of sitting for extended periods within a WebMD article: "The potential adverse health impact of prolonged sitting (which is something that we do on average for more than half of our day), is only just being realized. Our research highlights the importance of considering prolonged sedentary time as a distinct health risk behavior that warrants explicit advice in future public health guidelines."

Another scientist, Dr. James Levine, from the Mayo Clinic in Rochester, Minnesota, performs experiments in what he calls inactivity studies. He found over years of study that some people gain much more weight than do others even though they are strictly controlled in the number of **calories** they are given each day and with no **exercise** allowed. Levine found that some people just naturally move their bodies more than do others. These little movements each day add to more calories burned even when no formal exercises are done.

According to the *New York Times* article "Sitting a Lethal Activity?" the difference in calories expended (burned) was the amount of sitting performed each day. It compared two groups of people after they were given more food than usual in their daily diets: "Their bodies simply responded naturally by making

KEY TERMS

Cardiovascular—Relating to the heart and blood vessels.

High-density lipoprotein cholesterol—Abbreviated HDL cholesterol, a type of cholesterol often called "good" cholesterol.

Hypertension—The medical term for high blood pressure.

Obesity—Being excessively or extremely overweight.

Type 2 diabetes—Also called diabetes mellitus type 2, the type of diabetes that first occurs in adulthood and is characterized by high blood glucose, insulin resistance, and relative insulin deficiency. It often comes about due to being obese.

more little movements than they had before the overfeeding began, like taking the stairs, trotting down the hall to the office water cooler, bustling about with chores at home or simply fidgeting. On average, the subjects who gained weight sat two hours more per day than those who hadn't."

Preparation

Risks

Excessive sitting can lead to increased risk of a sore back, added extra pounds to the body weight, and other common ailments found in many people. However, sitting for long periods of time can also increase one's risk of cardiovascular disease, diabetes, and high blood pressure.

For instance, Dr. Marr Hamilton, from the Pennington Biomedical Research Center, in Raton Rouge, Louisiana, has been an inactivity researcher for several years. Hamilton stated that sitting for long periods results in the electrical activity within the body to drastically decrease; that is, muscles are not moving. When this happens, the metabolic system of the body also declines. A sitting person does not burn many calories; in fact, it is reduced to about one third of the metabolic rate if one was walking around. In an experiment Hamilton performed, he found that young, healthy adults had a 40% reduction in the ability of insulin to take in glucose after only 24 hours of being sedentary. This inactivity adversely affects the metabolic rate within these people.

Hamilton concluded that prolonged sitting, or any type of sedentary inactivity, leads to an increase risk of developing type 2 diabetes and obesity, and to the lowering of high-density lipoprotein (HDL,) cholesterol in the body, what is consider the "good" cholesterol.

Although in the past, it was assumed that exercising and eating a good diet could counter long periods of sitting, new research has come to light that long periods of inactivity are not alleviated with exercise

and healthy eating. Instead of sitting for long periods, medical professionals are now saying that it is necessary to periodically get up and move about when forced to sit for long periods, such as while at work during school, or even while riding in airplanes, trains, buses, or cars.

Results

It has been proven that sitting for prolonged periods of time is detrimental to health. It is beneficial to health, therefore, to avoid sitting for long periods. If forced by job, school, or general circumstances to long periods of sitting, it is better to stand up or walk around periodically throughout the day. For instance, answer a telephone call while standing up, or walk over to a work or school colleague rather than emailing them. If for no purpose than just to be healthier, stand up frequently when forced to sit long hours.

Sitting has been found to adversely effect health of humans. It can also lead to premature death. An American Cancer Society study, headed by American epidemiologist Alpa Patel, researched around 123,000 Americans between 1992 and 2006 with respect to their health. Patel and her colleagues found that men who spent six or more hours sitting each day had an average death rate that was 20% higher than men who sat for three hours or less. For women, the rate was even worse, at 40% higher.

Patel concluded that sitting over six hours a day reduces one's life span for a few years. In addition, in a related study performed in Australia, it was concluded that each additional hour of sitting each day increases the risk of dying by 11%. The study, headed by Dr. David W. Dunstan, was published on January 11, 2010, within the journal *Circulation* under the title "Television Viewing Time and Mortality."

Health officials in the United States recommend at least 30 minutes of moderate exercise daily. Walks in the park, hikes in the forest, or bike rides around the neighborhood are all good for physical and **mental health**. However, it is also important to stay active even if a job or school requires a lot of sitting. Rather than sitting sedentarily throughout the day, get out of the chair and stand or walk at least once an hour.

Dr. Toni Yancey, from the Kaiser Permanente Center for Health Equity at the University of California (San Diego), has written a book called "Instant Recess: Building a Fit Nation 10 Minutes at a Time." In it, Yancey states that sitting for long hours is not what the human body is used to doing. Sitting causes the body to shut down its metabolism—it stops burning calories. Even though one has a sedentary job or must sit at a desk while at school, motion can still be incorporated into these periods of inactivity. Simply stand up, move arms or legs while sitting, walk in place, bend, twist, and other simple exercises help the body to remain active so it continues to burn calories and, more importantly, to maintain a healthy and fit lifestyle. Yancey recommends just a few minutes of simple movements every hour will help to counter excessive inactive periods of sitting.

Resources

BOOKS

Plowman, Sharon A., and Denise L. Smith. *Exercise Physiology for Health, Fitness, and Performance*. Philadelphia: Wolters Kluwer Health/Lippincott Williams & Wilkins, 2011.

Sutton, Amy L, editor. *Fitness and Exercise Sourcebook*. Detroit: Omnigraphics, 2007.

Yancey, Toni. *Instant Recess: Building a Fit Nation 10 Minutes at a Time.*. Berkeley: University of California Press, 2010.

WEBSITES

Dunstan, D.W., et al. *Television Time and Mortality* Circulation. January 11, 2010, http://circ.ahajournals.org/content/121/3/384.abstract?sid=e7f04689-9dec-47b0-bdc6-1b26adb72296 (accessed September 6, 2011).

Exercise. Texas Heart Institute. (December 2010). http://www.texasheartinstitute.org/hic/topics/hsmart/exercis1.cfm (accessed June 6, 2011).

How Much Physical Activity Do You Need? Centers for Disease Control and Prevention. (March 30, 2011). http://www.cdc.gov/physicalactivity/everyone/guidelines/index.html (accessed June 6, 2011).

Neighmond, Patti. *Sitting All Day: Worse For You Than You Might Think* NPR. April 25, 2011, http://www.npr.org/2011/04/25/135575490/sitting-all-day-worse-for-you-than-you-might-think (accessed September 6, 2011).

Physical Activity. MedlinePlus. (March 20, 2011). http://www.nlm.nih.gov/medlineplus/ency/article/001941.htm (accessed September 13, 2011).

Sitting for Too Long Is Bad for Your Health. WebMD. (January 12, 2011). http://www.webmd.com/heart-disease/news/20110112/sitting-down-too-long-bad-health (accessed September 5, 2011).

Vlahos, James. *Is Sitting a Lethal Activity?* New York Times. April 14, 2011, http://www.nytimes.com/2011/04/17/magazine/mag-17sitting-t.html (accessed September 6, 2011).

ORGANIZATIONS

American Alliance for Health, Physical Education, Recreation and Dance, 1900 Association Drive, Reston, VA, 20191-1598, (703) 476-3400, (800) 213-7193, http://www.aahperd.org/.

National Coalition for Promoting Physical Activity, 1100 H Street, N.W., Suite 510, Washington, DC, 20005, (202) 454-7521, Fax: (202) 454-7598, http://www.ncppa.org/membership/organizations/.

President's Council on Fitness, Sports and Nutrition, 1101 Wootton Parkway, Suite 560, Rockville, MD, 20852, (240) 276-9567, Fax: (240) 276-9860, http://www.fitness.gov/.

William A. Atkins, BB, BS, MBA

Skateboarding

Definition

Skateboarding is a sporting activity in which an individual rides on a short, narrow board, usually made of some composite material, to which are attached a pair of small wheels at each end of the board. The rider propels himself or herself by place one foot on the board and pushing on the ground with the other foot. The rider typically stands in an upright or crouching position on the board, from which position any number of tricks can be performed.

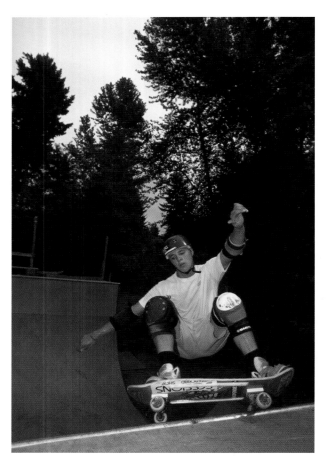

A male adolescent poises himself gracefully on the edge of a halfpipe. *(© Bettmann/Corbis)*

Purpose

People ride skateboards for a variety of reasons, including pure recreation, as a means of transportation, as a type of artistic display, or as a career as a professional skateboarder.

Demographics

The Sporting Goods Manufacturers Association (SGMA) conducts an annual survey of participation in more than 100 different sports. Its 2011 report showed that participation in skateboarding has declined significantly in recent years, falling from a total of 9,859,000 more-than-once participants in 2007 to 6,808,000 more-than-once participants in 2011, a decline of 30.9 percent. The largest one-year decline, from 2010 to 2011, occurred among so-called "frequent" riders, those who participated in the sport more than 52 times a year. Surveys tend to show that the vast majority of skateboarders are males. A 2009 survey conducted by the Board-Trac company, for

example, found that 93.3 percent of all "frequent" participants were male, and 6.7 percent, female. Among "infrequent" participants, the division was somewhat less pronounced, 80.7 percent male to 19.3 percent female. The sport is primarily one of young participants, with at least 85 percent of riders being under the age of 18. The most recent data suggest that the sport is becoming somewhat less popular among the mid-adolescent range (early teens), although it has begun to grow in popularity among the youngest age group, those between the ages of five and nine.

History

Most skateboarders date the beginnings of their sport to the end of the 1940s and early 1950s when a number of surfers began exploring ways of pursuing their sport in settings other than the ocean. They conceived the idea of putting wheels on strips of wood similar to surfboards and "surfing" city streets on these boards. The activity was given the name of "sidewalk surfing." For a decade, enthusiasm for the sport surged, and sales of wheeled surf boards surpassed the US$10 million mark by 1965. A year earlier, a specialty publication, Skateboarder Magazine, began publication, and also in 1965, the first international skateboarding championship was in Anaheim, California. The contestants were primarily 12 to 14-year-old boys, and the winner was 15-year-old Danny Bearer, later to become a skateboarding icon. By the early 1970s, skateboarding had begun to lose its appeal; sales of boards declined and Skateboarder Magazine went out of business.

Two events led to the revival of interest in skateboarding in the mid-1970s. First, manufacturers began to explore the use of alternative materials for the construction of boards. Plastics and composites were used to produce boards that were lighter and easier to maneuver than traditional wooden boards, which, nonetheless, continued to command a significant portion of the market. Second, riders migrated to the use of so-called vert ramps on which to practice their sport. At first, the primary and almost exclusive venue for skateboarding was city streets, parking lots, and other open, concrete areas. But in a few instances, riders were beginning to explore options to these open spaces, the most popular being vert ramps that are similar to the half pipe used in many extreme sports today. Reputedly, the first vert ramps were **swimming** pools that had been emptied by young men while their parents were on vacation, providing a more challenging site in which to practice their sport. A third factor may also have been the invention of a new maneuver on a skateboard, a so-called "ollie," in which a rider lifts the board and himself or herself into the air without the use of hands.

TONY HAWK (1968–)

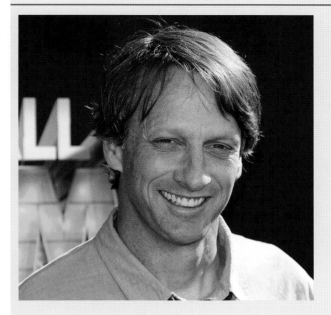

(© Allstar Picture Library/Alamy)

Tony Hawk is a California native who was instrumental in the evolution of skateboarding from the preppy recreation of the 1960s to the daring and extreme test of physical limits and mental creativity it has become. In seventeen years as a professional skateboarder, Hawk has invented more than eighty tricks and competed in an estimated 103 contests, winning seventy–three and placing second in nineteen. He quit competing in 1999 after landing the first-ever 900—two-and-a-half mid-air spins on the board.

When Hawk was nine years old, he found an outlet for his hyperactivity in a skateboard that his brother gave him. By 1980, he began competing but his family noticed it was difficult to help young Hawk cope with his own perfectionist expectations. Both of Hawk's parents were supportive of their son's athletic passion. His father was a regular part of Hawk's skateboarding life, driving Tony all over California to various skateboard competitions, and building countless skate ramps over the years. Frank Hawk founded the California Amateur Skateboard League in 1980 and the National Skateboarding Association (NSA) in 1983. The NSA organized many high-profile skateboarding competitions and was a key factor in the resurgence of skate culture that took place in the 1980s.

Hawk turned pro in 1982, at age fourteen, and placed third in his first professional contest. The fact that he was a professional skateboarder meant nothing to the bullies and jocks at school but his parents often excused him from class to travel to contests and demos.

When the skateboard industry plummeted in the early 1990s, Hawk raised enough money to start his own skate company, Birdhouse, with fellow Powell pro Per Welinder. The industry got a shot in the arm in 1995 when ESPN held its first Extreme Games that included bungee jumping, BMX riding, inline skating, and skateboarding. ESPN made Hawk the star of the games, which shot sales up for Birdhouse. By 1998, Birdhouse was one of the biggest companies in skateboarding, and Hawk was the sport's unofficial ambassador. Mainstream media latched onto Hawk and made him the most recognizable skateboarder in the world. He retained his superstar status in the skateboarding world, and starred in one of the most popular video game series ever, Tony Hawk's Pro Skater.

The ollie became a fundamental maneuver on which a whole host of other new tricks could be based.

The popularity of skateboarding crashed again in the late 1980s, partly because of safety issues related to the sport. Although vert skateboarding was thrilling, it was also very dangerous, as was the simpler form of the sport performed on public and private property. Soon insurance rates forced vert ramps to close down and property owners to ban skateboarding on their property. The sport soon evolved into an almost completely street-centered sport. With the arrival of the 1990s, interest in skateboarding once more began to increase, but this time it was often associated with the rise of a "punk" and "hard metal" culture in which riders took pride in being "out-of-the-mainstream." When the ESPN television channel held the first Extreme Games in 1995, a fission began to occur within the skateboarding community between those who saw an opportunity to move their sport into the mainstream (as a part of the ESPN X Games), and those who relished the underground aspects of skateboarding. Elements of that fission remain today as the sport continues to fluctuate in popularity both across the board and within its two main "mainstream" and "underground" elements.

Description

The basic concept that underlies skateboarding is simple, one stands on a skateboard and propels the board kicking with one foot, often performing a variety of tricks in the process. The precise nature of the activity, in addition to the site on which it is performed, differs widely, however, from version to

KEY TERMS

Boneless—A method of taking off and landing on the board while it is in the air.

Downhill skateboarding—A form of skateboarding in which riders travel down hills.

Endover—A skateboard maneuver that involves a 180 degree turn on the board.

Flatland skateboarding—A form of skateboarding that is done on a flat, hard-surface area.

Freestyle skateboarding—A form of skateboarding in which riders perform a variety of artistic and demanding maneuvers, often in accompaniment to music.

Ollie—A maneuver in which a rider lifts the board and himself or herself into the air without the use of hands.

Slalom skateboarding—A form of skateboarding in which racers travel downhill following a course laid out by cones.

Street skateboarding—A form of skateboarding in which the rider performs on the street, sidewalk, parking lot, shopping center, or other flat paved area.

Vert skateboarding—A form of skateboarding performed in a half-pipe.

Walking the dog—A series of endovers performed continuously

version. Some of the many variations of skateboarding include the following:

- Street skateboarding is a form of the sport in which the rider performs on the street, sidewalk, parking lot, shopping center, or other reasonably flat paved area. The rider attempts to overcome natural obstacles that are part of this environment, including curbs, steps, handrails, and ledges.

- Flatland skateboarding, as the name implies, is done on a flat, hard-surface area. It differs from street skateboarding in that it involves a very large variety of tricks that do not require the use of objects in the environment. Those tricks involve different kinds of flips, endovers (which involve a 180 degree turn on the board), kickflips (in which the board is flipped vertically into the air from the ground), walking the dog (a series of endovers performed continuously), and boneless (a method of taking off and landing on the board while it is in the air).

- Downhill skateboarding, as the name makes clear, downhill skateboarding is a form of the sport in which riders travel down hills, essentially to experience the thrill of a very fast race, often at speeds as great as 60 miles per hour.

- Slalom skateboarding is similar to slalom skiing. Racers travel downhill following a course laid out by cones around which they must move without displacing the cones. Five types of slalom skateboarding exist; they differ from each other in the length of the course and the spacing of the cones. In competitions, two racers may compete simultaneously against each other, or racers may complete the course one at a time, with each racer's time determining his or her final position in the contest. Slalom skateboarding is one of the most

highly organized forms of skateboarding with its own governing body, International Skateboard Slalom Racing, headquartered in Stockholm, Sweden.

- Freestyle skateboarding is regarded by some riders as the purest form of the sport, in which a rider uses only a board and a smooth surface on which to work. This variation of the sport is probably the most artistic form practiced, with connections to dance and gymnastics. The sport was popular in the early days of skateboarding, and then went into decline until the beginning of the twenty first century, at which point it experienced resurgence in popularity. In 2000, three Swedes, Daniel Gesmer, Bob Staton, and Stefan Åkesson founded the World Freestyle Skateboarding Association (WFSA) to ensure that there would always be competitions for men and women interested in the sport. The WFSA continues to exist today and to sponsor annual championships in the event. Its headquarters are in Stockholm, Sweden.

- Vert skateboarding, as described above, is practice in an oversized half-pipe in specially built facilities. The tricks that can be performed in the sport are so astounding and exciting that they have become a popular part of the ESPN X Games (along with other forms of skateboarding) aired annually on that television network.

Preparation

Sports medicine specialists generally recommend that a person who participates in any sport adopt some time of training and conditional program that will improve their strength, agility, endurance, balance, and other physical characteristics. In general, skateboard enthusiasts appear to have relatively little interest in these general training programs and tend to focus on increasing their skill levels in maneuvers that are specifically related to their sport, such as flips, aerials, grinds, and slides.

Equipment

Skateboarding requires a rather modest amount of equipment, most important of which is the skateboard itself. Experts recommend that a rider purchase the best board financially possible in order to provide the most useful and safest tool for the sport. In addition to the board, other essential equipment is a helmet, knee pads, elbow pads, and suitable shoes for the board. Experts recommend that the helmet, the most important piece of safety equipment, sit low on the forehead, have V-shaped side straps to protect the ears, has a buckle that makes the helmet fit tightly on the head, has installable pads that make the helmet fit tightly on the head, and that neither interferes with your movement while skateboarding nor moves about during the activity.

Training and conditioning

As mentioned above, most skateboarders appear to feel that their training and conditioning time is best spent on practicing the maneuvers required to carry out the variety of tricks they intend to demonstrate while doing their sport.

Risks

Studies on the incidence and nature of skateboard injuries have been sparse over the last decade. In 1998, research found that the rate of injuries among skateboarders was 8.9 per thousand participants, twice as great as it was for **inline skating** and half as great as it was for **basketball**. After declining from 1987 to 1993, the injury rate for the sport began to increase again and reached its highest level in the year of the study. The most common type of injury was ankle strain/sprain or wrist **fracture** (1.2 cases per 1,000 and 0.6 per 1,000, respectively). The most recent study on skateboarding injury was reported in 2010 and covered 100 skateboarders in Vienna. The study found that 97 percent of all respondents reported some type of injury from the sport, the most common of which affected the lower leg, ankle, or foot (32 percent of all injuries), followed by the forearm, wrist, or hand (16 percent). An interesting discovery was that only 13 percent of respondents reported using any type of protective gear. Another interesting finding from a number of surveys of skateboard injuries is that more than half resulted from uneven surfaces on which the sport was being conducted.

Results

Overall, it seems reasonable to conclude that skateboarding is a potentially risky sport that can be made safer by selecting a properly maintained practice surface and by wearing adequate protective equipment.

Resources

BOOKS

Louison, Cole. *The Impossible: Rodney Mullen, Ryan Sheckler, and the Fantastic History of Skateboarding.* Guilford, CT: Lyons Press, 2011.

Marcus, Ben, and Lucia Daniella Griggi. *The Skateboard: The Good, the Rad, and the Gnarly: An Illustrated History.* Minneapolis, MN: MVP Books, 2011.

Powell, Ben. *Skateboarding Skills: The Rider's Guide.* Richmond Hill, ON: Firefly Books, 2008.

Stutt, Ryan. *The Skateboarding Field Manual.* Richmond Hill, ON: Firefly Books, 2009.

Welinder, Per, and Peter Whitley. *Mastering Skateboarding.* Champaign, IL: Human Kinetics, 2012.

WEBSITES

Skateboard Science. Exploratorium. http://www.exploratorium.edu/skateboarding/ (accessed September 3, 2011).

SkateboardCity.com. http://www.skateboard-city.com/ (accessed September 3, 2011).

Slalom! International Skateboard Slalom Racing. http://www.slalomskateboarder.com/ (accessed September 3, 2011).

ORGANIZATIONS

International Association of Skateboard Companies, 22431 Antonio Pkwy, Suite B160-412, Rancho Santa Margarita, CA, 92688, 1 (949) 455-1112, Fax: 1 (949) 455-1712, http://skateboardiasc.org/contact/, http://www.skateboardiasc.org/.

International Skateboard Slalom Association, http://www.slalomskateboarder.com/.

Skate Park Association of the United States of America, 2118 Wilshire Blvd., #622, Santa Monica, CA, 90403, 1 (310) 495-7112, http://www.spausa.org/contact-us.php, http://www.spausa.org/.

David E. Newton, AB, MA, EdD

Skeletal system

Definition

The skeletal system is a living, dynamic, bony framework of the body, with networks of infiltrating blood vessels.

Description

Inside every person is a skeleton, a sturdy framework of about 206 bones that protects the body's organs, supports the body, provides attachment points for muscles to enable body movement, functions as a storage site for minerals such as calcium and phosphorus, and produces blood cells. Living mature bone is about 60% calcium compounds and about 40% collagen. Hence, bone is strong, hard, and slightly elastic. Humans are born with over 300 bones but some bones, such as those in the skull and lower spine, fuse during growth, thereby reducing the number. Although mature bones consist largely of calcium—70% calcium salts and about 30% organic matrix, mostly collagen

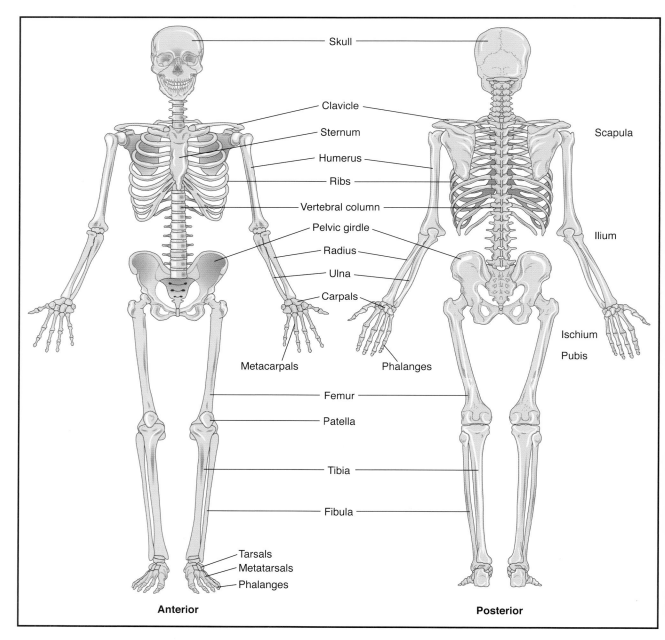

The skeletal system. (*Electronic Illustrators Group. © 2012 Cengage Learning.*)

fibers—most bones in the skeleton of vertebrates, including humans, began as cartilage. Cartilage is a type of connective tissue, and contains collagen and elastin fibers. The hard outer part of bones are comprised mostly of a proteins such as collagen, in addition to a substance called hydroxyapatite. This substance is composed primarily of calcium and other minerals, and stores much of the body's calcium; it is primarily responsible for the strength of bones. At the center of each bone is the marrow that is softer and less dense than the rest of the bone. The marrow contains specialized cells that produce blood cells that run through a bone, with nerves surrounding it.

Individual bones meet at areas called joints and are held in place by connective tissue. Most joints, such as the elbow, are called synovial joints, for the synovial membrane that envelopes the joint and secretes a lubricating fluid. Cartilage lines the surface of many joints and helps reduce friction between bones. The connective tissues linking the skeleton together at the joints are tendons and ligaments. Ligaments and tendons are both made up of collagen, but serve different functions. Ligaments link bones together and help prevent dislocated joints. Tendons link bone to muscle.

Because the bones making up the human skeleton are inside the body, the skeleton is called an endoskeleton. Some animals, such as the crab, have an external skeleton called an exoskeleton.

Types of bone

Bones may be classified according to their various traits, such as shape, origin, and texture. Four types are recognized based on shape. These are long bones, short bones, flat bones, and irregular bones. Long bones have a long central shaft, called the diaphysis, and two knobby ends, called the epiphysis. In growing long bones, the diaphysis and epiphysis are separated by a thin sheet of cartilage. Examples of long bones include bones of the arms and legs, the metacarpals of the hand, metatarsals of the foot, and the clavicle. Short bones are about as long as wide. The patella, carpels of the wrist, and tarsals of the ankle are short bones. Flat bones take several shapes, but are characterized by being relatively thin and flat. Examples include the sternum, ribs, hip bones, scapula, and cranial bones. Irregular bones are the odd-shaped bones of the skull, such as the sphenoid, the sacrum, and the vertebrae. The common characteristic of irregular bones is not that they are similar to each other in appearance, but that they cannot be placed in any of the other bone categories.

Bones may also be classified based on their origin. All bone (as well as muscles and connective tissue) originates from an embryonic connective tissue called mesenchyme, which makes mesoderm, also an embryonic tissue. Some mesoderm forms the cartilaginous skeleton of the fetus, the precursor for the bony skeleton. However, some bones, such as the clavicle and some of the facial and cranial bones of the skull, develop directly from mesenchyme, thereby bypassing the cartilaginous stage. These types of bone are called membrane bone (or dermal bone). Bone that originates from cartilage is called endochondral bone.

Finally, bones are classified based on texture. Smooth, hard bone called compact bone forms the outer layer of bones. Inside the outer compact bone is cancellous bone, sometimes called the bone marrow. Cancellous bone appears open and spongy, but is actually very strong, like compact bone. Together, the two types of bone produce a light, but strong, skeleton.

Structure

The human skeletal system is divided into two main groups: the axial skeleton and the appendicular skeleton. The axial skeleton includes bones associated with the body's main axis including:

- the skull
- the spine or vertebral column
- the ribs

The appendicular skeleton consists of the bones that anchor the body's appendages to the axial skeleton including:

- the pectoral girdle (shoulder area)
- the pelvic girdle (hip area)
- the upper extremities (arms)
- the lower extremities (legs)

AXIAL SKELETON. There are 28 bones in the skull. Of these, eight bones comprise the cranium and provide protection for the brain. In adults, these bones are flat and interlocking at their joints, making the cranium immobile. Fibrous joints, or sutures occur where the bony plates of the cranium meet and interlock. Cartilage-filled spaces between the cranial bones of infants, known as soft spots or fontanelles, allow their skull bones to move slightly during birth. This makes birth easier and helps prevent skull fractures, but may leave the infant with an odd-shaped head temporarily while the skull regains its shape. Eventually, the fontanelles in an infant's head are replaced by bone, and fibrous joints develop. In addition to protecting the brain, skull bones also support and protect the sensory organs responsible for sight, hearing, smell and taste.

The eight bones of the cranium are:

- frontal
- parietal (2)
- temporal (2)
- ethmoid
- sphenoid
- occipital

The frontal bone forms the forehead and eyebrows. Behind the frontal bone are the two parietal bones. Parietal bones form the roof of the cranium and curve down to form the sides of the cranium. Also forming the sides of the cranium are the two temporal bones, located behind the eyes. Each temporal bone encloses the cochlea and labyrinth of the inner ear, and the ossicles, three tiny bones of the middle ear that are not part of the cranium. The ossicles are the malleus (hammer), incus (anvil), and stapes (stirrups). The temporal bones also attach to the lower jaw, and this is the only moveable joint in the skull. Between the temporal bones is the irregular shaped sphenoid bone that provides protection for the pituitary gland. The small ethmoid bone forms part of the eye socket next to the nose. Olfactory nerves, or sense of smell nerves, pass through the ethmoid bone on their way to the brain. Forming the base and rear of the cranium is the occipital bone. The occipital bone has a hole, called the foramen magnum, through which the spinal cord passes and connects to the brain.

Fourteen bones shape the cheeks, eyes, nose, and mouth. These include:

- the nasal (2)
- zygomatic (2)
- maxillae (2)
- mandible

The upper, bony bridge of the nose is formed by the nasal bones and provides an attachment site for the cartilage making up the softer part of the nose. The zygomatic bones form the cheeks and part of the eye sockets. Two bones fuse to form the maxillae, the upper jaw of the mouth. These bones also form the hard palate of the mouth. The mandible forms the lower jaw of the mouth and is moveable, enabling chewing of food and speech. The mandible is the bone that connects to the temporal bones.

Located behind these facial bones are other bones that shape the interior portions of the eyes, nose, and mouth. These include:

- lacrimal (2)
- palatine (2)
- conchae (2)
- vomer bones

In addition to these 28 skull bones is the hyoid bone, located at the base of the tongue. Technically, the hyoid bone is not part of the skull but it is often included with the skull bones. It provides an attachment site for the tongue and some neck muscles.

Several of the facial and cranial bones contain sinuses, or cavities, that connect to the nasal cavity and drain into it. These are the frontal, ethmoid, sphenoid, and maxillae bones, all located near the nose. Painful sinus headaches result from the build up of pressure in these cavities. Membranes that line these cavities may secrete mucus or become infected, causing additional aggravation for humans.

The skull rests atop of the spine, which encases and protects the spinal cord. The spine, also called the vertebral column or backbone, consists of 33 stacked vertebrae, the lower ones fused. Vertebra are flat with two main features. The main oval shaped, bony mass of the vertebra is called the centrum. From the centrum arises a bony ring called the neural arch that forms the neural canal (also called a vertebral foramen), a hole for the spinal cord to pass through. Short, bony projections (neural spines) arise from the neural arch and provide attachment points for muscles. Some of these projections (called transverse processes) also provide attachment points for the ribs. There are also small openings in the neural arch for the spinal nerves that extend from the spinal cord throughout the body. Injury to the column of vertebrae may cause serious damage to the spinal cord and the spinal nerves, and could result in paralysis if the spinal cord or nerves are severed.

There are seven cervical, or neck, vertebrae. The first one, the atlas, supports the skull and allows the head to nod up and down. The atlas forms a condylar joint (a type of synovial joint) with the occipital bone of the skull. The second vertebra, the axis, allows the head to rotate from side to side. This rotating synovial joint is called a pivot joint. Together, these two vertebrae make possible a wide range of head motions.

Below the cervical vertebrae are the 12 thoracic, or upper back, vertebrae. The ribs are attached to these vertebrae. Thoracic vertebrae are followed by five lumbar, or lower back, vertebrae. Last is the sacrum, composed of five fused vertebrae, and the coccyx, or tail bone, composed of four fused bones.

The vertebral column helps to support the weight of the body and protects the spinal cord. Cartilaginous joints rather than synovial joints occur in the spine. Disks of cartilage lie between the bony vertebrae of the back and provide cushioning, like shock absorbers.

The vertebrae of the spine are capable of only limited movement, such bending and some twisting.

A pair of ribs extends forward from each of the 12 thoracic vertebrae, for a total of 24 ribs. Occasionally, a person is born with an extra set of ribs. The joint between the ribs and vertebrae is a gliding (or plane) joint, a type of synovial joint, as ribs do move, expanding and contracting with breathing. Most of the ribs (the first seven pair) attach in the front of the body via cartilage to the long, flat breastbone, or sternum. These ribs are called true ribs. The next three pair of ribs are false ribs. False ribs attach to another rib in front instead of the sternum, and are connected by cartilage. The lower two pair of ribs that do not attach anteriorly are called floating ribs. Ribs give shape to the chest and support and protect the body's major organs, such as the heart and lungs. The rib cage also provides attachment points for connective tissue, to help hold organs in place. In adult humans, the sternum also produces red blood cells as well as providing an attachment site for ribs.

APPENDICULAR SKELETON. The appendicular skeleton joins with the axial skeleton at the shoulders and hips. Forming a loose attachment with the sternum is the pectoral girdle, or shoulder. Two bones, the clavicle (collar bone) and scapula (shoulder blade), form one shoulder. The scapula rests on top of the ribs in the back of the body. It connects to the clavicle, the bone that attaches the entire shoulder structure to the skeleton at the sternum. The clavicle is a slender bone that is easily broken. Because the scapula is so loosely attached, it is easily dislocated from the clavicle, hence the dislocated shoulder injuries commonly suffered by persons playing sports. The major advantage to the loose attachment of the pectoral girdle is that it allows for a wide range of shoulder motions and greater overall freedom of movement.

Unlike the pectoral girdle, the pelvic girdle, or hips, is strong and dense. Each hip, left and right, consists of three fused bones, the ilium, ischium, and pubic. Collectively, these three bones are known as the innominate bone.

The innominates fuse with the sacrum to form the pelvic girdle. Specifically, the iliums shape the hips and the two ischial bones support the body when a person sits. The two pubic bones meet anteriorly at a cartilaginous joint. The pelvic girdle is bowl-shaped, with an opening at the bottom. In a pregnant woman, this bony opening is a passageway through which her baby must pass during birth. To facilitate the baby's passage, the body secretes a hormone called relaxin that loosens the joint between the pubic bones. In addition, the pelvic girdle of women is generally wider than that of men. This also helps to facilitate birth, but is a slight impediment for **walking** and **running**. Hence, men, with their narrower hips, are better adapted for such activities. The pelvic girdle protects the lower abdominal organs, such as the intestines, and helps supports the weight of the body above it.

The arms and legs, the upper and lower appendages of the body, are very similar in form. Each attaches to the girdle, pectoral or pelvic, via a ball and socket joint, a special type of synovial joint. In the shoulder, the socket, called the glenoid cavity, is shallow. The shallowness of the glenoid cavity allows for great freedom of movement. The hip socket, or acetabulum, is larger and deeper. This deep socket, combined with the rigid and massive structure of the hips, give the legs much less mobility and flexibility than the arms.

The humerus, or upper arm bone, is the long bone between the elbow and the shoulder. It connects the arm to the pectoral girdle. In the leg the femur, or thigh bone, is the long bone between the knee and hip that connects the leg to the pelvic girdle. The humerus and femur are sturdy bones, especially the femur, which is a weight bearing bone. Since the arms and legs are jointed, the humerus and femur are connected to other bones at the end opposite the ball and socket joint. In the elbow, this second joint is a type of synovial joint called a hinge joint. Two types of synovial joints occur in the knee region, a condylar joint (like the condylar joint in the first vertebra) that connects the leg bones, and a plane, or gliding joint, between the patella (knee cap) and femur.

At the elbow the humerus attaches to a set of parallel bones, the ulna and radius, bones of the forearm. The radius is the bone below the thumb that rotates when the hand is turned over and back. The ulna and radius then attach to the carpel bones of the wrist. Eight small carpel bones make up the wrist and connect to the hand. The hand is made up of five long, slender metacarpal bones (the palms) and 14 phalanges of the hand (fingers and thumb). Some phalanges form joints with each other, giving the human hand great dexterity.

Similarly, in the leg, the femur forms a joint with the patella and with the fibula and tibia bones of the lower leg. The tibia, or shin bone, is larger than the fibula and forms the joint behind the patella with the femur. Like the femur, the tibia is also a weight bearing bone. At the ankle joint, the fibula and tibia connect to the tarsals of the upper foot. There are seven tarsals of the upper foot, forming the ankle and the heel. The tarsals in turn connect to five long, slender metatarsals of the lower foot. The metatarsals form the foot's arch and sole and connect to the phalanges of the feet (toes). The 14 foot phalanges are shorter and less agile than the hand phalanges. Several types of synovial joints occur in the hands and feet, including plane, ellipsoid and saddle. Plane joints occur between toe bones, allowing limited movement. Ellipsoid joints between the finger and palm bones give the fingers circular mobility, unlike the toes. The saddle joint at the base of the thumb helps make the hands the most important part of the body in terms of dexterity and manipulation. A saddle joint also occurs at the ankles.

Bone development and growth

Since most bone begins as cartilage, it must be converted to bone through a process called ossification. The key players in bone development are cartilage cells (chondrocytes), bone precursor cells (osteoprogenitor cells), bone deposition cells (osteoblasts), bone resorption cells (osteoclasts), and mature bone cells (osteocytes).

During ossification, blood vessels invade the cartilage and transport osteoprogenitor cells to a region called the center of ossification. At this site, the cartilage cells die, leaving behind small cavities. Osteoblast cells form from the progenitor cells and begin depositing bone tissue, spreading out from the center. Through this process, both the spongy textured cancellous bone and the smooth outer compact bone forms. Two types of bone marrow, red and yellow, occupy the spaces in cancellous bone. Red marrow produces red blood cells, while yellow marrow stores fat in addition to producing blood cells. Eventually, in compact bone, osteoblast cells become trapped in their bony cavities, called lacunae, and become osteocytes. Neighboring osteocytes form connections with each other and thus are able to transfer materials between cells. The osteocytes are part of a larger system called the Haversian system. These systems are like long tubes, squeezed tightly together in compact bone. Blood vessel, lymph vessels, and nerves run through the center of the tube, called the Haversian canal, and are surrounded by layers of bone, called lamellae, that house the osteocytes. Blood vessels are connected to each other by lateral canals called Volkmann's canals. Blood vessels are also found in spongy bone, without the Haversian system. A protective membrane called the periosteum surrounds all bones.

Bone development is a complex process, but it is only half the story. Bones must grow, and they do so via a process called remodeling. Remodeling involves resorption of existing bone inside the bone (enlarging the marrow cavities) and deposition of new bone on the exterior. The resorptive cells are the osteoclasts and osteoblast cells lay down the new bone material. As remodeling progresses in long bones, a new center of ossification develops, this one at the swollen ends of the bone, called the epiphysis. A thin layer of cartilage called the epiphyseal plate separates the epiphysis from the shaft and is the site of bone deposition. When growth is complete, this cartilage plate disappears, so that the only cartilage remaining is that which lines the joints, called hyaline cartilage. Remodeling does not end when growth ends. Osteocytes, responding to the body's need for calcium, resorb bone in adults to maintain a calcium balance.

Function

The skeletal system has several important functions:

- It provides shape and form to the body, while allowing for body movement.
- It supports and protects vital organs and muscles.
- It produces red blood cells for the body in the bone marrow. Each second, an average of 2.6 million red blood cells are to replace worn out blood cells and those destroyed by the liver.
- It stores minerals including calcium and phosphorus. When excess are present in the blood, the bones will store minerals. When the supply in the blood runs low, minerals will be withdrawn from the bones to replenish the blood supply.

Common diseases and conditions

Even though bones are very strong, they may be broken. Most fractures do heal. The healing process may be stymied if bones are not reset properly or if the injured person is the victim of malnutrition. Osteoprogenitor cells migrate to the site of the **fracture** and begin the process of making new bone (osteoblasts) and reabsorbing the injured bone (osteoclasts). With proper care, the fracture will fully heal, and in children, often without a trace.

The joint between the mandible and the temporal bones, called the temporomandibular joint, is the source of the painful condition known as temporomandibular joint dysfunction, or TMJ dysfunction. Sufferers of TMJ dysfunction experience a variety of symptoms including headaches, a sore jaw, and a snapping sensation when moving the jaw. There are several causes of the dysfunction. The cartilage disk between the bones may shift, or the connective tissue between the bones may be situated in a manner that causes misalignment of the jaw. Sometimes braces on the teeth can aggravate TMJ dysfunction. The condition may be corrected with **exercise**, or in severe cases, surgery. Another condition, cleft palate, is due to the failure of the maxillary bones in the jaw to completely fuse in the fetus.

Bones are affected by poor diet and are also subject to a number of diseases and disorders. Some examples include scurvy, rickets, **osteoporosis**, **arthritis**, and bone tumors. Scurvy results from the lack of vitamin C. In infants, scurvy causes poor bone development. It also causes membranes surrounding the bone to bleed, forming clots that are eventually ossified, and thin bones that break easy. In addition, adults are affected by bleeding gums and loss of teeth. Before modern times, sailors were often the victims of scurvy, due to extended periods of time at sea with limited food. They consequently tried to keep a good supply of citrus fruits, such as oranges and limes, on board because these fruits supply vitamin C. By the twenty-first century, scurvy had become extremely rare in Western societies.

Rickets is a children's disease resulting from a deficiency of vitamin D. This vitamin enables the body to absorb calcium and phosphorus; without it, bones become soft and weak and actually bend, or bow out, under the body's weight. Vitamin D is found in milk, eggs and liver, and may also be produced by exposing the skin to sunlight. Pregnant women can also suffer from a vitamin D deficiency, osteomalacia, resulting in soft bones. The elderly, especially women who had several children in succession, sometimes suffer from osteoporosis, a condition in which a significant amount of calcium from bones is dissolved into the blood to maintain the body's calcium balance. Weak, brittle bones dotted with pits and pores are the result. Osteoporosis occurs most often in older people and in women after menopause. It affects nearly half of all those, men and women, over the age of 75. Women, however, are five times more likely than men to develop the disease. They have smaller, thinner bones than men to begin with, and they lose bone mass more rapidly after menopause (usually around age 50), when they stop producing a bone-protecting hormone called estrogen. In the five to seven years following menopause, women can lose about 20% of their bone mass. By age 65 or 70, though, men and women lose bone mass at the same rate. As an increasing number of men reach an older age, they are becoming more aware that osteoporosis is an important health issue for them as well.

Arthritis is another condition commonly afflicting the elderly. This is an often painful inflammation of the joints. Arthritis is not restricted to the elderly, and even young people can suffer from this condition. There are several types of arthritis, such as rheumatoid, rheumatic, and degenerative. Arthritis basically involves the inflammation and deterioration of cartilage and bone at the joint surface. In some cases, bony protuberances around the rim of the joint may develop. Most people will probably develop arthritis if they live to a significant older age. Degenerative arthritis is the type that commonly occurs with age. The knee, hip, shoulder, and elbow are the major targets of degenerative arthritis. A number of different types of tumors, some harmless and others more serious, may also affect bones.

Effect of fitness and nutrition

Most individuals take for granted good mobility and alignment. Getting out of bed in the morning, getting into the shower, and moving through every-day routines are managed in part, by a strong and healthy skeletal system.

Building and maintaining bone is important for everyone. The skeletal system needs to be "well maintained" in order to keep it strong and mobile. Strength exercises help bone density to remain intact, while **stretching** exercises help develop flexibility for continued good range of motion throughout the body. Doing **yoga**, **Pilates**, or working with resistance bands are also good forms of exercise for the skeletal system.

A fitness program should include strength training to improve balance and **energy**, prevent or minimize bone loss, and to minimize weight gain (which in turn, minimizes strain on bones). An exercise routine should include not only aerobic and strength training, but a warm up period as well. Doing so will give muscle groups added flexibility for use during more intense activity, and will help prevent injury. Stretching after a workout is also needed to move muscles and bones through an increased range of motion and allow for tissues to **cool down** gradually.

The use of weights is especially important in strengthening the skeletal system. It is important to use weights in a progressive manner, increasing the amount of weight as well as the number of repetitions, gradually and with safety in mind. Overdoing or overzealous weight lifting can lead to muscle injury, stress fractures, and early **fatigue**. It is best to have a goal in mind and work slowly and methodically toward that goal. A professional trainer may be of help when putting together an exercise schedule and routine.

Due to the reduction in estrogen levels, older women and menopausal women are especially at risk

KEY TERMS

Bone—Composed primarily of a non-living matrix of calcium salts and a living matrix of collagen fibers, bone is the major component that makes up the human skeleton. Bone produces blood cells and functions as a storage site for elements such as calcium and phosphorus.

Calcium—A naturally occurring element that primarily combines with phosphate to form the non-living matrix of bones.

Cartilage—A type of connective tissue that takes three forms: elastic cartilage, fibrocartilage, and hyaline cartilage. Hyaline cartilage forms the embryonic skeleton and lines the joints of bones.

Haversian system—Tubular systems in compact bone with a central Haversian canal that houses blood and lymph vessels surrounded by circular layers of calcium salts and collagen, called lamellae, in which reside osteocytes.

Marrow—A type of connective tissue that fills the spaces of most cancellous bone. It produces blood cells and stores fat.

Ossification—The process of replacing connective tissue such as cartilage and mesenchyme with bone.

Osteoblast—The bone cell that deposits calcium salts and collagen during bone growth, bone remodeling, and bone repair.

Osteoclast—The bone cell responsible for reabsorbing bone tissue in bone remodeling and repair.

Osteocyte—Mature bone cell whose main function is to regulate the levels of calcium and phosphate in the body.

Skeleton—Consists of bones and cartilage that are linked together by ligaments. The skeleton protects vital organs of the body and enables body movement.

Synovial joint—One of three types of joints in the skeleton and by far the most common. Synovial joints are lined with a membrane that secretes a lubricating fluid. Includes ball and socket, pivot, plane, hinge, saddle, condylar, and ellipsoid joints.

Vertebrates—Includes all animals with a vertebral column protecting the spinal cord such as humans, dogs, birds, lizards, and fish.

for osteoporosis so they should include strength training exercises in their fitness routine. Light weights will help add lean muscle (not bulk) and keep bones strong, reducing the chance for osteoporosis.

Some exercises and physical activities that enhance the skeletal system include:

- aerobics
- bicycling
- moderate or brisk walking
- rowing
- swimming
- water exercise

These exercises also promote cardiovascular fitness, including improved heart function and increased heart, lung, and muscle endurance.

In addition to good **bone health**, a balanced, systematic, and routine workout offers individuals numerous fitness benefits, as exercise helps to:

- Stimulate movement in the gastrointestinal tract to prevent constipation.
- Expand and oxygenate your lungs.
- Move blood throughout the circulatory system.
- Stimulate the lymphatic system.
- Relax and contract muscles throughout the entire body, increasing muscle tone and skin turgor.
- Promote and maintain good range of motion of the limbs.
- Accelerate a release of endorphins, improving mood, energy, and libido.
- Burn calories and aids in the reduction of body fat and, in turn, helps in weight control.
- Enhance heart health (especially aerobic exercise), aiding in the prevention of high cholesterol and high blood pressure. While cholesterol levels can be lowered by reducing weight and eating less saturated fatty foods, a key ingredient in a cholesterol lowering program is a regular and systematic physical training program.
- Maintain a healthy weight, avoiding propensity toward insulin resistance, diabetes, and resulting complications of diabetes.
- Give you more energy. Although you may feel tired after a good workout, you will have more energy in the long run.
- Make you feel good about yourself by taking charge of your weight, health, and well being.
- Reduce stress and aid in achieving a more restful night of sleep.
- Strengthen bones to help prevent osteoporosis.
- Stimulate white blood cell movement (especially brisk physical activity), making the immune system strong.

- Make you more aware of the food you eat— especially after having done a robust workout, potentiating a desire to make healthy food choices.

- Make you feel satisfied and rewarded about being disciplined in your choice to take time and take action, to be good to yourself, especially when achieving predetermined fitness goals along the way.

Bone strength is sustained not only through participation in a fitness program, but by good nutritional health as well. Vitamins, minerals and other nutrients help keep bones healthy. Calcium, potassium, phosphorus, magnesium, manganese, copper, zinc, and iron all contribute to good bone health. **Protein** provides amino acids, which are important for the build and development of bone growth. Vitamin D (found in fortified milk and fatty fish such as salmon and herring) promotes good bone health indirectly, by regulating calcium in the bloodstream, while boron helps maintain optimal levels of calcium throughout the body. Vitamin C (found in citrus fruits, strawberries and many green vegetables) helps stimulate enzymes responsible for cells that build bones. Vitamin K (found in leafy green vegetables) helps maintain bone density and strength.

With a decline in hormone production, the incidence of bone fracture is of concern as we grow older (especially for women, who have two to three times as many bone fractures as men) so for this reason, care must be taken to practice good nutritional habits to aid in skeletal structure and support, as well.

The American Heart Association recommends 30 minutes of exercise five times a week in conjunction with a heart healthy diet regimen. Remember to read food labels to examine not only calorie, fat, carbohydrate, and protein content, but also to determine serving size in relation to these numbers. Dieticians may be of assistance in understanding these food labels.

Making good nutritional choices and developing a healthy exercise regimen is beneficial to the skeletal system and the entire body as a whole. A strong and healthy skeletal system will support your wellness efforts. A well balanced fitness and nutrition regimen can improve not only the way you look and feel, but also have a positive impact on the health and quality of your life.

Resources

BOOKS

Bassey, Joan. *Strong Bones for Life.* London: Carroll & Brown, 2011.

Harper, Bob. *Are You Ready! Take Charge, Lose Weight, Get in Shape, and Change Your Life Forever.* New York: Broadway Books, 2009.

Kohlstadt, Ingrid. *Food and Nutrients in Disease Management.* Boca Raton, FL: CRC Press, 2009.

Manocchia, Pat. *Anatomy of Exercise: A Trainer's Inside Guide to Your Workout.* Richmond Hill, ONT: Firefly Books, 2009.

McDowell, Julie., ed. *Encyclopedia of Human Body Systems.* Santa Barbara, CA: Greenwood, 2010.

Plant, Jane., and Gill Tidey. *Eating for Better Health.* New York, NY: Virgin Books, 2010.

Reiner, Barti., and Bertha Frisch. *The Skeleton in Medicine,* 3rd ed. New York, NY: Springer, 2012.

Rizzo, Donald C. *Introduction to Anatomy and Physiology.* Clifton Park, NY: Delmar, 2011.

Schneider, Diane L, MD. *The Complete Book of Bone Health.* Amherst, NY: Prometheus Books, 2011.

Shils, Maurice E. *Modern Nutrition in Health and Disease,* 11th ed. New York, NY: Lippincott Williams & Wilkins, 2012.

PERIODICALS

Boskey, Adele L. "Musculoskeletal Disorders and Orthopedic Conditions" *Journal of the American Medical Association* 285 (2001): 619–623. http://jama.ama-assn.org/issues/v285n5/ffull/jsc00335.html.

Feder, G. et al. "Guidelines for the prevention of falls in people over 65." *British Medical Journal* 321 (2000): 1007–1011.

McClung, Michael R. et al. "Effect of Risedronate on the Risk of Hip Fracture in Elderly Women." *The New England Journal of Medicine* 344, no. 5 (2001): 333–40.

ORGANIZATIONS

Arthritis Foundation. 1330 W. Peachtree St., PO Box 7669, Atlanta, GA 30357-0669. (800) 283-7800. http://www.arthritis.org.

American Medical Association. 515 N. State Street, Chicago, IL 60654. Telephone: (800) 621-8335. http://www.ama-assn.org

National Center for Complementary and Alternative Medicine (NCCAM). 9000 Rockville Pike, Bethesda, MD, 20892. (888) 644-6226. http://nccam.nih.gov.

National Institutes of Health Osteoporosis and Related Bone Diseases-National Resource Center. 2 AMS Circle Bethesda, MD 20892-3676. (800) 624-BONE (2663). http://www.osteo.org.

National Osteoporosis Foundation. 1150 17th Street, Suite 500 NW, Washington, DC 20036-4603. (800) 223-9994. http://www.nof.org.

Crystal Heather Kaczkowski, MSc
Laura Jean Cataldo, RN, EdD

Skiing *see* **Winter sports**

Sling training

Definition

Sling training, also called sling fitness training and bodyweight suspension training, is a particular type of **exercise** program that uses the weight of the person exercising and the resistance of gravity, along with suspension equipment, to help develop balance, flexibility, joint stability, and strength in its users.

One of the websites touting the benefits of sling training is SuspensionExercise.com. Its home webpage states, "Suspension training is about harnessing your own body weight against gravity and performing suspended exercises to maximise strength development, stability, endurance and sculpt the body. This form of training is revolutionising workouts throughout the world as more people discover just how effective it is, and is being adopted by professional athletes and top trainers alike."

Purpose

The purpose of sling training is to exercise the entire body with the use of suspension devices in order to develop simultaneously better balance and coordination, flexibility and movability, joint stability, and strength. In addition, because this type of exercise program is so effective at improving the fitness of the participant, sling training also provides this improvement in many different types of exercises and intensity levels.

Demographics

Sling training can be performed by people of any **age** group and of any degree of fitness level. It is normally used as a compliment to traditional training programs.

Description

The program called sling training involves using the weight of the exerciser (that is as resistance to gravity) to perform all of the exercises. All that is needed is a device called a suspension trainer and a stable structure to attach the suspension trainer to, such as a door. A suspension trainer consists of resistance equipment. The basic equipment used for sling training consists of two handles, with lengths of adjustable webbing that can be fixed to a stationary object such as a wall, door, beam, bar, or any other stable structure. The handles are molded to be foot cradles or hand grips. Various exercises are possible under this method. The angle of inclination can be easily changed within each exercise, along with the intensity level.

The training consists of using one's own body weight and gravity to develop strength, balance, flexibility, and joint mobility—all at the same time. Individuals can customize the training to fit their own needs of difficulty and intensity. To do this, only the body position or angle at which the exercise is performed need be adjusted.

Because all sling training exercises involve a "suspended state" rather than positions found in traditional weight training equipment, the core muscles of the body (those within the trunk [torso]) are developed more fully. This is so because the body must work extra hard to stabilize its movements against the force of gravity while performing the exercises.

Some of the benefits of sling training are:

- total body strength workout
- superior core conditioning
- much better workout than balls, bands, and weight machines
- hundreds of exercises to choose, from beginning to expert levels
- easy to use for all fitness levels
- easy setup and easy to carry around
- helps to build functional strength for all types of sports
- increases balance for all levels of expertise

KEY TERMS

Biceps—Muscles in the upper arm, also called biceps brachii.

Calisthenics—Physical exercises that improve fitness and muscle tone, such as situps, pushups, and jumping jacks.

Cardiovascular—Relating to the heart and blood vessels.

Deltoids—Thick, triangular muscle that covers the shoulder joint.

Gluteals—Any of three muscles that form the buttocks in humans.

Gravity—The attraction due to the gravitational pull of the Earth to another body with mass.

Hamstrings—One of three muscles located on the back of the thigh that control leg movements.

Latissimus dorsi—Broad, triangular shaped muscles along the sides of the back.

Pectorals—Any of four flat muscles, positioned two on each side of the front of the chest, that help to move the upper arm and shoulder.

Quadriceps—A large muscle group at the front of the thigh that extends the leg.

Strength training—The use of resistance to muscular contraction to improve anaerobic endurance, muscle size, and overall body strength.

Triceps—Large muscle along the back of the upper arm that straightens the elbow.

Hundreds of sling training exercises are possible. The following are some of the more common ones used (along with their benefits, what muscles are primarily exercised, and the difficulty level):

- Back Row: builds strength and conditioning for the upper body, especially the middle and upper back; benefits the latissimus dorsi, posterior deltoids, biceps; beginner level of difficulty

- Balance Lunge: promotes good overall strength in the legs, one leg at a time, along with better coordination, stability, and balance; benefits the quadriceps, hamstrings, and gluteals; intermediate level of difficulty

- Bicep Curl: tones and shapes the biceps muscles with the use of curl movement, along with increasing overall body stability; benefits the biceps; beginner level of difficulty

- Chest Press: builds strength in the upper body, especially shoulder stability, while improving the core muscles; benefits the pectorals, triceps; intermediate level of difficulty

- Hamstring Curl: strengthens the hamstring muscles, along with overall strength, power, and balance of the legs; benefits the hamstrings; intermediate level of difficulty

- Hip Abduction: strengthens the lower back, increases stability and strength in the hips and back; benefits the gluteals (gluteus medius and gluteus minimus); beginner level of difficulty

- Oblique Leg Raise: builds strong, defined midsection dds to core muscle stability, and increases rotational strength and control; benefits traverse abdominal muscles and internal and external oblique muscles; intermediate level of difficulty

- Single Leg Squat: improves the entire lower body, especially adds strength, power, and stability to the hip extensor; benefits the quadriceps, hamstrings, and gluteals; intermediate level of difficulty

Preparation

Beginners to sling training should initially start with shorter workout times and longer rest periods in between each exercise. Make sure that the technique of each exercise is being performed properly. Be familiar with each exercise to make sure one is doing them correctly. As fitness levels increase, slowly increase the workout times and decrease the resting periods between exercises. Add more advances exercises into the workout program as one feels more comfortable with them. At the same time, increase resistance levels or increase the intensity of the workout as one's fitness levels increase.

Warming up is important because it helps to prepare the muscles before they are asked to do more strenuous work. A warm up period may consist of about five to ten minutes of light jogging, **walking**, or simple **calisthenics** like **jumping rope**. Let the body get accustomed to exercising. Do not overdo it at the beginning. Doing stretches are also recommended during the **warm-up** routine. However, do not stretch right at the start because one may pull a muscle.

Once sling training is completed, it is a good idea to spend about five minutes cooling down. Lightly jogging or walking helps the body to settle back down to its normal routine. More **stretching** exercises are also helpful.

Risks

There are always risk of injury while exercising in its various forms. However, these risks can be kept to a minimum by warming up before exercising and cooling down after finishing sling training. More importantly, the risks of not staying fit include becoming overweight or obese (excessively overweight), increasing one's risk for coronary heart disease, and an overall weakening of bones and muscles. To prevent this from happening, sling training is a good way to exercise all of the major muscle groups, stay fit, and reduce the risk of health problems.

For instance, the U.S. Department of Health and Human Services (HHS) recommends that healthy adults include aerobic exercise and strength training in their weekly fitness plans. The HHS states that these people perform at least 150 minutes of moderate aerobic exercise (or 75 minutes of vigorous aerobic activity) each week. In addition, the HHS states that strength training should be performed at least twice a week. Sling training is included within this strength training program.

Results

By doing sling training, athletes and other sports-minded individuals get stronger muscles, bones, and joints; become more physically fit; improve the **cardiovascular system** including the heart; reduce body fat; become more healthy, and improve flexibility, balance, and coordination.

Resources

BOOKS

Cook, Gregg, and Fatima d'Almeida-Cook. *The Gym Survival Guide: Your Road Map to Fearless Fitness.* New York: Sterling, 2008.

Plowman, Sharon A., and Denise L. Smith. *Exercise Physiology for Health, Fitness, and Performance.* Philadelphia: Wolters Kluwer Health/Lippincott Williams & Wilkins, 2011.

Schoenfeld, Brad. *Women's Home Workout Bible.* Champaign, IL: Human Kinetics, 2010.

Sutton, Amy L, editor. *Fitness and Exercise Sourcebook.* Detroit: Omnigraphics, 2007.

WEBSITES

Suspension Training. SuspensionExercise.com. http://suspensionexercise.com/index.php?page=Home (accessed September 28, 2011).

What is Bodyweight Suspension Training or Sling Fitness Training? Sling-Fitness.com. http://www.sling-fitness.com/what-ist-sling-training-about/bodyweight-suspension-fitness-training.html (accessed September 28, 2011).

ORGANIZATIONS

American Alliance for Health, Physical Education, Recreation and Dance, 1900 Association Drive, Reston, VA, 20191-1598, (703) 476-3400, (800) 213-7193, http://www.aahperd.org/.

American Council on Exercise, 4851 Paramount Drive, San Diego, CA, 92123, (888) 825-3636, support@acefitness.org, http://www.fitness.gov/.

National Coalition for Promoting Physical Activity, 1100 H Street, N.W., Suite 510, Washington, DC, 20005, (202) 454-7521, Fax: (202) 454-7598, http://www.ncppa.org/membership/organizations/.

National Strength and Conditioning Association, 1885 Bob Johnson Drive, Colorado Springs, CO, 80906, (719) 632-6722, Fax: (719) 632-6367, (800) 815-6826, http://www.nsca-lift.org/.

President's Council on Fitness, Sports and Nutrition, 1101 Wootton Parkway, Suite 560, Rockville, MD, 20852, (240) 276-9567, Fax: (240) 276-9860, http://www.fitness.gov/.

William A. Atkins, BB, BS, MBA

Snowboarding

Definition

Snowboarding is a winter sport that involves a rider going down a snowy or icy hill on a wide board in a position that resembles a surfer or skateboarder.

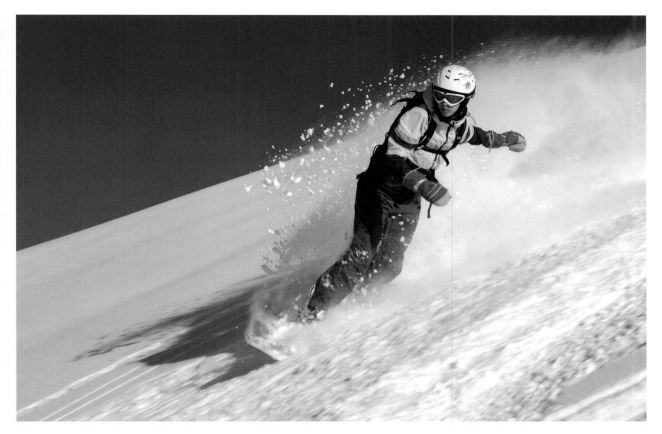

A snowboarder moves gracefully down a slope. *(© iStockPhoto.com/Konstantin Shishkin)*

Purpose

Most people ride snowboards for enjoyment. The sport is an alternative to skiing, often appealing to younger people who also love to skateboard or surf, but snowboard in the winter months. In alpine snowboarding, the purpose is to get down the hill using controlled turns. In competitive snowboarding, this may include controlled jumps and speed. Half-pipe and slopestyle involve airborne tricks, such as flips and twists, reaching down to grab the board, and combinations of these tricks. Contestants are judged on their technique, speed, and how high in the air they go.

Demographics

Participation in snowboarding increased more than 300 percent from 1998 to about 2010, to more than 6 million people in the United States. At the same time, fewer people were skiing. Part of the reason was the action involved in snowboarding, and part was that it costs less to get started in snowboarding

than in skiing. More men than women ride snowboards. In 2010, about 33% of people who rode snowboards were women. Snowboarders tend to be younger than skiers (averaging in the early 20s), and many ski and snowboard schools offer programs for children as young as three to five years old to begin learning The sport.

History

Snowboarding is a young sport compared with other **winter sports**. In 1965, an engineer named Sherman Poppen from Michigan bolted two skis side by side to make a toy for his daughter. He placed steel tracks on top to hold the rider's feet in place and added a rope for steering. His wife called the new board the "Snurfer" for its combination of snow and surfer, and the name stuck. Other inventors began working on similar designs soon after. An East Coast surfer named Dimitrije Milovich made snowboards based more on surfboards, but with metal edges, around 1970. A few years later, Bob

TOM SIMS (1950–)

Tom Sims is known as the creator of the snowboard. Sims grew up loving the sport of skateboarding. He built his own skateboards and he always preferred long boards, because they simulated surfboarding, which was another love of his. When the Sims family moved from California to New Jersey, Tom was frustrated that he was no longer able to skateboard during the harsh winter months. At the age of twelve, he built his first "Skiboard" out of wood. The following week, he made a bigger board and added aluminum to the bottom. That board can be found at the Colorado Ski Museum.

Sims quickly became known for his incredible carving ability, as well as his intensity and passion for the sport. He worked collaboratively with skateboarders and developed high-quality boards and bindings, and this research and development led to the creation of Sims Snowboards.

Webber tried to obtain a patent for a design he called a "skiboard." As these early pioneers continue to refine their designs, Milovich started production and his design was featured in a national magazine in 1975. The boards began to catch on around the world.

In 1979, Paul Graves put on a freestyle boarding demonstration at the annual Snurfer contest in Michigan by performing complete turns, dropping down to one knee while riding, and dismounting the board with a flip. Jake Burton Carpenter had been modifying Snurfer designs and also wanted to demonstrate his board. After some protest, he was allowed to enter a one-man competition at the event. Graves rode his Snurfer on television later that year in a North American commercial and magazines began running features about snowboarding.

In the 1980s, the first modern competitive snowboard competitions were held, including the first World Snowboarding Championships. Board design continued to improve, making boards turn on edge instead of through sliding. By the 1986 to 1987 season, the first soft boot had been invented. The first manual for snowboard instructors was developed in the same year. By 1993, there were 50 manufacturers in the United States marketing snowboards. The first halfpipe was ridden in Lake Tahoe, California. A rivalry between skiers and snowboarders followed much of this development, with a few ski resorts refusing to open their slopes to snowboarders. Suicide Six Ski Resort in Vermont was the first ski resort to welcome snowboarders in 1982. Only a handful did not allow snowboarders by the mid-2000s. Snowboarding no is a Winter Olympic event, including the halfpipe. Shaun White, (the "Flying Tomato") helped launch the popularity of snowboarding and especially halfpipe events, at the 2006 Winter **Olympics** and won gold again in 2010. In 2011, it was announced that slopestyle also will be included in the 2014 games.

Description

The sport of snowboarding has gained popularity in recent years and now nearly outranks the winter sport of skiing. Snowboarding takes place at ski resorts and special terrain parks during winter months. The sport grew from a combination of **skateboarding**, skiing, and surfing. Instead of the two skis used in skiing, snowboard riders use a single board that they ride in a fashion that is similar to skateboarding or surfing. Around the world, snowboarders now share ski runs with skiers and enjoy riding on some slopes of their own, along with doing special tricks in terrain parks with bumps, a U-shaped trench that is called a halfpipe, and other ways to challenge freestyling riders. Snowboarders can learn on very small and gentle slopes in ski and snowboard school yards with group instruction or private lessons. They can advance to beginning, intermediate, and advanced runs as they gain ability and confidence.

Technique

Riding a snowboard is different from skiing. Skiers generally shift their balance over their feet from side to side to control ski edges for turning and weight changes on the skis. The snowboarder shifts his or her weight from heel to toe. The stance and technique are similar to surfing or skateboarding. Shifting weight forward tends to make the board go downhill and shifting weight over the heels, or digging the heels into the edge of the board, drags it into the snow to stop. A regular stance on the board places the left foot in front of the right, and the goofy stance has the right foot ahead of the left.

Styles

There are several styles in snowboarding. Free-riding or all-mountain riding mean the boarder rides on whatever natural terrain is available. This most often is a groomed ski run, but the boarder may opt for moguls or off-trail riding, or may perform some aerial maneuvers. Freestyle or slopestyle is performing tricks using manmade structures, such as rails or boxes. The halfpipe is a U-shaped trench with high walls that help the rider get airborne to perform tricks such as twists and flips above the walls. Boardercross is a competitive race that combines snowboarding with elements of motocross for a race against other riders instead of just the clock.

Rules

Rules for recreational snowboarding vary, depending on ski resort policy. Usually, resorts have policies about riding their ski lifts, accepting risk, and safety to others. Other rules are really etiquette, but should be followed by riders to keep them and others safe. For example, skiers and snowboarders must look out for people on a trail when merging and always are responsible for seeing anyone before them on a run (the skiers or riders in front have the right of way). Riders always should be in control and should use a security leash so that if they crash, their riderless boards do not go sliding down the hill and crash into someone. Riders should observe rules that are posted at resorts. Competition rules vary depending on the event.

Preparation

Getting started in recreational snowboarding does not take a lot of preparation. It is a physically demanding sport, however, and can cause serious injuries to riders and other people on ski slopes if the riders do not learn how to use their boards. Snowboarding instructors recommend three half-day lessons before a rider heads out on his or her own. These lessons help teach the rider how to control the board, how to stop, and how to enjoy snowboarding more. The lessons help lessen chances of falling.

Equipment

Boots, bindings, and boards can be purchased or rented. It is advised to rent these items until deciding which style of boarding is preferred. All boarders need waterproof pants, jackets, and gloves. Goggles also are essential, and safety experts recommend wearing a helmet to prevent head injury.

KEY TERMS

Gluteal—Relating to the buttocks muscles.

Mogul—A mogul is a term for the bumps on certain ski runs (paths) and for the type of freestyle skiing that skis over the bumps and often involves aerial or acrobatic tricks.

Quadriceps—Large muscle group that runs down the front of the thigh.

Training and conditioning

Snowboarding uses foot and core muscles extensively. U.S. Snowboarding member Kevin Pearce says he works to keep his core and legs strong to be able to blast out of the half-pipe and perform aerial maneuvers. Recreational boarders also want to keep their quadriceps and gluteal muscles strong by lifting weights or doing squats. Calf raises will keep calf muscles strong to help with foot stability. Practicing balance with summer sports or on a balance board can help with snowboard balance. While at ski slopes, riders need to remember that they may be exercising at much higher altitudes than normal and drink plenty of water and other clear fluids. Healthy breakfasts with plenty of **carbohydrates** and a healthy lunch in the middle of the day that is not too heavy can help keep performance up. Riders also might want to keep a light **energy** snack in their jackets.

Risks

There are about 600,000 skiing and snowboarding injuries every year in North America, and many of these occur in children. Up to 20% of these injuries are head injuries. In fact, about 50% to 88 % of all deaths from skiing and snowboarding are caused by traumatic brain injuries. Wearing a helmet can reduce chance of a head injury. Other common injuries to snowboarders are wrist and elbow injuries that occur when snowboarders stretch out their arms to catch themselves when falling. Riders also need to take caution when exercising at high altitudes and in extremely severe weather. Avalanches and sudden winter storms are possible dangers for extreme snowboarders who hike to backcountry areas or ride on unmarked trails.

Results

Rising a snowboard demands that people be able to move well on the board and be able to **exercise** for long

- Is there any preparation I need to do before taking up snowboarding?
- Do I have any injuries or conditions that would prevent me from snowboarding?
- How can I prevent snowboarding injuries?

periods of time. For these reasons, it is an excellent way to improve physical fitness, especially in the winter months. About 45 minutes of snowboarding burns more than 280 **calories**. It also is a sport that people love for being in touch with nature. It gives riders a chance to be close to trees, mountains, and sometimes wildlife in the winter months. Renting or buying boots and bindings that fit properly and getting lessons from certified instructors make snowboarding more enjoyable and safer.

Resources

PERIODICALS

Joffe, Alain. "Use a Helmet with Skis and Snowboards." *Journal Watch Pediatrics and Adolescent Medicine* (October 6, 2010).

Johnson, Noah. "Time line: a Lesson in the History of the Shred." *Men's Fitness* 22 (December 2006):56.

"Orthopaedic Surgeons Offer Safety Tips for Winter Sports. "*Health and Beauty Close-up* (December 23, 2010).

Palmer, Lisa. "So You Want to Snowboard? How to Prepare for Winter's Graceful, Playful, Powder-shredding Sport. "*Muscle and Fitness/Hers* 8 (January-February 2007):24.

Rushlow, Amy. "Burn Calories Like an Olympian." *Women's Health* 7 (March 2010):25.

"Winter Activities that Can Land You in ER."*UPI News Track* (February 25, 2011).

"Workouts for Skiers and Snowboarders."*USA Today* 139 (October 2010):10.

WEBSITES

Watson, Stephanie. "How Snowboarding Works." Howstuffworks.com. http://www.howstuffworks.com/outdoor-activities/snow-sports/snowboarding.htm (accessed September 13, 2011.)

ORGANIZATIONS

United States Ski and Snowboard Association, 1 Victory Lane, Park City, UT, U.S., 84060, (435) 649-9090, Fax: (435) 649-3613, http://www.ussa.org.

Teresa G. Odle, BA, ELS

Soccer

Definition

Soccer, also known as association **football** or simply football, is a sport played with a spherical-shaped ball by two opposing teams whose players' purpose is to drive a ball into the opposing team's goal as many times as possible. Football, called soccer, is different from the football, also called American football, played in the United States and in other countries.

Purpose

The primary purpose of soccer is to drive a ball into the opposing team's goal so that at the end of the game (match) the team with the most points wins the match. Soccer also helps one to stay in good physical shape and fitness.

Demographics

In the twenty-first century, soccer is considered to be the most popular organized sport played in the world. It is estimated that over 250 million soccer players participate in the game in over 200 countries.

History

Soccer as it is recognized in the twenty-first century evolved through the ages from games played by kicking a ball. The earliest known kicking game is documented in a Chinese military manual from around the second or third centuries B.C. The modern rules of soccer are founded on the various forms of football played in England as early as the eighth century, and organized formally by the English in the nineteenth century. The "Laws of the Game" for soccer were first developed in England by the Football Association in 1863. Over the years, the game of soccer evolved so that today it is governed internationally by the International Federation of Association Football (FIFA, in French stands for the Fédération Internationale de Football Association). The premiere event for soccer in the world is the FIFA World Cup, which is held once every four years.

Description

The field

Soccer is played on a rectangular field with measurements of 100–120 yd (91.4–109.7 m) in length and 60–80 yd (54.9–73.2 m) of width. The middle of the field lengthwise is divided in half by the midfield line. In the center of the field (centered at the half-way point

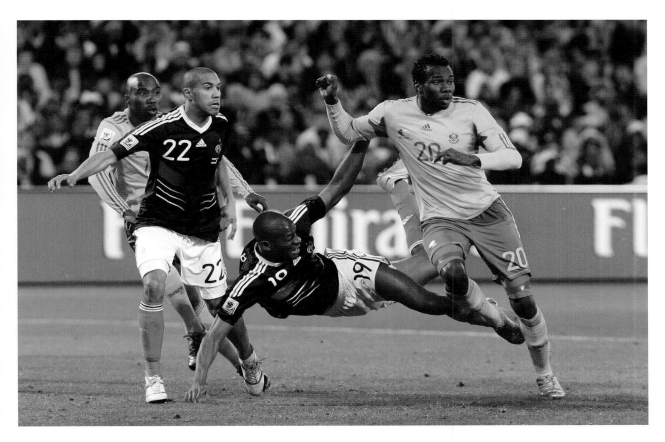

A match between France and South Africa during the 2010 FIFA World Cup in South Africa. *(© AP Images)*

of the midfield line) is a center circle, with a radius of 10 yd (9.1 m). This circle may not be entered into by defending players during the start of a kickoff. The field is composed of natural grass or artificial turf.

At the middle of the short dimension of the field is positioned the goals (between two posts, with a bar above and to the sides, and netting behind). A rectangular box, with outside dimensions of 44 yd (40.2 m) wide and 18 yd (16.5 m) deep and inside dimensions of 20 yd (18.3 m) wide and 6 yd (5.5 m) deep, is centered on the goal. It includes an arc that is 10 yd (9.1 m) from the penalty mark, which is inside the penalty area and 12 yd (11.0 m) from the end line. The rectangular box is the penalty area, and sometimes also called the penalty box. Penalties committed within this area may result in a penalty kick, which are kicked from the penalty mark. The goal area is a smaller rectangle inside the penalty area and centered on the goal. This area is where a goal kick must take place. The goal itself measures 24 ft (7.3 m) wide by 8 ft (2.4 m) high. In the four corners of the field is a one-yd (0.9 m) quarter circle that which is used by a player when kicking a corner kick.

The ball

The ball, called a football or a soccer ball, is a spherical ball that is approximately 28 in (71 cm) in circumference. Two teams of eleven players play on the field. A captain is appointed by each time, whose responsibility is to participate in the coin toss before a kick-off at the beginning of the game or for penalty kicks during the game.

Players

The only player position recognized by the Laws of the Game is the goalkeeper is. However, over time, certain informal positions, called outfield players, have been created. Forwards, or strikers, are used primarily to score goals. Defenders have the mission to prevent opponent players from scoring goals. Midfielders try to take the ball away from opposing players when they are in possession of the ball and also attempt to pass the ball to their forwards when their team controls the ball.

These outfielders are also divided according to the portion of the field they play. For instance, the central

PELE (1940–)

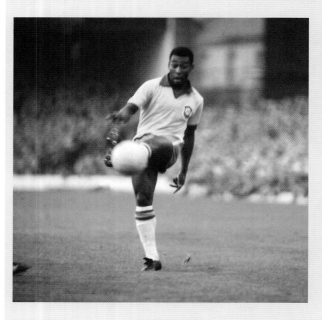

Pele grew up with a love for soccer. His parents could not afford a soccer ball so he kicked a sock filled with rags. At age eleven, one of Brazil's top players discovered him and trained him in secret. When he was seventeen, Pele was the youngest player in the World Cup tournament and he gained global attention by his skilled performance. Brazil had never won a World Cup before, even though soccer was very popular in the country. Pele's performance made him a national superstar.

Before his twentieth birthday, Pele had scored more than 400 goals. His love of the game was evident. He would shake the hand of the goalkeeper who stopped his shots, or salute the spectators when he scored a goal.

Pele's father told him to quit soccer when he was still on top, and Pele retired at age 34. He had scored 1,280 goals in 1,362 games.

(© Art Rickerby/Time & Life Pictures/Getty Images)

defenders play the central portion of the field, while the left midfielders play the left side of the middle part of the field. Even though these positions have been created, players are allowed to move between various positions during the match, often times depending if they are trying to score a goal (offensive) or are trying to defend their opponents from scoring (defensive).

All players, except the goalkeepers, are only allowed (during the play of the game) to use their feet to kick the ball or their bodies or heads (what is called "heading") to hit the ball as it flies through the air. They are not allowed to use their hands or arms except when throwing in the ball when re-starting game play, as when it is necessary after a penalty play.

The game

During playing of the match, players can play the ball in any direction. The team with control of the ball attempt to score a goal by dribbling or passing the ball to a teammate or by taking shots toward the goal. This goal is possessed by the opposing team and is guarded by its goalkeeper. At this same time, the opposing team is trying to gain possession of the ball by intercepting a pass or by tackling an opposing player who is in possession of the ball. Players can make physical contact onto opposing players only in certain situation. The referee

keeps the game going (time-wise) unless the ball exists the field or if a player violates a rule (the Laws of the Game).

The team that scores the most points at the end of the match will win the game. If the score is tied at the end of the regular match, then the game is declared a draw (tie), or the game continues into extra time or will be decided by a penalty shootout—such a conclusion is decided before the game begins.

Preparation

Warming up before playing soccer is essential. Muscles will be much more prepared to work if they are warmed up before soccer begins. Five or so minutes of light **exercise** will prepare the body for the demands inherent in soccer. **Stretching** exercises are also recommended during the **warm-up** routine. However, stretching should be done after other exercises so muscles are not injured. After playing soccer, spend another five minutes to cool-down. Light exercises or **walking** helps to restore the body to its resting state. Stretching afterwards is also recommended.

Risks

Soccer injuries range from minor ones (just aches and pains) to more serious ones (such as concussions

KEY TERMS

Calf muscle—The fleshy part of the back of the leg located below the knee.

Concussion—The most common type of traumatic brain injury.

Groin muscle—The muscle between the top of the thighs and the abdomen.

Hamstrings—One of two main tendons of the muscles behind the knees.

Laterally—Outwardly.

Quadriceps—The thigh muscle.

Shin splints—An aching, painful condition of the skin bone.

QUESTIONS TO ASK YOUR DOCTOR

- Am I in good enough physical shape to play soccer?
- What is the best way for me to become fit for soccer?
- Will soccer help me to become physically fit?
- Will I reduce the amount of fat on my body by playing soccer?
- What exercises should I perform to supplement my playing of soccer?
- How concerned should I be if I sustain a concussion playing soccer?
- How do I determine how hard to exercise with interval training?
- What type of physical fitness program should I use to prepare for soccer
- Where can I learn more about soccer?
- How often should I play soccer each week to become physically fit?
- Are there personal trainers locally that specialize in teaching soccer?
- Is there anything that would physically prevent me from playing soccer?
- What types of lifestyle changes will help while playing soccer?

and broken bones). Some of the most common injuries caused by playing soccer are head concussions; broken arms, legs, ankles, wrists, and noses; and sprains and tears to various muscles, tendons, and ligaments. Injuries to parts of the leg are the most frequent occurring injury in soccer. Specifically, knee injuries are the most frequent injury of the leg, followed by those of the ankle. Lateral (inside ligaments) sprains are more common than medial (outside ligaments) sprains, although, both occur on a regular basis. Other injuries include strains to the calf muscles, hamstrings, hip-abductor (groin) muscles, quadriceps, posterior cruciate ligament (ACL/PCL); and shin splints. Common injuries to the head, neck, and shoulder include: **concussion**; shoulder **fracture**, separation, or dislocation; whiplash or neck strain; and torn rotator cuff. Overall, injuries in soccer are some of the most frequent of any sport played around the world. **Dehydration** and exhaustion can also occur while playing soccer.

Results

Playing soccer adds strength to the upper and lower parts of the body. It also improves cardiovascular fitness and endurance. One's speed and agility also benefits from the playing of soccer. When soccer players are physically prepared to play soccer, they are much more likely to reduce their chances of having injuries. Bodies should be well conditioned and at their peak of fitness before the start of each soccer match. Muscles, tendons, ligaments, and bones must be ready to counter the assaults to the bodies that will take place while tackling, **running**, kicking, and jumping, during the game of soccer.

A three-year comprehensive study has been published in the *Scandinavian Journal of Medicine and Science in Sports*. Heading the research was Drs. Peter Krustrop and Jens Bangsbo, from the Department of Exercise and Sports Sciences at the University of Copenhagen. The project involved over 50 researchers from seven countries. They looked at men, women, and children from the ages of seven to 77 years, and their activities of soccer and running, along with a control group. As reported by the ScienceDaily.com article *Soccer Improves Health, Fitness and Social Abilities*, the conclusion of the article was: "Soccer is a pleasurable team sport that provides an all-round fitness and can be used as treatment for lifestyle-related diseases. Men worry less when playing soccer than when running. Women's soccer creates we-stories and helps women stay active."

Dr. Krustrup concluded: "Soccer is a very popular team sport that contains positive motivational and social factors that may facilitate compliance and contribute to the maintenance of a physically active lifestyle. The studies presented have demonstrated that soccer training for two-three hours per week causes significant cardiovascular, metabolic and musculoskeletal adaptations, independent on gender, **age** or lack of experience with soccer."

Resources

BOOKS

Blevins, Dave. *The Sports Hall of Fame Encyclopedia: Baseball, Basketball, Football, Hockey, Soccer.* Lanham, MD: Scarecrow Press, 2011.

Dobson, Stephen, and John Goddard. *The Economics of Football.* Cambridge: Cambridge University Press, 2011.

Hargreaves, Alan. *Skills and Strategies for Coaching Soccer.* Champaign, IL: Human Kinetics, 2010.

Hornby, Hugh. *Soccer.* New York: DK Publishing, 2008.

Lisi, Clemente Angelo. *A History of the World Cup, 1930–2010.* Lanham, MD: Scarecrow Press, 2011.

Micheli, Lyle J., editor. *Encyclopedia of Sports Medicine.* Thousand Oaks, CA: SAGE, 2011.

Moorman III, Claude T., and Donald T. Kirkendall, editors. *Praeger Handbook of Sports Medicine and Athlete Health.* Santa Barbara, CA: Praeger, 2011.

WEBSITES

Classic Football. FIFA.com. http://www.fifa.com/classic football/history/index.html (accessed August 23, 2011).

Soccer For Dummies. MSNBC. (May 23, 2010). http://nbcsports.msnbc.com/id/37304907/ns/sports-soccer/ (accessed August 23, 2011).

Soccer Improves Health, Fitness and Social Abilities. Science Daily.com. (April 7, 2010). http://www.sciencedaily.com/releases/2010/04/100406093524.htm (accessed August 23, 2011).

ORGANIZATIONS

American Alliance for Health, Physical Education, Recreation and Dance, 1900 Association Drive, Reston, VA, 20191-1598, (703) 476-3400, (800) 213-7193, http://www.aahperd.org/.

American Council on Exercise, 4851 Paramount Drive, San Diego, CA, \92123, (888) 825-3636, support@acefitness.org, http://www.fitness.gov/.

American Youth Soccer Organization, 19750 South Vermont Avenue, Suite 200, Torrance, CA, 90502, Fax: (310) 525-1155, (800) 872-2976, http://www.ayso.org/.

International Federation of Association Football, P. O. Box 8044, Zurich, Switzerland, 41 0 (43) 222-7777, Fax: 41 0 (43) 222-7878, http://www.fifa.com/.

National Coalition for Promoting Physical Activity, 1100 H Street, N.W., Suite 510, Washington, DC, 20005, (202) 454-7521, Fax: (202) 454-7598, http://www.ncppa.org/membership/organizations/.

President's Council on Fitness, Sports and Nutrition, 1101 Wootton Parkway, Suite 560, Rockville, MD, 20852, (240) 276-9567, Fax: (240) 276-9860, http://www.fitness.gov/.

William A. Atkins, BB, BS, MBA

Softball

Definition

Softball is a game played with a bat and a ball and, for the most part, its rules are the same as those played with **baseball**. However, it is different from baseball with respect to several significant factors such as the ball size, pitched ball speed, equipment, and field size. One of its most noticeable differences is that the ball is pitched underhand in softball, as opposed to overhand in baseball. Because softball is a physically active sport, it helps to provide good fitness to its participants.

Purpose

The purpose of softball is to win the game over the competition. However, the performance of the sport also provides people a good way to stay healthy. The game helps to strengthen muscles and provide for good overall cardiovascular health. Because softball involves so much **running** it also helps to produce strong leg muscles. Balance and coordination is also necessary in softball, so the game also improves these abilities.

Demographics

Both men and boys and women and girls regularly play softball. Youth software is played separately from adult-played softball. Softball is considered the most popular sport in the United States, with an estimated 40 million Americans playing at least one softball game during the year. In addition, Senior Softball USA states that over 1.5 million seniors play softball annually. Over the world, softball is played in well over one hundred countries.

Description

Types

Three main types of softball occur. They differ in reference to the speed of the pitched ball. The three types of softball are fast-pitch, slow-pitch, and modified pitch (a combination of fast- and slow-pitch). In slow-pitch, the ball is released at a moderate speed and delivered with a very noticeable arc, reaching regulated heights from 6 to 12 ft. (1.8 to 3.6 m). The umpire can call a pitch illegal if it is too high or low. However, in fast-pitch, the pitcher throws the ball as fast as possible, so little arc is visible. In modified-pitch, there are no regulations for the ball's arc. Slow-pitch is considered the most popular type of softball However, fast-pitch softball, which is most similar to baseball, is popular with some groups such as girls.

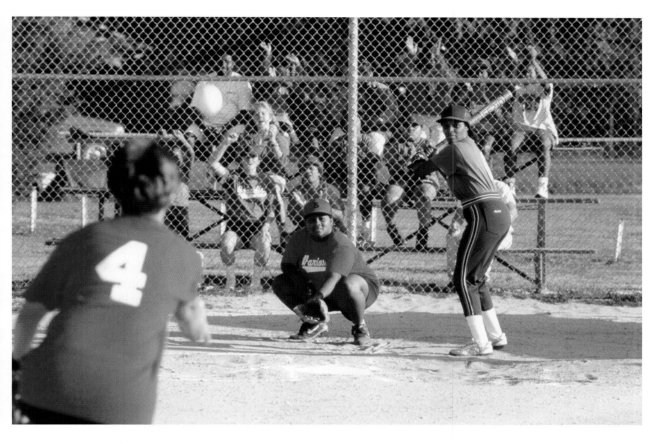

All eyes are on the softball as it leaves the pitcher's hand. *(© Ariel Skelley/Corbis)*

Umpire

Umpires are in charge of the rules of softball and controls how the game proceeds. The number of umpires can range from one to seven. A plate umpire calls balls and strikes at home plate. Base umpires can be positioned at each of the three other bases, and another three umpires can be scattered about in the outfield. However, most games of softball use only two or three umpires.

Field

Softball is played on a large field, sometimes called a diamond, which is smaller than a baseball field, though in the same arrangement. The field is divided into an infield and outfield. The infield, which is square shaped (and tilted to look like a diamond), includes the four bases (home plate, first base, second base, and third base) with home plate furthest away from the outfield, followed by first base to the right, second base at the top, and third base on the left. The infield is usually composed of dirt, or a combination of dirt and brick dust, paralleling the bases with grass sometimes in the center (except for the pitching area). However, the infield can also be composed entirely of one substance, such as dirt, grass, artificial turf, asphalt, or other materials. The outfield is usually composed of grass but it, too, can be other materials. The bases are usually 40 to 65 ft. (12.2 to 19.8 m) apart. Near the center of the square is a pitcher's circle or mound, and inside is a small, flat rectangular area called the "rubber," which is used by the pitcher when pitching the ball toward the plate.

The average distances from home plate to the center, left, and right field fences of a softball field is around 220 to 250 ft. (67 to 75 m). The infield played in fast-pitch softball usually measures 60 ft. (18.3 m) apart between all of the three bases and home plate. Similarly, the bases for modified-pitch softball are usually 65 ft. (19.8 m) apart, while the bases for slow-pitch can vary between 60 and 65 ft. (18.3 and 19.8 m). The distance between the pitcher's mound and the home plate also depends on how the game is played. In men's fast-pitch and modified-pitch the distance is 46 ft. (14 m), while in women's fast-pitch and modified-pitch, this distance is 40 ft. (12.2 m). In both men's and women's slow-pitch, the distance is 50 ft. (15.2 m).

KEY TERMS

Calf muscle—The fleshy portion of the back of the leg, located below the knee.

Concussion—The most common type of traumatic brain injury.

Contusions—Bruising.

Groin muscles—The muscles located between the top of the thighs and the abdomen.

Hamstring muscle—The muscle located at the back of the thigh that controls certain leg movements.

Laceration—Irregular tear-like wound.

Quadriceps muscles—A group of four muscles located at the front of the thigh.

Tendinitis—Inflammation of a tendon, usually after excessive use.

Teams

Usually nine or ten players play on each team, depending on the softball type. The team at bat—those players hitting the ball— are on offense. The other team is in the field (defensive), and its players are positioned at its various positions. Ten players per team is used in slow-pitch softball, but fast-pitch and modified-pitch play use nine-player teams. In a nine-player team, the infielders consist of the pitcher, catcher, first baseman, second baseman, shortstop, and third baseman, while the outfielders are made of the left fielder, center fielder, and right fielder. In slow pitch softball there is an extra outfielder (tenth player) called a roamer because this player moves around ("roams") the entire outfield.

Game

The game is played for a specific number of innings, usually six or seven, but sometimes up to nine. Each team gets to play offense and defense, once each inning. One team will play offense (batting) in the top half of the inning, while the other team plays defense (in the field). During the bottom half of the inning the teams reverse positions. The game is usually begun by tossing a coin to see who begins first on offense and defense. Sometimes this arrangement is determined by whom is the home and visiting teams.

The offensive team attempts to score runs when its players, one at a time, try to hit the ball, while standing next to home plate inside the batter's box, as it is thrown by the opposing team's pitcher while on the pitching mound. When the ball it hit by a member of the offensive team, the defensive team tries to make "outs" in numerous ways. Conversely, the offensive team keeps on trying to make "runs" until three outs occur. Three outs mean the offensive team has ended its time at bat and that half of the inning is over. It is now time for the teams to switch their offensive and defensive roles.

The game starts with one player (first in the batting order) going to the batter's box next to home plate. The pitcher throws the ball towards home plate with an underhanded motion. The batter may attempt to hit the ball with a softball bat as it crosses the plate. If the batter swings but does not hit the ball, then the throw is classified a strike. If the batter does not swing, then two things can happen: (1) if the ball is outside the strike zone (predetermined by the plate's width and the height of the armpits and knees of the batter), then it is classified as a "ball" or (2) if it is inside the strike zone then it is a "strike". Three strikes means the batter is out (a strikeout), and four balls means the batter is permitted to go to first base (a walk).

If the batter, instead, hits the ball within the boundaries of the playing field, then the defensive players attempt to catch the ball either in the air (a fly ball) or while it bounces over the ground (a ground ball). If one of the players catch the ball in the air (whether it is in bounds or not), the batter is out. If the ball is caught while traveling on the ground, then the player catching the ball must throw the ball to first base before the batter can reach it while running. The player can touch (tag) the runner or touch the first base bag before the runner get there—in both cases for an out. However, if the runner gets to first base before being tagged or before the first-baseman gets the ball, then the runner is safe, and remains on first base.

After the first player is finished being a batter, the next player in the batting order (predetermined before the game, but may change with substitute players) comes to the plate. The same sequence occurs for this new batter, and each player in his/her assigned order will come to the plate as a batter. Any given half inning will continue until the defensive team gets three outs. During this time, the offensive team tries to score as many points (runs) as possible. This is done by advancing players on the bases, going (counterclockwise) from home plate to first, second, third, and finally back to home plate in order to score one run. Players are advanced on the bases by hitting the ball while as a batter and not being called out, **walking** to first base as a batter after being pitched to and receiving four balls (pitched balls outside the strike zone), or being hit by a pitched ball. While running around the bases, the player is called a base runner or runner.

Generally, only one runner may occupy any base at any one time, and the runners cannot pass each other. When a ball is batted into fair play, the runners on base must attempt to advance if there are no unoccupied bases behind them. As such, a runner on first base must run to second base if the batter hits the ball into the playing field. The defensive players can throw to second play and force the lead runner out. The defensive team can also throw to first place. If they do both successfully, then a double play occurs (that is, two outs occur).

Many other rules also are applied to softball. The official rules of softball, as provided by the International Softball Federation, are found at: http://www.internationalsoftball.com/english/rules_standards/Rulebook_2002.pdf

Ball

The ball used in softball is called the "softball.". It is larger than the size of the ball used in baseball. It can be made from various regulated materials, including silky fiber, rubber, cork, and a polyurethane mixture. It is wound with a twisted yarn. The inside of the ball is then covered with latex or rubber cement. The exterior of the ball is finally covered with white or yellow leather in two pieces, which is in an approximate shape of a figure-8. These two pieces are sewn together with thread.

Two sizes of balls are used. A 12-inch ball, which is used in all games except slow-pitch, measures between 11.88 and 12.13 in (30.2 and 30.8 cm) in circumference and has a weight of between 6.25 and 7 oz (177.2 and 198.4 g). In fast-pitch and modified-pitch a 16 in (40.6 cm) ball in circumference is used.

Bat

The softball bat is made of wood or composite materials such as carbon fiber. It is restricted to being no more than 34 in (86.4 cm) in length and no more than 38 oz (1,077.3 g) in weight. Other regulated performance standards are also applied to the softball bat.

Preparation

Warming up before playing softball is critical so muscles can be best prepared for all of the activities involved in the game. Five or so minutes of light **exercise** will prepare the body for the physical actions found within softball. **Stretching** exercises are also recommended. However, stretching should be done after other exercises so muscles are not injured. After playing softball, spend another five minutes to cooldown. Light exercises or walking helps to return the body to its resting state. Stretching afterwards is also recommended.

Risks

Softball injuries can happen. They range from minor aches and pains to more serious ones such as concussions and broken bones. Some of the common injuries include sprains, contusions, or lacerations to various muscles, tendons, and ligaments. Knee, ankle, back, shoulder, forearm, wrist, and hand injuries occur sometimes in softball. Other specific injuries in softball include strains to the calf muscles, hamstrings, groin muscles, quadriceps, and shin splints.

Pitchers are more likely to sustain an injury to their pitching arm, wrist, or forearm, along with their shoulder, neck, or back, because of the repetitious and forceful nature of the arm's motion while pitching. One of the most common injuries to pitchers is shoulder **tendinitis** (an inflammation of the tendon within the shoulder).

For catchers, the back and knee are common problems caused by their position crouching behind the plate. However, all players of softball are at risk of sustaining injuries while playing their chosen position and while being a batter and runner. The more physically fit one is, the less likely one will sustain a serious injury. However, some injuries are not avoidable, and are not dependent on one's degree of fitness

Results

Playing softball helps to increase strength to the upper and lower parts of the body, especially the lower body. It also improves cardiovascular fitness. One's speed and agility also is increased from the playing of softball. Overall, softball is a good way to stay fit and maintain a healthy lifestyle.

Resources

BOOKS

Cross, Rod. *Physics of Baseball and Softball*. New York: Springer, 2011.

Garman, Judi, and Michelle Gromacki. *Softball Skills & Drills.*. Champaign, IL: Human Kinetics, 2011.

Hanlon, Thomas W. *The Sports Rules Book*. Champaign, IL: Human Kinetics, 2009.

Martens, Rainer, and Julie S. Martens. *Complete Guide to Slowpitch Softball*. Champaign, IL: Human Kinetics, 2011.

WEBSITES

Historical Facts about Softball. AthleticsScholorships.net. http://www.athleticsscholarships.net/history-of-softball.htm (accessed September 8, 2011).

How It All Started. Senior Softball USA. http://seniorsoftball.com/ssusa.php (accessed September 9, 2011).

How to Play Softball. Ehow.com. http://www.ehow.com/how_2048949_play-softball.html (accessed September 8, 2011).

Softball.com. Web Site. http://www.softball.com/home.jsp (accessed September 8, 2011).

U.S.A. Softball. Web Site. http://www.usasoftball.com/ (accessed September 8, 2011).

ORGANIZATIONS

Amateur Softball Association of America, 2801 N.E. 50th Street, Oklahoma City, OK, 73111, (405) 424-5266, http://www.asasoftball.com/.

Independent Softball Association, 680 East Main Street, Suite 101, Bartow, FL, 33830, (863) 519-7127, Fax: (863) 533-4290, http://isasoftball.com/.

National Softball Association, P. O. Box 7, Nicholasville, KY, 40304, (859) 887-4114, Fax: (859) 887-4874, nsahdqtrs@aol.com, http://www.playnsa.com/.

United States Sports Specialty Association, http://www.usssa.com/sports/.

William A. Atkins, BB, BS, MBA

Somatic nervous system *see* **Nervous system, somatic**

Sore muscles *see* **Delayed onset muscle soreness**

Spin class *see* **Indoor cycling class**

Sports nutrition

Definition

The term sports nutrition refers to the dietary selections that a person makes in order to achieve peak performance for some physical activity, whether it be recreational **exercise** or participation in a competitive sport.

Purpose

The purpose of sports nutrition is to support athletes towards optimum performance be it skill, power, strength, speed or endurance, all of which requires physical training and the correct nutrition is essential to the training effect.

Demographics

Any person who engages in any type of physical activity, whether it is personal workout just to improve one's general fitness or preparation for a major professional sporting event, can benefit from a better understanding of the role of good nutrition.

History

Sports historians often point to the Greek fighter Milo of Crotona, who competed in five Olympic Games between 532 and 516 bce as an ancient example of early interest in sports nutrition. Records indicate that Milo ate 9 kilograms (20 pounds) of meat, 9 kilograms (20 pounds) of bread, and more than 8 liters (18 pints) of wine every day while preparing for a fight. This tidbit of information tells us almost nothing about the history of sports nutrition other than that competitors obviously knew that their diet would have some effect on their athletic performance. Any form of scientific basis for that simple-minded belief, however, was largely lacking until the early twentieth century. At that point in history, scientists had begun to develop specific information as to the ways in which carbohydrates, proteins, fats, and other nutrients affect a person's strength, speed, endurance, and other physical properties.

KEY TERMS

Carbohydrate—A complex organic compound consisting of carbon, hydrogen, and water that is the primary energy source for the human body.

Electrolyte—An inorganic ion, such as sodium, potassium, or calcium ion, that is essential for normal body functions.

Fat—An organic compound that has a number of functions in the body, one of which is the production of energy when carbohydrate supplies are depleted.

Nutritional supplement—A substance, such as a vitamin, mineral, amino acid, or herb, taken to compensate for the lack of some essential nutrient in one's daily diet.

Protein—A complex organic compound that can be used as a source of energy for the body, but that is primarily used for the construction of cells and tissues, for the production of enzymes in the body, and for other functions.

The earliest scientific studies on the physiology of exercise can be traced to the mid-nineteenth century, when the first monograph on the topic was published by William H. Byford, then a physician and professor at the Rush Medical School in Chicago. His monograph was entitled "On the Physiology of Exercise," the first time those two words had occurred together in the title of a journal article. Byford's article had little impact, however, and it was more than 30 years before the first textbook on the topic was published, On the Physiology of Exercise, by E. M. Hartwell, of Johns Hopkins University. A few years later, in 1892, George W. Fitz established the first formal laboratory of exercise physiology at Harvard University, a laboratory that was to remain in operation in one form or another for another half century. Upon the dawn of the twentieth century, then, the first fundamental research on the relationship between human physiology and exercise had begun, and some basic facts were in place for continued study throughout the next century. An essential step in that process occurred in 1954 with the creation of the American College of Sports Medicine, which has been one of the leading institutions in the study of sports nutrition ever since.

Description

The human body requires certain nutrients in order to stay alive and function normally. These nutrients are **carbohydrates**, proteins, **fats**, vitamins, and minerals. The body also requires additional substances that, while not classified as nutrients, are still essential to good health. Adequate fluid levels are an example. When a person engages in some type of physical activity, the body experiences a greater demand for one or more nutrients. For example, one of the most common deficiencies that develop during physical exercise is **dehydration**, or a reduction in the amount of one's body fluids. Dehydration is one of the most common causes of decreased performance by an athlete. It can result in an increase in one's body temperature, an inability to concentrate, increased levels of lactic acid in the muscles (that leads to **muscle pain**), increase heart rate, and a decrease in strength. These symptoms can largely be avoided if a person remembers to continuing hydrating during exercise or a sporting event. The American Dietetic Association (ADA) has listed a number of benefits associated with proper nutritional practices, including:

- making it possible for a person to train for longer periods of time at higher intensity;
- delaying the onset of fatigue;
- promoting recovery from a physical activity;
- helping the body to adapt to a particular type of exercise or activity;
- improving one's overall health and body strength;
- enhancing one's coordination;
- helping to maintain a healthy immune system;
- reducing the chance of injury; and
- reducing the risk of other physical problems, such as muscle cramps and stomach aches.

The specific nutritional recommendations for any athlete depending on a number of factors, including one's sex, **age**, general physical health, skill level, and level of commitment to exercise or sport. Most individuals benefit from consulting with a coach, trainer, nutritionist, sports physician, dietitian, or other expert in deciding the type of diet one should pursue before, during, and after a physical activity. Generally speaking, most experts believe that the ideal dietary program for an athlete requires similar nutrients as that of the average person , oftentimes they have higher **energy** requirements. Athletes who discover that they are deficient in one or more nutrients are in that condition, usually, not because of their participation in athletics, but because they have chosen an inadequate diet for their normal daily lives. Anyone who understands and follows the general guidelines for a healthy everyday diet will also be nutritionally fit for almost any normal type of exercise or sporting activity.

Many athletes have come to depend heavily on the use of so-called nutritional supplements to enhance their physical skills. The term nutritional supplements refers to substances that one takes in order to supplement a diet that is otherwise inadequate in one or more vital nutrients, such as vitamins or minerals. People take nutritional supplements for many reasons, one of which, for athletes, is to improve their overall health and strength and enhance their performance in some particular sport. Today, there are hundreds of nutritional supplements available at almost every type of store, supporting a multi-billion dollar business in the United States alone. Considerable controversy surrounds the use of nutritional supplements to enhance physical performance, at least partly because most healthy Americans ingest all of the nutrients they need to remain strong and healthy if they pursue a healthy diet. The evidence for the effectiveness in using nutritional supplements to enhance one's physical performance is very thin indeed, and the risks associated with some such supplements do exist.

Types

The nutritional recommendations for exercise and sports are often sub-divided into three general categories: pre-exercise nutrition; during-exercise nutrition; and post-exercise nutrition. Nutritionists often suggest carbohydrates as the primary component of pre-exercise meals, with relatively smaller amounts of **protein** and fat. Carbohydrates provide the energy stores needed for any exercise or sporting event. A diet recommended by the American Dietetic Association, for example, calls for items such as fruits, oatmeal, peanut butter, honey, lean hamburger, yogurt, turkey, and cheese three to four hours before exercise, and a sports drink and additional fruit up to a half hour before the exercise.

Nutrition during exercise, according to the ADA, should consist primarily of the carbohydrates and electrolytes needed to replace lost stores during the exercise. A sport drink, such as Gatorade (that was developed just for this purpose) is almost ideal for such a situation. Small amounts of fruits, jams, honey, and bread can also be consumed during exercise.

The goal of post-exercise nutrition is to replace those nutrients lost during the exercise. Recovery nutrition should begin very soon after completion of the

QUESTIONS TO ASK YOUR DOCTOR

- Can you help me devise a dietary plan to make sure that I receive an adequate amount of nutrients for a person of my age engaged in my favorite sporting activity?
- How can I know if I am receiving the proper amount of nutrients in my daily life and in the sporting activities in which I participate?
- Are there signs or symptoms that would indicate that I am receiving insufficient levels of nutrients during an exercise or sporting activity?

exercise, as soon as 15 minutes and no later than an hour after the exercise has ended. Again, foods that produce quick carbohydrates are preferable, such as sports drinks, smoothies, fruits, and bread or crackers. A main meal should include protein as well as carbohydrate supplements, such as turkey, vegetables, tofu, vegetables, lean steak, and brown rice. (See the detailed and complete ADA recommendations at http://www.eatright.org/Public/content.aspx?id = 7056.)

Risks

There are no risks associated with ingesting a health diet consisting of the proper amount of all nutrients. On the other hand, there may be some risks associated with the use of nutritional supplements. Nutritional supplements are not monitored by government agencies such as the Food and Drug Administration (FDA), as are foods and drugs. Supplement manufacturers, then, have greater latitude in the claims they can make for their products and the standards they follow in producing those supplements. Some supplements are certainly beneficial to one's health and athletic performance, many have no effect at all on either health or performance, and some may actually have harmful (and in a small number of instances, life-threatening) effects. Anyone who chooses to use a nutritional supplement as part of a training program should seek professional advice from a trainer or medical professional before starting to use such a substance.

Resources

BOOKS

Bean, Anita. *Anita Bean's Sports Nutrition for Young Athletes.* London: A. & C. Black, 2010.
Bernadot, Dan. *Advanced Sports Nutrition*, 2nd ed. Leeds, UK: Human Kinetics, 2012.

Clark, Nancy. *Nancy Clark's Sports Nutrition Guide Book*, 4th ed. Champaign, IL: Human Kinetics, 2008.

Dunford, Marie, and J. Andrew Doyle. *Nutrition for Sport and Exercise.* Belmont, CA: Wadsworth Cengage Learning, 2012.

Williams, Melvin H. *Nutrition for Health, Fitness & Sport*, 9th ed. Boston: McGraw-Hill, 2010.

WEBSITES

Fitness and Sports Nutrition. National Agricultural Library. http://fnic.nal.usda.gov/nal_display/index.php?info_center=4&tax_level=2&tax_subject=257&topic_id=1358 (accessed October 18, 2011).

Questions Most Frequently Asked about Sports Nutrition. http://www.fitness.gov/faq.pdf (accessed October 18, 2011).

Sports Nutrition American Dietetic Association. http://www.eatright.org/Public/content.aspx?id=7055 (accessed October 18, 2011).

ORGANIZATIONS

International Society of Sports Nutrition, 600 Pembrook Dr., Woodland Park, CO, 80863, Fax: (719) 687-5184, (866) 740-4776, issn.sports.nutrition@ gmail.com, http://www.sportsnutritionsociety.org/.

David E. Newton, AB, MA, EdD

Sprain *see* **Muscle strain**

Sprinting *see* **Running**

Squash

Definition

Squash is a racquet sport placed by two players in a four-walled court with a small, hollow rubber ball. It is similar to the game of **racquetball**, although distinct differences exist between the two games. Because the game of squash involves intense competition between its two players, it is an excellent **exercise** activity, one that is good for the **cardiovascular system**, including the heart.

Purpose

The goal in squash is to score more points and, thus, win the game over the opposing player. However, its performance also provides for a good cardiovascular workout. A player can expend ("burn") from 600 to 1,000 cal. (3,000 to 4,000 kJ) per hour in a hearty game of squash. Because of this, it is a good aerobic workout. A typical game will find players exerting themselves at about 80% of their maximum heart rate as they travel from corner to center court and then returning to another corner or back wall, repeatedly, as play progresses throughout the game. Short bursts of speed are intermingled with short recovery periods, making for a high level of aerobic fitness.

The game also helps to improve anaerobic fitness as its activities help to strengthen and tone muscles, especially helping to strengthen the leg muscles with all of its **running**, and the muscles in the upper body, especially the muscles within the arms, shoulders, chest, and back. Balance and coordination are also improved in squash, as players must be agile as they quickly change directions and speeds throughout the game.

Demographics

Squash is played in at least 188 countries and territories around the world. Countries where squash is especially popular include Australia, Canada, Egypt, France, Germany, Malaysia, the Netherlands, Pakistan, South Africa, Spain, the United Kingdom, and the United States,

Description

Squash is played with a small, hard rubber ball in a court with two opposing players. When the game was first created, it was patterned after a game called racquets (or hard racquets), which is similar to today's **handball**. Because the floor area was so small when played inside a racquets court, the ball bounced very quickly off the wall, making it very difficult to hit. Somewhere along the line, the ball was intentionally (or maybe accidently) punctured with the hope it would not move quite so fast. Thereafter, the ball became "squashed" when it hit against the wall, gaving it its name: squash racquet or, today, simply squash.

Court

The playing dimensions of a squash court, according to international standards, is 32 ft (9.75 m) long and 21 ft (6.4 m) wide. The front wall contains a horizontal "out line" that is 15 ft (4.57 m) off the floor. It continues along the two side walls, slanting downward, until reaching the "out line" on the back wall, which returns to being horizontal. The out line on the back wall is 7 ft. (2.13 m) above the floor. Shots hitting above or on the out line are considered out of bounds.

The front wall also contains a "service line" that is 6 ft (1.83 m) above the floor and a "tin," which is a sheet of metal that begins on the floor and extends

19 in (480 mm) upward from the floor. When the ball hits the tin, it produces a distinctive metallic ping, telling the players that the ball is out of bounds.

The floor is marked with a "front line" that goes across the width of the floor, separating the front and back of the court. It also contains a "half-court" line, which is parallel to the side walls, and separates the left and right hand sides of the back portion of the court. It is divided in half by two rear "quarter courts" that contain two smaller "service boxes"—the first one in the upper-left quadrant of the back-left quarter court and the second one in the upper-right quadrant of the back-right quarter court (as facing the front wall). The floor markings are used only for serves within squash.

Equipment

Squash players use a racquet and a ball to perform their activities on the squash court. The structure of the racket is usually made of composite materials or metals such as boron, graphite, Kevlar, or titanium. The maximum dimensions of racquets are 27.0 in. (686 mm) long by 8.4 in. (215 mm) wide. The maximum weight for the racquet is 9 oz. (255 g), however most racquets usually weigh between 4 and 7 oz. (110 and 200 g). The head of the racquiet is usually strung with synthetic strings, although natural materials were used in the past.

The ball used in squash has a diameter of between 1.56 and 1.59 in. (39.5 and 40.5 mm), and a weight of 0.81 to 0.88 oz. (23 to 25 g). It is made of two pieces of a rubber compound that is glued together to form a hollow sphere. Different types of balls are used depending on various factors such as player experience and expertise, atmospheric conditions, and court temperature. Because of these different types of ball, they are color coded to indicate different speeds and

bounce. The colors and related speeds and bounce intensity are:

- blue (fast speed and very high bounce intensity)
- red (medium and high)
- green or white (medium to slow and average)
- yellow (slow and low)
- double yellow (slow and very low)
- orange (super slow and super low).

Eye protection is also used by squash players to avoid injuries from speeding balls and swinging racquets in the closed quarters of the court.

Game

The two players playing a game of squash usually start with a decision as to who serves first. Frequently, this is accomplished by spinning a racket and seeing which player correctly guesses whether the logo ends up or down after the racket stops spinning. The winning (serving) player starts by deciding whether to serve from the left or right service box. In either case, he/she begins by placing both feet within the box without touching its lines. When served the ball must hit the front wall above the service line and below the out line. When it bounces past the front wall, the ball must land in the opposite quarter court. The receiving player then volleys the ball, and the volley continues until one of the players misses or the ball goes out of bounds. When serve changes players, it is called "hand out." Only one serve per volley is allowed in squash.

During other hits (besides the serve), the ball must hit against the front wall, below the out line and above the tin. The ball is permitted to hit the back wall or side walls at any time during play, with the only restriction being that it must hit below the out line. In addition, the ball must not strike the floor between bouncing off the racket and hitting the front wall. Further, a ball touching either the tin or the out line is considered to be out. After the ball hits the front wall, it is allowed to bounce only once on the floor (and, as stated before, any number of times against the side or back walls) before a player must hit it against the front wall.

Players may move anywhere around the court. However, intentionally or unintentionally hindering the movements of another player is not permitted. Players typically return to the center of the court after making a shot—the most advantageous position for returning the ball. If the server wins the point, the serving player continues to serve until he/she loses the volley, at which time the receiving player becomes the serving player. Therefore, points are scored only when serving the ball.

A game is completed when the first player reaches 9, 11, or 21 points, whatever is decided by the players before the game starts. Scoring to 11 is today considered the official number of points for the completion of a game. If played to 9 points and the game is tied at 8 points, then the receiving player can state "set 1" or "set 2", meaning the games will proceed to 9 or 10 points, respectively. Games played in competitions or tournaments usually are decided by the "best" of five games—three games out of five must be won to win the match. A referee usually officiates games when played as part of a squash league or during competitions or tournaments.

Preparation

Warming up before starting a squash is important so muscles can be prepared for all of the intense motions and movements involved in the game. Five or more minutes of low to moderate exercise will prepare for the activities in squash. **Stretching** exercises are also recommended, but after other exercises are completed, so muscles are less likely to be injured. After playing squash, take about five minutes to cooldown. Light exercises or **walking** should be included. Stretching afterwards is also recommended.

Risks

Squash injuries can happen. Tennis elbow, what is medically called lateral epicondilvtis, is a common squash injury due to excessive use of the muscles and tendons in the forearm. Injuries to the lumbar region,

knee, ankle, and general muscles problems are some of the other more common injuries that occur when playing squash.

Results

Playing squash helps to increase strength to the upper and lower parts of the body, especially the lower body. It also improves cardiovascular fitness. One's speed and agility also is increased from the playing of squash Overall, squash is a good way to stay fit and maintain a healthy lifestyle.

Forbes magazine ranked various sports as to their health benefits. Squash was rated as the number one sport of those considered by the magazine. The categories were: cardiovascular endurance, muscular strength, muscular endurance, flexibility, **calories** per 30 minutes, and injury risk. The first four categories were ranked, from 1 to 5, with 1 = nothing special, 2 = not bad, 3 = good, 4 = darn good, and 5 = excellent. The fifth category, injury risk, was rated on a scale consisting of 1 = low, 2 = so-so, and 3 = high. The category calories per 30 minutes was based on the **energy expenditure** of a 190-lb. (86.2 kg) person over a 30-minute time period, as provided by the American College of Sports Medicine. Squash ranked 4.5 in cardiovascular endurance, 3 in muscular strength, 5 in muscular endurance, 3 in flexibility, 5 in calories per 30 minutes, and 2 in injury risk— for an overall score of 22.5 that was good enough for the healthiest sport in the survey, including **rowing**, **rock climbing**, **swimming**, cross-country skiing, **basketball**, cycling, running, modern pentathlon, and **boxing**.

Forbes states in its article: "The preferred game of Wall Street has convenience on its side, as 30 minutes on the squash court provides an impressive cardio respiratory workout. Extended rallies and almost constant running builds muscular strength and endurance in the lower body, while lunges, twists and turns increase flexibility in the back and abdomen. For people just getting into the game, it's almost too much to sustain, but once you get there, squash is tremendous."

Resources

BOOKS

White, Colin. *Projectile Dynamics in Sport: Principles and Applications.* Abingdon, Oxon, England: Routledge, 2011.

Yarrow, Philip, and Aidan Harrison. *Squash: Steps to Success..* Champaign, IL: Human Kinetics, 2010.

Hanlon, Thomas W. *The Sports Rules Book.* Champaign, IL: Human Kinetics, 2009.

WEBSITES

Squash Healthiest Sport Says Forbes Magazine. Squash-Player.co.uk. http://www.squashplayer.co.uk/sp_latest/forbes_survey.htm (accessed September 9, 2011).

Squash Injuries. SquashRacquetReviews.com. (September 3, 2010). http://www.squashracketreviews.com/Squash-Injuries/Squash-Injuries/ (accessed September 12, 2011).

Squash Racquets: Early History. HickokSports.com. http://hickoksports.com/history/squashrackets.shtml (accessed September 9, 2011).

ORGANIZATIONS

Professional Squash Players Association, 123 Cathedral Road, Cardiff, Wales, CF11 9PH, 44 29 (2038) 8446, Fax: 44 29 (2022) 8185, psa@psa-squash.com, http://www.psa-squash.com/.

U.S. Squash, 555 Eighth Avenue, Suite 1102, New York, NY, 10018-4311, (212) 268-4090, Fax: (212) 268-4091, office@ussquash.com, http://www.ussquash.com/.

World Squash Federation, 25 Russell Street, Hastings, East Sussex, United Kingdom, TN34 1QU, 44 0 (1424) 447440, Fax: 44 0 (1424) 430737, http://www.worldsquash.org/.

William A. Atkins, BB, BS, MBA

Stability training

Definition

Stability training is a type of **exercise** training program that helps to strengthen and steady the body's core muscles so that all other extremity movements (arms and legs) are more easily performed. It is sometimes called core stability training or stability training because such training concentrates on the core muscles of the upper body, excluding the neck, head, and arms. The completion of stability training provides for increased muscle endurance, along with added tendon and ligament strength and better range of motion for joints and muscles. Generally, stability training is used as a foundation to a larger fitness program, one that provides for enhanced performance, added muscular strength, and reduced risk from injuries.

Purpose

The general purpose of stability training is to provide the human body with the best possible ability to move freely about in its daily activities. Foremost, it is a good foundation for a strong body. The body is able to better control its movements in any direction, shift its body weight, and transfer **energy** from the trunk to the outer extremities. stability training provides the body with dynamic balancing of the joints, and a properly aligned and stable posture. stability training makes for a strong set of core muscles so people can develop a physically fit body for both daily activities and sports-related performance.

Demographics

Stability training is appropriate for anyone interested in maximizing the fitness of their core muscles. As such, stability training lends itself as an excellent supplement for other exercise programs, such as those including aerobic and anaerobic exercises.

Description

Stability training is used to stabilize the muscles of the torso so that the spine, pelvis, and shoulders are all stabilized. The torso muscles (those of the upper body) attach to the spine, pelvis, and shoulders, such as the scapula, the muscle that attaches to the back of the shoulder. With such stabilization of the torso, the extremities are provided with a good foundation in which to move. stability training is also used to provide the best posture possible for the human body.

One type of exercise for stability training is called abdominal bracing. This technique uses exercises, such as abdominal crunches (commonly called ab crunches) and sit-ups to contract the abdominal muscles. Specific programs or devices used to develop core strength include medicine balls, stability balls, kettle bells, wobble boards, **Yoga**, and Pilate's.

The core muscles located throughout the torso include:

- Erector spinae: Also named sacrospinalis, this group of muscles and tendons runs vertically from the neck and through to the lower back; they lie within a groove on the side of the vertebral column.
- External obliques: Also called external abdominal oblique muscles, these three flat muscles are located on the side and front of the abdomen (also called the lateral anterior abdomen).
- Gluteus maximus: Also abbreviated as glutes, it is the largest of the three gluteal muscles, and makes up the largest portion of the buttocks.
- Gluteus medius: One of the three gluteal muscles, it is a broad, thick muscle located on the outer surface of the pelvis.
- Gluteus minimus: One of the three gluteal muscles, it is the smallest of the gluteal muscles, located just under the gluteus medius.

KEY TERMS

Aerobic exercises—Exercises that speed up respiration and heart rate, such as walking, running, bicycling, and swimming.

Anaerobic exercises—Exercises high enough in intensity that oxygen is required at a greater rate than it can be supplied, for instance heavy weight training and sprinting.

Cardiovascular—Relating to the heart and blood vessels.

Tendon—The inelastic band of connective tissue that attaches a muscle to a bone or other body part.

- Hip adductors: A group of adductor muscles on the thigh, consisting of the adductor brevis, adductor longus, adductor magnus, adductor minimus, pectineus, gracilis, and obturator externus.

- Hip flexors: Located in front of the pelvis and the upper thigh; the muscles that make up the majority of hip flexors include psoas major, psoas minor, illiacus, rectus femoris, pectineus, sartorius, and tensor fasciae latae.

- Internal obliques: Situated under the external obliques, but running in the opposite direction.

- Multifidus: Located under the erector spinae along the vertebral column, these muscles extend and rotate the spine.

- Rectus abdominis: Often referred to as the "six-pack" muscle, it is located along the front of the abdomen.

- Transverse abdominis: Positioned under the obliques, it is the deepest of the abdominal muscles (muscles of the waist) and wraps around the spine for protection and stability

Equipment often used with stability training includes:

- Body weight: Push-ups, pull-ups, abdominal crunches, and similar exercises do not need equipment, only one's body weight.

- Resistance tubing: Inexpensive and lightweight tubing provides resistance when performing resistance exercises.

- Free weights: Barbells and dumbbells are often used when performing stability exercises.

- Weight machines: This equipment can be used for stability training, and is commonly found in fitness centers and gymnasiums; and often can be purchased for home use.

Stability training exercises should work all the muscles in the torso, either simultaneously or with several exercises that focus on isolated muscle groups. Popular exercises for stability training include:

- Plank: While staying in the downward position (closest to the floor), do a push-up with the body's weight on the forearms, elbows, and toes; also called front hold or abdominal bridge.

- Side plank: While lying on the side with legs straight and one foot on top of the other; straighten the bottom arm and place the other hand on the hip; flex the feet and balance while on the sides of the feet.

- Push-up: While using the common push-up exercise, lower the body using the arms.

- Squat: While standing up straight, move back to a crouching position (like sitting back in a chair) with the knees bent and the buttocks on or near the heels.

- Back bridge: While laying on the back with the hands by the sides and the knees bent and the feet flat on the floor, tighten the abdominal and buttock muscles while raising the hips to form a straight line from the knees to the shoulders.

- Hip lift: While laying on the back with the arms by the sides and the palms facing up, raise up both legs to they are straight up toward the ceiling and perpendicular to the torso; now lift up the hips a few inches off the floor while keeping the legs pointed straight up.

Preparation

Warming up is important, as it is with any type of exercise or physical activity, because it helps to prepare the muscles before they do more difficult work. Exercises involving stability training place the muscles under extra tension for longer periods than normal for most other exercises, so a **warm-up** period is critical before beginning this training. A warm-up period may consist of about five minutes of light exercise or **walking**. Stretches are also recommended during the warm-up routine.

Once stability training is completed, it is a good idea to spend about five minutes cooling down. Light exercise or walking helps the body to settle back down to its normal routine. More **stretching** exercises are also recommended.

Risks

Performing stability training exercises poses some health risks to the body. It is important to use proper form and technique while performing the exercise. Stop any exercises if pain is present. It is important to breath continuously (and not hold one's breath) during the performance of stability training exercises.

Results

The major benefits of stability training include:

- better management of chronic medical problems
- increased stamina
- development of strong bones
- enhanced athletic performance
- extended and improved movement of the extremities, such as the arms and legs
- improved proper posture and reduced strain on the spine
- reduced or eliminated back pain
- minimized chance of injuries
- stabilization of the spine

Resources

BOOKS

Cook, Gregg, and Fatima d'Almeida-Cook. *The Gym Survival Guide: Your Road Map to Fearless Fitness.* New York: Sterling, 2008.

Plowman, Sharon A., and Denise L. Smith. *Exercise Physiology for Health, Fitness, and Performance.* Philadelphia: Wolters Kluwer Health/Lippincott Williams & Wilkins, 2011.

Schoenfeld, Brad. *Women's Home Workout Bible.* Champaign, IL: Human Kinetics, 2010.

Siff, Mel Cunningham. *Supertraining.* Denver: Supertraining Institute, 2004.

Sutton, Amy L, editor. *Fitness and Exercise Sourcebook.* Detroit: Omnigraphics, 2007.

WEBSITES

Louriero, Felipe. *Benefits of Core Stability Training.* AmateurEndurance.com. http://www.amateurendurance.com/triathlon-training/article/benefits-of-core-stability-training/ (accessed November 10, 2011).

Quinn, Elizabeth. *The Best Core Exercises.* Sportsmedicine. about.com. (September 3, 2011). http://sportsmedicine.about.com/od/abdominalcorestrength1/a/NewCore.htm (accessed November 10, 2011).

Strength Training: Get Stronger, Leaner, Healthier. WebMD. (June 30, 2010). http://www.mayoclinic.com/health/strength-training/HQ01710 (accessed November 10, 2011).

ORGANIZATIONS

American Alliance for Health, Physical Education, Recreation and Dance, 1900 Association Dr., Reston, VA, 20191-1598, (703) 476-3400, (800) 213-7193, http://www.aahperd.org.

American Council on Exercise, 4851 Paramount Dr., San Diego, CA, 92123, (888) 825-3636, support@acefitness.org, http://www.acefitness.org.

National Coalition for Promoting Physical Activity, 1100 H St., NW, Suite 510, Washington, DC, 20005, (202) 454-7521, Fax: (202) 454-7598, http://www.ncppa.org.

President's Council on Fitness, Sports and Nutrition, 1101 Wootton Parkway, Suite 560, Rockville, MD, 20852, (240) 276-9567, Fax: (240) 276-9860, http://www.fitness.gov.

William A. Atkins, BB, BS, MBA

Stationary bicycle

Definition

The stationary bicycle, also known as the **exercise** bicycle or exercise bike, is an indoor exercise machine that is pedaled like a bicycle. It has a seat, handlebars, pedals, and usually has a device to adjust tension or resistance.

Purpose

The stationary bicycle provides a low-impact, aerobic workout for people who want to exercise indoors. People who choose this option include individuals seeking a cardiovascular workout, those who want to lose weight, people participating in physical therapy like a knee rehabilitation program, and those whose exercise options are limited because of pain in their lower backs, hips, or joints.

Exercise bicycles are also used by busy people trying to fit exercise into their schedules. They can ride the bicycle in their homes or at a gym, and

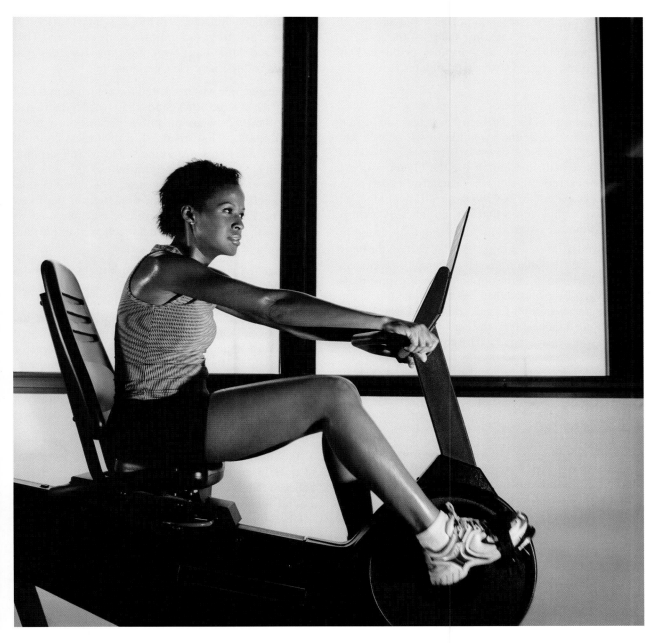

A woman burn calories on a stationary bicycle. *(© Jon Feingersh/Getty Images)*

read a book or watch TV. Stationary bicycles also add to the learning experience in elementary schools that implemented programs where students pedal exercise bikes and read books and magazines, or work on class assignments. In addition, bicyclists use exercise bicycles to train for events and to cycle when weather conditions prevent them from riding outdoors.

Pedaling a stationary bicycle is a nonweight-bearing exercise, one done when a person is not standing. The exercise strengthens muscles in the lower body in areas including the back, legs, and thighs. Exercising on a stationary bicycle is an aerobic workout that benefits the heart and lungs. Furthermore, the **calories** burned help with **weight loss**. Those benefits are increased when working out on a dual-action exercise bicycle; one that usually has moveable handlebars. The person grips the handlebars for an upper body, cardiovascular workout.

Some machines are equipped with a computer board that measures actions such as the calories burned, pedaling speed, and distance pedaled. This device is often referred to as an ergometer.

History

The concept of the stationary bicycle could be said to have come before the invention of the bicycle. On September 30,1796, inventor Francis Lowndes received a patent in London for the Gymanasticon, an indoor exercise machine. Sir Richard Phillips published that patent in a 1796 issue of *The Monthly* magazine, a publication that carried items of interest from around the world.

Lowndes' invention to exercise "all parts of the body at once" consisted of a frame large enough to contain a person. There was also the option to exercise some parts of the body. People used their feet to operate treadles in the Gymanasticon that turned cranks and wheels. The cranks were handheld, and the person could, talk, read, or write while exercising at a pace equal to "two or even ten miles" per hour, according to the patent. While designed for someone to stand for exercise "similar in its effect to **walking** or running", an unhealthy person could sit and exercise in the Gymanasticon.

Early bicycles

Standing was also the posture for using the *draisine*, the two-wheeled walking machine that German Baron Karl von Drais invented in 1817. Similar to a scooter, the *draisine* was the forerunner of the bicycle. When Kirkpartick Macmillan of Scotland put pedals on the *draisine* in 1839, he created the bicycle.

Modifications to the bicycle included the 1865 velocipede, also known as the boneshaker because it was made of wood. Later models were wood with metal tires. The public enjoyed riding velocipedes at indoor rinks called riding academies.

In 1866, French mechanic Pierre Lallemont, took out the first United States patent on bicycle with pedals. Although it is not clear who first invented the stationary bicycle, Exercycle company records showed the invention of that exercise machine in 1932.

The Exercycle

According the 1938 United State patent, New Yorker Howard J. Marlowe renewed the patent for his nonmotorized exercising machine. It was designed to exercise the muscles used when bicycling, horseback riding, and using a **rowing** machine. The 1940 patent granted to New York mechanical engineer Gordon Bergfors described improvements to Marlowes'

exercising machine to provide a greater variety of exercises. Bergfors also motorized the machine. That patent and later ones were filed by Bergfors and assigned to the Exercycle Corporation.

The machine was marketed for home use and sold during the 1930s, 1940, and 1950s. Sales increased during the 1960s when the public became more interested in fitness. That trend led to the fitness boom of the 1980s and 1990s, according to David St. Germain. He bought Exercycle Corporation in in 1993 and serves as president of Theracycle. The name change in 1996 reflected St. Germain's redesign of the Exercyle. The Thereacycle is an exercise machine used by people with movement disorders such as multiple sclerosis and Parkinson's disease.

Over the years, notables who bought Exercycles included Presidents Franklin Roosevelt, Dwight Eisenhower, Richard Nixon, John Kennedy, and Ronald Reagan. The Exercycle was shown in the 1988 movie *Working Girl*, and celebrities who used the exercise machine included the movie's director Mike Nichols, Barbra Streisand, John Wayne, and Jane Fonda.

Lifecycle

In 1968, America chemist Keene Dimick invented a stationary bicycle that he equipped with electronics to track his progress exercising. He and his wife Adele believed that bicycling could make people more fit and extend their lives, so they named his invention the Lifecycle.

The chemist planned to sell the Lifecycle to business people and invested a million dollars in that plan. He did not succeed and sold rights to the cycle to Ray Wilson around 1973. Sales were slow, so his partner Augie Nieto suggested they send free Lifecyles to 50 major health club owners and managers in the United States. The strategy worked and sales were brisk.

Schwinn

Partners Ignaz Schwinn and Adolph Arnold launched Schwinn in 1895 in Chicago. The company began manufacturing an upright exercise bike in 1967, and unveiled the Airdyne stationary bike in 1978. While resistance in stationary bicycles was created through the use of brake pads and a flywheel, the Airdyne featured air resistance generated by a fan installed in the exercise bike. In addition, the Aridyne provided an upper body workout because the pedals were connected to the handlebars.

Description

The headline in a 1960 *New York Times* advertisement proclaimed that "now millions can enjoy youthful **energy** after 35" by using the " Exercycle with Bergfors All Body-Action." According to the ad, some people seemed to lose "vim and vitality" after age 35, and one reason for that was that they lacked the right kind of exercise.

In the 21st century, people in almost every age group can ride stationary bicycles. Nonmotorized exercise bicycles are designed for riders as young as 2 years old. For youths and adults, the offerings include the traditional upright stationary bicycle and the recumbent stationary bicycle. The upright machine resembles a bicycle.

The recumbent stationary bicycle has a bucket-like seat that provides back support. The pedals are in front, and the person sits in a reclining (recumbent) position with legs extended to pedal. The seat is larger and may be more comfortable for some riders. Fully recumbent bicycles are completely reclined; semi-recumbent machines are partially reclined.

Although the knee motion range is the same as that of an upright bicycle, the direction of the recumbent machine causes less force on the knee joints. This could be helpful for people undergoing knee rehabilitation and those with knee and back problems.

Stationary bicycle features

Dual-action bicycles add upper body exercise to the lower body workout. Some upright and recumbent machines have an ergometer, a computer system that tracks information such as time, speed, distance pedaled, and calories burned. In addition some machines are equipped with a heart-rate monitor.

Resistance

The resistance mechanism on a stationary bicycle allows the person to adjust the resistance to the pedals in order to have a more intense workout. The types of resistance include the:

- flywheel. This is similar to the outdoor bicycle that a person pedals.
- manual tension is changed by adjusting a device on the bicycle.
- air resistance involves pedaling against the wind generated by a fan.
- magnetic resistance controlled by magnets is said to provide a smooth workout.

Stationary bicycle selections

The range of stationary bicycles included the following models, with list prices in September 2011.

EXERCISE BICYCLES FOR CHILDREN. Some upright models for preschoolers included educational features so that the children learned while they pedal. Offering included the Fisher-Price Smart Cycle Racer for ages 3 to 6. Priced at US$85, the stationary bicycle was also a learning center and an arcade game system.

The Redmon Happy Bike costing US$129.99 had an odometer that measured elements such as time, distance, and calories burned.

Furthermore, elementary school Kids Read and Ride programs rely on the donation of larger stationary bicycles. The exercise machines were placed in classrooms where students read books and magazines in class while exercising on the bikes.

UPRIGHT STATIONARY BICYCLES. Upright exercise bicycles included these models from Marcy, Schwinn, and Life Fitness:

- Marcy Upright Magnetic Resistance Bike ME710 priced at $459.99 had an adjustable seat and a computer screen that displayed speed, distance, time, and calories burned.
- Schwinn Airdyne Exercise Bike cost US$750. The dual-action machine could be used for a total workout or to separately exercise the lower body. The computer measured time, distance, calories, and resistance level, and could be set for different elevations.
- Life Fitness C1 upright Lifecycle priced at US$1,199 had contact heart-rate hand sensors, a water bottle holder, and reading rack. The price included the Basic Workout console. Settings included manual adjustment, the hill mode with hills and valleys that increased in difficulty, and a random setting that included combinations of hills and valleys.

RECUMBENT EXERCISE BICYCLES. Recumbent stationary bicycles included these models from Marcy, Schwinn, and Life Fitness:

- Marcy Magnetic Recumbent Bike costing US$499.99 and had an adjustable seat and a computer screen that displayed speed, distance, time and calories burned.
- Schwinn 220 Recumbent Bike priced at US$499 had feedback features include eight workout programs, six course profiles, a fitness test, and 16 resistance levels. The bicycle had a heart rate monitoring systems, holders for magazines, and an adjustable seat and handlebars.

- Life Fitness R1 recumbent Lifecycle costing US$1,399 had contact heart-rate hand sensors, a water bottle holder, and reading rack. The price included the Basic Workout console. Settings included manual adjustment, the hill mode with hills and valleys that increased in difficulty, and a random setting that included combinations of hills and valleys.

Benefits

A stationary bicycle is easy to use for nearly age group and is generally safe to use. The exercise bicycle provides a low-impact aerobic workout for the healthy as well as people with conditions such as back or joint pain. Pedaling an exercise bike strengthens muscles in the legs and glutes; it is also beneficial to the heart and lungs. A dual-action machine adds to the upper body workout.

In addition to those benefits, riding an exercise bike burns calories and should lead to weight loss. The amount of calories burned depends on factors such as the person's weight and how fast the individual pedals. Someone who weighs 150 lb. (68 kg) will burn 250 calories when pedaling at a moderate rate for 30 minutes. At a brisk pace, the person burns 375 calories.

In addition, school Kids Read and Ride programs make learning fun while giving children the opportunity to exercise.

Risks

Home stationary bicycles are usually not stored, and parents need to be aware that young children may climb on them and fall. In addition, care should be taken with youngsters and child-sized bikes because some cycle parts could pose a choking hazard.

For older riders, stationary bicycles are generally safe. However, it is important to consult with a doctor before beginning any exercise program. This is especially important for people who are obese or have conditions including **hypertension** and cardiocirculatory problems. The medical professional can help to establish a safe program for using an exercise bike.

Resources

WEBSITES

American College of Sports Medicine "Selecting and Effectively Using A Stationary Bicycle." ACSM.org. http://www.acsm.org/AM/Template.cfm?Section = brochures 2&Template = /CM/ContentDisplay.cfm&ContentID = 8108 (accessed September 15, 2011).

"Exercise Equipment." *Consumer Reports* 74, no. 2 (February 2009): 33–37.

Kids Read and Ride Program. http://www.kidsreadandride.com/index.html (accessed September 15, 2011).

"Life Fitness: a history of innovation." *The Journal on Active Aging* 14, no. 6 (March April 2002): 40–42. http://www.icaa.cc/1-Organizationalmember/member-articles/lifesfitness2.pdf (accessed September 15, 2011).

Liz Swain

Step aerobics

Definition

Step aerobics is an aerobic **exercise** that is performed by stepping onto and off of an elevated platform while doing upper body movements. Also known as step training, the choreographed moves are done as a moderate to high-intensity cardiovascular workout.

Purpose

The word aerobic means "with air," and aerobic exercises consist of movements of a specific intensity that are done for a specific amount of time. The intensity and time exercising force the heart and lungs to work harder. The aerobic workout requires more oxygen than is present in the body. As the lungs take in more oxygen from the air, the heart rate increases and breathing becomes more rapid. Aerobic exercises also burn fat.

Aerobic activities involve the repetitive movements of large muscles including those in the legs. The activity level varies from the moderate to high intensity pace. During a moderate-intensity exercise such as **walking** briskly; the person sweats, breathing increases, and the heart rate increases. The person is able to converse while exercising. Higher intensity exercises include jogging and **running**.

Step aerobics is described as low impact in terms of stress on the body because one foot is always on the ground. Other aerobic exercise workouts may have been low intensity, but the activities placed stress on the knees. The step workout involves repeatedly stepping onto and off of a platform for a

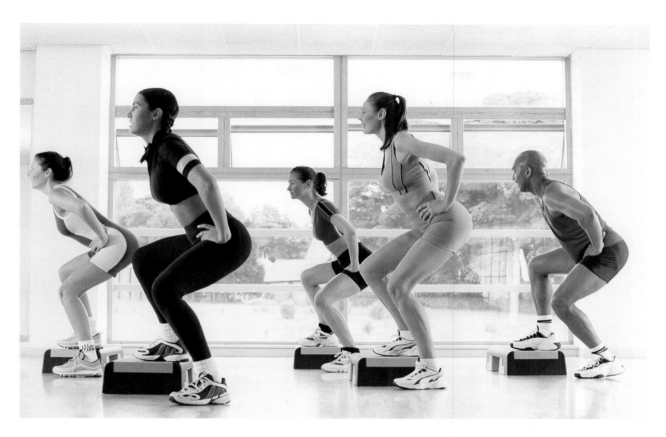

A group doing lateral lunges during a step aerobics class. (© *Stockbyte/Jupiterimages*)

cardiovascular workout. Methods of changing the intensity level of the workout level include increasing the height of the platform. Adjustable equipment allows people to work at the beginner level at 4 in. (10.16 cm) height, an advanced level at 8-in. (20.32 cm) height, and more advanced heights of 10 (25.4) to 12 in. (30.48 cm).

Demographics

During the 1990s, step aerobics was one of the most popular forms of exercise in the United states, according to publications including the *Boston Globe*. A February 8, 1993 headline in the Massachusetts newspaper declared, "In just 7 years, step aerobics has conquered the fitness industry."

While other aerobics classes consisted primarily of women, there was an increase in male enrollment for step training classes, according to an August 17,1990 *Chicago Tribune* article. Health club director Lisa Faremouth told reporter Steve Dole that men considered step aerobics to be "less dancey" than other **dance** exercise classes. They also appreciated the "tough workout."

By September 2011, there were step aerobic classes and workout materials like DVDs for adults and children. Aerobics is in the category of vigorous intensity exercises recommended for adolescents by the United States Centers for Disease Control and Prevention. (CDC)

History

Step aerobics resulted from some 20th Century fitness concepts and an injured knee. American Gin Miller, who is credited with developing step training, pointed out on her website that coaches trained athletes by having them run up and down stadium stairs.

During World War II, Harvard University developed a fitness test that involved the test subject stepping on and off of a 20. in. (50.8 cm) tall bench. The Harvard Step Test required the person to step 30 times for a minute, with the subject tested for from one to three minutes. The person's resting pulse rate was taken before the test and measured again after the test.

In 1968, American Kenneth Cooper, MD, MPH; introduced the world to a new exercise concept with his bestselling book, *Aerobics*. Cooper coined the word

DENISE AUSTIN (1957–)

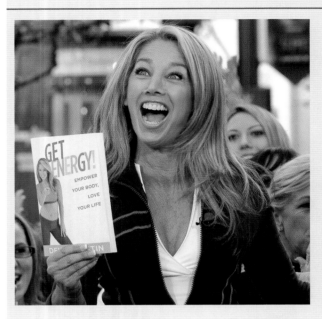

(© Noel Vasquez/Getty Images)

Born February 13, 1957, Denise Austin is one of the most visible fitness gurus in the United States. As the former resident fitness advisor on the "Today" show, the host of several top-rated daily workout television programs, and the creator of countless exercise videos, Austin has appeared on the television screens of millions. Athletics run in Austin's family. Her father was a pitcher for the St. Louis Browns major league baseball team in the 1940s, and her mother was once the New York State champion in jump roping. So it was no surprise when Austin showed an aptitude for gymnastics as a child. She competed internationally in her teens and was ranked in the top ten in the United States by the National Collegiate Athletic Association (NCAA) in 1976. After graduating from college (which she attended on a gymnastics scholarship), she founded her own fitness company that designed exercise programs for workplaces and health clubs. The company was so successful that Austin had to hire some of her friends to help her out; after Austin was discovered by television fitness show host Jack LaLanne and hired by him as a cohost, launching her media career, Austin gave the company to her friends completely.

In her books and videos, Austin "gives the basic commonsense advice we all need to hear: fad diets don't work, and successful weight loss means cutting calories and increasing exercise," Los Angeles Times reviewer Jane E. Allen wrote, referring specifically to Lose Those Last 10 Pounds: The 28–Day Foolproof Plan to a Healthy Body.

aerobics and advocated for the relationship between cardiovascular fitness and health and longevity.

Step therapy

An injured knee in 1986 led aerobics instructor Gin Miller to develop step training. A physical therapist advised her to step up and down on a milk crate to strengthen her knee muscles. She didn't have a crate, so Miller used the porch step at her Georgia home. When the repetitions became boring, she put some aerobic music on the stereo. While stepping to the music, Miller was inspired to create an exercise form that repeatedly lifted the body's weight.

She wanted to share the workout with others and had a bench built around the perimeter of the aerobics room at Gold's Gym in Marietta. The step exercises were so popular that the bench was cut into smaller pieces so more people could do the step workout.

Miller's efforts to market the training led her to Reebok in 1989. That year, the footwear company created the Step Reebok shoe, and Miller created programming and trained instructors for the Step Reebok program. She also served with other fitness professionals on the National Step Reebok Training program.

Early workouts sometimes involved holding hand weights while stepping. That practice was discontinued because of the possible risk of injuring the shoulder and elbow joints, Miller wrote on her website. Instead, **weightlifting** was incorporated in another way. In 1991, the Step Reebok Circuit Workout was unveiled. Workouts alternated between step training and weight training.

As of September 2011, Miller continued to head a business that sells her instructional DVDs and equipment for step training and other activities.

Description

Step aerobic routines are easy to learn for most people, and workouts are designed for a range of fitness levels. Step aerobics are usually done to music that ranges from 120 to 127 beats per minute, and the goal of the workout is to exercise within the target heart range for a certain amount of time. The **target heart rate** is the rate that the heart should pump during exercise to achieve the maximum cardiovascular benefit. The rate is based on a percentage of the maximum heart rate, a figure based on factors including **age** and fitness level.

Since platform height contributes to the exercise intensity, beginners should start with a 4 in. (10.16 cm) platform. The 8 in. (20.32 cm) platform is recommended for the intermediate level and is used by someone who is fit and has done step training for eight weeks. The 10 in. (25.4) platform is for the advanced stepper, and the 12 in. (30.48 cm) platform is used by an athlete who is tall, very fit, and proficient at stepping. The workout starts with a **warm-up** and ends with a cool-down.

Before beginning the exercises, the body should be aligned so that the shoulders are relaxed, the pelvis is slightly tilted, and the knees are slightly bent. Steps are done with the feet pointing forward. When stepping, the entire foot lands on the surface; landing on the heel could result in pain or injury. The person steps on to the center of the platform, and all of the foot is on the platform.

Step patterns

Step patterns include the:

- basic right and left. The basic right starts with the person stepping onto the platform with the right foot, and then brings the left foot. The person then steps down with the right, and then the left. For the basic left, the pattern starts with the left foot.
- alternating knee lift. The person steps onto the platform with the right foot. The left leg is raised to form a 90-degree angle with the knee. The left leg is lowered to the floor. The right foot is returned to the floor, and the left foot steps onto the platform. The right leg is raised to form a 90-degree angle with the knee, and then the foot is lowered to the floor.
- biceps curl. This pattern that could be done with the basic right, basic left, or alternating knee lift step patterns. The pattern starts with arms straight and hands clenched in fists. The elbows bend as the arms are curled towards the chest when the foot is on the platform. The arms are straightened when both feet are on the platform. Arms are curled as the first foot steps down, and curled when both feet are on the floor.

Preparation

Before beginning a step aerobics program, people should consult with their doctors to make sure that they are healthy enough for this type of exercise. This is especially important for women who are pregnant. Aerobic shoes should be worn, and step aerobics should not be done when a person is barefooted. For those who want to work out at home, the next step is

usually the purchase of a platform and acquiring a workout DVD or book with instructions. Before buying a book or DVD, it could be worthwhile to check these materials out at the library or rent the DVD.

Aerobic shoes

The American Academy of Podiatric Sports Medicine (APSMA) recommends aerobic shoes that provide enough cushioning and shock absorption to compensate for the pressure on the foot that much greater than that done when walking. That impact affects the 26 bones in each foot, according to the APSMA.

The shoes should provide stability for side-to-side motion and an arch design that compensates for those forces. In addition, a "sufficiently thick" upper leather or strap support provides good medial-lateral (side-to-side) stability. The shoe should also have a toe box high enough to prevent irritation of the toes and nails, according to the APSMA.

Step platforms

Step platforms are usually rectangular and made of hard plastic. Some platforms have a slip-resistant surface made of a material like rubber. The equipment may have risers that are used to adjust the platform height. The scope of platforms sold in September 2011 included the:

- Reebok Incline Step with DVD. Priced at US$79.99, the three-in-one platform consisted of a flat step for a basic step workout, an incline step for balance training for increased muscular activity, and a flat-to-incline bench for use as an all-in-one strength and core-conditioning tool.
- Stamina Aerobic Step. Sold for US$70, the platform came with a DVD and could be adjusted for 4-in. (10.16 cm) and 6-in (15.24 cm) levels. It could be used flat or at an incline.
- The Step Original Health Club Step Aerobic Trainer. The platform marketed by The Step was priced at US$109.99 and adjusted to 4-in. (10.16 cm), 6-in (15.24 cm), and 8-in. (20.32 cm) heights.

Step training DVDs

Step aerobic DVDs include numerous Gin Miller titles and DVDs featuring other instructors. In September 2011, the DVDs included:

- Gin Miller titles sold on her website. These included *Simply Step Classic Moves*, *Step Aerobic Extreme Step*, and *Step Reebok The Power Workout*. Each sold for US$19.95.

- Shapely Girl: *Let's Get Stepping with Debra Mazda: Beginner Step Cardio Workout*. Priced at US$19.99, the DVD is part of the ShapleyGirl DVD series. The DVD includes a bonus toning track and step tutorial.
- *Step and Tone Workout*. Fitness expert Gilad Janklowicz leads a workout that involves stepping and light hand weights to combine fat burning and toning in the DVD that cost US$14.95.

Risks

Step aerobics is not suitable for all people. Once the doctor clears a person for step training, it is important to do the steps properly and avoid hyperextending the knee. In addition, people should pace themselves when they are doing step aerobics in a class or at home. The instructor and others in the class or on the DVD may be more physically fit or younger, so it is not necessary or safe to try to keep up with them.

Moreover, pregnant women should use caution when doing step aerobics. They should not exercise until they feel exhausted.

Results

Step aerobics provides the health benefits of an aerobic workout without the adverse affects of that high-impact that acitivity. Stepping benefits the heart and lungs while burning **calories**. In addtion, step training shapes and tones DQ-upper and lower body muscles, especially those in the buttocks, thighs, and legs.

Resources

BOOKS

Webb, Tamilee. *Tamilee Webb's Step Up Fitness Workout.* New York: Workman Publishing, 1995.

WEBSITES

American Orthopaedic Foot and Ankle Society. "Shoes." AAOS.org.http://orthoinfo.aaos.org/topic.cfm?topic = a00143 (accessed September 21, 2011).

Miller, Gin. "Step Training History, Evolution & Guidelines." GinMiller.comhttp://www.ginmiller.com/gmf06/instructor/step_history/introduction.html (accessed September 21, 2011)

ORGANIZATIONS

American Council on Exercise, 4851 Paramount Drive, San Diego , CA, 92123-1449, (858) 576-6500, Fax: (858) 576-6564, support@acefitness.org, http://www.acefitness.org/.

Liz Swain

Steroids *see* **Anabolic steroids and anabolic steroid use; Performance-enhancing drugs**

Stomach exercises *see* **Core training**

Strain *see* **Muscle strain**

Stress fracture *see* **Fracture**

Stretching

Definition

Stretching involves extending the limbs, lengthening and relaxing muscles, and moving joints through their range of motion, to maintain and improve muscle and joint flexibility.

Purpose

Stretching can improve flexibility, ease movement, and relieve muscle tension. It may improve posture, balance, coordination, strength, and physical performance, and increase blood flow to muscles. Regular stretching may lengthen muscle fibers so that they contract more vigorously during **exercise**. It can relax muscles and may help prevent soreness or stiffness. Some researchers believe that muscle cramps may be caused by inadequate stretching that leads to abnormalities in the control of muscle contraction. Stretching can help joints move through their full range of motion, improving biomechanics and athletic performance, reduce **fatigue**, and help prevent overuse injuries.

For many people, stretching is an enjoyable activity that can be performed anywhere at any time. It can be a pleasant way to begin and conclude a workout. Stretching can also relax muscles that are contracted due to emotional tension and stress, especially back and neck muscles. Chronically tensed muscles are a risk factor for pain and injury. Gentle stretching can also relax the mind.

Description

Stretching can be either dynamic, involving smooth, gentle movements, or sustained or static—holding a stretch without moving. Dynamic stretching should follow a **warm-up** and static stretching should follow a **cool down**. Stretching also can be performed as an independent routine or incorporated into exercise. Stretching is an integral part of practices such as **yoga**, **Pilates**, and tai chi. A muscle-stretching floor program, called body sculpting, is sometimes part of aerobic workouts. Stretching routines may involve a rope or strap, a partner, or a machine.

Stretching is usually directed at major muscle groups—the calves, thighs (hamstrings and quadriceps), hips, lower, middle, and upper back, arms (biceps, triceps, and forearms), shoulders (deltoids and rotator cuffs), and neck—as well as other muscles and joints that are used regularly. Stretching should always be balanced, with the right and left sides stretched for the same amount of time. Stretching should be performed regularly—at least two or three times per week—since any benefits are quickly lost if it is discontinued.

Stretches appear to be most beneficial if they are sport- or activity-specific, focusing on the muscles used in the activity. For example, **soccer** players are more at risk for hamstring sprains, so stretching should focus on the hamstrings—the muscles of the back of the thigh. **Baseball** players might focus on shoulder stretches for throwing or forearm stretches for batting. Activity-specific movements, such as a front kick in **martial arts**, can be performed slowly, at low-intensity, and gradually speeded up over the course of a warm-up.

Dynamic stretches

Dynamic stretches help prepare the body for an active workout or competition. They are slow, controlled movements that can be as simple as arm circles, hip rotations, **walking** or jogging exercises, or yoga movements. Dynamic stretches generally include several repetitions of about 30 seconds each, performed at a comfortable pace:

- Sun salutations are yoga movements that stretch various body parts.
- The yoga pose downward-facing dog can be made dynamic by lifting alternate legs or pedaling the feet.
- Knee lifts or high-knee walking or jogging flex the hips and shoulders and stretch the gluteus muscles

(glutes), quadriceps (quads), and lower back. They can include spinal twists.
- Butt-kicks can be combined with walking, jogging, or running to stretch the quads and hip flexors.
- Walking with straight-leg kicks (goose-step marching) stretches the hamstrings, glutes, calves, and lower back.
- Walking lunges or walking with high-knee lunges stretches the glutes, hamstrings, hip flexors, and calves.
- Walking side lunges stretch the groin, glutes, hamstrings, and ankles.
- Running carioca steps—crossing the legs in front of each other by twisting the hips, with the shoulders square—stretches the ankles, abductors, adductors, glutes, and hips.
- Back pedalling—short choppy steps followed by open strides with kick-backs—stretches the hip flexors, quads, and calves.
- Scorpions—kicking the feet toward the opposite outstretched arms while lying facedown—stretch the quads, hip flexors, glutes, lower back, abdominals, and shoulders.
- Hand-walking stretches the shoulders, core, and hamstrings.
- Side bends stretch the triceps, upper back, abdominals, and obliques.

There are many sport-specific dynamic stretches. Runners often perform squats, lunges, and buttock kicks. Sports that require moving rapidly in different directions, such as soccer, tennis, and **basketball**, use dynamic stretches such as the spider-man—crawling on the hands and feet as if climbing a wall.

Static stretches

Total body static stretches should be performed for four to six minutes after a workout or competition, to lengthen muscles and increase flexibility. Each stretch should be performed slowly and steadily, held for about 30 seconds without bouncing, and repeated three or four times:

- back of the calf—leaning into a support and extending the back leg with the heel pressed down
- standing and seated hamstring stretches
- quadriceps—pulling the foot toward the buttocks
- inner thighs, hips, and groin—seated with heels together in front or cross-legged and pushing down the inner thighs
- hip flexors and groin—one knee on the floor and other leg forward and bent at the knee and the hips lowered or forward

- iliotibial band (ITB)—standing with one leg crossed over the other at the ankle and reaching overhead with the arm
- lower back—flattening the lower back to the floor or knee-to-chest
- upper back—pulling the shoulder blades together or pushing the arms up and back with the fingers interlaced
- triceps—with the arms overhead, pulling a bent elbow up and behind the head
- rotator cuff—stretching one arm across the body with the other arm
- internal shoulder rotators—grasping a towel with one hand behind the back and the other overhead, pulling the top hand toward the ceiling
- neck—pulling the head gently toward the shoulder

PNF and rope stretching

Proprioceptive neuromuscular facilitation (PNF) was developed in the 1940s and 1950s as physical therapy for paralysis. During the 1980s, sports therapists and trainers adapted some of its techniques for increasing range of motion. PNF stretching combines passive and active stretches. Both isometric muscle contraction ("hold") and concentric muscle contraction ("contract"), followed immediately by a passive stretch, facilitate a reflex relaxation called autogenic inhibition. Reciprocal inhibition is a reflex relaxation or stretching in the muscle opposing the muscle that is stimulated.

Three PNF stretches for the hamstrings illustrate these principles. Each stretch begins by lying on the back with one leg on the floor and the other extended straight up. A partner moves the extended leg to the point of mild discomfort and holds it in a passive stretch for ten seconds before one of the following stretches:

- For hold-relax, the hamstrings are contracted isometrically by pushing against the partner's hand for six seconds, then relaxed back to the passive stretch for 30 seconds. With the next stretch, the leg should move farther because of greater hip flexion due to autogenic inhibition in the hamstrings.
- For contract-relax, the hamstrings are contracted concentrically by pushing against the partner's hand, as the leg is pushed to the floor through its full range of motion, followed by a 30-second passive stretch. Again, the leg should be able to move farther due to autogenic inhibition.
- For hold-relax with opposing muscle contraction, the hamstrings are contracted isometrically, with the partner applying enough force that the leg

remains static for six seconds, to initiate autogenic inhibition. For the 30-second passive stretch, the hip is flexed to pull the leg in the same direction that it is being pushed, initiating reciprocal inhibition, and again enabling the leg to move further.

Rope stretching is similar to PNF stretching but with a rope instead of a partner. Like PNF, active isolated stretching (AIS) is based on the theory that working one muscle group, such as the biceps, relaxes and lengthens the opposing muscle group, in this case the triceps. Each active stretch lasts only a few seconds and is repeated about ten times. Although special stretching ropes are available, a jump rope or dog leash is also suitable.

Precautions

Proper stretching technique is extremely important. Incorrect stretching is not only ineffective, it may cause injury. Muscles must be warmed up—cold muscles should never be stretched. Stretching cold muscles can directly contribute to pulled and torn muscles. Movements also must always be carefully controlled.

Dynamic stretches can be performed before a workout, since they do not illicit an inhibitory reaction. However they should not cause pre-workout fatigue.

Static stretching should only be performed after exercise because it elicits a neuromuscular inhibitory response that can last up to 30 minutes and decrease muscle strength by as much as 30%. Stretches should be performed slowly and gently, with deep relaxed breathing to prevent muscle tension. Stretches should never be forced and should never cause pain. Most stretches should be held for ten to 30 seconds. Holding them for less time will not sufficiently lengthen muscle. Static stretching should always be sustained rather than ballistic (bouncing or bobbing). Bouncing can cause small muscle tears that leave scar tissue, further tightening muscles, decreasing flexibility, and potentially causing pain. Stretching does not speed the removal of waste products from muscles, as is sometimes claimed. Some proponents of active stretching, such as PNF or AIS, argue that static stretching cuts off blood flow to muscle and provokes a protective reflex.

PNF stretching is not recommended for anyone under age 18. Only one PNF exercise should be performed on a muscle group in a single session and there should be at least 48 hours between sessions. PNF stretching should not be performed on the day of a competition.

Some traditional stretches, such as the hurdler's stretch and the yoga plow, are now considered ill-advised because they put excessive pressure on the knees and back, respectively. Other stretches should

KEY TERMS

Active isolated stretching (AIS)—A stretching technique that relaxes and lengthens a muscle group by working the opposing group, usually with a rope or strap.

Adductor—Any of the three strong triangular muscles of the inside of the thigh.

Autogenic inhibition—Reflex relaxation that occurs when a passive stretch immediately follows an isometric or concentric muscle contraction; used for PNF stretching.

Biceps—The large flexor muscle of the front of the upper arm.

Concentric contraction—Muscle contraction in which the muscles shorten while generating force, as when lifting a weight.

Deltoid—The large triangular muscle that covers the shoulder joint and laterally raises the arm.

Dynamic stretching—Stretching with smooth, gentle. continuous movements.

Glutes, glutei—The three muscles of each buttock, especially the outermost gluteus maximus that extends and laterally rotates the thigh.

Hamstrings—The three muscles at the back of the thigh that flex and rotate the leg and extend the thigh.

Hip flexors—The group of muscles that flex the thigh bone toward the pelvis to pull the knee up.

Iliotibial band (ITB)—The fibrous tissue along the outside of the hip, thigh, and knee that stabilizes the knee and helps to flex and extend the knee, and is a common problem for runners and other athletes.

Isometric—Muscular contraction against resistance without significant change in muscle fiber length.

Obliques—The two flat muscles on each side that form the middle and outer layers of the lateral walls of the abdomen.

Proprioceptive muscular facilitation (PNF)—A type of stretching with a partner designed to increase range of motion; used by occupational and physical therapists, chiropractors, and sports therapists and trainers.

Quadriceps—The large muscle of the front of the thigh.

Reciprocal inhibition—Reflex relaxation or stretching in the muscle opposing the tensed muscle.

Rotator cuff—A supporting and strengthening structure of the shoulder joint.

Static stretching—Sustained stretching of muscles without movement.

Sun salutations—Total body yoga warm-up exercises.

T'ai chi—An ancient Chinese discipline involving controlled movements specifically designed to improve physical and mental well-being.

Triceps—The muscle of the back of the arm.

not be performed by people with certain medical conditions. For example, knee-to-chest stretches should not be performed by anyone with **osteoporosis**, since it can increase the risk of compression fractures of the vertebrae.

Preparation

The most important preparation for stretching is warming up for five–ten minutes, since stretching cold muscles can cause injury. The warm-up may be brisk walking, light jogging, cycling, **jumping rope**, or other total body movements. The warm-up increases blood flow to muscles, raises their temperature, increases the elasticity of muscle fibers, and lubricates joints. Loosening up the knees is particularly important. PNF stretching should be preceded by a five-to-ten-minute light aerobic warm-up and dynamic stretches.

Aftercare

Static stretching should only be performed after workouts. No other aftercare is usually required.

Complications

Stretching may cause further injury, for example, to a strained muscle. People with chronic medical conditions or injuries should consult their physician or physical therapist about stretching techniques or adaptations.

Results

Stretching may be beneficial. For example, one study of a static reach-and-hold hamstring stretch found that stretching every day for four weeks increased hamstring flexibility by about 20 degrees. Continuing to stretch two or three days a week for another four weeks added another four degrees, whereas not continuing to stretch led to a loss of seven degrees of flexibility. However other studies have shown no benefit and the static stretching remains controversial.

Although dynamic stretching before a workout is generally believed to increase power, flexibility, and range of motion, it is unclear whether it helps prevent injury. A 2011 study found that stretching before **running** neither caused nor prevented injury. However changing one's routine—starting to stretch or giving up stretching before a run—put runners at risk for injury. This was especially true for those who were used to stretching before a run and gave it up.

Resources

BOOKS

Anderson, Bob, and Jean Anderson. *Stretching*. 30th anniversary ed. Bolinas, CA: Shelter, 2010.

Armiger, Phil. *Stretching for Functional Flexibility*. Philadelphia: Wolters Kluwer Health/Lippincott, Williams, & Wilkins, 2010.

Bakewell, Lisa. *Fitness Information for Teens*. 2nd ed. Detroit, MI: Omnigraphics, 2009.

Berg, Kristian. *Prescriptive Stretching*. Champaign, IL: Human Kinetics, 2011.

Blahnik, Jay. *Full-Body Flexibility*. 2nd ed. Champaign, IL: Human Kinetics, 2011.

Haas, Jacqui Greene. *Dance Anatomy*. Champaign, IL: Human Kinetics, 2010.

Martin, Suzanne. *15 Minute Stretching Workout*. New York: DK, 2010.

PERIODICALS

Dawson-Cook, Susan. "How's Your Posture? Identifying and Remediating Common Postural Anomalies." *American Fitness* 29, no. 3 (May/June 2011): 24–29.

Halverson, Ryan. "Flexibility Differences Among Men and Women." *IDEA Fitness Journal* 8, no. 6 (June 2011): 15.

Perrier, Erica T., et al. "The Acute Effects of a Warm-Up Including Static or Dynamic Stretching on Countermovement Jump Height, Reaction Time, and Flexibility." *Journal of Strength and Conditioning Research* 25, no. 7 (July 2011): 1925–31.

Puentedura, Emilio J., et al. "Immediate Effects of Quantified Hamstring Stretching: Hold-Relax Proprioceptive Neuromuscular Facilitation Versus Static Stretching." *Physical Therapy in Sport* 12, no. 3 (August 2011): 122–26.

Rancour, Jessica, Clayton F. Holmes, and Daniel J. Cipriani. "The Effects of Intermittent Stretching Following a 4-Week Static Stretching Protocol: A Randomized Trial." *Journal of Strength and Conditioning Research* 23, no. 8 (November 2009): 2217–22.

Trotter, Kathleen. "Flexibility: Never Underestimate the Value of a Good Stretch! These Four Moves Will Help Keep Injuries Away, Relax Your Mind and Soothe Sore Muscles." *Chatelaine* (May 2011): 88.

WEBSITES

American Academy of Orthopaedic Surgeons. "Warm Up, Cool Down and Be Flexible." Your Orthopaedic Connection. http://orthoinfo.aaos.org/topic.cfm?topic=A00310 (accessed August 28, 2011).

Bain, Julie. "New Ideas on Proper Stretching Techniques." WebMD Feature. October 25, 2010. http://www.webmd.com/fitness-exercise/features/new-ideas-on-proper-stretching-techniques (accessed September 1, 2011).

Douglas, Scott. "Peace Through Strength." *Running Times* (September 2011): 46–50. http://www.whartonperformance.com/assets/Running%20Times.pdf (accessed August 28, 2011).

Mayo Clinic Staff. "Stretching: Focus on Flexibility." Mayo Clinic. February 23, 2011. http://www.mayoclinic.com/health/stretching/HQ01447 (accessed August 28, 2011).

McHugh, M.P., and C.H. Cosgrove. "To Stretch or Not to Stretch: The Role of Stretching in Injury Prevention and Performance." *Scandinavian Journal of Medicine and Science in Sports* 20, no. 2 (April 2010): 169–81. http://onlinelibrary.wiley.com/doi/10.1111/j.1600-0838.2009.01058.x/full (accessed August 30, 2011).

"PNF Stretching." Sports Fitness Advisor. http://www.sport-fitness-advisor.com/pnfstretching.html (accessed August 28, 2011).

Reynolds, Gretchen. "Stretching: The Truth." *New York Times*. October 31, 2008. http://www.nytimes.com/2008/11/02/sports/playmagazine/112pewarm.html (accessed September 1, 2011).

"Stretching." TeensHealth. April 2009. http://kidshealth.org/teen/food_fitness/exercise/stretching.html# (accessed August 28, 2011).

"Stretching Before a Run Does Not Prevent Injury." American Academy of Orthopaedic Surgeons. February 17, 2011. http://www6.aaos.org/news/pemr/releases/release.cfm?releasenum=974 (accessed August 28, 2011).

ORGANIZATIONS

American Academy of Orthopaedic Surgeons, 6300 North River Road, Rosemont, IL, 60018-4262, (847) 823-7186, Fax: (847) 823-8125, orthoinfo@aaos.org, http://www.aaos.org.

The AAOS provides musculoskeletal education to orthopaedic surgeons and others throughout the world.

It supports various medical and scientific publications and publishes consumer information.

American Orthopaedic Society for Sports Medicine, 6300 North River Road, Suite 500, Rosemont, IL, 60018, (847) 292-4900, Fax: (847) 292-4905, (877) 321-3500, info@aossm.org, http://www.sportsmed.org.

The AOSSM provides a forum for education and scientific research for sports medicine professionals. It is primarily concerned with the effects and impacts of exercise on people of all ages, abilities, and fitness levels.

Margaret Alic, PhD

Sudden cardiac death related to exercise or sport

Definition

Sudden cardiac death (SCD) related to **exercise** or sports is generally defined as sudden cardiac death occurring during or within one hour of exercise or sport participation.

Description

Sudden cardiac death related to sport or exercise means that the exerciser suffers a cardiac arrest during exercise/sport, or within one hour of stopping. While sometimes the SCD is due to a known cause, or a trauma, often times, the cardiac arrest is completely unexpected in an athlete who was presumably healthy and fit. Sometimes there are warning signs and symptoms leading up to the cardiac arrest, such as syncope during or after exertion, but often times, the athlete was performing his sport seemingly without symptoms or issues.

Demographics

Sudden cardiac death during exercise or sports is uncommon. Specifically, in US high- school and college athletes (age 12-24 years), the incidence of SCD has been found to be 0.5/100 000 participants per year. However, because there is not a mandatory, national registry for recording all deaths related to sport and exercise, this number may be underestimated.

Statistics re: sudden death related to exercise and sport vary with the sub-group studied. A recent study of NCAA college athletes suggests that the highest rates of SCD occur in **basketball** and **football**. At the high school level, there appears to be a higher rate of SCD in football, basketball, **baseball**, **lacrosse**, and **soccer**. For athletes older than 35 years, sudden death is most commonly related to **running**, rather than sports participation.

Sport-related SCD is more common in men than women, which partially reflects the greater rate of sport participation in men. It is more common in African Americans than Caucasians.

Causes and symptoms

The most common etiologies of sport/exercise-related sudden cardiac death vary by age. Older athletes (typically defined as older than 35 years) are most likely to suffer cardiac arrest as a result of unsuspected coronary artery atherosclerosis. In this case, the athlete may have a positive family history for pre-mature heart disease, or other cardiac risk factors, such as high **cholesterol**, high **blood pressure**, diabetes, **obesity**, or a smoking history. Older individuals with known or unknown atherosclerosis performing higher intensity exercise they are not accustomed to, particularly in extreme environments, such as snow shoveling, may have a particularly high risk. The older athlete/exerciser may have warning signs and symptoms, such as chest tightness with exertion, feeling out of breath, or as if they are going to pass out, or may be asymptomatic leading up to the arrest.

For athletes younger than 35 years of age, non-traumatic sudden cardiac death is usually a result of congenital or acquired cardiac disturbance. The most common causes of non-traumatic sudden cardiac death in the United States are:

• hypertrophic cardiomyopathy
• dilated cardiomyopathy
• right ventricular cardiomyopathy
• myocarditis
• abnormalities of the heart's electrical conduction system (i.e., ion channelopathies (long-QT syndrome, catecholaminergic polymorphic ventricular tachycardia, and Brugada syndrome) Wolff-Parkinson White)
• coronary anomaly
• Marfan's syndrome

Regardless of underlying pathology, the cause of SCD is typically a sudden lethal arrhythmia, though in the case of Marfan's syndrome, the cause of death may be sudden dissection of the aorta.

Sudden cardiac arrest in younger athletes can also be caused by commotio cordis. Commotio cordis is when a blunt trauma to the chest, such as that caused by a baseball, hockey puck, or lacrosse ball, strikes the chest at an electrically vulnerable period, causing sudden ventricular fibrillation or another dangerous

AED—Automatic external defibrillator.

Arrhythmia—Irregular, abnormal heart rhythm.

Atherosclerosis—Narrowing of arteries due to plaque build up.

Athlete's heart—An enlarged heart due to chronic exercise training that is physiological (normal), not pathological.

Brugada's syndrome—Inherited heart condition that results in an arrhythmia.

Cardiac arrest—Sudden death due to lack of heart beat.

Commotio cordis—Non-penetrating blow to the chest that interrupts a heart beat and causes sudden cardiac death or other serious heart arrhythmia.

Coronary anomaly—Congenital anatomical abnormality in coronary arteries.

Dilated cardiomyopathy—Enlarged, floppy weak heart that does not pump blood effectively and can be due to many different causes, including a virus.

Echocardiogram—Ultra sound examination of the heart that provides information about the heart's chambers and valves.

EKG—Test that examines the electrical conduction of the heart.

Hypertrophic cardiomyopathy (HCM)—Pathological, excessive thickening of the heart muscle and the most common cause of sudden death in American athletes.

Hyponatremia—Low sodium level often due to excessive sweating and replacement of fluid with water rather than a sodium-containing solution.

Marfan's syndrome—Genetic connective tissue disorder that increases risk of sudden death by dissection of the aorta.

Myocarditis—Inflammation of the heart muscle usually due to viral or bacteria infection.

NSAIDS—Non-steroidal anti-inflammatory drugs.

Platelet activation—Blood clotting.

Syncope—partial or complete loss of consciousness.

Ventricular tachycardia—Abnormal, rapid heart beat.

Ventricular fibrillation—Severely abnormal heart arrhythmia that will result in death without prompt treatment.

Wolff Parkinson White—Abnormal electrical conduction of heart's signal to beat which can increase the risk of developing an arrhythmia.

---

arrhythmia. The tragedy here is that these athletes have normal hearts, and are simply "in the wrong place at the wrong time."

Recently, another sub-group of exercise-related deaths has been making headlines. Anecdotally, it appears that there is an increase in sudden cardiac death related to (running) races, particularly those of a 10k distance or greater. It is unclear whether there is an actual increase in deaths, or whether the increase simply reflects better tracking. Assuming the death rate has indeed increased, one likely explanation is the "mainstreaming" of marathons and other races, meaning less fit, older, and potentially less healthy individuals are participating.

There remains a possibility that even healthy runners are at greater risk during or immediately following a challenging race. The prevailing theory is that the musculoskeletal trauma of running and other types of endurance exercise release muscle enzymes, which may activate platelets and produce a thrombus (blood clot), inducing cardiac ischemia (lack of oxygen) and subsequently, an arrhythmia.

Thus, the guidelines recently issued by the International **Marathon** Medical Directors Association suggests a baby aspirin the morning of a training run or race of 10k distance or greater. Their full recommendations for runners of 10 k distances or greater are:

- take a baby aspirin the morning of the training run/race

- avoid NSAIDS before or during a race

- drink sports drinks instead of plain water (for thirst) during and after the run/race to avoid hyponatremia

- avoid sprinting at the end of the race unless they have trained this way

- avoid attempting a distance they are not prepared to do

- have a yearly physical in which they discuss their training with their physician

Finally, though not all athletes will suffer warning signs and symptoms, it is important to realize that many do. Athletes, coaches, trainers, and physicians should be aware of "red flags" that could indicate an underlying cardiac problem: chest pain or tightness during or after exertion; unusual shortness of breath during or after exertion; pre syncope or syncope during or after exercise; palpitations or an irregular heart beat during or after exercise. In addition, a family history of sudden cardiac death, particularly at a young age, should be considered a risk factor and may necessitate further testing.

Diagnosis

An athlete who is noted to become suddenly unconscious and pulseless during or after exercise or sport is diagnosed as having suffered a SCD.

Treatment

An athlete who has suffered a SCD needs immediate cardiopulmonary resuscitation and defibrillation. This requires an emergency plan that provides a prompt response by trained personnel, and transport to a medical center for more advanced testing and treatment. The use of AEDs at sports arenas, gyms, health clubs, and finish lines has increased the survival rate of athletes who suffer sudden cardiac death.

Prognosis

The prognosis depends on the speed of CPR, defibrillation, and the EMS response, as well as the underlying cause of the SCD. Suffering SCD with an AED present dramatically increases the odds of survival.

Prevention

There is considerable debate over prevention of SCD in athletes. In part this is because the death rate is already low and these instances are considered rare. Currently, the America Heart Association recommends a screening exam by a trained professional, paying particular attention to family history, report of symptoms, blood pressure, pulse, and heart sounds. A pre-participation EKG is not routinely performed in the U.S, though it is in many European countries. It is not entirely clear that requiring Ekgs would save lives, though some studies have shown it be both life saving and cost effective. An issue is that many athletes have abnormal EKGs due to "athlete's heart," and thus it takes a highly trained professional to understand which changes are physiological versus pathological. In a recent paper addressing this issue, Pelici et al suggested that athletes' ECG abnormalities be divided into two groups: common and training-related; uncommon and training-unrelated. This classification is based on prevalence, relation to exercise training, association with an increased cardiovascular

---

QUESTIONS TO ASK YOUR DOCTOR

- Is there any reason why I should not exercise intensely?
- Would an EKG be helpful to have?
- Is my training plan a good fit for me?

risk, and need for further clinical investigation to confirm (or exclude) an underlying **cardiovascular disease**.

On the other hand, the main cause of SCD in the U.S. is HCM, and estimates suggest that 90-95% of individuals with HCM have an abnormal ekg. The specific EKG changes seen in HCM are not changes typically seen in "athlete's heart," though there is overlap. In countries where an ekg is required, such as Italy, the death rate during sport decreased considerably after a policy was instituted requiring EKGs. But there are some major differences between the U.S. and Italy. First, their death rate was higher to begin with. Second, all screenings are performed by physicians trained in sports cardiology. In the U.S, screening procedures and requirements vary considerably at current, and thus mandating EKGs presents a logistical challenge.

Resources

PERIODICALS

Borjesson M and Pelliccia A. "Incidence and etiology of sudden cardiac death in young athletes: an international perspective." *Br. J. Sports Med* 43, 2009.

Corrado A, Biffi, D, Basso C, Pelliccia A, and Thiene G. "12-lead ECG in the athlete: physiological versus pathological abnormalities *Br. J. Sports Med.* 43, 2009

Harmon KG, Irfan, MA, Klossner D, and Drenzer, JA. "Incidence of Sudden Cardiac Death in National Collegiate Athletic Association Athletes / Clinical Perspective ." *Circulation.* 123, published online before print April 4, 2011

Link MS, Estes NA. "Athletes and Arrhythmias." *J Cardiovasc Electrophysiol* 21, Oct 2010.

Maron BJ et al. *Recommendations and Considerations Related to Preparticipation Screening for Cardiovascular Abnormalities in Competitive Athletes: 2007 Update: A Scientific Statement From the American Heart Association Council on Nutrition, Physical Activity, and Metabolism: Endorsed by the American College of Cardiology Foundation/ Circulation* 115; 14–18, March 12, 2007

WEBSITES

IMMDA's Health Recommendations For Runners &
Walkers. http://www.aimsworldrunning.org/
immda.htm/ accessed November 3, 2011.

Lisa Womack, PhD

Sunburn

Definition

Sunburn is damage to the skin occurring as a
result of exposure to the sun's ultraviolet (UV) rays.
Sunburn is usually noticeable within three hours after
exposure and results in red, painful skin that may feel
warm to the touch. The condition generally takes
several days to heal and may result in blistering or
peeling of the skin. Sun exposure, especially repeated
experiences of sunburn, can lead to certain diseases of
the skin including skin cancer.

Description

Sunburn, which occurs after exposure to the sun's
UV rays, most often results in first-degree burning of
the skin. In first-degree sunburn, pain, redness, and
some swelling may be experienced, and the skin may
feel warm when touched. The symptoms of second-
degree sunburn may result after more prolonged sun
exposure and when negligible or no sunscreen has been
used to prevent sun damage. The symptoms of second-
degree sunburn include the symptoms of first degree
(pain, redness, swelling, hot to the touch) wherein the
symptoms are more severe and include blistering of the
skin. In second-degree sunburn, deeper layers of the
skin including nerve endings have been damaged. This
degree of sunburn takes longer to heal than first-
degree burning.

Sunburn is used to describe a condition resulting
in exposure to the sun's natural UV rays, or to artificial UV rays experienced after exposure to sunbed
tanning lamps. Sunbeds are artificial tanning devices
that may offer a supposedly faster, safer alternative to
more dangerous natural sunlight, however research
indicates that the UV radiation exposure acquired
from sunbed tanning still leads to skin damage, and
can contribute to skin cancer.

Sometimes the term "sun poisoning" is used, however the sun does not actually poison the skin. Sun
poisoning refers to a very severe case of sunburn in
which overexposure to ultraviolet radiation causes all
the symptoms of sunburn (redness, pain, swelling,
warmth, blistering) along with fever, chills, headache,
nausea, and/or dizziness. **Dehydration** is also a common
factor in severe cases of sunburn, or "sun poisoning."

Causes and Symptoms

Beyond pain, redness, swelling, warmth-to-the-
touch, and blistering, UV radiation can lead to other
physical complications. Repeated UV exposure leads
to aging, spotting, and wrinkling of the skin, known as
photoaging. Skin spots - also called age spots, liver
spots, or solar lentigines, result after years of prolonged ultraviolet light exposure when the melanin of
the epidermis becomes clustered together, or is
produced by skin cells in high concentrations.

A condition known as actinic keratosis—or solar
keratosis—may arise after repeated sun or UV exposure.
An actinic keratosis is a rough, dry, scaly, or warty patch
of skin usually appearing on the face, hands, arms, or

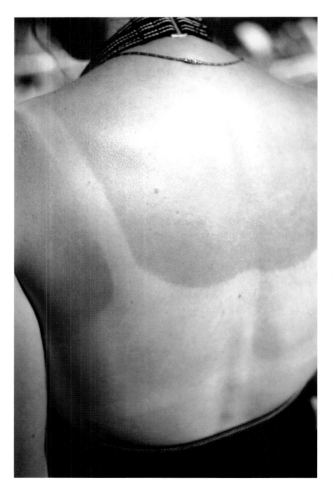

Woman with a sunburn. (© *Michelle Del Guercio/Photo
Researchers, Inc.*)

shoulders—areas of the body most exposed to the sun. An actinic keratosis usually begins as a small spot or patch and generally takes several years to develop. These patches are usually treated as precancerous, however, as they frequently result in malignancy.

Damage to the eyes is a complication of exposure to ultraviolet light, either by sunlight or tanning beds or bulbs. Inflammation to the cornea, known as photokeratitis, and inflammation to the conjunctiva, called photoconjunctivitis, may result. These conditions are usually temporary and can easily be prevented with protective eyewear—UV-filtered sunglasses.

Long-term effects to the eye caused by exposure to ultraviolet light may also result. One such consequence of repeated UV exposure to the unprotected eye is cataracts. Cataracts form when the lens, and the transparent layer surrounding the lens, become increasingly clouded and opaque. Cataracts impair vision and may lead to blindness.

Another consequence of UV radiation overexposure on the eyes is pterygium, a condition in which thickened conjunctiva grows from the inner side of the eyeball usually covering part of the cornea. The mass of conjunctiva is usually fleshy and creamy in nature, and results in inhibited vision.

Overexposure to ultraviolet radiation has been linked to immune suppression. Low doses of UV-B exposure can compromise the immunological response of animals and humans, and excessive UV-B exposure can lead to overall immunological suppression. When immunity is compromised by ultraviolet radiation, the skin's ability to respond to allergic triggers and other compromising factors are limited. People with the herpes simplex virus experience a greater number of outbreaks of cold sores after exposure to UV radiation.

The leading cause of skin cancer is exposure to UV radiation, especially a history of repeated or prolonged exposures. Sun over-exposure in childhood and adolescence is linked to the occurrence of skin cancer later in life. The World Health Organization reports that one in three diagnosed cancers is a skin cancer; the most fatal of these is malignant melanoma.

Skin cancers are classified under two types: melanomas and nonmelanomas. Melanomas are formed when changes occur to melanocytes—cells of the epidermis responsible for the production of melanin. Basil cell carcinoma is linked to ultraviolet radiation and is a nonmelanoma. It is the most common form of skin cancer in the U.S. where, according to the American Cancer Society, 75% of all cases of skin cancer are basil cell carcinomas.

KEY TERMS

Actinic keratosis—A condition of premalignant lesions resulting from excessive sun damage and usually occurring after middle age. It lesions are flaky, scaly, or warty in nature and may result in malignancy.

Cataract—A clouding that develops in the lens of the eye or the surrounding transparent membrane that inhibits the passage of light.

Epidermis—The upper, nonvascular layer of the skin.

Melanocytes—A cell of the epidermis that produces melanin.

Melanoma—A usually malignant tumor of the melanin-forming cells that is known to metastasize rapidly.

Photoaging—The effects of long-term exposure to ultraviolet light, either by sunlight or artificial UV light, resulting in wrinkling and spotting of the skin.

Photoconjunctivitis—Swelling of the conjunctiva of the eye as a result of exposure to ultraviolet light.

Photokeratitis—Swelling of the cornea of the eye as a result of exposure to ultraviolet light.

Pterygium—Thickened growth of the conjunctiva, fleshy and creamy in nature, growing from the inner side of the eyeball and usually covering part of the cornea. Pterygium results in inhibited vision.

Solar lentigines—Spots appearing on the epidermis due to repeated exposure of the skin to ultraviolet rays, either from the sun or from sunbed tanning. Also called age spots or liver spots.

The majority of basil cell carcinomas occur on areas of the skin that commonly receive sun exposure—the face, neck, forearms, shoulders, tops of the hands, or scalp. These skin cancers are slow-growing and painless, and develop in the epidermis, or top cell layer of the skin. Basil cell carcinomas may appear as a new skin growth that does not heal, or that bleeds frequently or easily.

At one time basil cell carcinomas were common in people over age 40, but now they are appearing in younger people. People with fair skin, light colored eyes (blue or green), blonde or red hair, or who are frequently exposed to x-ray radiation may be at a higher risk for these skin cancers. Basil cell skin cancer rarely metastasizes, however if left too long untreated, it may spread into surrounding tissue or even bone.

Another type of nonmelanoma skin cancer that is linked to UV radiation exposure is squamous cell carcinoma. In its earliest stages, squamous cell carcinoma is called Bowen's disease, or squamous cell in situ. In this stage, it has not yet spread to surrounding tissues. Actinic keratosis is a flaky, patchy, or warty skin lesion that can also lead to squamous cell carcinoma.

A squamous cell cancer may appear as a round, reddish patch—usually larger than 1 inch in diameter—that is rough or scaly on the surface and that does not heal. Squamous cell cancers are more likely to occur in places where a person experiences sun exposure—such as the face, neck, arms, and hands—and on people who are fair-skinned, fair or red haired, blue or green eyed, and with a history of repeated sunburns early in life. They may also appear on people with a history of x-ray radiation exposure, or who have had chemical exposures.

Melanoma is the most dangerous form of skin cancer and accounts for the leading cause of death among diseases of the skin. Melanomas are formed when changes occur to melanocytes—cells of the epidermis responsible for the production of melanin. Melanomas may occur in normal appearing skin, or in moles or other skin areas that have changed shape or appearance over time. More infrequently, melanomas can appear in the iris of the eye, the retina, or other areas inside the body. People most at risk for melanomas are the same individuals as those at risk for nonmelanomas, but all people can get this or other types of skin cancers.

Treatment

Once sunburn has occurred, there is no treatment that can successfully remedy it, but there are measures that can be taken to help soothe the discomfort and help the healing process.

- Cold compress — Place a cool, damp cloth over the affected area or areas, or submerge sunburned skin in a cool bath.
- Moisturize—Consistently apply aloe vera gel (best when cooled) or other moisturizers over the affected areas. Be certain to avoid any gels or creams with alcohol as an ingredient, as alcohol will further dry out the skin.
- Pain Reliever—If necessary, take an OTC non-steroidal anti-inflammatory drug (NSAID) such as Advil or Motrin in cases where pain or fever persists.

It is important to remember that peeling skin may still be sensitive, and to treat it gently. Attempting to rush the peeling process may cause tearing of new skin, and may lead to infection. Also, **blisters** should be left alone, or covered in gauze. Attempting to break or

QUESTIONS TO ASK YOUR DOCTOR

- Considering my skin type, what level of SPF should I be wearing?
- Considering my skin type and usual activities, how often should I be applying SPF?
- Are any of the moles and marks on my skin in need of biopsy?
- Considering my past sun, UV radiation, x-ray radiation, or chemical exposure, how likely am I to be diagnosed with any of the types of skin cancers? What should I be looking for?

squeeze blisters interferes with the body's natural healing process and may lead to infection.

Basil cell carcinomas are treated most frequently by types of surgical excision, or they may be frozen or irradiated. Squamous cell cancers are treated in the same manner as basil cell carcinomas, however Bowen's disease—early stage squamous cells—may be treated with photodynamic therapy, wherein a combination of photosensitizing medication and a light therapy are used to kill cancer cells.

Prevention

Whenever going out of doors, summer or winter, one should protect skin from ultraviolet radiation with the use of protective sunscreen of at least a factor of 15, although a sun protection factor (SPF) of 30 or above is recommended. When going out of doors, apply sunscreen liberally and often to all areas of the body, especially those areas that will be in direct sunlight. Wear protective sunglasses—those shades with UV filtering. Limit the amount of time you will spend in sunlight, and stick to the shade whenever possible. Avoid tanning beds, as the ultraviolet radiation from the bulbs in these beds does contribute to skin damage like burning, aging, and wrinkling, as well as all types of skin cancers.

Resources

BOOKS

van der Leun, J. C., and F. R. de Gruijl. "Influences of Ozone Depletion on Human and Animal Health." *UV-B Radiation and Ozone Depletion: Effects on Humans, Animals, Plants, Microorganisms, and Materials* (New York: Ann Arbor 1993), 95-123.

WEBSITES

"Basil Cell Carcinoma." PubMed Health. Ncbi.nlm.nih.-gov, last modified, February 2008. (accessed October 11, 2011).

"Health effects of overexposure to the sun." EPA.gov, last modified, July 2010. (accessed October 10, 2011).

"Squamous Cell Carcinoma." PubMed Health. Ncbi.nlm.nih.gov, last modified, July 2011. (accessed October 11, 2011).

"Sunbeds, tanning, and UV exposure." WHO.int, last modified April 2010, (accessed October 10, 2011).

"Sunburn." Mayoclinic.com, last modified August 02, 2011, (accessed October 10, 2011).

"Ultraviolet radiation and human health." WHO.int, last modified, December 2009. (accessed October 10, 2011).

ORGANIZATIONS

American Cancer Society, 250 Williams ST NW #6000, Atlanta, GA, 30303, (800) 227-2345, http://www.cancer.org/index.

The Skin Cancer Foundation, 149 Madison Avenue, Suite 901, New York, NY, 10016, (212) 725-5176, http://www.skincancer.org/.

Julie Jordan Avritt

Surfing *see* **Ocean sports**

Suspension training *see* **Sling training**

Swimming

Definition

Swimming for fun, **exercise**, and competition is popular among people of all ages and physical conditions.

Purpose

Swimming is excellent aerobic exercise for improving and maintaining physical and **mental health**. Water supports the weight of the body—preventing impact on and straining of muscles, bones, and joints—while the resistance of the water forces the muscles to work hard, building strength. This makes swimming an appropriate exercise for older people and those with chronic illnesses and disabilities. It is recommended exercise for people with **arthritis** and joint replacements and those requiring physical therapy. Injured athletes, especially those with leg injuries, often use swimming for rehabilitation and to maintain fitness. Many people report that they enjoy swimming more than land-based exercise.

Demographics

Swimming is the second most popular exercise activity and the third most popular sport among Americans. There are nearly nine million residential and public-use swimming pools in the United States:

- 17% of adult Americans swim at least six times per year.
- 7% of adult males swim for exercise, including 10% of those aged 18–29 and more than 1% of those aged 75 and older.
- 6.2% of women swim for exercise, including 8% of 18–29-year-olds and 1.5% of those aged 75 and older.

Pediatric

Swimming is the most popular exercise activity of American children:

- An estimated 5–10 million infants and preschool children participate in water-instruction programs.
- Almost all children between the ages of 8 and 12 (97%) report that they have been swimming in the past year.
- Among children between the ages of 7 and 17, 41% report swimming at least six times every year.

History

Humans have been swimming throughout recorded history. Swimming associations, clubs, and competitions appeared in the nineteenth century. In the twenty-first century most towns in the United States have public pools and many have indoor pools for year-round swimming.

Description

Swimming is low-impact, non-weight-bearing exercise that can be enjoyed by the entire family and continued throughout life. U.S. Masters Swimming has competitions for all **age** groups, including those aged 100–104. People can swim in pools, ponds, rivers, lakes, and oceans. Most public pools, fitness centers, and private clubs offer swimming lessons.

The crawl, also called freestyle, is the most popular swimming stroke and the easiest to learn. Breaststroke and butterfly are less popular since they are more difficult and require precise timing. The butterfly also requires strength.

Adapted aquatics modifies swimming techniques to accommodate individual abilities. People with almost any physical disability can exercise by swimming with an appropriate flotation device. Flotation

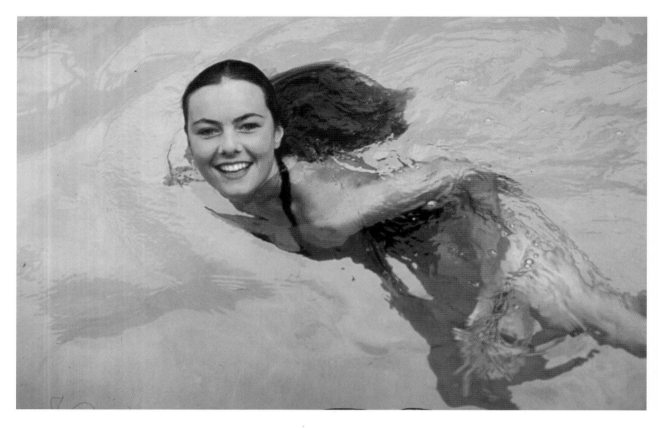

A woman swimming. (© *Custom Medical Stock Photo, Inc. Reproduced by permission.*)

devices also are used for learning to swim, practicing specific strokes, and adding resistance for building muscle strength and tone. These devices include:

- kickboards for practicing kicks and resting the arms
- pull buoys to float the legs while working the upper body
- fins for working the legs and swimming faster

Preparation

A general exercise program that strengthens the shoulder and upper back muscles can help prevent shoulder pain from the repetitive motion of swimming. Swimming should be preceded by a three- to five-minute **warm-up** of jumping jacks, stationary biking, or **walking** or **running** in place, followed by slow and gentle **stretching**, holding each stretch for 30 seconds.

Equipment

No special equipment is needed for swimming. Optional equipment includes bathing caps to keep hair dry, goggles for eye protection, and swim fins to increase motion in the water. Face masks and snorkels are often used when swimming in lakes or oceans to view underwater aquatic life.

Swimmers should dry off or shower immediately after swimming, so a towel or place to shower is beneficial.

Training and conditioning

Swimming may be a relatively high-intensity activity and lap swimming or swimming fast can be very vigorous exercise. Swimming for cardiovascular fitness should raise the heart rate to its target level for at least 20 minutes. Workout schedules for improving cardiorespiratory endurance recommend at least 20–30 minutes of swimming three–five days per week. **Interval training** involves swimming 50 yards followed by a 10-second rest, then swimming 100 yards and resting 10 seconds, and so on up to 300 yards of swimming, and then reversing the pattern. Varying strokes can help prevent boredom. An after-swim cool-down can involve slowing down the stroke or switching to a more leisurely stroke. Water that is warmer than body temperature relaxes muscles, whereas cooler water prevents overheating during a strenuous workout.

MICHAEL PHELPS (1985–)

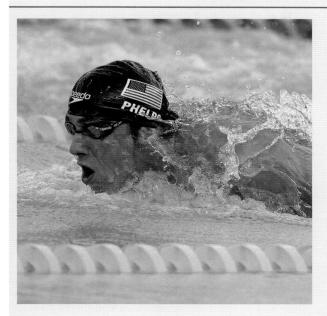

(© MARKA/Alamy)

Born June 30, 1985, in Baltimore, Maryland, Michael Phelps, the youngest man to break a swimming world record. Phelps took to swimming when he was seven years old, finding that some of his normal awkwardness, caused by being hyperflexible, vanished in the water. At eleven, Phelps began training with Bob Bowman, who saw immediately that Phelps had Olympic potential. Bowman encouraged Phelps to train to a degree where he could watch the 2000 Olympics, but Phelps pushed himself harder. At 15, Phelps placed in the Olympic trials and became the youngest member of the American team for the Sydney Olympics. Then at 16, Phelps became the youngest American male swimmer to become a professional.

In the 2004 Olympic trials, Phelps became the first swimmer to qualify in six individual Olympic events. Given the intensity of the scheduling, Phelps chose to participate in only five events, racing 17 different times, creating the opportunity for him to challenge Mark Spitz's record of seven gold medals in one Olympics. At his first event, the results were promising: Phelps won the 400 meter individual medley by a full three–and–a–half seconds, setting a world record. But breaking the gold–medal record at the 2004 Olympics was not to be. The American team placed third in the 4x100 freestyle relay, and Phelps took a bronze in the 200 meter free-style, losing to Australian Ian Thorpe, who had beaten him in the 100 meter butterfly at the 2003 World Championships. When Bowman took the head coach position for the University of Michigan's swimming team after the 2004 Olympics, Phelps went with him, enrolling for classes and continuing to train with him in Ann Arbor. Due to his status as a professional, he was unable to race for the university, and instead served as a volunteer assistant coach under Bowman. Phelps continued to train all 365 days of the year—including Christmas morning—typically swimming between 7 and 12 miles per day.

At the 2008 Games in Beijing, Phelps raced 17 times in nine days, taking the gold medal in all eight of the events he raced and succeeding in his goal of breaking Spitz's record as well as tying the record of gymnast Aleksander Dityatin for eight medals at a single Olympics. The games brought Phelps' career totals of world records to four individual world records and two team world records. To enhance the visibility of swimming, Phelps founded a social networking site, SwimRoom.com and is the founder of the Michael Phelps Foundation that promotes health and activity, primarily for children, through the sport of swimming.

Swimming may also be enjoyed for leisure and fun with family and friends, whether at the beach or in a pool. Many people choose to enjoy a calm and restful swim as a means of relaxation after work or a stressful day.

Risks

Since water cushions the joints, it greatly reduces the incidence of athletic injury. Nevertheless, according to the U.S. Consumer Product Safety Commission, there were almost 172,000 swimming-related injuries treated in emergency rooms, physicians' offices, and clinics in 2007. The most common swimming injury is shoulder pain from repetitive motion. Other swimming risks include:

- sunburn
- falling in and around concrete pools
- being trapped by weeds or grass in ponds and lakes
- recreational water illnesses (RWIs), especially diarrhea caused by parasites such as *Giardia* or *Cryptosporidium*, bacteria such as *Shigella* or *Escherichia coli* O157:H7, or noroviruses
- swimmer's itch, or cercarial dermatitis, a skin rash caused by parasites from infected snails
- swimming-pool granuloma, a chronic skin infection caused by *Mycobacterium marinum*

- stings from jellyfish or a Portuguese man-of-war
- spinal cord injuries, permanent brain damage, or death from diving into shallow water or hitting a diving board

Two of the biggest swimming dangers are panicking and becoming too tired to swim. Jumping into cold water can raise **blood pressure** and heart rate and slow down muscles. Swimmers should:

- learn to swim
- wear personal flotation devices (PFDs) if inexperienced
- swim in designated areas with lifeguards
- never swim alone
- never swim at night
- get out of the water if a cramp develops
- never swim during storms, fog, or high winds
- never swim when fatigued, too cold, or overheated
- not swim strenuously when ill
- never jump or dive into shallow or murky water
- never swim in a lake or river after a storm if there is flooding or the water appears to be rising
- wear sunscreen
- avoid alcohol

Ocean swimming requires special precautions, including:

- avoiding piers
- watching for flags or messages about strong waves
- facing toward waves
- never running into waves headfirst
- swimming parallel to shore before heading in if caught in a undercurrent or riptide (rip current)

Various measures can make swimming more pleasurable:

- Goggles protect the eyes from chlorine in pools and bacteria in lakes and ponds and make it easier to keep the eyes open underwater.
- Rinsing the eyes with sterile eyewash or artificial tears can reduce redness and discomfort from chlorine.
- Wetting and conditioning hair before swimming and washing with specially formulated swimmer's shampoo and conditioning afterwards can help protect hair from chlorine damage.
- Bathing caps protect hair from chlorine and reduce resistance in the water.
- Footwear can protect against jagged rocks, broken bottles, or trash in lakes or ponds.

Swimmer's ear or otitis externa, an infection of the outer and/or inner ear canal often caused by *Pseudomonas aeruginosa*, may be prevented by:

- wearing earplugs
- drying the ear canal with a towel or a hair dryer (swabbing with cotton can scratch the ear canal, encouraging infection)
- using alcohol-based eardrops to clear water from the ear
- avoiding polluted water

Precautions for preventing RWIs include:

- not swallowing swimming water
- showering with soap before and after swimming
- washing hands after using the toilet or changing diapers

Pediatric

Drowning is the second most common cause of death from unintentional injury among children and teens:

- Drowning can occur in less than two minutes after going underwater.
- Children aged one to four are most at risk for drowning in swimming pools.
- Older children and teenagers are most at risk for drowning in unsupervised quarries, ponds, lakes, rivers, or oceans.
- Children with seizure disorders are at a much higher risk for drowning.
- Alcohol is a factor in many teenage drownings.

The American Academy of Pediatrics (AAP) suggests that children be taught to swim between the ages of five and eight and cautions that children younger than four may not be developmentally ready to learn to swim. However, a recent study suggests that swimming lessons may help prevent drowning in one–four-year-olds. In addition:

- Children should swim only with adult supervision and with a buddy.
- Children under age five should be under "touch supervision"—within arm's reach.
- Children should use a Coast Guard-approved PFD when learning to swim.
- Toys should never be used as flotation devices.
- Children should be washed thoroughly with soap before swimming.
- Small children should have frequent bathroom breaks or have their swim diapers checked often.
- Swallowing too much pool water can sicken a child.
- Infants and toddlers should be in swimming programs with their parents and should not put their heads underwater because they may swallow too much water.
- Children with ear tubes in the middle ear may need to wear ear plugs.

Results

Many people swim as one component of a weight-loss program. Swimming can also speed up **metabolism** that may contribute to **weight loss**. The number of **calories** burned by swimming depends on stroke efficiency and buoyancy:

- Efficient swimming burns fewer calories.
- Body fat increases buoyancy and reduces calorie burning.
- A 150-lb (68-kg) woman swimming laps for one hour at 25 yd (23 m) per minute burns about 275 calories. At 50 yd (46 m) per minute she burns about 500 calories.
- It has been estimated that swimming—regardless of the stroke—burns only about 11% fewer calories than running and 3% fewer than biking.

There are numerous health benefits associated with swimming. Swimming at a comfortable pace is a good way for a sedentary person to begin exercising, because it is less strenuous than many other types of exercise and increases one's fitness without causing strain.

Swimming helps to improve cardiovascular fitness, breathing, the heart muscle, and circulation.

The rhythmic motion of swim strokes promotes controlled, deep breathing, utilizing the diaphragm and increases lung volume. The heart is strengthened and increases its efficiency. People with **hypertension** benefit from swimming because the blood vessels expand and increase blood volume, which can lower blood pressure. Circulation in general improves because water pressure on the legs and feet moves blood upward through the veins.

Endurance, muscle strength, joint flexibility, and balance are enhanced with swimming. Almost all the major muscle groups, especially the arm, shoulder, and chest muscles are used during the exercise. Men who completed an eight-week swimming program had a 23.8% increase in triceps strength.

Studies have show that many chronic illnesses can be decreased with 150 minutes of swimming each week. Swimming can also reduce risk of death by about one-half compared to sedentary people. It is a beneficial form of exercise for people with heart disease and diabetes, and can maintain or improve bone density in post-menopausal women. The intensity and frequency of migraine headaches has also been show to decrease with swimming. Older adults may show a decrease in disability and improved quality of life. It can even improve the physical and mental health of pregnant women and the health of their unborn babies.

Mental health benefits of swimming include improving mood in both women and men, and providing an opportunity for quiet contemplation. Children with developmental disabilities often find swimming very therapeutic as well.

Swimming has been found to increase sustained cardiorespiratory endurance—the delivery of oxygen and nutrients to tissues and removal of waste products. Twelve weeks of swim training improved maximal oxygen consumption by 10% in a group of sedentary middle-aged men and women. It increased their stroke volume—the amount of blood pumped per beat, a measure of heart strength—by up to 18%.

Resources

BOOKS

Hines, Emmett W. *Fitness Swimming,* 2nd ed. Champaign, IL: Human Kinetics, 2008.

Jendrick, Megan Quann, and Nathan Jendrick. *Get Wet, Get Fit: A Complete Guide to a Swimmer's Body.* New York: Fireside, 2008.

Montgomery, Jim, and Mo Chambers. *Mastering Swimming.* Champaign, IL: Human Kinetics, 2009.

Salo, Dale, and Scott A. Riewald. *Complete Conditioning for Swimming.* Champaign, IL: Human Kinetics, 2008.

PERIODICALS

"A Sport for All Seasons." *Harvard Health Letter* 35, no. 1 (November 2009): 4.

Chase, N. L., X. Sui, and S. N. Blair. "Swimming and All-Cause Mortality Risk Compared with Running, Walking, and Sedentary Habits in Men." *International Journal of Aquatic Research and Education* 2, no. 3 (2008): 213-223.

Peterson, Judy. "Get in the Swim!" *Current Health 2* 52, no. 4A (July/August 2009): 18.

Redford, Gabrielle DeGroot. "Lap It Up." *AARP The Magazine* 35, no. 8 (April/May 2009): 8-11.

WEBSITES

"Healthy Swimming/Recreational Water." *Centers for Disease Control and Prevention.* July 25, 2011. http://www.cdc.gov/healthywater/swimming/ (accessed October 18, 2011).

Mayo Clinic Staff. "Children's Swimming: Keep Health Risks at Bay." *MayoClinic.com.* May 25, 2011. http://www.mayoclinic.com/print/childrens-health/CC00003/METHOD = print (accessed October 18, 2011).

"Swimming." *KidsHealth.* June 2011. http://kidshealth.org/kid/watch/out/water.html (accessed October 18, 2011).

"Swimming Injury Prevention." *Your Orthopaedic Connection.* June 2011. http://orthoinfo.aaos.org/topic.cfm?topic = A00116 (October 18, 2011).

Weil, Richard. "Swimming." *MedicineNet.*http://www.medicinenet.com/swimming/article.htm (accessed October 18, 2011).

ORGANIZATIONS

American Academy of Orthopaedic Surgeons, 6300 North River Rd., Rosemont, IL, 60018-4262, (847) 823-7186, Fax: (847) 823-8125, orthoinfo@aaos.org, http://www.aaos.org.

American Academy of Pediatrics, 141 Northwest Point Blvd., Elk Grove Village, IL, 60007-1098, (874) 434-4000, Fax: (874) 434-8000, kidsdocs@aap.org, http://www.aap.org.

Arthritis Foundation, P.O. Box 7669, Atlanta, GA, 30357-0669, (800) 283-7800, http://www.arthritis.org.

U.S. Centers for Disease Control and Prevention (CDC), 1600 Clifton Rd., Atlanta, GA, 30333, (800) CDC-INFO (232-4636), cdcinfo@cdc.gov, http://www.cdc.gov.

U.S. Masters Swimming, P.O. Box 185, Londonderry, NH, 03053-0185, (800) 550-SWIM, Fax: (603) 537-0204, http://www.usms.org.

USA Swimming, 1 Olympic Plaza, Colorado Springs, CO, 80909, (719) 866-4578, Fax: (719) 866-4669, http://www.usaswimming.org.

Margaret Alic, PhD
Laura Jean Cataldo, RN, EdD

T

Table tennis

Definition

Ping pong is a game in which two or four players hit a light, hollow ball back and forth across a net stretched across the center of a table. The game is more commonly known as table tennis, reflecting its origin as an indoor modification of the sport of lawn **tennis**. The term Ping pong is a federally registered trademark for the game first issued to Parker Brothers, Inc., in 1901, and now owned by Escalade Sports, of Evansville, Indiana.

Purpose

The purpose of the game is for each player to hit the ball in such a way that his or her opponent is unable to return the ball legally. For each such occasion, the successful player is awarded one point. The player reaching 11 points first wins the game, except that in games tied at 10 points each, one player must gain a lead of two points to be declared the winner. Official competitions usually consist of an odd number of games, of which one person must win the majority (3 games out of 5, 4 out of 7, or 5 out of 9, for example)

Demographics

Anyone old enough to hold a table tennis paddle (racket) can play the game. Local, regional, national, and international competitions often have categories for boys and girls under the age of 15 (cadets) and under the age of 18 (juniors), as well as categories for men and women, with singles, doubles, and team events at most ages. USA Table Tennis currently claims to have more than 240 associate clubs with a total of more than 8,000 members in the United States. In 2000, the North American Association of Sports Economists estimated that about 38,000 people played table tennis regularly in the United States, making it the 26th most popular sport in the nation, just below

badminton and just above **handball**. By some estimates, more than 300 million people play table tennis worldwide, with a very large fraction of that number residing in East Asia, especially China, where the sport is said to be the third most popular sport in the country. More than 300 million people in China watched the 2008 Summer **Olympics** men's table tennis final between two Chinese players.

History

Table tennis is generally thought to have originated in England in the 1880s. The rapidly growing popularity of lawn tennis at the time led a number of individuals to consider ways in which the sport could be imported to the indoors, allowing it to be played year around. One of the earliest versions of table tennis actually consisted of a doll-house-type, scaled down model of a tennis court, with tiny replicas of lawn tennis rackets, net, and balls. Before long, however, inventors became more imaginative and began making simplified versions of the lawn tennis model, using simply a flat table with a low net stretched across the middle, with players using small rackets and a ball made out of rubber or cork. The ball proved to be the greatest hindrance in the development of the game, since neither rubber nor cork was suitable for producing the type of bounce needed for a successful game.

A major breakthrough occurred in 1901 when a British table tennis enthusiast, James Gibb, discovered that an American novelty item, celluloid balls, were the perfect substitute for rubber and cork balls previously used in the sport. At almost the same time, an Englishman by the name of E. C. Goode decided to cover the wooden paddle used in table tennis with a dimpled rubber coating, producing a racket very similar to the one still used today. With these improvements, table tennis took off rapidly as a popular sport both in England and the United States. Players began to write, sell, and buy books about table tennis, the game

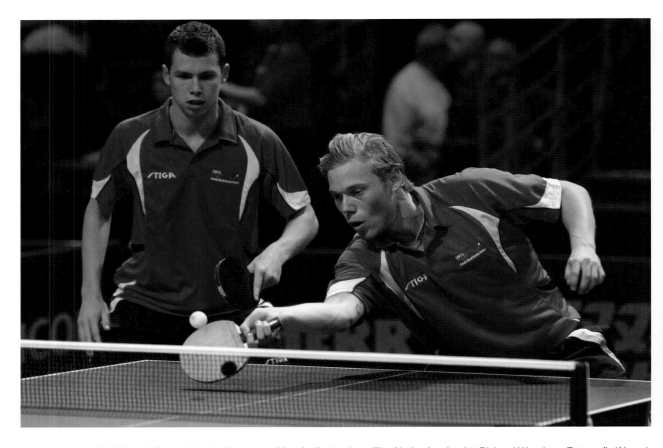

A match at the 2011 World Cup table tennis competition in Rotterdam, The Netherlands. *(© Richard Wareham Fotografie/Alamy)*

spread to China and other parts of the Far East, and the first unofficial world championship was held in 1902.

The first national governing body for the sport of table tennis was created in 1921 with the founding of the Table Tennis Association in Great Britain. Five years later, an international organization, the International Table Tennis Federation (ITTF), was founded in Berlin by eight European nations, Austria, Czechoslovakia, Denmark, England, Germany, Hungary, Sweden and Wales. ITTF sponsored the first official world table tennis championship in the same year, 1926, with all championships being won by individuals or teams from Hungary. The men's champion was Roland Jacobi, the women's champion was Mária Mednyánszky, and both men's and mixed doubles were also won by teams from Hungary. The ITTF continues to be the international governing board for the sport. The United States Table Tennis Association was founded in 1933, although it has since changed its name to USA Table Tennis (USATT).

Table tennis has been an Olympic sport since 1988, during which time Asian individuals and teams have dominated the sport. At the 2008 Summer Olympics in Beijing, members of the Chinese team won all four gold medals in the sport, as well as the silver and bronze medals in both men's and women's singles. The German team was the only non-Asian team to win a medal (silver) in the table tennis competition. The World Championship is held on a biennial basis, most recently in 2011 in Rotterdam. Individuals and teams from China have won all 20 gold medals in the last four World Championships.

Description

A singles table tennis match involves two individuals facing each other on opposite sides of a wooden or wood-like table 9 ft. (2.7 m) long, 5 ft. (1.5 m) wide and 30 in. (76.2 cm) high. A net 6 in. (15 cm) high stretches across the center of the table. The table is bisected along its long dimension by a white line. Play begins when the person who has won the right to serve first throws the ball at least 6 in. (15 cm) into the air with his or her free hand, the hand not holding the racket. The "six inch high" rule is commonly disregarded during informal recreational games, but is enforced strictly in formal competition. The player then strikes the ball as

KEY TERMS

Block—A defensive shot made simply by placing one's racket in front of an opponent's shot, returning at a speed nearly equal to its original speed.

Chop—A defensive shot in which a player strokes downward on the ball, giving it a high degree of topspin.

Flip—A shot made with a short flick of the wrist, rather than a full arm's swing at the ball.

Lob—A defensive shot made by hitting the ball high into the air, allowing the defending player to recover position.

Loop—A stroke in which the ball has a great deal of topspin, causing it to jump upward after hitting the table.

Racket—The paddle with which one hits the ball in table tennis.

Smash—A rapid, powerful stroke at a ball which has been returned with a significant arc above the table.

Speed drive—A stroke in which the ball is propelled forward at high speed.

it descends from the highest point in its arc such that it hits his or her side of the net once before entering the opponent's side of the table. The opponent then attempts to return the ball to the server after the ball has struck his or her side of the table once, and once only. Play continues back and forth in this way until one player makes an illegal return, which can involve the ball hitting into the net or leaving the table on any side before having struck the table once.

Rules for doubles play differ slightly from those for singles play. First, the server must make the ball strike the right-hand side of his court (the reason for the white line down the center of the table) before it passes over the net, after which it must hit the right-hand side of the receiver's court. After the first hit, players may return the ball anywhere on the table. Players on each team take turn returning the ball, and the same player can not hit the ball twice in succession. A number of rules also determine the sequence in which each individual is either server or receiver at various points in the game. Team play involves some combination of singles and doubles events, with the team winning the greater number of individual events being declared the winner of the match.

Table tennis play involves a highly sophisticated combination of strokes in which the ball can be delivered without any spin or with a number of types of spin, including backspin, topspin, sidespin, and corkscrew spin. These spins can be combined with a variety of shot styles, such as a speed drive, loop, flip, smash, chop, block, or lob. Penalty points are assessed for a variety of infractions, such as hitting the ball with any part of the racket not covered by rubber, touching the table with the hand not holding the racket, striking the ball twice in succession, or obstructing the ball with one's body or clothing.

Preparation

As is often the case, table tennis players should prepare for their sport by training in the specialized skills needed in the sport itself (such as forehand and backhand shots and offensive and defensive play), but also in general physical skills, such as weight training, agility improvement, and endurance development. The level of preparation needed is generally a function of the level at which one expects to perform; with individuals who are interested primarily in a game from time to time have to be much less concerned about training and conditioning than those who play competitively at an international level.

Equipment

Table tennis requires a minimum of equipment, which includes a racket and ball, a jersey, shorts, and suitable athletic shoes.

Training and conditioning

Books and articles on training and conditioning programs for table tennis strongly emphasize foot-work and shot-making skills that are essential to the game. Training schedules for national teams often have players at a table practicing a variety of shots for at least two hours a day, as often as five days a week. Increasingly, table tennis coaches are emphasizing training to develop strength, agility, and endurance. A member of the United States national team, for example, is expected to do weight training three days out of the week. By contrast, a Chinese training camp places greater emphasis on fitness exercises, such as push-ups, sit-ups, and rope jumping. The last of these exercises is especially important because it achieves two goals at the same time: improving one's agility and endurance. Trainers also encourage athletes to cross-train in sports that improve their aerobic endurance, such as **swimming**, cycling, and **running**. **Stretching** is also an important part of most training programs because of its role in preparing one's muscles for the stresses to which they will be exposed. An overview of training for table tennis is available at http://www.usatt.org/news1/Champion_Physical_Training.pdf.

Risks

Table tennis is generally regarded as a very safe sport, with few serious injuries. Few scientific studies have been conducted on the specific risks one faces in playing table tennis. A 2009 review of the available evidence found that, in one study, the largest percentage of injuries affected the waist (25.1% of all injuries), followed by damage to the shoulder (15.7%) and the knees (9.3%). A second study had somewhat different results, with the greatest fraction of injuries affecting the shoulder (23.3%), followed by the knee and ankle (9.3% each). A number of coaches and trainers have pointed to the relatively high risk posed by non-competition events, such as inadequate or poor training or poor "housekeeping" practices. The latter category includes injuries sustained when a player steps on balls that have been left on the floor, causing her or him to slip and fall.

Results

Avoiding injuries in table tennis involves not only the usual need for well-planned conditioning and training, but also alertness to environmental factors that may pose non-competition risks to one's health and well-being.

Resources

BOOKS

Charyn, Jerome. *Sizzling Chops & Devilish Spins: Ping-pong and the Art of Staying Alive.* New York: Four Walls Eight Windows, 2002.

Geske, Klaus, and Jens Mueller. *Table Tennis Tactics: Your Path to Success.* Aachen, Germany: Meyer & Meyer Sport, 2010.

McAfee, Richard. *Table Tennis: Steps to Success.* Champaign, IL: Human Kinetics, 2009.

Pollisco, Roy R. *Superior Table Tennis: The Science and Art.* Seattle: CreateSpace, 2009.

WEBSITES

The Sport of Table Tennis. Oracle ThinkQuest. http://library.thinkquest.org/20570/facts.html (accessed August 20, 2011).

Table Tennis General Information and History of Table Tennis. Table Tennis Links. http://www.bydewey.com/info.html (accessed August 20, 2011).

Table Tennis Rules. Pongworld. http://www.pongworld.com/more/rules.php (accessed August 20, 2011).

ORGANIZATIONS

International Table Tennis Federation, 11, Chemin de la Roche, 1020 Lausanne, Switzerland, 4121 340 7090, Fax: 4121 340 7099, ittf@ittf.com, http://www.ittf.com.

USA Table Tennis, One Olympic Plaza, Colorado Springs, CO, 80909-5769, (719) 866-4583, Fax: (719) 632-6071, usatt@usatt.org, http://www.usatt.org/.

David E. Newton, AB, MA, EdD

Tae kwon do

Definition

Tae kwon do, also spelled taekwondo or taekwon-do, is a martial art; it is also the national sport of South Korea. The name *tae kwon do* comes from three Korean words that mean "to strike with the foot," "to strike with the fist," and "the way" or "the art." Thus, the name of the sport can be loosely translated as "the art of kicking and punching."

Purpose

The purpose of traditional tae kwon do is self-defense, specifically, to render opponents unable to inflict harm by striking them with the legs and feet. The purpose of professional or semi-professional tae kwon do is to win a match against an opponent or compete at the Olympic level. Amateurs may participate in the contemporary sport in order to learn self-defense or for overall physical fitness rather than to compete in formal matches; tae kwon do helps to develop the student's strength, speed, balance, flexibility, and stamina. It is also part of formal military training for the South Korean army. More recently, some researchers are investigating tae kwon do as a form of **exercise** for seniors to lower their risk of falls, as the sport has been shown to improve flexibility and balance in older adults.

Demographics

Tae kwon do is the most popular martial art worldwide in terms of the number of participants; one American source gives a figure of 30 million practitioners in 123 countries as of 2008, with 3 million qualified at the black belt level. A South Korean source maintains that there are 70 million practitioners of tae kwon do in 190 countries. After entering the Olympic Games as a demonstration event in 1988, tae kwon do became an official Olympic sport in 2000. It is one of only two **martial arts** included in the **Olympics**, judo being the other. Tae kwon do is practiced by women as well as men and by people in all **age** groups except for very young children. A few dojangs (schools) accept children as young as two years of age; however, most do not enroll "little tigers" below the age of four or five.

History

There is some disagreement among historians about the origins of contemporary tae kwon do. Some elements of it can be traced back as far as the Three Kingdoms period (37 B.C.–A.D. 668), when Korea was divided among three rival powers. Silla, the least powerful of the warring kingdoms, had an elite corps of warriors known as Hwarang, who cultivated a style of unarmed self-defense techniques known as subak. As the Hwarang were recruited from the sons of noble families, they were taught philosophy, history, and a code of ethics as well as martial arts and horsemanship, and it is thought that the ethical code of contemporary tae kwon do is a descendant of this ancient tradition of education.

The unarmed combat techniques and other martial skills fell into disuse in Korea when Confucianism became the dominant philosophy. Under the Joseon Dynasty (A.D. 1392–1910), any skill or activity that was not related to academic subjects was devalued. The military lost its former prestige, while the older techniques of self-defense survived only in the army. When the Japanese occupied Korea from 1910 to 1945, they banned all aspects of native Korean identity, from religion and traditional dress to folk

customs and even names. Martial arts training was forbidden; however, some forms of subak survived and were taught underground. Meanwhile, some Koreans studied in Japan during the occupation period; there they were exposed to karate and other Japanese martial arts. Some even attained black belt status in Japanese karate schools.

After the defeat of Japan and the liberation of Korea at the end of World War II, schools of martial arts were opened all over Korea. Some claimed to teach the traditional Korean art of subak while others taught various combinations of subak, karate, and kung fu. Nine different kwans (schools) of martial arts emerged in the early 1950s. In order to achieve some degree of standardization, then-President Syngman Rhee instructed the kwans in 1955 to adopt the single name of tae kwon do for the martial art they were teaching and to begin to unify their various styles. Although the Korea Taekwondo Association (KTA) was formed in 1959 to carry out the unification of the various styles taught by the postwar kwans, standardization is still not complete as of 2011.

Description

Tae kwon do resembles karate and kickboxing in that it is a martial art that relies on the use of the legs and feet more than the arms or hands because the human leg is stronger and has a greater reach than the arm. In general, tae kwon do utilizes kicks aimed at the opponent from a moving stance combined with blocks, kicks, punches, and open-handed strikes. Some forms of tae kwon do also permit grabbing, taking down, or throwing the opponent in techniques borrowed from judo, or allow the use of pressure points.

Practitioners of tae kwon do wear a uniform known as a dobok (the Korean word for "robe" or "training clothes"), traditionally made of cotton and usually either white or black. The dobok consists of a jacket-like top and wide-legged pants. It is worn with a belt denoting the athlete's grade or rank. The first belt is typically white, followed by yellow, green, blue, red, and then black to indicate increasing proficiency. Some schools of tae kwon do award brown belts in place of red.

Although there is no single pattern followed by all tae kwon do schools worldwide, most teach students some or all of the following:

• Basic instruction in the techniques and rules of tae kwon do.

• An aerobic workout that includes stretching exercises.

KEY TERMS

Dobok—The uniform worn to practice tae kwon do. Traditionally made of cotton and usually white or black, the dobok has a jacket-like top and wide-legged pants. It is worn with a belt whose color indicates the student's rank.

Dojang—The Korean word for a tae kwon do school or training hall.

Hogu—The Korean word for the chest protector worn in sport tae kwon do.

Hyeong—The Korean word for the patterns or forms of movement sequences that are a major component of tae kwon do practice. It is also spelled hyung.

Subak—The style of unarmed self-defense techniques taught in ancient and medieval Korea.

- Patterns (hyeong), sometimes called forms, that are systematic sequences of movements intended to promote endurance and the ability to focus the mind as well as condition the body. Patterns are one of the events in tae kwon do competitions, where the athletes are judged on their speed, precision, energy level, and control in performing the movements. While Chong-Ji, the first pattern learned by the beginner, consists of 19 movements, some patterns have as many as 68 or 72 distinct movements.

- Self-defense techniques.

- Sparring with a partner.

- Relaxation and meditation techniques.

- Breaking objects—usually boards, but may also involve bricks, tiles, or blocks of ice—as part of training or martial arts demonstrations.

- Examinations for promotion to the next rank. Promotion tests typically include demonstrating proficiency in performing patterns, in sparring with a partner, in breaking boards (or other objects), and answering verbal questions about the history, concepts, and philosophy of tae kwon do. Higher-level black belt tests may require submitting a research paper as well as demonstrating physical proficiency.

- Instruction in ethical and mental discipline, self-respect, courtesy to others, and a commitment to justice.

Types of tae kwon do

There are two basic types of tae kwon do as of 2011—traditional and sport, although each has numerous variations.

TRADITIONAL. Traditional tae kwon do emphasizes the martial art as a way of life, not just an athletic exercise. In the traditional approach, the student is expected to understand "how Tae Kwon Do can help them and others in their everyday lives, not just in the *dojang* (training hall)." The five tenets of tae kwon do are taught to students as part of their total development, the qualities of mind and character they should cultivate in order to become true masters of the martial art. These five tenets are courtesy, integrity, perseverance, self-control, and "indomitable spirit."

In traditional tae kwon do, students are expected to recite a student oath at the opening and closing of every class session. The International Tae Kwon Do Association states, "Reciting the Student Oath instills a sense of responsibility and self-discipline as well as respect for one's self and others." The oath is as follows:

- I shall observe the tenets of tae kwon do.

- I shall respect all instructors and seniors.

- I shall never misuse tae kwon do.

- I shall be a champion of freedom and justice.

- I shall strive to build a more peaceful world.

SPORT. Sport tae kwon do is the form of the art represented in the Olympics and such other competitions as the Asian Games. Most tae kwon do competitions include patterns, breaking, and self-defense techniques as well as sparring; in the Olympics only sparring matches are judged. Competitors in sparring matches wear a hogu (chest guard) in addition to protective gear for the shins and forearms. The hogu also serves as a point of reference in the scoring system, as a kick or punch to the hogu counts as one point, a blow to the hogu that turns the opponent's body around counts as two points, and a kick that knocks the opponent down is awarded three points.

Matches take place in rings that are about 30 ft (9 m) square. Each match has three rounds, with one-minute rest periods between rounds. At the end of three rounds, the competitor with the higher number of points wins the match. Blows are full-force; if one competitor is knocked out by a legal blow, the opponent automatically wins the match. There are two age groups in sport tae kwon do matches: 14- to 17-year olds; and 18 years and older.

Preparation

Preparation for tae kwon do begins with enrollment in a dojang or school to learn the basic techniques of the art and its underlying philosophy of character building as well as physical conditioning. Most schools in the United States have separate classes for adults and children.

Equipment

No specialty equipment is required for tae kwon do.

Training and conditioning

Individuals should train with a qualified instructor. Due to the physical nature of tae kwon do and the need to use multiple muscle groups and limbs, participants should be physically fit, be able to move quickly, and have a good sense of balance.

Tae kwon do instructors often give commands in the Korean language during class sessions, and students may be required to show that they understand these words as part of their promotion examinations.

Risks

Tae kwon do can lead to significant injuries; it is estimated that about 8% of those who participate in sport competition are injured, without regard to sex, age, or level of skill. A study of injuries among athletes in the 2008 Olympic Games classified tae kwon do as one of the riskiest sports, along with **weightlifting**, **soccer**, hockey, and **boxing**. Most tae kwon do injuries are minor, however. Bruising is common, with the leg being the most common location of injury. Tae kwon do participants are also at risk for injuries to the foot and ankle from the twisting and impact mechanisms involved in kicking the opponent and pivoting on the ankle joint.

As with any form of physical exercise, a person interested in tae kwon do should consult their primary care doctor first to make sure that they do not have any previously undiagnosed conditions that might make martial arts workouts risky or unsuitable. Those with a history of leg, knee, or ankle injuries from other sports or from accidents should be particularly careful to have a checkup before enrolling in a tae kwon do class. The sport emphasizes the use of the legs and feet, and injuries to these parts of the body are common during practice or competition.

Participants injured during a competition match should seek immediate medical attention, particularly if they have been kicked in the head or been knocked out.

QUESTIONS TO ASK YOUR DOCTOR

- What is your opinion of tae kwon do as a form of exercise for older adults as well as for adolescents and young adults?
- Do any of your other patients practice tae kwon do? Do they enjoy it?
- What are the risks of serious injury in tae kwon do?
- Have you ever visited a tae kwon do class?

Results

People who enjoy tae kwon do usually report improved muscular strength, endurance, agility, and coordination as well as overall physical fitness. Studies of the benefits of tae kwon do as a method of fall prevention for seniors differ in their findings.

Resources

BOOKS

Park, Yeon Hee, Yeon Hwan Park, and Jon Gerrard. *Tae Kwon Do: The Ultimate Reference to the World's Most Popular Martial Art*, 3rd ed. New York: Facts On File, 2009.

Park, Yeon Hwan. *Tae Kwon Do: My Life and Philosophy*. New York: Checkmark Books, 2009.

Yates, Keith D. *The Complete Guide to American Karate and Tae Kwon Do*. Berkeley, CA: Blue Snake Books, 2008.

PERIODICALS

Callahan, L.F. "Physical Activity Programs for Chronic Arthritis." *Current Opinion in Rheumatology* 21 (March 2009): 177–82.

Cromwell, R.L., et al. "Tae Kwon Do: An Effective Exercise for Improving Balance and Walking Ability in Older Adults." *Journals of Gerontology, Series A: Biological Sciences and Medical Sciences* 62 (June 2007): 641–46.

Jones, K.D., and G.L. Liptan. "Exercise Interventions in Fibromyalgia: Clinical Applications from the Evidence." *Rheumatic Diseases Clinics of North America* 35 (May 2009): 373–91.

Junge, A., et al. "Sports Injuries during the Summer Olympic Games 2008." *American Journal of Sports Medicine* 37 (November 2009): 2165–72.

Kang, C., et al. "Acetabular Labral Tears in Patients with Sports Injury." *Clinics in Orthopedic Surgery* 1 (December 2009): 230–235.

Lystad, R.P., et al. "Epidemiology of Injuries in Competition Taekwondo: A Meta-analysis of Observational Studies." *Journal of Science and Medicine in Sport* 12 (November 2009): 614–21.

Matsushigue, K.A., et al. "Taekwondo: Physiological Responses and Match Analysis." *Journal of Strength and Conditioning Research* 23 (July 2009): 1112–1117.

Vormittag, K., et al. "Foot and Ankle Injuries in the Barefoot Sports." *Current Sports Medicine Reports* 8 (September-October 2009): 262–66.

OTHER

Hee-Sung, Kim *Taekwondo: A New Strategy for Brand Korea.* Ministry of Culture, Sports, and Tourism of the Republic of Korea (MCST). December 21, 2009. http://www.mcst.go.kr/english/issue/issueView.jsp?-pSeq = 1401 (accessed October 18, 2011).

International TaeKwon-Do Association (ITA). *Chon-Ji.* http://www.itatkd.com/aa_form1.html#top (accessed October 18, 2011).

ORGANIZATIONS

American College of Sports Medicine (ACSM), P.O. Box 1440, Indianapolis, IN, 46206, (317) 637-9200, Fax: (317) 634-7817, http://www.acsm.org/.

International Taekwon-do Federation (ITF), Via Cesare Pascoletti 29, scala A2, interno F, Rome, Italy, 00163, 390645443165, Fax: 390645443165, itfadmhq@fastwebnet.it, http://www.tkd-itf.org.

United States Taekwon-Do Federation (USTF), 6801 W. 117th Ave., E-5, Broomfield, CO, 80020, (303) 466-4963, Fax: (303) 466-3587, rsereff@rmi.net, http://www.ustf-itf.com.

World Taekwondo Federation (WTF), 4th floor, Joyang Bldg. 113, Samseong-dong, Gangnam-gu, Seoul, Korea, 822566-2505, Fax: 822533-4728, wtf@wtf.org, http://www.wtf.org.

Rebecca J. Frey, PhD
Laura Jean Cataldo, RN, EdD

T'ai chi

Definition

T'ai chi is an ancient Chinese **exercise** with movements that originate in **martial arts** practice. While used as a type of self-defense in its most advanced form, t'ai chi is practiced widely for its health and relaxation benefits. "Chinese shadow boxing," another name for T'ai chi, is one of the most popular low-intensity workouts around the world for people in search of well being and a way to combat stress.

Purpose

Also known as t'ai chi ch'uan (pronounced *tie-jee chu-wan*), the name comes from Chinese characters

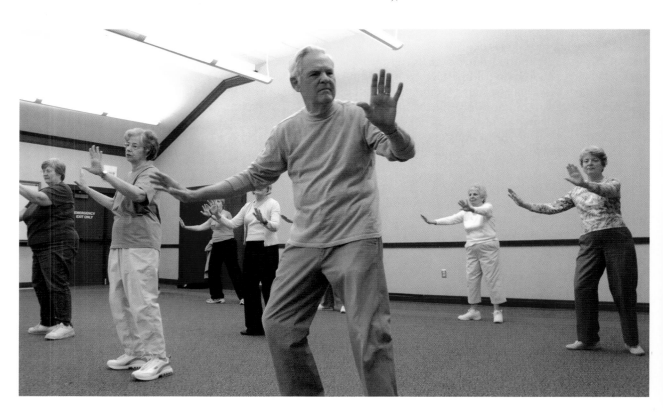

Seniors share a t'ai chi experience. *(© AP Images/Steve Rouse)*

LAO TZU

Lao Tzu (sixth century B.C.) is believed to have been a Chinese philosopher and the reputed author of the *Tao te ching*, the principal text of Taoist thought. He is considered the father of Chinese Taoism.

The main source of information on Lao Tzu's life is a biography written by the historian Ssu-ma Chien (145-86 B.C.) in his *Records of the Historian*. Lao Tzu is not really a person's name and is only an honorific designation meaning old man. It was common in this period to refer to respected philosophers and teachers with words meaning old or mature. It is possible that a man who assumed the pseudonym Lao Tzu was a historical person, but the term Lao Tzu is also applied as an alternate title to the supreme Taoist classic, *Tao te ching* (Classic of the Way and the Power).

An important quality of the tao is its "weakness," or "submissiveness." Because the tao itself is basically weak and submissive, it is best for man to put himself in harmony with the tao. Thus, the *Tao te ching* places strong emphasis on nonaction (*wu wei*), which means the absence of aggressive action. Man does not strive for wealth or prestige, and violence is to be avoided. This quietist approach to life was extremely influential in later periods and led to the development of a particular Taoist regimen that involved special breathing exercises and special eating habits that were designed to maintain quietude and harmony with the tao.

that translated mean "supreme ultimate force." The concept of t'ai chi, or the "supreme ultimate," is based on the Taoist philosophy of yin and yang, or the nature of when opposites attract. Yin and yang combine opposing, but complementary, forces to create harmony in nature. By using t'ai chi, it is believed that the principal of yin and yang can be achieved. A disturbance in the flow of chi (qi), or the life force, is what traditional Chinese medicine bases all causes of disease in the body. By enhancing the flow of chi, practitioners of t'ai chi believe that the exercise can promote physical health. Students of t'ai chi also learn how to use the exercise in the form of meditation and mental exercise by understanding how to center and focus their cerebral powers.

In the traditional Chinese understanding of health and well-being, t'ai chi is not regarded as a self-sufficient compartment of a person's life, as physical exercise often is viewed by Westerners. Instead, t'ai chi is considered part of an overall way of healthful living that includes massage, proper diet, meditation, and herbal medicines as needed.

Demographics

Surveys, including a 2007 inquiry by the National Center for Complementary and Alternative Medicine (NCCAM) report that an estimated 2.3 million people use t'ai chi in the United States, many of whom report to use t'ai chi for health-related benefits including:

- an improvement in balance and muscle strength
- diminished pain and stiffness in joints and muscles
- a low-impact form of exercise
- to help decrease the risk of falls
- to calm and relax, promoting more restful sleep

Of particular interest, is a change in acceptance and popularity of t'ai chi among men in the United States. In the 1970s and 1980s, many adult males regarded t'ai chi as a form of exercise that was not challenging enough for "real men." Since the late 1990s, however, more men have begun practicing t'ai chi in order to relieve stress or as a form of cross-training with another sport.

While the additional benefits of t'ai chi remain to be studied, it continues to be widely practiced in the United States and other Western countries. The ancient art maintains its prominence in China, where many people incorporate it into their daily morning routine.

History

The origins of t'ai chi are rooted deep in the martial arts and Chinese folklore, causing its exact beginnings to be based on speculation. The much-disputed founder of t'ai chi is Zhang San-feng (Chang San-feng), a Daoist (Taoist) monk of the Wu Tang Monastery, who, according to records from the Ming-shih (the official records of the Ming dynasty), lived sometime during the period from 1391–1459. Legend states that Zhang happened upon a fight between a snake and a crane, and, impressed with how the snake became victorious over the bird through relaxed, evasive movements and quick counterstrikes, he created a fighting-form that shadowed the snake's strongest attributes. With his experience in the martial arts, Zhang combined strength, balance, flexibility, and speed to bring about the earliest form of t'ai chi.

Historians also link Zhang to joining yin-yang from Taoism and "internal" aspects together into his exercises. The feeling of inner happiness remains a primary goal for those who practice t'ai chi. Although its ancient beginnings started as a martial art, t'ai chi was modified in the 1930s to the relaxing, low-intensity exercise that continues to have the potential to be transformed into a form of self-defense, similar to karate or kung-fu.

Description

Zhang created a combination of movements and beliefs that led to the formation of the fundamental "Thirteen Postures" of his art. Over time, these primary actions have transformed into soft, slow, relaxed movements, leading to a series of movements known as the form. Several techniques linked together create a form. Proper posture is a key element when practicing t'ai chi to maintain balance. All of the movements used throughout the exercise are relaxed with the back straight and the head up.

Just as the movements of t'ai chi have evolved, so have the various styles or schools of the art. As the form has grown and developed, so has the difference in style along with the different emphasis from a variety of teachers. A majority of the different schools or styles of t'ai chi have been given their founder's surnames.

The principal schools of t'ai chi include:

• Chen style
• Hao (or Wu Shi) style
• Hu Lei style
• Sun style
• Wu style
• Yang style
• Zhao Bao style

Many of the most commonly used groupings of forms are based on the Yang style of t'ai chi, developed by Yang Pan-Hou (1837–1892). Each of the forms has a name, such as "Carry the Tiger to the Mountain," and as the progression is made throughout the many forms, the participant ends the exercise almost standing on one leg. While most forms, like "Wind Blows Lotus Leaves," has just one movement or part, others, like "Work the Shuttle in the Clouds," have as many as four. While the form is typically practiced individually, the movement called "Pushing Hands" is a sequence practiced by two people together.

Preparation

Masters of t'ai chi recommend that those who practice the art begin each session by doing a **warm-up** of gentle rotation exercises for the joints and gentle **stretching** exercises for the muscles and tendons. Other suggestions for preparing the mind and body include: gaining a sense of body orientation; relaxation of every part of the body; maintaining smooth and regular breathing; gaining attention or feeling; being mindful of each movement; maintaining proper posture; and moving at the same pace throughout each movement. The main requirement for a successful form of t'ai chi is to feel completely comfortable while performing all of the movements.

Equipment

There is no **age** limitation for those who learn t'ai chi, and there is no special equipment needed for the exercise. Participants are encouraged to wear loose clothing and soft shoes.

Training and conditioning

Participants should select a qualified t'ai chi instructor. It is beneficial to consider the type of training and number of years of experience, whether or not the instructor specializes in a particular type of t'ai chi, and if the instructor is a member of a professional organization. Some instructors have their own website to offer information about their classes, and to provide information on the practice of t'ai chi.

Masters of t'ai chi are trained extensively in the various forms of the art by grandmasters who are extremely skillful of the exercise and its origins. For those who wish to learn t'ai chi from a master, classes are taught throughout the world in health clubs, community centers, senior citizen centers, and official t'ai chi schools. Before entering a class, the instructor's credentials should be reviewed, and they should be questioned about the form of t'ai chi they teach.

It is important for individuals to be shown the proper form to avoid strain, imbalance, and possible injury. In addition, they should know what parts of the body might be stressed by a particular posture, and be able to maintain their balance without undue limitations. Some of the more rigorous forms of the art may be too intense for older people, or for those who are not confident of their balance. Participants are encouraged to get a physician's approval before beginning any t'ai chi program.

Risks

Although t'ai chi is not physically demanding, it requires close attention to one's posture. Those who want to practice the exercise should notify their physician before beginning. The physician will caution the patient if they are taking medications that might interfere with balance, or if they have a condition that could make a series of t'ai chi movements dangerous.

KEY TERMS

Aerobics—Any of various forms of sustained vigorous exercise, such as jogging, calisthenics, or jazz dancing, intended to stimulate and strengthen the heart and respiratory system.

Cortisol—A steroid hormone released by the cortex (outer portion) of the adrenal gland when a person is under stress.

Fibromyalgia—A chronic disease syndrome characterized by fatigue, widespread muscular soreness, and pain at specific points on the body.

Qi—The traditional Chinese term for vital energy or the life force. Also spelled "ki" or "chi" in English translations of Japanese and Chinese medical books.

Taoism—A Chinese religion and philosophy based on the doctrines of Laotse that advocates simplicity and selflessness.

Results

The art of t'ai chi is many things to the people who practice it. To some, it is a stretching exercise that incorporates a deep-breathing program. To others, it is a martial art—and beyond this, it is often used as a **dance** or to accompany prayer. While the ways in which it is used may vary, one of the main benefits for those who practice it remains universal—t'ai chi promotes good health. This sense of well being complements t'ai chi's additional benefits of improved coordination, balance, and body awareness, while also calming the mind and reducing stress. Those in search of harmony between the mind and the body practice dynamic relaxation.

While the reasons why t'ai chi is practiced vary, research has uncovered several reasons why it may help many medical conditions. For example, people with rheumatoid **arthritis** (RA) are encouraged to practice t'ai chi for its graceful, slow sweeping movements. Its ability to combine stretching and range-of-motion exercises with relaxation techniques work well to relieve the stiffness and weakness in the joints of RA patients. An ongoing research program at Stanford University in California is evaluating the beneficial effects of t'ai chi on patients with fibromyalgia. A study of fibromyalgia patients in Georgia reported in 2003 that t'ai chi brought about significant improvement in the patients' control of their symptoms.

T'ai chi has also been shown to benefit patients with osteoarthritis (OA). A group of Korean researchers found that women diagnosed with OA showed significant improvement in their balance and abdominal muscle strength after a 12-week program of Sun-style t'ai chi.

In 1999, investigators from Johns Hopkins University in Baltimore, Maryland, studied the effects of t'ai chi on those with elevated **blood pressure**. Sixty-two sedentary adults with high-normal blood pressure or stage I **hypertension** who were aged 60 or older began a 12-week aerobic program or a light-intensity t'ai chi program. The exercise sessions both consisted of 30-minute sessions, four days a week. The study revealed that while the aerobics did lower the systolic blood pressure of participants, the t'ai chi group's systolic level was also lowered by an average of seven points—only a point less than the aerobics group. Interestingly, t'ai chi hardly raises the heart rate while still having the same effects as an intense aerobics class.

In addition to lowering blood pressure, research suggests that t'ai chi improves heart and lung function. The exercise is linked to reducing the body's level of a stress hormone called cortisol, and to the overall effect of higher confidence for those who practice it. As a complementary therapy, t'ai chi is also found to enhance the mainstream medical care of cancer patients who use the exercise to help control their symptoms and improve their quality of life.

Physical therapists investigated the effects of t'ai chi among 20 patients during their recovery from coronary artery bypass surgery. The patients were placed into either the t'ai chi group or an unsupervised control group. The t'ai chi group performed classical Yang exercises each morning for one year, while the control group walked three times a week for 50 minutes each session. In 1999, the study reported that after one year of training, the t'ai chi group showed significant improvement in their cardio respiratory function and their work rate, but the unsupervised control group displayed only a slight decrease in both areas.

T'ai chi is also used to keep people from falling—something that happens to one in three people over age 65 each year. Researchers from Emory University in Atlanta, Georgia, had dozens of men and women in their 70s and older learn the graceful movements of t'ai chi. The study discovered that those who learned to perform t'ai chi were almost 50% less likely to experience falls within a given time frame than subjects who simply received feedback from a computer screen on how much they swayed as they stood. Those who fall experience greater declines in everyday activities than those who do not fall, and are at a greater risk of

QUESTIONS TO ASK YOUR DOCTOR

- In what way do you think t'ai chi will benefit me?
- What other treatment options do you recommend?
- What tests or evaluation techniques will you perform to see if t'ai has been beneficial for me?
- Will performing t'ai chi interfere with my current medications?
- Do I have any physical limitations that would prohibit my undertaking t'ai?

requiring placement in a nursing home or other type of assisted living. Researchers recommend the use of t'ai chi for its ability to help people raise their consciousness of how their bodies are moving in the environment around them. By raising awareness of how the body moves, people can focus on their relationship to their physical environment and situations they encounter everyday.

In addition to studying the cardiovascular and range-of-motion benefits of t'ai chi, researchers are investigating its positive effects on the **immune system**. A team of scientists in California reported in 2003 that t'ai chi boosts the resistance of older people to the shingles virus—a virus that is both more common and more severe in the elderly.

Some research done in the United States focuses on the emotional and psychological benefits of t'ai chi. One recently discovered advantage of t'ai chi is its ability to hold people's interest longer than many other forms of exercise. One study in Oregon found that only 20% of people enrolled in a six-month t'ai chi program dropped out before the end, compared to an average of 55% for other forms of exercise. With regard to depression, a study of college students found that those who were taking t'ai chi classes had a lower rate of depression than students enrolled in other fitness programs.

While the martial arts offer very vigorous physical workouts and often result in injuries, the practice of t'ai chi is a good alternative to these sports without overstraining the body. Patients with bad backs have found t'ai chi eases their discomfort.

Resources

BOOKS

Austin, Andrew. *Tai Chi for Beginners*. New York: Rosen Publishing Group, Inc., 2011.

Docherty, Don. *Tai Chi Chuan: Decoding the Classics for the Modern Martial Artist*. Wiltshire, UK: The Crowood Press, 2009.

Gilligan, Peter, A. *What Is 'Tai Chi'?* London: Jessica Kingsley Publishers, 2010.

Herman, Kauz. *Tai Chi Handbook*. New York: Overlook Press, 2009.

Stone, Justin. *T'ai Chi Chih! Joy Thru Movement*, 3rd ed. Boston: Good Karma Publishing, Inc., 2009.

PERIODICALS

Christou, E. A., Y. Yang, and K. S. Rosengren. "Taiji Training Improves Knee Extensor Strength and Force Control in Older Adults." *Journals of Gerontology, Series A: Biological Sciences and Medical Sciences* 58 (August 2003): 763–766.

Cooper, Bob. "An Exercise in Vitality: Put Away Your Prejudices—T'ai Chi Ain't Just for Senior Citizens and Vegans." *Men's Fitness* 18 (September 2002): 86–91.

Filusch Betts, Elaine. "The Effect of T'ai Chi on Cardiorespiratory Function in Patients with Coronary Artery Bypass Surgery." *Physical Therapy* (September 1999).

Irwin, M. R., J. L. Pike, J. C. Cole, and M. N. Oxman. "Effects of a Behavioral Intervention, T'ai Chi Chih, on Varicella-Zoster Virus Specific Immunity and Health Functioning in Older Adults." *Psychosomatic Medicine* 65 (September-October 2003): 824–830.

Li, F., K. J. Fisher, P. Harmer, and E. McAuley. "Delineating the Impact of T'ai Chi Training on Physical Function Among the Elderly." *American Journal of Preventive Medicine* 23 (August 2002): 92–97.

Song, R., E. O. Lee, P. Lam, and S. C. Bae. "Effects of T'ai Chi Exercise on Pain, Balance, Muscle Strength, and Perceived Difficulties in Physical Functioning in Older Women with Osteoarthritis: A Randomized Clinical Trial." *Journal of Rheumatology* 30 (September 2003): 2039–2044.

Taggart, H. M., C. L. Arslanian, S. Bae, and K. Singh. "Effects of T'ai Chi Exercise on Fibromyalgia Symptoms and Health-Related Quality of Life." *Orthopaedic Nursing* 22 (September-October 2003): 353–360.

ORGANIZATIONS

American Association of Oriental Medicine, 5530 Wisconsin Avenue, Suite 1210, Chevy Chase, MD, 20815, (301) 941-1064, http://www.aaom.org.

Canadian Taijiquan Federation, P.O. Box 421, MiltonOntario, Canada, L9T 4Z1, http://www.canadiantaijiquanfederation.com.

National Center for Complementary and Alternative Medicine (NCCAM), 9000 Rockville Pike, Bethesda, MD, 20892, (888) 644-6226, http://nccam.nih.gov.

Patience T'ai Chi Association, 2620 East 18th St., Brooklyn, NY, 11235, (718) 332-3477, http://www.patiencetaichi.com.

Rebecca J. Frey, PhD
Laura Jean Cataldo, RN, EdD

Tap *see* **Dance**

Target heart rate

Definition

The target heart rate range is a helpful guide for monitoring **exercise** intensity. It should take into account an individual's fitness level, habitual exercise level, medical history, goals, and overall program. The target heart range, also called training heart range, is calculated based on age-predicted maximal heart rate, and desired level of exercise effort. For most people, a level of effort at or about 50-85% of maximal heart rate is suggested. Factoring in resting heart rate, which allows one to calculate a "heart rate reserve," tends to be a little more accurate.

Purpose

Exercise increases the demands on the body and heart, which causes the heart to beat faster. Target heart rate range is a guide to how quickly the heart should beat during exercise. Calculating a target heart rate range allows an individual to work out more safely and effectively. Once the target heart rate range has been calculated, pulse should be monitored during exercise and compared to the range to make sure the exercise effort is appropriate. The exercise intensity can then be adjusted accordingly.

For example, if an individual has calculated a target heart rate range of 130-160 beats per minute, and checks his pulse during exercise and finds it is lower than 130 beats per minute, the exercise is probably not challenging enough to be very beneficial. Depending on his medical history and fitness level, heart rates over 160 beats per minute might be too high to be safe. Thus, the target heart rate range is used to guide the intensity of the exercise program.

Description

In general, the higher the heart rate, the more challenging the exercise, and the greater the metabolic demands on the body. This holds true for most types of cardiovascular exercise, such as **running**, **walking**, biking, stair climbing, hiking, and many types of indoor exercise equipment, such as ellipticals and stationary cycles. Target heart rate is not an appropriate method to monitor the intensity of a weight lifting program.

While a recommended intensity range of 50-85% of maximum heart rate is safe and effective for most people, there are some notable exceptions. Highly fit athletes, who have performance goals and not just fitness goals, perform much of their exercise at heart rates near the top of or above the target heart rate range. **Interval training** programs, which are characterized by work/rest ratios, call for brief bouts of intense exercise at 80-95% of maximal heart rate, followed by active rest intervals at a low enough intensity to allow for recovery. Unfit individuals and those with medical conditions should exercise at low to moderate intensities until they have become more conditioned. This will correspond to heart rates at the lower end of the target heart rate range. Exercising more moderately when untrained confers less risk than exercising intensely.

Determining target heart range

In order to accurately estimate target heart rate range, two pieces of information are needed: **age**, and resting pulse.

- To monitor pulse, turn the palm up, and place two fingers on the thumb side of the wrist. Count the pulse for 60 seconds after resting quietly or first thing in the morning. This value is resting heart rate.
- To estimate maximal heart rate, the American College of Sports Medicine suggests this equation: max heart rate is 206.9 − (age x .67).
- To calculate training heart range, subtract resting heart rate from maximal heart rate, then multiply by 50-85%, and then add back in resting heart rate. Example for a 30 year old with a resting heart rate of 70 beats per minute: 206.9 − (30 x 0.67) = 187 beats per minute (this is the estimated maximal heart rate) 187 − 70 (resting heart rate) x 0.50-0.85 + 70 = a training heart rate range of 129 to 169 beats per minute.
- If resting heart rate is not known, maximal heart rate can be estimated using the same equation, and the individual simply multiples this number by the desired intensity to get an estimate of what the heart rate should be. In the case of a 30 year old: 206.9 − (30 x .67) = maximal heart rate of 187 beats per minute, 187 x .60 -.90 = 112 − 168 beats per minute.

Generating the equation without factoring in resting heart rate is a little less accurate.

How to use the target heart rate range

After several minutes of warm up, and once the desired exercise level is achieved, pulse is monitored. While continuing to exercise, pulse is counted for 10 seconds and multiplied by six. This number equals heart rate in beats per minute, and should fall within the target heart rate range. If it is below the range calculated, the exercise may be too easy. If it is higher than the range, the exercise might be too challenging

KEY TERMS

Atrial fibrillation—An irregular heart beat.

Beta blockers—Medications prescribed to patients with heart disease or high blood pressure that lower heart rate at rest and during exercise.

Cardiovascular exercise—Exercise that uses the larger muscles of the body, increases the demand for oxygen, increases the heart rate, and can be sustained for longer than several minutes.

Diabetic autonomic neuropathy—A complication of long-standing diabetes that results in a altered heart rate response; generally characterized by a high resting heart rate and blunted maximal and exercise heart rates.

Estimated age-predicted maximal heart rate—Determined using the equation: 206.9 − (age x 0.67).

Exercise intensity—The difficulty of the exercise as defined by the increase in oxygen demand and heart rate.

Pulse—Heart rate.

Target heart rate range—A high and low heart rate range based on a percentage of maximal heart rate.

to be sustained or safe. This process should be repeated periodically throughout the workout, and anytime the type of exercise is changed (i.e., goes from a **treadmill** to a bike).

It is important to realize that exercise intensity (which is gauged by heart rate) and exercise duration (minutes spent exercising) are interrelated. Target heart rate is a range, not one number, and likewise, the exercise program parameters are best thought of as a spectrum. For example, exercising for 50 minutes at the lower end of the target heart rate is beneficial, but so is exercising for 20 minutes at the higher end. Because intensity and duration are interrelated, both need to be considered in the exercise prescription.

This means that a runner going out for 4-mi. (6.4 km) run may shoot for a heart rate near 85% of his maximum by increasing his pace, but may run at a slower pace that elicits 60% of his maximum when he is out for a 10-mi.(16-km) run.

Precautions

In certain cases, age-predicted maximal heart rates and/or target heart rate ranges are not appropriate. Age-predicted maximal or training heart rates

should not be used for individuals taking beta blockers or other medications that lower heart rate; people who are diabetic with autonomic neuropathy; or individuals who have an irregular heart rate, such as atrial fibrillation. Pregnant women should be cautious about using a target heart range to gauge exercise intensity due to the wide variability of heart rate when pregnant.

Age-predicted maximum heart rate is an estimation, not an exact science. While this calculation works well for most people, it is not exact for all people. The only way to know an individual's maximal heart rate with certainty is by having a maximal exercise test.

Individuals using target heart rate range to guide exercise intensity should not be misled by heart rate charts posted on equipment and gym walls. Many of these charts and posters incorrectly designate a "fat burning zone" at the lower end of the target heart rate range. In actuality, more total **calories** and fat are burned at higher exercise intensities (higher heart rates). This is because higher exercise intensity places a greater metabolic demand on the body both during and after exercise.

Preparation

To use the target heart rate correctly, an individual must practice counting their pulse while exercising. Waiting until exercise is over to count pulse is not advised as heart rate tends to drop quickly and this could lead the individual to think that the intensity needs to be increased even when it does not. Alternatively, a heart rate monitor can be purchased and worn during exercise. These devices usually employ a chest strap or watch and provide a constant heart rate during exercise.

Complications

An individual using heart rate range to guide exercise intensity must be able to monitor pulse correctly. If the exercise feels very difficult but the heart rate is low, the individual may not be measuring correctly, or may be waiting until exercise is over before measuring. Some studies indicate that heart rate decreases about five beats per minute every 10 seconds after stopping exercise. Even people who have received instruction on pulse palpation take 15-20 seconds to obtain heart rate after they stop exercising. Therefore, counting pulse during exercise is recommended if at all possible.

Results

Using a target heart rate range allows an individual to guide intensity during exercise so that the program is safer and more effective. As fitness improves, it takes harder exercise to elicit the same heart rate. In this regard, monitoring heart rate is a great way to see progress, and to know when the program needs to be updated.

Resources

BOOKS

ACSM's Guidelines for Exercise Testing and Prescription. 8th ed. Philadelphia: Lippincott Williams & Wilkins, 2010.

ACSM's Resource Manual for Guidelines for Exercise Testing and Prescription. 6th ed. Philadelphia: Lippincott Williams & Wilkins, 2010.

PERIODICALS

Dinesh, J., G.A. Sforzo, and T. Swensen. "Monitoring Heart Rate Using Manual Palpation." *ACSM's Health & Fitness Journal* 11, no. 6 (November/December 2007): 14–18.

Thompson, D.L. "Improving VO$_2$ $_{max}$." *ACSM Health Fitness Journal* 9, no. 5 (September/October 2005): 4.

WEBSITES

"Get Moving!" American Heart Association. http://www.heart.org/HEARTORG/GettingHealthy/PhysicalActivity/Physical-Activity_UCM_001080_SubHomePage.jsp (accessed August 23, 2011).

ORGANIZATIONS

American College of Sports Medicine, 401 W. Michigan St., Indianapolis, IN, 46206-1440, (317) 637-9200, Fax: (317) 634-7817, http://www.acsm.org.

American Council on Exercise, 4851 Paramount Dr., San Diego, CA, 92123, (858) 576-6500, Fax: (858) 576-6564, (888) 825-3636, resource@acefitness.org, http://www.acefitness.org.

American Heart Association, 7272 Greenville Avenue, Dallas, TX, 75231, (800) 242-8721, Review.personal.info@heart.org, http://www.heart.org.

Lisa S. Womack, MEd

Tendinitis

Definition

Tendinitis is the inflammation of a tendon, a tough rope-like tissue that connects muscle to bone.

Description

Tendinitis usually occurs in individuals in middle or old **age** because it is often the result of overuse over a long period. Tendinitis can occur in younger individuals from acute overuse.

Tendons that commonly become inflamed include:

- tendons of the hand
- tendons of the upper arm that effect the shoulder
- Achilles tendon and the tendon that runs across the top of the foot
- tendons attached to the kneecap

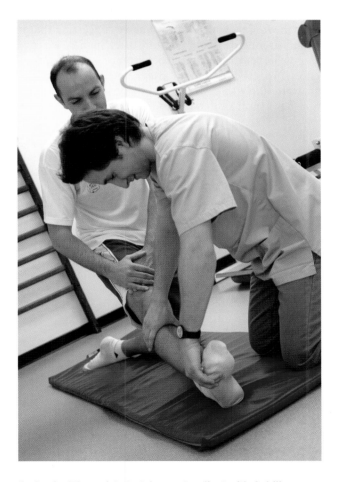

A physical therapist stretches out a client with Achilles tendonitis. (© *Phanie/Photo Researchers, Inc.*)

Demographics

Tendinitis is a very common injury, especially among individuals who participate in professional or recreational sports and fitness activities and individuals whose jobs involve physical activity. Achilles tendinitis is believed to occur at a rate of somewhere between 6 and 37 cases per 100,000 people; about four out of five injuries of this kind occur during athletic or fitness activities. Bicipital tendinitis is estimated to occur at a rate of 1.2 injuries per 100,000 population.

Tendinitis occurs much more frequently in men than in women, with some estimates suggesting that it occurs as much as six times more often in men. It is not clear whether this increased occurrence is due to differences in participation in sports and other activities that are likely to cause tendinitis or if it is related to another aspect of gender. Individuals over the age of 30 are at an increased risk of tendinitis, with most injuries occurring in individuals age 40–60.

Athletes are at an increased risk of tendinitis compared to the general population. Sports that require repeated movements are the most likely to lead to tendinitis. These include:

- tennis
- running
- golf
- bowling
- baseball
- dancing
- bicycling
- swimming

Causes and symptoms

Tendonitis is caused in one of two ways. Sudden onset tendinitis can be caused by a sudden overexertion of the tendon. This type of tendinitis is not as common as progressive tendinitis. Progressive tendinitis is caused over time by repeated movements that stretch the tendon. Both sudden **stretching** and repeated overuse injure the connection between the tendon and the muscle to which it is attached. The injury is largely mechanical, but when it occurs, the body tries to heal it by initiating an inflammatory reaction. Inflammation increases the blood supply, bringing nutrients to the damaged tissues along with **immune system** cells to combat infection. The result is swelling, tenderness, pain, heat, and redness if the inflammation is close to the skin.

Diagnosis

A diagnosis of tendinitis is made after a medical history is taken, including information about what sports and professional activities the individual commonly engages in. Often, this information can be very suggestive of tendinitis without additional tests being necessary. For example, an elbow problem in an individual who plays many hours of tennis each week is quite likely to be extensor tendinitis (tennis elbow).

Some tendon injuries are superficial and easy to identify through a simple manual examination. These include extensor tendinitis over the outside of the elbow, and Achilles tendinitis just above the heel. Several tendons in the shoulder can be overused or stretched; often the shoulder has more than one injury simultaneously. Tendinitis in the biceps, the infraspinatus, or the supraspinatus tendon may accompany a tear of the shoulder ligaments or an impingement of one bone or another. Careful pressure testing and movement of the parts is often all that is necessary to identify the tendinitis.

Situations where tendinitis cannot be diagnosed using only a history and physical examination require x rays and/or magnetic resonance imaging (MRI) to determine the underlying problem. X rays do not show tendons; however, they are useful for ruling out other possible causes of the pain and inflammation. MRIs are useful at determining if a tendon has torn.

Treatment

Rest, ice, compression, and elevation (RICE) is typically the recommended method to treat the acute condition. The best way to apply ice is in a bag with water. The water applies the cold directly to the skin. Chemical ice packs can get too cold and cause frostbite. Compression using an elastic wrap minimizes swelling and bleeding in an acute injury. Splinting may help rest the limb. Pain and anti-inflammatory medications (e.g., aspirin, naproxen, ibuprofen) can help reduce pain and swelling. Sometimes the inflammation lingers and requires additional treatment. Injections of cortisone-like drugs often relieves chronic tendinitis, but should be reserved for resistant cases since cortisone can occasionally cause undesirable side effects.

If tendinitis is persistent and unresponsive to nonsurgical treatment, surgery to remove the afflicted portion of tendon can be performed. Surgery is also done to remove calcium buildup that comes with persistent tendinitis.

Prognosis

Generally, tendinitis heals if the provoking activity is stopped. In some cases, such as when an occupation-related activity is the cause of the injury, making even minor changes to the way in which the activity is performed can help give the tendinitis time to heal and prevent future problems. If a sports activity is causing the tendinitis, small changes in posture or hold can sometimes be beneficial.

Prevention

If given enough time, tendons will strengthen to meet the demands placed on them. They grow slowly because of their poor blood supply, so adequate time is required for good conditioning. Occupational and physical therapists can help an individual identify ways to change posture, stance, and hold in order to reduce the risk of recurrence.

Resources

BOOKS

Anderson, Marcia K., and Gail P. Parr. *Fundamentals of Sports Injury Management,* 3rd ed. Baltimore: Wolters Kluwer/Lippincott Williams & Wilkins, 2011.

Hutson, Mike, and Cathy Speed, eds. *Sports Injuries.* New York: Oxford University Press, 2011.

Marcovitz, Hal. *Sports Injuries.* Detroit: Lucent Books, 2010.

Wilk, Kevin E., Michael M. Reinold, and James R. Andrews, eds. *The Athlete's Shoulder,* 2nd ed. Philadelphia: Churchill Livingstone/Elsevier, 2009.

PERIODICALS

Carcia, Christopher, R., et al. "Achilles Pain, Stiffness, and Muscle Power Deficits: Achilles Tendinitis." *Journal of Orthopaedic and Sports Physical Therapy* 40, no. 9 (September 2010): A1–26.

Williams, Isaiah, W., and Byron S. Kennedy. "Texting Tendinitis in a Teenager." *Journal of Family Practice* 60, no. 2 (February 2011): 66–67.

WEBSITES

Diseases & Conditions: Achilles Tendonitis Overview. The Cleveland Clinic. http://my.clevelandclinic.org/disorders/tendonitis/hic_tendonitis.aspx (accessed November 13, 2011).

Tendinitis. The Mayo Clinic. (November 8, 2011). http://www.mayoclinic.com/health/tendinitis/DS00153 (accessed November 13, 2011).

ORGANIZATIONS

American College of Sports Medicine, P.O. Box 1440, Indianapolis, IN, 46206-1440, (317) 637-9200, Fax: (317) 634-7817, http://www.acsm.org.

National Academy of Sports Medicine, 5845 E. Still Circle, Suite 206, Mesa, AZ, 85206, (818) 595-1200, Fax: (480) 656-3276, (800) 460-6276, http://www.nasm.org.

J. Ricker Polsdorfer, MD
Tish Davidson, AM

Tennis

Definition

Tennis is a sport that is played on a court with either two competing players (singles) or two pairs of players (doubles). Each player has a strung racquet that is used to hit a hollow, felt-covered, rubber ball over a net into the opponent's court.

Purpose

Tennis is played worldwide for recreation and cardiovascular exercise. It is also an Olympic sport and a popular spectator sport played by celebrity professionals, with four Grand Slam tournaments: the Australian Open, the French Open, Wimbledon, and the U.S. Open.

Demographics

Tennis is played by millions of people around the world, of all ages, both genders, and every ethnic and socioeconomic class. Among Americans, 3.7% of males report playing tennis, including 5.7% of those

ROGER FEDERER (1981–)

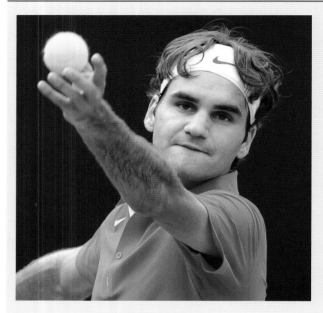

Swiss professional tennis player Roger Federer. *(Massimo Cebrelli/Getty Images.)*

Born in Basel, Switzerland, on August 8, 1981, Roger Federer started playing tennis at age eight. His parents, who were weekend amateurs, got him interested in the game, but he took it to another level. In 1998, Federer won the Wimbledon junior title and finished that year as the number–one junior in the world. He also reached the finals at the U.S. Open and semifinals at the Australian Open, and took the title and the Orange Bowl in Miami, Florida. In 1999, he was the youngest player—at 18 years, four months—to finish in the top 100. He advanced to his first Association of Tennis Professionals (ATP) semifinals in Vienna, Austria, and went on to quarterfinals in Marseille, France; Rotterdam, Netherlands; and his hometown of Basel. In 2000, he was the number–two–ranked tennis player in Switzerland and lost the bronze medal at the Olympic Games that year to Arnaud Di Pasquale.

In 2001, Federer broke seven–time champ Pete Sampras's 31–match Wimbledon winning streak in the fourth round. Up to this point, Federer had never made it past quarterfinals at a Grand Slam tournament. Also, his stunning performances were often followed by massive upsets. For instance, after showing up Sampras, he lost three first–round matches at majors, including at Wimbledon in 2002, the Australian Open in January of 2003, and the French Open in May of 2003. The Wimbledon loss was a huge setback, because it was in straight sets against Mario Ancic, ranked number 154 in the world. However, he snagged a Tennis Masters Series shield in Hamburg, Germany, in 2002 and qualified for the Tennis Masters Cup later that year in Shanghai, China. He reached the semifinals with a

aged 18–29, and 2% of American females play tennis, including 3.1% of those aged 18–29.

History

Tennis in some form dates back several thousand years. Older forms of tennis were played on an indoor court and are sometimes referred to as real tennis or royal tennis. It was considered one of the "sports of kings." Modern tennis originated in Birmingham, England, in the 1860s, when Major Henry Gem and Augurio Perera combined the game of indoor racquets with the Spanish ball game pelota and adapted it for play on a croquet lawn. In 1874 they founded the first tennis club at Leamington Spa, England. Originally popular with upper-class English-speaking peoples, tennis eventually spread around the world. The rules of the game have changed very little since the 1890s.

Description

Tennis is a two- or four-person, non-contact, weight-bearing, high-impact activity. Singles tennis is considered vigorous or heavy exercise—exercise during which it is possible to say only a few words before catching one's breath. Doubles tennis is considered moderate exercise—exercise during which it is possible to talk, but not sing. Tennis is a sport that requires sharp sudden turns, called cutting activities. It is less helpful for improving cardiovascular endurance than some other exercises, since it involves a great deal of starting and stopping. It is not necessary to play a game of tennis to reap its exercise benefits: an individual can practice serving and hitting a tennis ball against a wall and perform tennis drills.

Preparation

A thorough warm-up should precede a game of tennis, such as jogging around the court for 5–10 minutes, followed by warm-up play. Gradual stretching exercises for the wrist, such as wrist curls, are excellent exercises for tennis.

Equipment

A tennis racquet and tennis ball are necessary pieces of equipment for all players. Some individuals

perfect 3–0 record before losing to eventual victor Lleyton Hewitt in three close sets.

Federer captured four titles in the first half of 2003 at Marseille, France; Dubai, United Arab Emirates; Munich, Germany; and Halle, Germany. The 2003 Wimbledon win finally put an end to questions of whether he could overcome his anxiety to capture a major title. After beating fifth–seeded Andy Roddick, he advanced to his first Grand Slam final. On July 6, 2003, he triumphed over Mark Philippoussis, 7–6 (5), 6–2, 7–6 (3). Following Wimbledon 2003, Federer lost to David Nalbandian at the U.S. Open in September in their fourth–round match. Later that month, he fell to Hewitt at the Davis Cup final as well. However, in October he bounced back by successfully defending his CA Trophy against Spain's Carlos Moya. This was his sixth ATP title of the year, and he set a new record for ATP best season with 67 wins, 14 losses. In addition, it put Federer in a three–way tie with Roddick and Spaniard Juan Carlos Ferrero for the year–end ATP number–one spot.

Federer won the Stefan Edberg Sportsmanship Award for five straight years and was selected as the favorite player in a fan poll for the sixth consecutive year. In 2006 he was appointed a "goodwill ambassador" for UNICEF and made his first trip for the organization to tsunami–ravaged Tamil Nadu. In 2007, Federer appeared in a series of commercials for Gillette razors with golfer Tiger Woods and French soccer player Thierry Henry. On April 11, 2009, Federer married Miroslava "Mirka" Vavrinec in Switzerland. On July 23, 2009, they became the parents of twin daughters, Charlene Riva and Myla Rose. In Federer's hometown, Basel, the St. Jakobshalle tennis building was renamed in his honor. Federer finished as ATP World Tour Champion for the fifth time in six years in 2009. He became the all–time leader in men's tennis with 15 Grand Slam singles titles with his seventh straight Wimbledon final, defeating Roddick. He also took four titles in the season and earned his fifteenth ATP World Tour Masters 1000 crown in Madrid and his sixteenth in Cincinnati, Ohio.

During the 2010 season, Federer took five titles and finished in the top two. He won his sixteenth Grand Slam at the Australian Open but lost at Wimbledon in the quarter-finals. In August he won his seventeenth ATP World Tour Masters 1000 trophy in Cincinnati, tying Agassi. He lost in September at the U.S. Open, but won his sixty–fourth tour–level title in Stockholm. He took another title in his hometown and ended the season with the title at Barclays ATP World Tour in London. Federer opened the 2011 season with a January win in Doha, his third win there. He lost at the Australian Open and tournaments in Dubai, Indian Wells, Miami, and Monte Carlo, then went onto the clay courts of Madrid, hitting a personal best 25 aces on clay, though falling in the semifinals. He continued in this vein, losing at Wimbledon, Montreal, Cincinnati, and the U.S. Open. The week after the U.S. Open, however, he helped Switzerland gain a place in the 2012 Davis Cup World Group with a victory over Australia.

choose to wear loose fitting clothes designed for tennis activity, and many wear sweatbands during play, as well. Good fitting rubber soled footwear is necessary to be worn on the court surface.

Tennis courts can be indoors or outdoors. Most communities in the United States have public tennis courts as well as private tennis clubs. Professional tennis is played on four types of surfaces: clay; hard surfaces such as acrylic, asphalt, or concrete; grass; and carpet or artificial turf. Each of these surfaces differs in the speed and height of the ball's bounce. The tennis court also includes a specially designed net, which divides the playing area.

Training and conditioning

Tennis can be played by anyone who can hold a racquet. It can be adapted for children and adults of almost any age and type of disability, including those in wheelchairs.

Risks

There are some risks of injury associated with tennis. These injuries often occur because:

- The player did not adequately warm up.

- A beginner overdid it, especially if their technique is poor.

- A player does not have proper equipment. For example, playing with a racket that is too tightly or too loosely strung or with worn-out shoes can be dangerous. A handle with a good grip is particularly important. An improperly fitted tennis racquet can contribute to tennis elbow.

To avoid these and other risks tennis players should:

- wear tennis shoes with good supports to prevent ankle injuries

- wear two pairs of socks or support socks for added ankle support

- if possible, avoid playing on "no-give" surfaces such as cement, asphalt, or synthetic courts

- use heel inserts on hard-surface courts to absorb shocks and help prevent lower back injuries

- dry the racket handle with sawdust or powdered chalk to prevent blisters on the hands

KEY TERMS

Achilles tendon—The strong tendon joining the calf muscles to the heel bone.

Aerobic—Strenuous physical exercise that results in a significant increase in respiration and heart rate.

Biceps—The large flexor muscle of the front of the upper arm.

Bursitis—Inflammation of a bursa, the fluid-filled sacs located between tendons and bones in the joints.

Calorie—A unit of energy supplied by food.

Endorphins—A class of peptides in the brain that are produced during exercise and bind to opiate receptors, resulting in pain relief and pleasant feelings.

Plantar fasciitis—Inflammation and pain under the heel.

Repetitive stress or strain injury (RSI)—A musculoskeletal injury, such as tendonitis, caused by cumulative damage to muscles, tendons, ligaments, nerves, or joints from highly repetitive movements and characterized by pain, weakness, and/or numbness.

Tendonitis—Inflammation of a tendon.

Tennis elbow—Inflammation and pain over the outside of the elbow, usually resulting from excessive strain on and twisting of the forearm; also called lateral epicondylitis or tendonitis of the elbow.

- drink plenty of fluids before, during, and after play to avoid stiffness and cramps
- have a first-aid kit on hand

Repetitive stress injuries (RSIs) or overuse injuries are a major risk of playing tennis. Tennis elbow or tendonitis of the elbow is inflammation and soreness or pain on the outside (lateral) side of the upper arm near the elbow from the repeated motion of the wrist or forearm. Tennis elbow is often caused by damage to a specific muscle of the forearm. There may be partial tearing of the tendon fibers that connect muscle to bone at or near their point of origin on the outside of the elbow. For example, during a groundstroke in tennis when the arm is straightened, the extensor carpi radialis brevis (ECRB) muscle of the forearm helps stabilize the wrist. When the ECRB becomes weakened from overuse, microscopic tears can form in the tendon.

Other types of tennis RSIs include:

- rotator cuff tendonitis or tennis shoulder—an inflammation of the tendons in the shoulder caused by repeatedly moving the arm over the head

- Achilles tendonitis of the heel
- bursitis—inflammation of the bursa in a joint from repetitive joint motions such as serving

Techniques for avoiding tennis injuries include:

- When serving or making an overhead shot, the player should bend at the knees and raise the heels, so that the upper body weight is evenly balanced over the heels and the back does not arch unnecessarily.
- Serving should be performed with a bent arm. Serving with a straight arm and wrist transfers all of the shock from the wrist to the elbow.
- Players with tennis elbow should not serve overhand.
- On forehand shots the arm should be bent so that the force of the swing is taken by the biceps and shoulder rather than the elbow.
- Backhand swings should begin from the shoulder and the thumb should not be placed behind the grip of the racquet for added support.
- A two-handed backhand can help prevent tendonitis.
- When hitting ground strokes, excessive top spin should not be put on the ball.
- Quick starts and stops can cause mild ankle sprains.
- Landing on the ball of the foot can injure the Achilles tendon.
- A tennis shoe with a medial arch support or heel cup can sometimes relieve the pain of plantar fasciitis that results from overuse of the foot, although rest is the best cure.

Athletes who play tennis are at risk for stress fractures. These are small cracks in a bone resulting from the repeated stress of the feet striking the ground. A change in the playing surface, such as switching from a grass court to a clay court, increases the risk of a stress fracture.

Results

Tennis is a weight-bearing, bone-building exercise. It is an aerobic activity that works the large muscles of the arms, legs, and hips and raises the heart and respiratory rates. A 160-lb (73-kg) person burns about 584 calories in one hour of singles tennis. A 200-lb (91-kg) person burns about 728 calories and a 240-lb (109-kg) person burns about 872 calories in one hour of tennis. Tennis can increase production of endorphins—brain chemicals that create feelings of pleasure and reduce stress.

Resources

BOOKS

American Sports Education Program. *Coaching Youth Tennis,* 4th ed. Champaign, IL: Human Kinetics, 2008.

Drewett, Jim. *How to Improve at Tennis.* New York: Crabtree, 2008.

Powell, Mike. *A Game to Love: In Celebration of Tennis.* New York: Abrams, 2011.

Roetert, Paul, and Mark Kovacs. *Tennis Anatomy.* Champaign, IL: Human Kinetics, 2011.

Sampras, Pete, and Peter Bodo. *A Champion's Mind: Lessons from a Life in Tennis.* New York: Crown, 2008.

Woods, Kathy, and Ron Woods. *Playing Tennis After 50.* Champaign, IL: Human Kinetics, 2008.

PERIODICALS

Charles, Katie. "How to Ace Tennis Elbow." *New York Daily News* (October 21, 2009): 22.

Levitan, Paul. "African Americans Enriched Tennis." *Philadelphia Tribune* 125, no. 26 (February 10, 2009): 7I.

Pluim, B. M., et al. "Consensus Statement on Epidemiological Studies of Medical Conditions in Tennis, April 2009." *British Journal of Sports Medicine* 43, no. 12 (November 2009): 893.

Tagliafico, Alberto Stefano, et al. "Wrist Injuries in Nonprofessional Tennis Players: Relationships with Different Grips." *American Journal of Sports Medicine* 37, no. 4 (April 2009): 760.

ORGANIZATIONS

American College of Sports Medicine. P. O. Box 1440, Indianapolis, IN 46206-1440. (317) 637-9200. Fax: (317) 634-7817. http://www.acsm.org.

American Council on Exercise. 4851 Paramount Dr., San Diego, California 92123. (888) 825-3636. http://www.acefitness.org/default.aspx.

American Medical Association. 515 N. State St., Chicago, IL 60610. (800) 621-8335. http://www.ama-assn.org.

President's Council on Fitness, Sports & Nutrition. 1101 Wootton Pky., Ste. 560, Rockville, MD 20852. (240) 276-9567. http://fitness.gov/index.html.

OTHER

"Tennis Court Safety." *Your Orthopaedic Connection.* http://orthoinfo.aaos.org/topic.cfm?topic = A00133.

"Tennis Elbow." *MedlinePlus.* http://www.nlm.nih.gov/medlineplus/ency/article/000449.htm.

"Tennis Elbow (Lateral Epicondylitis)." *Your Orthopaedic Connection.* http://orthoinfo.aaos.org/topic.cfm?topic = A00068.

ORGANIZATIONS

American Academy of Orthopaedic Surgeons, 6300 N. River Road, Rosemont, IL, 60018-4262, (847) 823-7186, Fax: (847) 823-8125, orthoinfo@aaos.org, http://www.aaos.org.

American Orthopaedic Society for Sports Medicine, 6300 N. River Road, Suite 500, Rosemont, IL, 60018, (847) 292-4900, http://www.sportsmed.org.

International Tennis Federation, Bank Lane, Roehampton, London, UK, SW15 5XZ, + 44 (0)20 8878 6464, Fax: + 44 (0)20 8878 7799, http://www.itftennis.com.

United States Tennis Association, 70 West Red Oak Lane, White Plains, NY, 10604, (914) 696-7000, http://www.usta.com.

Margaret Alic, PhD
Laura Jean Cataldo, RN, EdD

Thermal injuries

Definition

A thermal injury is any damage to the skin caused by contact with a hot object, as in exposure to a flame, or scalding with a hot liquid; by exposure to a source of radiation, such as a **sunburn** or contact with a radioactive material; through contact with an electrical charge; or by exposure to a corrosive chemical, such as lye or strong acid. Frostbite is sometimes classified as a thermal injury, although it does not result from contact with a hot or corrosive material, because its initial symptoms are similar to those of thermal injury.

Description

The most common type of thermal injury is one in which the skin is heated to an abnormally high temperature. Studies indicate that human skin normally is not damaged at temperatures less than 111°F (44°C) if exposure does not exceed six hours. At temperatures ranging from 111–124°F (44–51°C), the rate of skin damage doubles with every one degree Celsius increase in temperature. Above 185°F (70°C), serious damage occurs in less than one second. Individuals respond somewhat differently to thermal injuries depending on certain characteristics of the skin, including moisture content of the skin; degree of pigmentation; presence of insulating materials, such as hair and skin oil; and efficiency of blood circulation in the affected area.

Skin cells damaged by thermal injury may experience one of three fates. Those most directly affected by the injury die almost immediately. The region in which this damage occurs is called the zone of coagulation because cells die when the materials of which they are made clump together and lose their ability to function normally. Cells that are somewhat more distant from the source of heat may also be damaged, but not so severely as to result in their death. With prompt and proper treatment, they may survive and continue functioning as normal cells. The region covered by cells of this type is known as the zone of stasis. Cells in the general region of a thermal injury, but at still greater distances from its main source, are likely to recover within a matter of about seven days provided that infection does not develop or shock does not occur. This area of cells is known as the zone of hyperemia, a term that means an increase of blood supply because cells in this region produce a more abundant supply of blood in response to the thermal injury.

The human body responds in a complex variety of ways in response to a thermal injury, as an attempt to protect and heal the damaged body part. At the site of the injury, biochemical changes occur that make the capillaries more porous, dumping their contents into the intercellular fluid and causing the accumulation of liquids at the site of the damage. Elsewhere in the body, the vascular system becomes more resistant to the flow of blood so that blood returns to the heart more slowly and the heart pumps blood more slowly. First, there is a redistribution of blood flow following thermal injury whereby some organs experience an increased resistance to blood flow while others a decreased resistance to blood flow. Second, the reduction in cardiac output would only occur with severe thermal injury and not in all instances as it is insinuated with the current statement. Simultaneously, a number of other changes occur in the body in response to the thermal injury, including the destruction of red blood cells, death of muscle tissue, hyperventilation as a means of increasing the rate of **metabolism**, gastrointestinal disturbances that may result in nausea and vomiting, increased release of essential neurotransmitters such as **epinephrine** and norepinephrine, and a change in the **immune system** that makes the body more susceptible to infection.

Injuries caused by chemicals, radiation, electrical current, and very low temperatures all produce similar cellular and biochemical responses at the site of injury although the precise mechanism of cell destruction varies. For example, exposure to any chemical substance that has the potential for coagulating cellular contents can produce a burn-like response in the skin. Substances in this category include strong acids and bases, whose low or high pH, respectively, can damage and destroy cells, as well as a number of organic compounds that can also cause coagulation of cell contents. Electrical charges and radiation attack biochemical molecules directly, destroying them and interrupting the normal metabolic functions of a cell. For example, ultraviolet radiation in sunlight causes blood vessels in the skin to dilate, allowing a larger volume of blood to flow through the area, resulting in the characteristic pink or red color associated with sunburn. Extended exposure to sunlight increases the risk of damage to cells in the affected region, which initiates the host of immune responses that are also associated with other types of thermal injury.

Another group of thermal injuries include those that are not directly related to exposure to a source of heat, chemicals, radiation, or electrical current, but that develop as the result of exposure to extended or abnormal periods of heat and humidity without benefit of rehydration. The simplest of such injuries are heat cramps, characterized by severe **muscle pain** and cramping, usually after extended periods of **exercise** in high heat. A somewhat more serious condition resulting from the same cause is **heat exhaustion**, characterized by dizziness, nausea, and general body weakness resulting from a loss of liquids and electrolytes. The most serious consequence of heat exhaustion is that it may lead to heat stroke (also known as sunstroke), a potentially life-threatening condition in which the body is no longer able to cool itself adequately with symptoms such as a temperature of more than 104°F, nausea, vomiting, headache, rapid heartbeat, **fatigue**, confusion, lethargy, stupor, and, eventually, coma and death.

Demographics

Probably the most complete set of data on burn injuries in the United States is produced annually by the American Burn Association (ABA). In the ABA's report for 2009, the most common type of thermal injury for which treatment was sought in medical facilities was contact with fire or flames, accounting for 40% of all cases for which an etiology was known. The second most common source of burns was scalding, accounting for 30% of such cases. Other sources of thermal injury were contact with a hot object (9%), electrical injuries (4%), and chemical burns (3%). Other and non-specified etiology accounted for the remaining portion of thermal injuries. Seventy one percent of burn victims in 2009 were males and 29%, females. Burns occurred most commonly among males in the age groups 20-30 (16.5%), 31-40 (15.1%), and 41-50 (15.4%), and among females in the age groups 5-16 (11%), 21-30 (11.3%), and 41-50 (12.3%). Whites accounted for the largest fraction of burn victims, 60.0 percent in this study, followed by African Americans (16.5%), Hispanics (12%), and Asian Americans (2%). These data are somewhat incomplete because the overall distribution of burn victims by gender, age group, ethnicity, and other characteristics was not reported.

Additional findings of the ABA study for 2009 included:

- Almost two thirds of all reported burn cases occurred in the home and were defined as non-work related.

- The mortality rate from all kinds of burns was 4.0% for males and 4.6% for females.

- The most common cause of death associated with a burn injury was pneumonia.

- The most common cause of a burn injury for children under the age of five was scalding.

- The danger of dying from a burn increases with the age of the patient and the amount of body area covered by the burn.

- For patients under the age of 60, smoke inhalation increases the chance of death from thermal injury by a factor of 15.

- The average length of hospital stay for a burn victim is one day for each one percent of body area covered by the injury.

Causes and symptoms

Thermal injuries are caused by exposure to or contact with hot objects, such as irons, stoves, curling irons, steam, chemicals, electrical current, and radiation. Extended exposure to sunlight can also cause certain types of thermal injuries, such as sunburn, heat cramps, heat exhaustion, and heat stroke.

The symptoms of a burn differ according to the severity of the injury. For the least damaging burns, the only symptoms may be a reddening and swelling of the skin and some discomfort or pain. In more serious burns, redness, swelling, and pain are likely to increase, and **blisters** may begin to form. In the most severe burn cases, the skin may turn a whitish or black, charred, color with numbness and a leathery or shiny appearance. Other, systemic symptoms may also be observed with more serious burns, the most dangerous of which is shock. Symptoms of shock include pale, clammy skin; general bodily weakness; and bluish lips and fingernails. Since the early stages of shock may be nearly asymptomatic, caregivers must be alert for this complication in burn victims.

Diagnosis

Thermal injuries are usually easily diagnosed because patients can describe the circumstances that led to their injury: they spilled scalding water on their arm, placed their hand on a hot stove, touched a live wire, spilled a chemical on their lap, or played too many sets of tennis on a hot day. Visual inspection of the injured site provides important direct information as to the injury that has occurred. No blood or imaging tests are typically required to confirm a thermal injury.

Most thermal injuries can be classified according to the degree of damage to the skin. The skin consists of three major layers, the outer layer (epidermis), middle layer (dermis), and inner layer (subcutaneous layer). Burns that damage, but do not penetrate, the epidermis are known as first degree burns. First degree burns may be painful and unsightly, but they are not life-threatening and usually resolve with first aid treatment within a week. Burns that destroy a portion of the epidermis and penetrate to the dermis are called second degree burns. They are characterized not only by swollen, red skin, but also by the appearance of blisters formed from liquid released by damaged cells in the dermis. Burns that penetrate to the subcutaneous layer are called third degree burns. Skin that has been damaged may turn white or black and develop a leathery feel, although there may be little or no pain. The most serious burns are those that penetrate all three layers of the skin and reach into muscle and nerve tissue. These fourth degree burns may produce skin that looks very much as if it has been set on fire, with a black, charred appearance.

Treatment

Burn treatment depends to a considerable extent on the classification scheme. The vast majority of first degree burns resolve on their own with little or no special care. The use of skin moisturizers, such as aloe vera cream, or an antibiotic or pain-suppressant cream may reduce the pain associated with the burn and increase the rate at which it heals. Pain killers such as acetaminophen can also be used to reduce pain and discomfort. Second degree burns require more aggressive treatment that includes cooling the burned area with a cold compress and covering the burned area to reduce the risk of infection. Use of an analgesic to reduce pain and discomfort is also warranted. Third degree burns are serious medical emergencies that require professional treatment. The only first aid involved is getting the patient to a medical care facility as quickly as possible. Care may then involve a number of procedures, including a tetanus shot (since burned skin is especially at risk for a tetanus infection),

KEY TERMS

Baux score (or index)—A measure used by medical workers to estimate the prognosis for recovery from a burn injury. The Baux is equal to the age of the patient plus the portion of the body damaged by the burn injury.

Dermis—The middle of three major layers of the skin.

Epidermis—The outermost of three major layers of the skin.

Heat cramp—A condition characterized by cramping and pain caused by too much exercise in hot conditions.

Heat exhaustion—A condition more serious than heat cramp caused by overexercise in hot conditions, characterized by dizziness, nausea, and general bodily weakness.

Heat stroke—The most serious stage of overexercise, heat-related medical conditions in which the body is no longer able to disperse heat faster than it is being produced; a potentially life-threatening condition.

Subcutaneous layer—The innermost of three major layers of the skin.

Zone of hyperemia—The region on the skin most distant from the actual burn site where cells continue to function normally.

Zone of coagulation—The region on the skin at which a burn actually occurs.

Zone of stasis—The region on the skin adjacent to the zone of coagulation where cells may be affected, but not necessarily destroyed by, the causative agent of the burn.

IV **hydration** (to replace water lost as a result of the burn), IV administration of antibiotics (to reduce the risk of infection), debridement and excision (to remove dead and damaged skin), and possible skin grafting (to replace lost and damaged skin). Fourth degree burns are life-threatening conditions that require more aggressive treatment, which may include amputation of a damaged limb.

Prognosis

Prognosis for a thermal injury depends to a large extent on three factors: the severity of the burn, the area of the body covered by the burn, and the age of the victim. A common measure for determining a patient's prognosis from burn is the Baux score, which is equal to the age of the patient added to the percent of the patient's body surface area covered by the burn. Traditionally, a burn victim with a Baux score of more than 100 was thought to be at high risk for death from the burn injury, while a patient with a Baux score over 130 was thought to be beyond the means of medical science for survival. In recent years, a number of adjustments in the Baux score have been suggested. These changes reflect the fact that the care available for a burn victim has improved dramatically in the last few decades, making possible the chance of survival for many patients who, in earlier years, would probably have died from their burns.

First degree burns resolve with little or no treatment in a matter of a few days or few weeks, depending on the severity of the burn. A second degree burn often requires between one to three weeks for full recovery, usually after debridement or excision has been used. Third degree burns often require a skin graft, which may require three weeks or more to heal.

The healing process often depends to a considerable degree on the speed and expertise with which the patient is treated. ABA has listed a number of instances in which a burn victim should be transported as soon as possible to a specialized burn center, including:

- patients under the age of ten or over the age of 50 with burns over more than 10% of their bodies
- patients of any age with third degree burns over more than 5% of their bodies
- patients with burns on the hands, feet, face, or groin area
- burns accompanied by inhalation injury
- chemical burns
- electrical burns
- scalds
- tar burns
- radiation burns

Prevention

According to some studies, as many as 85% of all cases of thermal injury could have been prevented. A number of organizations have recommended a variety of steps that individuals and families can take to reduce the risk of thermal injury in the home. These include:

- not smoking in bed, or even better, not smoking anywhere
- placing smoke alarms throughout the house and making sure their batteries are always functioning

- having a plan for escaping from fires in the home
- avoiding fireworks
- keeping matches and flammable materials away from children
- keeping hot foods and liquids out of the reach of children
- properly insulating and isolating electrical cords
- storing cleaning supplies and other potentially harmful household chemicals out of the reach of children
- wearing proper clothing (short sleeves) and protective gear (oven mitts) when cooking
- teaching young children not to use stoves, ovens, microwaves, curling irons, irons and other potentially harmful equipment
- teaching children about the potential burn risks posed by fireplaces and wood stoves
- not holding or carrying a child while you, yourself, are holding a hot drink or hot food
- adjusting the temperature on your water heater to prevent water from becoming hot enough to scald someone

Resources

BOOKS

Herndon, David N. *Total Burn Care*. Edinburgh: Saunders Elsevier, 2007.

Hettiaratchy, Shehan, Remo Papini, and Peter Dziewulski. *ABC of Burns*. Malden, MA: BMJ Books, 2005.

PERIODICALS

Falk, Bareket, and Raffy Dotan. "Temperature Regulation and Elite Young Athletes." *Medicine and Sport Science* 56 (2011): 126-149.

Yarmolenko, Pavel S., et al. "Thresholds for Thermal Damage to Normal Tissues: An Update." *International Journal of Hyperthermia*, 27 (4; 2011): 320-343.

WEBSITES

First Aid for Burns. "MedicineNet." http://www.medicinenet.com/burns/article.htm (Accessed on September 5, 2011).

Thermal Burns: Rapid Assessment and Treatment. "EB Medicine." http://www.ebmedicine.net/topics.php?paction=showTopicSeg&topic_id=111&seg_id=2135 (Accessed September 5, 2011).

ORGANIZATIONS

American Burn Association, 311 S. Wacker Dr., Suite 4150, Chicago, IL, USA, 60606, 1(312) 642-9260, Fax: 1(312) 642-9130, info@ameriburn.org, http://www.ameriburn.org.

Burn Prevention Foundation, 236 N. 17th St., Allentown, PA, USA, 18104, 1(610) 969-3930, Fax: 1(610) 969-3940, burnprev@fast.net, http://www.burnprevention.org/.

David E. Newton, A.B., M.A. Ed.D.

Thigh exercises *see* **Hip and thigh exercises**

Track and field

Definition

The term "track and field" applies to a group of **running**, jumping, and throwing events, such as various types of sprints, middle- and long-distance runs, hurdles, relays, hammer and discus throw, and long and triple jump. Along with cross-country, racewalking, and road running, track and field constitutes the umbrella sport known as "athletics."

Purpose

The purpose of all track and field events is for a competitor to perform better than any of his or her fellow athletes. Runners attempt to cover some given distance in the shortest time of all competitors; jumpers jump higher or farther than other competitors; and throwers propel an object at a greater distance than any one else in the competition.

Demographics

The demographic structure of various track and field events varies with the type of activity. Some sports, such as pole vault, tend to be limited to males in their late adolescence or early adulthood. Other sports, such as discus and shot put, have seen successful competitors in their fourth decade. A triple jump competition, for example, could at least in theory

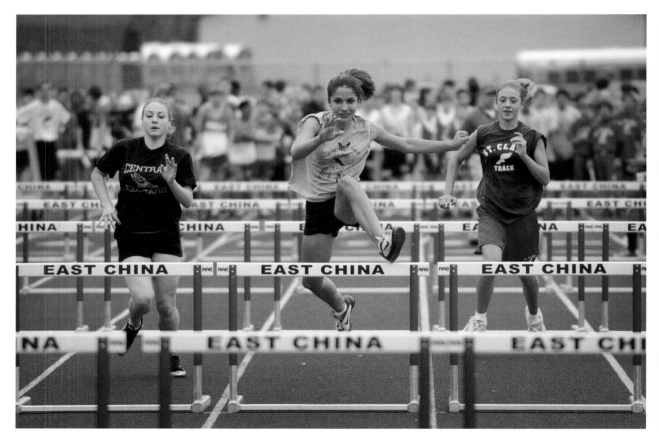

Runners compete in a track and field event. *(© Ilene MacDonald/Alamy)*

include men ranging in age from 18 to 40. Because of the popularity of track and field in junior high and high school, USA Track and Field (USATF) has established two junior divisions for boys and girls under the age of 11 and 11 to 18. These age groups are further divided into two-year divisions known as sub-bantam, bantam, midget, youth, intermediate, and young. The USATF also sponsors an annual Junior Olympic program in which 70,000 young athletes participated in 2011.

History

Given that most track and field events require a minimal amount of special equipment and involve the most basic of human activities—running, jumping, and throwing—it is difficult to imagine that people have not been engaged in such activities since the earliest centuries of human civilization. Many historians trace the beginning of track and field to the first Olympic Games, held in Greece in 776 BCE. Those games involved a single event, the stadion footrace from one side of the stadium to the other. Still, most

historians acknowledge that events similar to those that constitute modern track and field were being held centuries before the first Olympiad. For example, some archaeological remains suggest that Olympic-like contests may have been held in Greece as early as the tenth century BCE. Other studies point to equally ancient origins of track and field in other parts of the world. One example is the Tailteann Games held in County Meath, Ireland, from 1829 BCE to 554 BCE. Written records indicate that these games included a number of events similar to modern-day track and field, including pole vaulting, stone throwing, triple jump, and wheel throwing.

The history of track and field is closely associated with the history of the Olympic Games, of which they have been a part since the first modern Olympic Games of 1896. Those games were the first instance at which athletes from around the world came together to compete against each other. They included contests in 100-, 400-, 800-, and 1500-meter running races; 110-meter hurdles; long-, high-, and triple-jump; pole vault; discus; and shot put.

Prior to the first Olympiad, sporting events in track and field were organized primarily by sporting clubs, military organizations, or educational institutions. By the last quarter of the nineteenth century, however, groups of interested athletes were beginning to establish national organizations for the creation of rules, regulations, and standards for track and field events; for sponsoring competitions and national championships; and for promoting the sport within their home country. The first of these organizations was the Amateur Athletic Association, established in England in 1880. Comparable associations were created in the United States in 1888, the Amateur Athletic Union, and in France in 1889, Union des sociétés françaises de sports athlétiques. In 1912, representatives of 17 national track and field associations met in Stockholm, Sweden, to found the first international governing organization for the sport, the International Amateur Athletics Federation, later to become the International Association of Athletics Federation, still the international governing body for the sport.

The Amateur Athletic Union (AAU) remained the governing body for track and field in the United States until 1979, when the AAU was restricted from presiding over more than one sport in the United States. In that year, a new organization, The Athletics Congress/USA (TAC/USA), was created to replace the AAU's governance role for track and field. In 1992, TAC/USA changed its name to USA Track and Field (USATF), by which it is still known. USATF currently claims to have almost 100,000 individual members, as well as organizational members that include the U.S. Olympic Committee, the National Collegiate Athletic Association (NCAA), Road Runners Club of America, Running USA, and the National Federation of State High School Associations. The federation sanctions more than 4,000 events nationwide each year and supervises the activities of more than 2,500 local clubs through 57 state chapters. It also sponsors a large number of national championships in events such as the 100 Mile Trail Championship, the Masters Throws Championship, the PanAmerican Race Walk Cup, the 100 km Trail Championship, and the Indoor Heptathalon Championship.

Description

Track and field events are typically held in outdoor stadiums that feature an oval track 400 m in circumference on which running events are held. Other events, such as jumping and throwing events, are generally held in the grassy area within the oval. Indoor track and field events are also popular, with a setting similar to that for outdoor track and field,

except that the oval track is usually 200 m in length. The number of lanes within the oval track varies from venue to venue, ranging from four to six on indoor tracks to six to eight on outdoor tracks.

The events included in track and field can be classified into a number of distinct categories, the first of which is sprint. Sprint races are short races that emphasize a quick start and rapid acceleration by participants. The most widely run sprints are 100-, 200-, and 400-m sprints, which equates to 110-, 220-, and 440-yd. sprints. Races are sometimes run at other distances also, including 60 m, run most often on indoor tracks, as well as 50-, 300-, and 500-m sprints. Middle-distance events include the 800- and 1500-m and one mile runs. The 3,000-m run is included less commonly. Runners in the 800-m race start from a staggered position, in order to equalize the distance run by competitors. The most common long-distance races are the 5,000- and 10,000-m races, although the 3,000-m race may also be included in this category.

The only team events included in track and field are the relays, which are run by four-person teams against each other. Each member of the team runs a predetermined distance, such as 100 m, before handing off a baton to the next member of the team. The two most common relay events are the 4x100- and 4x400-m relays, meaning that each runner in the first instance runs 100 m, while each member of a team runs 400 m in the second instance.

The only other events held on the track oval are the hurdles, races in which participants are required to leap over bars during a race of 110 m and 400 m (for men) and 100 m and 400 m for women. The hurdles are 3 ft. (1 m) in height for men and 2.5 ft. (0.8 m) high for women. A variation of the hurdles race is steeplechase, in which runners must jump over a variety of hurdle-like barriers as well as one or more water barriers. Although different distances are possible, the most common length of the steeplechase is now 3,000 m.

The four jumping events in track and field are the long jump, high jump, triple jump, and pole vault. In the long jump, an athlete runs down a runway at least 131 ft. (40 m) in length and kicks off a rectangular launch pad before landing in a sandy pit. The jumper who covers the greatest distance without fouling (e.g., by stepping beyond the launch point) is the winner. In the high jump, a competitor runs down a short approach lane, launches upward off the ground, and falls over a horizontal bar. The competitor who jumps over the bar at its highest setting without fouling (such as knocking the bar off its supports) is the winner. The

KEY TERMS

Athletics—A term that includes traditional track and field events, as well as a few other sports, such as road running and race walking.

Combined events—Track and field events in which a competitor takes part in a number (usually five, seven, or ten) of events, with the winner being the person with the highest total score for those events.

Pylometrics—A type of exercise designed to produce fast, powerful movements by strengthening the ability of muscles to expand and contract more quickly and efficiently.

Relay—A track and field event in which two or more teams consisting of four members each race against each other.

triple jump was formerly called the hop, skip, and jump, which describes the three activities required to complete the activity. A competitor runs down the runway, hops once on the same foot, then performs a skip before launching off a marked area, as in the long jump. In the pole vault, the athlete gains speed and momentum by running down a track carrying a long pole. As she or he approaches the bar, the pole is thrust into the ground and the athlete is projected into the air over the bar. The athlete who "clears" the bar at its highest point without fouling (such as knocking off the bar) is the winner of the event.

Throwing events differ from each other primarily in the object that is thrown, a 16-lb. (7.25-kg) metallic sphere for men (8.8-lb. [4-kg] sphere for women) in the shot put; a 4.4-lb. (2-kg) metallic disc (for both men and women) in the discus; a metal-tipped wooden spear 8.5–8.9 ft. (2.6–2.7 m) in length for men (7.2–7.5 ft. (2.2–2.3 m) for women) in the javelin; and a 16-lb. (7.25-kg) metal ball attached to a wire between 3.85 and 3.98 ft. (1.175 and 1.215 m) in length for the hammer throw.

The final set of events found in track and field are combined events, in which a man or women participates in some set of events, with the winner being the person who has the highest total score for all events added together. The most common combination events are the pentathalon (five events), the heptathalon (seven events), and the decathalon (ten events). As an example, the women's heptathalon includes the 200- and 800-m run, the 100-m hurdles, the long and high jump, the shot put, and the javelin. The men's heptathalon substitutes the 110-m hurdles for the 100-m hurdles, the 60-m sprint for the 100-m sprint, the 1,000-m run for the 800-m run, and the pole vault for the javelin throw.

Preparation

Preparation for track and field events is dictated to a large extent by the specific event itself, with some events, such as the 100-m sprint, emphasizing speed; while others, such as the mile run, endurance; and yet others, such as the shot put, strength.

Equipment

Some track and field events, such as races and hurdling, require no equipment beyond a shirt, shorts, and suitable shoes. Other events require the use of specialized equipment whose characteristic features are described in detail by the governing body for the sport. For example, USA Track and Field provides a handbook describing in detail the precise weight and length measurements permitted for each type of equipment, such as the javelin or discuss. Each item listed in the handbook has separate legal measurements depending on the type of competition involved and age and gender of participant.

Training and conditioning

Each event in track and field has its own regimen in developing the specific skills needed for that sport. For runners, a training program for the 100-m dash emphasizes topics such as proper positioning for the beginning of the race, proper methods for rising and accelerating as the race begins, achieving maximum acceleration and speed as the race develops, and maintaining maximum speed through the final stages of the race. But, as with most sports, a variety of other training and conditioning exercises not directly involved in the sport can be used to help a person prepare for an activity. As an example, the following training tips have been offered by one authority in the field in helping to prepare for the pole vault:

- a series of step-ups onto a box 12–18 in. (30–46 cm) in height to simulate the steps taken during take-off for the vault
- running in place for ten seconds at a time, repeated two or three times, to increase runway speed
- dribbling a basketball, to improve hand-eye coordination

- one-step jump ups, to increase strength and power needed for take-offs for a vault
- short jump ups into a sand pit, first on one foot, then on the other, increasing in height each time, to improve take off power for the vault
- fast skips for a distance of about 65 ft. (20 m), to lengthen one's stride on the runway
- fast hops, first on one foot then on the other, for a distance of about 65 ft. (20 m), to improve strength, power, and coordination

Experts in each separate track and field event have developed training and conditioning programs such as this one to improve an athlete's overall strength, endurance, agility, coordination, and balance, as well as the specific skills required in that event.

Risks

The U.S. Consumer Products Safety Commission (CPSC) conducts an annual survey on injuries associate with various types of activities and equipment used by people in the United States. The most recent data available (for 2007) show that track and field is one of the safest sporting activities in which Americans participate, with an average of 6.6 injuries per 100,000 participants. Comparable rates for some other sports are 92.1 for **baseball** and **softball**, 150.9 for **football**; 26.0 for horseback riding; and 18.9 for **volleyball**. The highest injury rate for track and field events were for those in the 5–14 age group (21.5/100,000) and the 15–24 age group (22.8/100,000). Women were slightly more likely to be injured in track and field than were men (7.0 versus 6.2 per 100,000). The vast majority of injuries that were reported resulted in immediate treatment and release (6.4 per 100,000) compared to those who needed hospital care (0.2 per 100,000).

Relatively little research has been done on the nature of injuries experienced in track and field. A 2005 survey of such research found nine studies on track and field injuries in boys and girls under the age of 18. It found that the vast majority of injuries involved the lower extremities, ranging from 64% to 87% in the five most relevant studies. Of these, the most common locations for injuries were the lower leg (in three studies), the knee (one study), and the upper leg (one study). The most common type of injury was inflammation of tissue (in three or four studies) and strains (in one study). Overall, strains, sprains, and inflammation were the most common types of injuries found in all track and field participants for which available data were available.

Results

All commentators on track and field injuries emphasize the importance of proper preparation in avoiding injuries associated with the sport. A program of **warm-up** and stretching loosens muscles and prepares them for the stress placed on them by an activity. A good general program in strength training is also recommended as a way of avoiding injuries resulting from repetitive and overuse of body parts involved in a sport. Pylometric exercises help develop power and bursts of strength. Proper shoes for a particular track and field event are also important. A wide variety of athletic shoes are available, and participants should find exactly the right type of shoe for the event in which they are involved. Finally, trainers and conditioners emphasize the importance of good nutrition and, in particular, of **hydration** before participation in a track and field event.

Resources

BOOKS

Bowerman, William J., and William Hardin Freeman. *Bill Bowerman's High-performance Training for Track and Field*. Monterey, CA; Coaches Choice, 2009.

Henderson, Jason. *Field Events*. London: Carlton, 2011.

Matthews, Peter. *Athletics 2011: The International Track and Field Annual*. Cheltenham, UK: SportsBooks, 2011.

Morgan, Kevin. *Athletics Challenges: A Resource Pack for Teaching Athletics*. New York: Routledge, 2011.

USA Track & Field 2011 Competition Rules. Indianapolis, IN: USA Track and Field, 2011.

WEBSITES

All Track & Field Training & Coaching Articles. Everything Track and Field. http://www.everythingtrackandfield. com/catalog/matriarch/MultiPiecePage.asp_Q_PageID_ E_155_A_PageName_E_ArticleListingPage (accessed September 6, 2011).

Track and Field. About.com. http://trackandfield.about. com/ (accessed September 6, 2011).

World-Track.org. http://world-track.org/ (accessed September 6, 2011).

ORGANIZATIONS

International Association of Athletics Federation, 17 rue Princesse Florestine BP 359, Monaco, Monaco, MC98007, 37793 10 8888, Fax: 37793 15 9515, http:// www.iaaf.org/aboutiaaf/contacts/feedback.html, http://daegu2011.iaaf.org/.

USA Track and Field, 132 East Washington St., Suite 800, Indianapolis, IN, 46204, (317) 261-0500, Fax: (317) 261-0481, http:// www.usatf.org.

David E. Newton, AB, MA, EdD

Treadmill

Definition

A treadmill is a piece of **exercise** equipment that has a belt that loops around, driven by a motor. The continuous loop allows a person to walk or run on the treadmill in place.

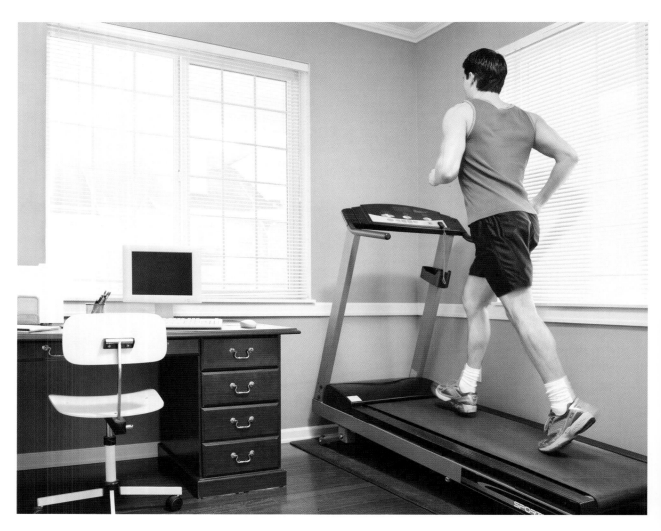

A man uses a treadmill in his home. (© Anderson Ross/Jupiterimages)

Purpose

Treadmills are used mostly for home or gym exercise. More than 50 million people in America use them, a 40% increase over the past 10 years. Some have the treadmills for convenience, so that they can exercise while at home with their children, or while watching their favorite television programs. Others have them as alternatives to outdoor activity when weather keeps them inside. Gym treadmills are used as part of exercisers' aerobic workouts or to warm up before participating in strength training.

The benefits of **walking** and **running** have been shown in many studies. When done in moderation, this sort of regular exercise can help keep bones and muscles strong, and burn **calories** to keep weight in check or help people lose weight, and improve health. Still, many children and adults are inactive and families purchase treadmills to help provide an exercise option at home. Another problem adding to **obesity** and health problems is that many Americans have jobs that require them to sit at desks and computers all day, and trying to fit in exercise in their spare time. New desks fitted for treadmills help office workers, and even home computer users, walk at slow speeds on their treadmills instead of **sitting**.

Treadmills have other uses, especially in health care. An exercise stress test is used to check heart function and signs of disease. Physicians strap electrodes on the patient's chest and have him or her walk on a treadmill and then perform an electrocardiogram, or ECG, to measure how the heart performs when under stress, or when pumping to the patient's exercising lungs and muscles. Treadmills may be used in physical or cardiac therapy to help the patient gain back physical or heart function under the direction and watchful eye of the therapist.

History

Most historians can trace the roots of the treadmill's use with humans to early in the nineteenth century. The idea was meant to teach prisoners not to be idle. Sir William Cubit was the man credited with the invention that saw its way to 44 prisons in England. The British had adopted treadmills to provide hard labor for inmates and to grind grain on some "treadwheels." Some American prisons also used the treadmill to work their prisoners, but only from 1822 to 1824. The prisoners had to grind grain on the treadmills for 10 hours a day, with only 20 minutes off each hour. The public could come and watch them from a special viewing house.

For many years, the machines were used only by prisoners and animals (for milling or to power butter churners). The animals walked on an uphill belt set in motion by a series of gears. The mechanics of the treadmill were improved to become devices such as assembly-line conveyor belts. The first medical use of a treadmill was in 1949, when cardiologist Robert Bruce and Dr. Paul Yu of the University of Rochester worked together to develop an early treadmill exercise test. This test has stood the test of time. Though bikes also are used, and the technology is more advanced, the basic stress test is in place 60 years after its invention.

Many manufacturers worked to provide treadmills for home and gym use. Throughout the years, they have added features to them and made different types so that the equipment can be more affordable for consumers. The typical treadmill for a home gym costs about US$1,000–2,000, but basic and used models can cost less. Motorized treadmills lead sales of all exercise equipment, and even when sales of equipment decreased 3.5% from 2008 to 2009, the decrease in sales of treadmills was only 1%. In the 2000s, treadmills have entered the water and gone space age. A new portable and submersible treadmill can be used in **swimming** pools to help people with rehabilitation and aquatic therapy. NASA has a treadmill on the International Space Station that astronauts use to work out regularly. It helps them get exercise in the small space of the station, and also helps stop some of the bone loss that occurs when living in zero gravity.

Description

The treadmill allows a user to walk or run in place on the machine on a belt that moves underneath the feet in a continuous loop. The walker or runner sets the belt to a desired speed, usually measured in miles per hour or kilometers per hour. A motor turns the belt; most have 1.5–3 horsepower. Most treadmills go up to a maximum speed of about 10 miles per hour. That equals six minutes per mile, which is a fast running speed. The deck is the main body of the machine, including a frame that supports the belt and the weight of the exerciser. It has to be strong enough to support the walker's weight when he or she is still, but also the shock of the exerciser's weight when moving, much like a shock absorber in a car. Steel frames are much stronger than plastic ones. Rollers turn the belt, and should be large and heavy enough to last for many turns or uses. The belt should be two-ply and strong. Most are 14–24 in. (36–61 cm) wide and about 3.7–5.3 ft. (1.1–1.6 m) long. People who are larger may want a wider belt, but being tall in particular can affect

KEY TERMS

Aerobic—Any activity intended to increase the body's oxygen consumption and improve the functioning of the cardiovascular and respiratory systems.

Cardiovascular—Relating to the heart and blood vessels.

Electrocardogram—Also called an ECG or EKG, it is a recording of the electrical activity in the heart to determine if there are problems or diseases.

belt size. Tall people have longer stride, or step, lengths and may need longer decks and belts to ensure they do not accidentally step off the back of the treadmill while walking or running. The deck also has arms that come from the front partway down the side so that walkers can hold or grab them when necessary. Most treadmills incline up to 10%, which is enough for most exercisers, although special models may incline up to 15%.

Treadmills typically come with control panels, or electronics. These displays and controls help the user set speed, incline (walking or running at an angle, as if going uphill) and preset programs that can take the user through changing speed or incline options aimed at specific goals, such as burning fat or improving cardiac fitness. Displays show information such as time exercised, time left in a program, calories burned, and steps or miles walked. The control panel also has emergency stop buttons and "keys" that can attach to the walker or runner so that if he or she falls, the key should pull a tripper that stops the belt. Most units also have monitors that the walker can wear, usually on his or her finger, to monitor pulse and heart rate. Almost every treadmill has some sort of lip to hold a book or magazine and a water bottle holder. Many home models have decks that fold up to move out of the way when not used.

Most treadmills in gyms and newer consumer models come with high-tech tools and perks. For example, many have input jacks for MP3 players. Some gym treadmills have televisions, DVD players, or other media built in to the displays that work with fitness software programs. In fall 2011, a new model announced a Wi-Fi connection that provided routes using satellite technology via the Internet. The model sells for about US$2,000.

Benefits

The health benefits of walking have been proven in numerous studies. Studies have shown that just an hour of walking a week can reduce risk for stroke, heart disease, and overall **cardiovascular disease**. The

2008 guidelines on physical activity for Americans suggest at least 2.5 hours a week of moderate-intensity exercise (such as brisk walking). They suggest that more exercise, or exercising at higher intensity, helps even more. A treadmill offers the opportunity to exercise indoors, which can provide convenience and safety for some walkers and runners. Walking also is beneficial to bone and joint **disease prevention** and treatment, and often is done under the supervision of a doctor or therapist. Patients may be sent home with instructions to begin a walking program and gradually increase their time and speed. A treadmill helps them easily measure both. Treadmill workouts are used to help people manage diabetes, and specially designed treadmills with extra-long decks are used to help people in rehabilitation after strokes or injuries.

There are numerous reasons why people are less active than they should be, but one of the main reasons is time. A treadmill is one form of exercise that allows people to be at home if they need to stay home, and to perform another task while walking. People who like to watch television can at least do so while moving instead of sitting, which can improve health tremendously. Studies have associated poor health with inactivity. Employers are trying to improve their workers' health. Combining a treadmill and computer workstation gives employees the chance to move while they work instead of sitting for eight or more hours straight. These office walkers walk at speeds from 1 to 3 mph after becoming used to working a computer while walking on the treadmill several hours a day, and burn many more calories than they would sitting. They have specially adapted desks.

Risks

Treadmills are the most popular piece of exercise equipment, but also the most dangerous. According to the Consumer Product Safety Commission, 19,000 people visited emergency rooms in 2009 for treadmill injuries, and 6,000 of them were children. The injuries included broken bones, concussions, and amputated

QUESTIONS TO ASK YOUR DOCTOR

- Is there any health condition or disease that would prevent me from using a treadmill?
- How can a treadmill prevent diseases I am at risk for?
- Can using a treadmill help me recover from an injury or illness?

fingers. The reason most people are injured is that they become distracted. People who use multimedia, computers, read, or talk to friends and family while on treadmills should be cautious. They should set the appropriate speed and constantly be aware of where their feet are on the deck. Sometimes, when running in particular, the exerciser drifts to the back of the belt. Stepping off the back could cause serious injury. It also is possible to step off the side of the belt. Turning and moving the arms can cause imbalance or inattention to the feet. When entering and exiting the treadmill, the walker always should pause or stop the motor. Hands should always be near the handrail, or one hand on the rail for balance when performing tasks such as drinking, wiping with a towel, or other tasks.

Resources

BOOKS

Murphy, Wendy. *Weight and Health*, Minneapolis, MN: Twenty-first Century Books, 2008.

PERIODICALS

"A Treadmill You'll Want to Use." *Shape* 29, no. 8 (April 2010): 114.

Levine, James A., and Jennifer M. Miller. "The Energy Expenditure of Using a 'Walk and Work' Space for Office Workers with Obesity." *British Journal of Sports Medicine* 41 (2007): 558-61.

"Rollable Underwater Treadmill for Pools." *Rehabilitation Management* (August-Septmber 2010): 32.

"What Exercise Can Do for You." *Exercise (Harvard Special Health Report)* (2007): 9.

WEBSITES

"2008 Sporting Goods Sales Reach $53.4 Billion." NSGA.org. http://www.nsga.org/i4a/pages/index.cfm?pageID=4207 (accessed September 21, 2011).

CBS News. "Treadmills: Danger at Our Feet." CBSNews.com. http://www.cbsnews.com/stories/2011/09/05/earlyshow/health/main20101692.shtml (accessed September 21, 2011).

Editors of PureHealthMD. "Choosing a Treadmill." DiscoveryHealth.com. http://health.howstuffworks.com/wellness/diet-fitness/exercise/choosing-a-treadmill.htm/printable (accessed September 21, 2011).

"How Do Treadmills Work?" EHow.com. http://www.ehow.com/how-does_4569789_treadmills-work.html (accessed September 22, 2011).

Sanders Polin, Bonnie, and Frances Towner Geidt. "Walking the Treadmill: An Easy Exercise for People with Diabetes." DiabeticLifestyle.com. http://www.diabeticlifestyle.com/exercise/walking-treadmill (accessed September 21, 2011).

U.S. Department of Health and Human Services. "2008 Physical Activity Guidelines for Americans." Health.gov. http://www.health.gov/paguidelines/pdf/paguide.pdf (accessed September 21, 2011).

ORGANIZATIONS

President's Council on Sports, Fitness, and Nutrition, 1101 Wootton Parkway, Suite 560, Rockville, MD, 20852, (240) 276-9567, Fax: (240) 276-9860, fitness@hhs.gov, http://www.fitness.gov.

Teresa G. Odle, BA, ELS

Triathlon *see* **Ironman**

Type 2 diabetes *see* **Diabetes mellitus**

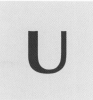

U

U.S. President's Council on Fitness, Sports, & Nutrition

Definition

The U.S. President's Council on Fitness, Sports, & Nutrition (PCFSN) advises the U.S. President on developing accessible, affordable, and sustainable programs for physical activity, fitness, sports, and nutrition, for the benefit of all Americans.

Purpose

The purpose of the PCFSN is to assist the President's administration in providing information and developing programs and initiatives that help empower all Americans to adopt healthy lifestyles through regular physical activity, fitness, participation in sports, and good nutrition. The PCFSN places specific emphasis on:

- increasing public awareness of and interest in fitness, sports, and nutrition
- encouraging and enhancing coordination of programs among public and private sectors
- improving the availability of research-based information and access to guidance
- increasing the access and participation of all Americans—especially children, teens, and populations and communities with specific health risks and/or disparities

Demographics

Lack of physical activity and **exercise**, poor physical fitness, and poor nutrition are growing concerns in the United States and other parts of the developed world. Some 34 million American adults are considered obese, with a **body mass index** (BMI) of 30 or higher. Over the past three decades, childhood **obesity** rates have tripled for adolescents and nearly doubled for younger children. Almost one in three American children is now overweight or obese. Among black and Hispanic American youth, almost 40% are overweight or obese. The incidence approaches 50% among American Indian and Alaskan Native youth. Once almost nonexistent in young people, the incidence of type 2 diabetes in youth is increasing at alarming rates and 75% of children and teens with type 2 diabetes are obese. These young people are much more likely to develop serious diabetes-related complications as adults. If these trends continue, it is estimated that one-third of all children born in 2000 will eventually develop diabetes, in addition to other chronic lifestyle-related conditions, such as **asthma**, high **blood pressure**, heart disease, and cancer.

These trends are attributed to physical activity levels and eating habits that have changed drastically in recent decades. Children are much less likely to walk or bike to and from school than in the past. Only one-third of high-school students maintain the recommended levels of physical activity. Budget cuts and the pressures of high-stakes academic testing have led to reductions in or the complete elimination of school recess and physical education programs. More than 28% of schools do not have regularly scheduled **recess** in grades one through five. According to the Centers for Disease Control and Prevention (CDC), only 8% of elementary schools, 6.4% of middle schools, and 5.8% of high schools require daily physical education classes. After-school sports and outside play have been replaced with television, video games, and the Internet. Youth aged eight to 18 now spend an average of 7.5 hours per day using entertainment media. Only 35% of adults aged 18 and older engage in regular leisure-time physical activity and 33% engage in no leisure-time physical activity at all. Home-cooked meals have been replaced with snacks, fast food, sugary beverages, and larger portion sizes. Americans are averaging caloric intakes that are 31% higher than they were 40 years ago, and include 56%

more **fats** and oils and 14% more sugar and sweeteners, adding up to an extra 15 lb (7 kg) of sugar annually, compared with 1970.

Description

Origins

In the 1950s, research by Hans Kraus and Bonnie Prudden documented a decline in physical fitness among American children, with almost 58% of students failing at least one fitness test component, such as leg lifts, sit-ups, trunk lifts, or toe touches. As a result, in 1956, President Dwight D. Eisenhower, at the urging of several prominent politicians and athletes, formed the President's Council on Youth Fitness. Over the years, the President's Council supported research and provided resources and motivation to increase physical education in schools. After its re-branding as the President's Council on Physical Fitness and Sports, its mission expanded to include the promotion of physical activity for all Americans. In June 2010, President Barack Obama issued an executive order that added the word "Nutrition" to the Council's title and further expanded its mission to include the promotion of healthy eating habits for all Americans.

The PCFSN is a committee composed of up to 25 volunteers who, through the Secretary of Health and Human Services, advise the U.S. President. The Council includes professional and Olympic athletes, physicians, and other experts on and advocates for fitness and healthy lifestyles. For 2010–2012, the Council Co-chairs were New Orleans Saints quarterback and Super Bowl XLIV Most Valuable Player Drew Brees and Olympic gymnast Dominique Dawes. PCFSN programs and initiatives are carried out through partnerships with private- and public-sector organizations at the national, state, and local levels that are focused primarily in the areas of education, parks and recreation, fitness, and sports.

Physical activity initiatives

A major focus of the PCFSN are three annual national promotions: the National Physical Fitness & Sports Month in May, the National Great Outdoors Month in June, and the July National Park and Recreation Month. The PCFSN also partners with the U.S. Department of the Interior on America's Great Outdoors interagency initiative that supports community-based efforts to better conserve and utilize outdoor space and connect Americans with outdoor activities.

The **President's Challenge**, America's foremost physical activity and fitness initiative, is a cornerstone of the PCFSN that administers it through a co-sponsorship agreement with the Amateur Athletic Union (AAU). The President's Challenge is a free program open to all Americans aged six and older, aimed at encouraging regular physical activity and fitness. The individual challenges include the:

- youth physical fitness test
- adult fitness test
- Presidential Activity Lifestyle Award (PALA), a six-week program for jump-starting a regular fitness routine
- Presidential Champions Award, a point-based online program for physically active children and adults who have completed the PALA and want to increase the intensity and frequency of their activities

The PCFSN is a sponsor of Let's Move!, First Lady Michelle Obama's ambitious campaign to solve the problem of childhood obesity within a generation. Let's Move! aims to make nutritious, affordable food available to all Americans. It supports parents and schools in their efforts to serve healthier foods and help children become more physically active. There are four pillars to Let's Move!

- Healthy Choices provides parents with the information and tools to improve their children's nutrition. Its initiatives include front-of-package food labeling, a partnership with the American Academy of Pediatrics to promote BMI tracking at well-child physician visits, and public education partnerships with Disney and NBC
- Healthier Schools increases funding for the Child Nutrition Act to enroll more children in free and reduced-price school meals and to improve the nutritional quality of school meals.
- Access to Affordable Healthy Food encourages the relocation of grocery stores and farmer's markets to "food deserts"—the communities in which 23.5 million Americans lack access to supermarkets.
- Physical Activity promotes the President's Challenge, in partnership with the PCFSN and most sports leagues, with special emphasis on the PALA and fitness screening and physical education in schools.

Although Let's Move! hopes to engage students in healthy eating and physical activity at home, it views schools as key to solving the problems of childhood inactivity and obesity, since children spend such a large proportion of their time there. Let's Move! promotes the incorporation of nutrition education and physical education into school curricula. It also helps

KEY TERMS

Body mass index (BMI)—A measure of body fat; the ratio of weight in kilograms to the square of height in meters.

Diabetes, type 2—The most common form of diabetes, usually developing in obese adults, but becoming increasingly common in young people; characterized by high blood sugar (hyperglycemia) due to impaired insulin utilization, sometimes coupled with an inability to increase insulin production.

Health disparities—Differences in health, health care, and/or health outcomes between different racial and ethnic groups, genders, and geographical locations within a single population.

Let's move!—First Lady Michelle Obama's initiative for combating childhood obesity.

Obesity—Excessive weight due to accumulation of fat, usually defined as a body mass index of 30 or above or body weight greater than 30% above normal on standard height-weight tables.

Overweight—A body mass index between 25 and 30.

Presidential activity lifestyle award (PALA)—A component of the President's Challenge, the PALA is a six-week commitment to daily physical activity, designed for everyone from young children to seniors.

President's challenge—America's foremost physical activity and fitness initiative and a cornerstone of the U.S. President's Council on Fitness, Sports, & Nutrition.

---

school leaders develop low- or no-cost physical activity programs—including before-, during-, and after-school activities, school recesses, clubs, intramural and interschool sports, walks, and bike rides—to supplement physical education classes.

The PCFSN is an affiliate of the U.S. National Physical Activity Plan. This is a comprehensive set of policies, programs, and initiatives for increasing physical activity among all segments of the American population. The plan involves hundreds of private- and public-sector organizations, with the aim of creating a national culture of physical activity for the improvement of health, the prevention of disease and disability, and enhanced quality of life. The PCFSN is involved with partner organizations in the education and parks, recreation, fitness, and sports sectors.

The PCFSN was involved in the steering committee, the writing group, and communications teams for the 2008 Physical Activity Guidelines for Americans (PAG). Based on a report by a scientific advisory panel of experts in physical fitness and public health, the PAG was the first such work to be published by the federal government. It will be updated every five years. The Council also collaborates with the Communication Research Database of the Office of Disease Prevention and Health Promotion and with the Office of Public Health and Science, both of which are within the U.S. Department of Health and Human Services (HHS).

The *PCFSN Research Digest* is published quarterly. It covers a variety of physical fitness topics, including means of promoting fitness, physical

education in schools, and physical fitness with regard to youth, families, and seniors, and conditions such as pregnancy, asthma, and breast cancer.

Nutrition initiatives

The PCFSN is involved with Dietary Guidelines for Americans (DAG), which is updated every five years by the Departments of Agriculture (USDA) and Health and Human Services. The DAG forms the cornerstone of the government's science-based nutrition policies and educational activities.

The Council also partners with the USDA to sponsor:

• Nutrition.gov, a food and human nutrition information source for consumers from the National Agricultural Library

• Eat Smart, Play Hard, a program to educate children, parents, and caregivers about the importance healthy eating and daily physical activity

• the Food and Nutrition Service that provides children and low-income populations with access to healthy food and nutrition information

• MyPyramid.gov that provides personalized eating plans and interactive tools based on the DAG

Other partnerships

The PCFSN collaborates with the U.S. Department of Education and with various other agencies within the HHS, including:

QUESTIONS TO ASK YOUR DOCTOR

- What is my body mass index (BMI)?
- How much physical activity should I get?
- What physical activities do you recommend for me?
- Am I healthy enough to take part in the President's Challenge?
- How can I promote physical activity and good nutrition at my child's school?

- the Substance Abuse and Mental Health Services Administration (SAMHSA) that works to reduce the impacts of substance abuse and mental illness

- the CDC's Behavioral Risk Factor Surveillance System that has tracked health conditions and risky behaviors throughout the United States and its territories since 1984

- the CDC's Body and Mind (BAM!) program that provides kid-friendly information on food, nutrition, physical activity, and safety

- the National Bone Health Campaign that encourages girls to become physically active and consume more calcium and vitamin D for preventing osteoporosis later in life

- Girlshealth.gov, for promoting healthy, positive behaviors in girls aged 10–16

- Healthfinder that provides online information and tools for staying healthy

- the Health Resources and Services Administration (HRSA), the primary federal agency for improving access to health care for uninsured, isolated, and medically vulnerable populations

- Healthy People 2020, a decade-long, large-scale public health initiative

- the Office of the Surgeon General

- the Office on Women's Health that promotes health equity for girls and women, as well as the Quick Health Data Online for state- and county-level health data

- within the National Institutes of Health (NIH), the National Heart, Lung and Blood Institute, the National Institute of Diabetes and Digestive and Kidney Diseases, the National Institute on Drug Abuse's Anabolic Steroid Abuse program, and the Weight-Control Information Network (WIN)

Awards

The PCFSN confers awards for national and local contributions to physical activity, fitness, and sports. Since 2006, its Lifetime Achievement Award (LAA) has recognized individuals for their significant contributions to the advancement of physical activity and fitness. Annual Community Leadership Awards recognize up to 50 individuals for their contributions to physical activity, fitness, or sports programs in their communities. The Council also confers a Science Board Honor Award.

Resources

PERIODICALS

Newbell, Trillia. "Fitness Gets Presidential." *American Fitness* 29, no. 3 (May/June 2011): 52.

Vargas, Vianesa. "Fighting the Weight of Our Nation." *American Fitness* 28, no. 6 (November/December 2010): 21.

WEBSITES

"Exercise and Weight Control." President's Council on Fitness, Sports, & Nutrition. http://www.fitness.gov/resources-and-grants/resources/exercise-weight.html (accessed July 25, 2011).

"Learn the Facts." Let's Move! http://www.letsmove.gov/learn-facts/epidemic-childhood-obesity (accessed July 25, 2011).

Let's Move! America's Move to Raise a Healthier Generation of Kids. http://www.letsmove.gov (accessed July 24, 2011).

"Obama Administration Releases National Prevention Strategy." June 16, 2011. http://www.hhs.gov/news/press/2011pres/06/20110616a.html (accessed July 25, 2011).

President's Council on Fitness, Sports, & Nutrition. June 23, 2010. http://www.fitness.gov/pcfsn-overview-2010.pdf (accessed July 25, 2011).

The President's Council on Physical Fitness and Sports. "Fast Facts About Sports Nutrition." Council Publications. July 25, 2011. http://www.fitness.gov/fastfacts.htm (accessed July 25, 2011).

The President's Council on Physical Fitness and Sports. "Fitness Fundamentals: Guidelines for Personal Exercise Programs." Council Publications. July 25, 2011. http://www.fitness.gov/fitness.htm (accessed July 25, 2011).

The President's Council on Physical Fitness and Sports. "10 Tips to Healthy Eating and Physical Activity for You." Council Publications. July 25, 2011. http://www.fitness.gov/10tips.htm (accessed July 25, 2011).

ORGANIZATIONS

American Academy of Pediatrics, 141 Northwest Point Blvd., Elk Grove Village, IL, 60007-1098, (847) 434-4000, Fax: (847) 434-8000, http://www.aap. org; http://www.healthychildren.org.

Centers for Disease Control and Prevention, 1600 Clifton Road, Atlanta, GA, 30333, (800) CDC-INFO (232-4636), cdcinfo@cdc.gov, http://www.cdc.gov.

President's Challenge, 501 North Morton St., Suite 203, Bloomington, IN, 47404, Fax: (812) 855-8999, (800) 258-8146, preschal@indiana.edu, http://www. presidentschallenge.org.

President's Council on Fitness, Sports, & Nutrition, 1101 Wootton Parkway, Suite 560, Rockville, MD, 20852, (240) 276-9567, Fax: (240) 276-9860, fitness@ hhs.gov, http://www.fitness.gov.

Margaret Alic, PhD

Unstructured play *see* **Recess and unstructured play**

Upper body exercises

Definition

Upper body exercises are for the chest, back, shoulders, sides, and arms. They are designed to tone and strengthen the upper body muscles: trapezius and deltoids (shoulder); pectoralis (chest); trapezius, rhomboids, and lower back (back); biceps, triceps, and brachioradialis (arms); and latissimus dorsi (sides and back).

Purpose

Upper body **exercise** can either tone or increase muscle mass and contribute to overall health and fitness. Most fitness routines in North America incorporate upper body exercises as part of a whole-body workout. Fitness magazines regularly contain articles on upper body exercises, from mild **yoga** movements to violent karate chops. Some people do upper body exercises to tone or strengthen muscles. A smaller number do it as part of a **bodybuilding** routine that greatly strengthens muscles and increases muscle size (known as **muscle hypertrophy**), often to enter body-builing competitions, including ones for teenagers, women, and older adults (age 50 and above.)

Demographics

Upper body exercises are done by both men and women, adults, and teenagers.

History

Regular exercise as a way of promoting health can be traced back at least 5,000 years to India, where yoga originated. In China, exercises involving **martial arts**, such as tai chi, qi gong, and kung fu, developed at least 1,500 years ago. The ancient Greeks had exercise programs 2,500 years ago that led to the first Olympic games in 776 B.C. Olympic sports geared towards the upper body include javelin throw, shot put, archery, **rowing**, canoeing, and kayaking. Nearly all general fitness programs have an upper body component. Within the last 100 years the scientific and medical communities began documenting the benefits that even light but regular exercise has on physical and mental well-being.

Although weight training became popular with a small number of people in the 1940s, it was not until the 1960s that regular exercise programs began to flourish throughout North America and Europe, with much emphasis of upper body exercises, primarily for the upper arms and chest. Gymnasiums, once used mainly by male bodybuilders and boxers as training facilities, now are common throughout the United States, Canada, and other industrialized nations. Modern day gyms and health and fitness clubs offer a wide-range of exercise activities for men and women that can fit every lifestyle, age group, and exertion level. Most have exercise machines, along with barbells and **dumbbells** that target specific upper body muscles.

Description

Exercise comes in many forms but there are three basic types: resistance, aerobics, and **stretching**. These are generally classified in three areas: upper and lower body and the abdomen. Most upper body exercises consist of stretching and resistance. Yoga and martial arts are basically muscle stretching routines and **weightlifting** is resistance exercise. Upper body exercises are usually part of any general fitness routine, whether it is simply to tone the muscles or to bulk them up. The primary upper body muscles are trapezius and rhomboids (upper back); deltoids and rotator cuff (shoulders); pectorals (chest); biceps, triceps, and forearm muscles (arms); erector spinae (lower back); and obliques and latissimus dorsi (sides and back). Most yoga and martial arts routines incorporate upper body exercises and movements, from slow and gentle (**t'ai chi** and yoga) to fast and aggressive (karate and kung fu).

Upper body exercises can be divided into three types: stretching, resistance with machines and weights, and resistance without machines or weights. Stretching is usually done for five to ten minutes before and after an exercise regimen. Specific upper body stretches include neck rolls, shoulder shrugs, arm circles, side stretches, wrist curls, torso twists, and overhead triceps stretches.

KEY TERMS

Aerobic exercise—Any brisk exercise or physical activity that requires the heart and lungs to work harder and promote better oxygen circulation in the blood. Running, jogging, swimming, and cycling are aerobic exercises.

Hypertension—High blood pressure.

Martial arts—Various methods of armed and unarmed combat, using the arms, hands, feet, and legs as weapons, that originated centuries ago in Asia, primarily China, Japan, Korea, and the Philippines. The most popular styles include karate, kung fu, jujitsu, judo, aikido, t'ai chi, and tae kwon do.

Osteoporosis—A disease in which the bones become very brittle, porous, break easily, and heal slowly, especially in post-menopausal women.

Yoga—A system of exercises that originated in India 5,000 years ago involving breathing exercises and postures based on Hindu yoga.

Upper body exercises using machines include t-bar rows (back, sides, arms, and shoulders), vertical bench press (chest, arms, shoulders), military press (shoulders), back extension (lower back), reverse preacher curls (biceps), and lat pulldowns (back and upper body). Non-machine upper body exercises include routines that use a medicine ball, barbell, dumbbells, and exercise bands. Among non-machine exercises are push-ups (upper arms and chest), pull-ups (arms), reverse grip chin-ups (back, sides, and biceps), dumbbell bent-over row, barbell curls, snatch (back and shoulders), dumbbell or barbell bench press (chest and upper arms), and dumbbell pullovers (chest).

Preparation

Anyone considering a regular exercise program should consult first with a physician. Persons with serious health problems, such as heart disease, **diabetes**, AIDS, **asthma**, and **arthritis** should only begin an exercise regimen with their doctor's approval. Any upper body exercise routine should generally be preceded with a **warm-up** of five to ten minutes. When **exercising at home** or the gym, loose and comfortable clothes and athletic shoes are helpful. Any exercise program should end with 5-10 minutes of stretching and cool-down exercises.

Risks

For most people, the main risk associated with upper body exercises is overexertion. This can lead to muscle and tendon strains, sprains, tears, and other injuries. Upper body exercise does not need to be strenuous to be beneficial. People with certain chronic health problems should take special precautions. People with diabetes should closely monitor their glucose levels

QUESTIONS TO ASK YOUR DOCTOR

- Do I need to have a stress test or other diagnostic procedure before I begin an exercise program?
- How much do I need to exercise each day?
- What types of upper body exercises do you recommend for me based on my health?
- Am I healthy enough to engage in exercise?
- What medical and health aspects should I consider before starting an upper body exercise program?

before and after upper body exercises. Individuals with heart disease should never exercise to the point of chest pain or angina. Upper body exercise can induce asthma. It is essential for people with asthma to get their doctor's permission before starting an exercise program.

The primary adverse side effect of upper body exercising can be sore muscles and stiff joints a day or two after beginning an exercise routine and lasting for several days.

Results

Results usually depend on goals and determination. Regular upper body workouts using light weights or no weights are good for toning and firming muscles, especially in the upper arms and chest. Workouts that use heavier weights and gradually increase the amount of resistance weight over weeks and months increase muscle mass, resulting in larger and leaner biceps, triceps, chest, forearms, and shoulders. Exercises that use the side muscles (latissimus dorsi) can lead to an "hourglass" shape, especially in males, with firm, concave sides.

Upper body exercise promotes overall good health and well-being. Hundreds of studies during the past several decades link regular exercise to reduced risks for heart disease, stroke, diabetes, **obesity**, depression, **hypertension**, and **osteoporosis**.

Resources

BOOKS

Faigenbaum, Avery, and Wayne Westcott. *Youth Strength Training: Programs for Health, Fitness, and Sport.* Champaign, IL: Human Kinetics Publishers, 2009.

Knopf, Karl. *Healthy Shoulder Handbook.* Berkeley, CA: Ulysses Press, 2010.

Schlosberg, Suzanne, and Liz Neporent. *Fitness for Dummies.* Hoboken, NJ: For Dummies Publishing, 2010.

Wuebben, Joe, and Jim Stoppani. *Stronger Arms and Upper Body.* Champaign, IL: Human Kinetics Publishers, 2008.

PERIODICALS

Bornstein, Adam. "Bulletproof Your Upper Body." *Men's Health* (April 2010): 36.

Clements, French. "Strengthening Your Upper Body." *Dance Magazine* (June 2009): 36.

Hartman, Bill. "Strong Shoulders Ahead." *Men's Fitness* (November 2009): 106.

Nilsson, Nick. "The Best Arm Exercises You've Never Heard Of." *Joe Weider's Muscle & Fitness* (February 2010): 50.

Unke, Sarah. "Upper Body Builders." *Tennis* (May 2009): 97.

Wilson, Eboni. "Eboni Wilson's Back Routine." *Flex* (July 2011): 84.

WEBSITES

Belleme, Gina. *Upper Body Exercise Routine for Women.* LiveStrong.com. (June 9, 2011). http://www.livestrong.com/article/467351-upper-body-exercise-routine-for-women/ (accessed October 30, 2011).

Increase Upper Body. Men's Fitness. http://www.mensfitness.com/fitness/strength-training/increase-upper-body (accessed October 30, 2011).

Rogers, Chris D. *Upper Body Stretches.* Love To Know: Exercise.http://exercise.lovetoknow.com/Upper_Body_Stretches (accessed October 30, 2011).

Upper Body Strength Exercises. Department of Kinesiology and Health, Georgia State University. (January 22, 1998). http://www2.gsu.edu/~wwwfit/upperbod.html (accessed October 30, 2011).

ORGANIZATIONS

American Council on Exercise, 4851 Paramount Dr., San Diego, CA, 92123, (858) 576-6500, Fax: (858) 576-6564, (888) 825 = 3636, support@acefitness.org, http://www.acefitness.org.

Canadian Association of Fitness Professionals, 110-255 Consumer Rd., Toronto, Canada ON, M2J 1R4, 1(416) 493-3515, Fax: (416) 493-1756, (800) 667-5622, info@canfitpro.com, http://www.canfitpro.com.

National Association for Health and Fitness, 65 Niagara Square, Room 607, Buffalo, NY, 14202, (716) 851-4052, Fax: (716) 851-4309, wellness@city-buffalo.org, http://www.physicalfitness.org.

The President's Council on Physical Fitness and Sports, Dept. W, 200 Independence Ave. SW, Room 738-H, Washington, DC, 20201-0004, (202) 690-9000, Fax: (202) 690-5211, fitness@hhs.gov, http://www.fitness.gov.

Ken R. Wells

Urinary system

Definition

The urinary system consists of organs, muscles, tubes, and nerves that are responsible for producing, transporting, and storing urine. The major structures of the urinary system include the kidneys, the ureters, the bladder, and the urethra.

Description

The kidneys

The two kidneys are located lateral (to each side) to the spinal column, along the posterior (back) wall of the abdominal cavity. Each kidney is bean-shaped and approximately the size of one's fist (4–5 in, or 10–13 cm in length). The hilus is the indentation found along the medial side (the side closest to the midline of the body) of the kidney and is the point at which blood vessels (the renal artery and renal vein), nerves, and the ureter enter and exit the organ. The outer layer of the kidney is called the renal cortex, and the inner region of the organ is called the renal medulla.

The individual filtering unit of the kidney is called a nephron, of which there are approximately one million in each kidney. Each nephron extends from the renal cortex into the renal medulla and empties into the funnel-like reservoir of the kidney called the renal pelvis. There are three major components of the nephron: Bowman's capsule, the glomerulus (plural, glomeruli), and the renal tubule. Bowman's capsule is a structure that contains the glomerulus, a cluster of capillaries that is the main filtering device of the nephron. The afferent arteriole brings blood from the branches of the renal artery into Bowman's capsule, where fluid is filtered through the glomerulus. Blood

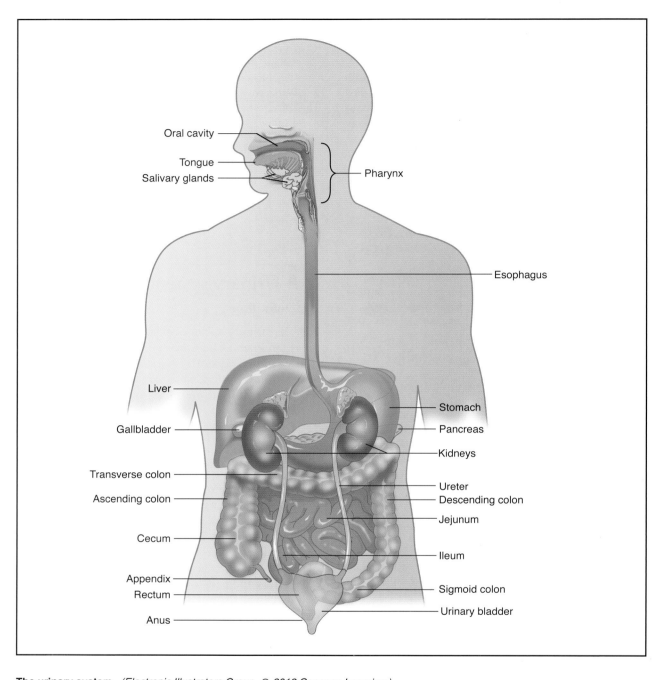

Oral cavity

Tongue

Salivary glands

Pharynx

Esophagus

Liver

Gallbladder

Transverse colon

Ascending colon

Cecum

Appendix

Rectum

Anus

Stomach

Pancreas

Kidneys

Ureter

Descending colon

Jejunum

Ileum

Sigmoid colon

Urinary bladder

The urinary system. *(Electronic Illustrators Group. © 2012 Cengage Learning.)*

exits the glomerulus by way of the efferent arteriole, passing through the persitubular capillaries and eventually entering the renal vein. The renal tubule has four main sections: the proximal tubule, the loop of Henle, the distal tubule, and the collection tubule. The end closest to Bowman's capsule is called the proximal tubule. The loop of Henle extends from the proximal tubule in the renal cortex to the medulla and back to the cortex, into the distal tubule. The distal tubule empties into a collecting duct that in turn empties into the renal pelvis.

The ureters

Urine is transported from the renal pelvis of each kidney to the urinary bladder by way of a thin muscular tube called the ureter. The ureter of an adult is typically 8–10 in (21–26 cm) long and approximately 0.25 in (0.75 cm) in diameter. The walls of the ureter are muscular and help to force urine toward the bladder, away from the kidneys.

The bladder

The urinary bladder is a hollow organ with flexible, muscular walls; it is held in place with ligaments attached to the pelvic bones and other organs. Its primary function is to store urine temporarily until urination occurs, when urine is discharged from the body. When the bladder is empty, its inner wall retracts into many folds that expand as the bladder fills with fluid. The bladder of a healthy adult can typically hold up to 2 cups (0.5 L) of urine comfortably for two to five hours. Circular muscles called sphincters are found at bladder openings—from the ureters and to the urethra—and control the flow of urine out of the bladder by closing tightly around the opening.

The urethra

The urethra is a tube that leads from the bladder to the body's exterior. In females, the urethra is typically about 1.5 in (4 cm) in length and carries only urine; its opening is found anterior (in front of) the opening to the vagina. In males, the urethra is much longer—approximately 8 in (20 cm) in length—and extends from the bladder to the tip of the penis. It passes through the prostate gland; semen is directed into the urethra via the ejaculatory ducts of the prostate. The male urethra alternately transports urine (during urination) and semen (during ejaculation).

Function

Production and transport of urine

Urine is a fluid composed of water and dissolved substances that are in excess of what the body needs to function, as well as various wastes that are by-products of **metabolism**, such as urea, a nitrogen-based waste. These substances are transported into the bloodstream that enters the kidney by way of the afferent arteriole, a branch of the renal artery.

The blood is filtered from there through the glomerulus, where glucose, minerals, urea, other soluble substances, and water pass through to the renal tubule. This fluid is called filtrate. Filtered blood leaves the glomerulus through the efferent arteriole that branches into the renal vein. The filtrate is transported through the renal tubule where, under normal circumstances, most of the water (about 99%), glucose, and other substances are reabsorbed into the

bloodstream through the peritubular capillaries. Urine is what remains at the distal end of the renal tubule.

The urine is transported from the distal and collections tubule to a collection duct and into the renal pelvis. It enters the ureter and is transported to the bladder; a small amount of urine is carried from the renal pelvis to the bladder via the ureter every 10 to 15 seconds. As the bladder fills with urine, pressure from the accumulating fluid stimulates nerve impulses causing the muscles in the wall of the bladder to tighten. Simultaneously, the sphincter muscle at the opening to the urethra is signaled to relax, and urine is forced out of the bladder through the urethra.

Role in human health

The kidneys filter impurities from the bloodstream as waste material and fluid get excreted via urine. Therefore, it is important to maintain a healthy urinary system.

If kidney function becomes compromised, blood creatinine tends to rise and the urinary removal of creatinine may become inefficient. Although the reasons are unclear, studies among athletes suggest that those who engage in regular **exercise** may help preserve and retain good kidney function. Regular exercise appears to have an effect on keeping creatinine levels low, helping improve creatinine clearance through the bloodstream.

In addition, exercise helps maintain overall health and prevention of conditions that have a negative effect on the kidneys including diabetes and high **blood pressure** that damage blood vessels within the kidney nephrons and damage the filtering ability of glomeruli, contributing to renal insufficiency. Additional health risk factors for renal insufficiency include a family history of renal disease, **obesity**, coronary artery disease, and **peripheral vascular disease**.

Exercise puts increased stress on the kidneys so care must be taken to drink water at regular intervals during a workout in order to prevent **dehydration**. While exercising, the amount of blood flow to the kidneys decreases while at the same time, the rate of waste filtration increases. Dehydration diminishes blood flow to the kidneys, negatively impacting removal of creatinine; therefore, it is crucial that fluids are consumed before, during, and after exercising to adequately maintain **hydration** levels.

In order to control the flow of urine, muscles of the urinary system around the urethra and bladder areas must be able to contract and relax. These pelvic muscles must stay strong to work effectively, and are impacted by exercises that strengthen the core. These muscles can be weakened from childbirth, smoking, **age**, surgery in the pelvic region, and some medications.

Exercises that strengthen these, and other muscles of the core include:

• aerobics
• yoga
• moderate or brisk walking
• rowing
• swimming

In addition to good urinary system health, a balanced, systematic, and routine workout offers individuals other fitness benefits:

• Stimulate movement in the gastrointestinal tract to prevent constipation.
• Expand and oxygenate the lungs.
• Move blood throughout the circulatory system.
• Stimulate the lymphatic system.
• Relax and contract muscles throughout the entire body, increasing muscle tone and skin turgor.
• Promote and maintain good range of motion of the limbs.
• Accelerate a release of endorphins, improving mood, energy, and libido.
• Burn calories and aid in the reduction of body fat that helps in weight control.
• Enhance heart health (especially aerobic exercise), aiding in the prevention of high cholesterol and high blood pressure. While cholesterol levels can be lowered by reducing weight and eating less saturated fatty foods, a key ingredient in a cholesterol lowering program is a regular and systematic physical training program.
• Maintain a healthy weight, avoiding propensity toward insulin resistance, diabetes, and resulting complications of diabetes.
• Reduce stress and aid in achieving a more restful night of sleep.
• Strengthen bones to help prevent osteoporosis.
• Stimulate white blood cell movement (especially brisk physical activity), making the immune system strong.

The American Heart Association recommends 30 minutes of exercise five times a week in conjunction with a heart healthy diet regimen. A regular exercise routine and nutritious diet will also help in weight management. Read food labels to examine not only calorie, fat, carbohydrate, and **protein** content, but

---

KEY TERMS

Creatinine—A waste product of metabolism. Kidney function is measured in part by its ability to filter and remove creatinine from the body. High levels of creatinine often reflect poor kidney function.

Cystitis—Inflammation of the urinary bladder.

Dialysis—A medical procedure in which waste products are filtered from the bloodstream by a machine.

Filtrate—The fluid that results when blood is filtered through the glomerulus; a precursor to urine.

Hilus—The indentation found along the medial side of the kidney; the point at which blood vessels (the renal artery and renal vein), nerves, and the ureter enter and exit the organ.

Nephritis—Inflammation of the kidney.

Nephron—The individual filtering unit of the kidney; consists of Bowman's capsule, the glomerulus, and the renal tubule.

Renal cortex—The outer layer of the kidney.

Renal medulla—The inner region of the kidney.

Renal pelvis—The funnel-like reservoir of a kidney that empties to the ureter.

Sphincters—Circular muscles that control the flow of urine in to/out of openings to/from the bladder.

---

also to determine serving size in relation to these numbers. Dieticians may be of assistance in understanding food labels.

Nutrition has an impact on urinary system function, including how this system eliminates waste, cleans the body of impurities, removes toxins, and cleans the blood. Diet intake, including food, fluids, vitamins, and minerals, play an active role in a healthy urinary system:

• Fruits and vegetables such as blueberries, blackberries, red grapes, eggplants, purple cabbage, and plums, are high in phenolic antioxidants that help decrease inflammation and promote good urinary tract function.

• Yogurt and yogurt products containing probiotic bacteria promote growth of "good bacteria" and keep growth of "bad bacteria" to a minimum that aids the prevention of urinary tract infections.

- Coriander helps soothe irritations associated with urinary tract infections.
- Garlic has been found to enhance antioxidant activity and help minimize problems due to decreased blood supply to kidneys.
- Celery, watermelon, and asparagus help flush the urinary system, and aid in the elimination of toxins.
- Cranberry extract has been shown to help purify the urinary tract and aid in preventing bladder infections.
- Water intake, drinking six-to-eight 8-oz glasses of water every day can help keep the urinary system flushing toxins and filtering properly.

High levels of alcohol necessitate the urinary system to have to work harder to eliminate toxins associated with alcohol ingestion, so care should be taken to keep alcohol consumption at a minimum.

Making good nutritional choices and developing a healthy exercise regimen is beneficial to the urinary system and the entire body as a whole.

Common diseases and conditions

Kidney diseases and other urinary system disorders affect millions of Americans to some degree. An estimated 8.4 million new urinary conditions occur each year, including infections of the kidneys, urinary tract, bladder, and others. Urinary tract stones prompt over 1.3 million visits annually to the doctor's office with over 250,000 hospital stays. Urinary incontinence is estimated to affect 13 million adults in the United States. In 1998, approximately 398,000 individuals were diagnosed with end-stage renal disease (ESRD), of which over 63,000 died. In that same year, 245,910 patients utilized dialysis services—a medical procedure in which waste products are filtered from the bloodstream by a machine.

Some common diseases and conditions of the urinary system include:

- Nephritis (also called glomerulonephritis): Nephritis is an inflammation of the kidneys. It may be caused by a bacterial infection (pyelonephritis) or an abnormal immune response. Chronic nephritis may result in extensive damage to the kidneys and eventual kidney failure.
- Urinary tract infection (UTI): This broad term includes infections of the urethra and/or bladder (lower UTI) or the kidneys and/or ureters (upper UTI). UTIs may be caused by bacteria, fungi, viruses, or parasites.
- Cystitis: More commonly known as a bladder infection, cystitis is common in women and may be caused by bacteria introduced into the urethra

---

QUESTIONS TO ASK YOUR DOCTOR

- What are the indications that I may have a problem with my urinary system?
- What diagnostic tests are needed for a thorough assessment?
- What treatment options do you recommend for me?
- What dietary changes, if any, would you recommend for me?
- What measures can be taken to prevent urinary system problems?

from the vagina. Cystitis in males may result from a prostate infection. It can be treated successfully with antibiotics.

- Urinary incontinence: This is defined as involuntary urination. Urinary incontinence may involve an urgent desire to urinate followed by involuntary urine loss (urge incontinence); an uncontrolled loss of urine following actions such as laughing, sneezing, coughing, or lifting (stress incontinence); loss of small amounts of urine from a full bladder (overflow incontinence); continual leakage of urine (total incontinence); or a combination of problems (mixed incontinence).
- Kidney/urinary tract cancers: Cancer may develop in any of the structures of the urinary system. Kidney cancer accounts for approximately 2% of cancers diagnosed in adults, more often affecting males than females. Bladder cancer may also occur, with smoking being the most significant risk factor.
- Urinary tract stones: Urinary calculi or urinary tract stones may be called kidney stones or bladder stones, depending on the site of their formation. They may form because of an excess of salts or a lack of stone-formation inhibitors in the urine. Urinary tract stones may cause bleeding, pain, urine obstruction, or infection.

Resources

BOOKS

McDowell, Julie, ed. *Encyclopedia of Human Body Systems*. Santa Barbara, CA: Greenwood, 2010.

Rizzo, Donald C. *Introduction to Anatomy and Physiology*. Clifton Park, NY: Delmar, 2011.

Schmitz, Paul G. *Renal: An Integrated Approach to Disease*. New York: McGraw–Hill Medical, 2011.

PERIODICALS

Johnson, Sarah T. "From incontinence to Confidence." *American Journal of Nursing* (February 2000): 69–74.

ORGANIZATIONS

American Association of Kidney Patients, 3505 E. Frontage Rd., Suite 315, Tampa, FL, 33607, (800) 749-2257, http://www.aakp.org.

American Urological Foundation, 1000 Corporate Blvd., Linthicum, MD, 21090, (410) 689-3990, http://www.urologyhealth.org.

National Institute of Diabetes and Digestive and Kidney Diseases, 31 Center Dr., MSC 2560, Bethesda, MD, 20892-2560, http://www2.niddk.nih.gov.

National Kidney Foundation, 30 East 33rd St., New York, NY, 10016, (800) 622-9010, http://www.kidney.org.

U.S. Renal Data System (USRDS), 914 S. 8th St., Suite S-206, Minneapolis, MN, 55404, (612) 347-7776, http://www.usrds.org.

Stéphanie Islane Dionne
Laura Jean Cataldo, RN, EdD

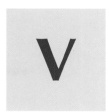

Vinyasa yoga

Definition

Vinyasa **yoga** refers to a way of doing yoga that emphasizes the union of breath and movement, usually involving a gradual progression from one asana (pose) to the next so that the poses are smoothly connected. The word *vinyasa* comes from two Sanskrit words that mean "to place" and "in a special way." Sometimes called the "breathing system," vinyasa is not a distinctive tradition but a technique that can be incorporated into ashtanga, Iyengar, and other schools of yoga.

Vinyasa is sometimes used to refer to vinyasa flow, a style of yoga developed by Bryan Kest in the Los Angeles area in the 1990s. Kest, a student of Pattabhi Jois and the originator of **power yoga**, was followed by such other instructors as Erich Schiffmann, Shiva Rea, and Seane Corn, each of which has put his or her individual stamp on vinyasa practice. In vinyasa flow classes, students are taught to synchronize the breath with a series of body postures that flow into one another, and also to practice transitional vinyasas between sustained asanas.

Purpose

There are several reasons why yoga practitioners may practice vinyasa:

- To increase body heat.
- To change the energy pattern of the practice so that the student can feel the energy of different asanas more fully. Each asana is thought to have its own distinctive energy pattern. Many vinyasas consist of counterposes to the asana just performed. The counterposes bring the body's energy back to neutral, so to speak, in preparation for the next asana.
- To help the body release impurities. In the ashtanga tradition, vinyasa is thought to increase the fire of the digestive process and clear the mind of disturbing thoughts; as well as speed up the body's removal of wastes.
- To develop internal awareness or mindfulness, and improve the ability to concentrate the mind.
- To increase the student's sensitivity to the body's internal sensations and messages.

Another reason for practicing vinyasa is that it teaches practitioners of yoga to extend the mindset of vinyasa practice to all of their activities. Specifically, vinyasa requires paying attention to the entire structure of one's practice: its beginning, its gradual building to a peak level of activity, its completion, and its integration. Extending this approach to one's entire life means giving proper attention to the beginning of any course of action, following through in a series of linked steps, and bringing the action to completion.

Demographics

According to a survey taken by *Yoga Journal* in 2008, 16.7% of the 16 million Americans who practice yoga practice some form of vinyasa. Although vinyasa is incorporated into some forms of yoga instruction for children, most vinyasa classes are geared to older teenagers and adults.

History

Vinyasa yoga is usually traced back to Tirumalai Krishnamacharya (1888–1989), an Indian teacher of yoga who founded an influential school in Mysore. Krishnamacharya never left India over the course of his long life; however, his pupils carried many of his teachings to the West. They include B.K.S. Iyengar, the founder of **Iyengar yoga**; K. Pattabhi Jois, the founder of ashtanga yoga; and several other noted yoga teachers, including Krishnamacharya's three sons.

According to Srivatsa Ramaswami (1939–), a teacher of yoga who studied with Krishnamacharya from 1955 to 1988, it was Krishnamacharya's insistence on coordinating movement with breathing that struck Ramaswami as something new—even though this approach to yoga is widely taken for granted in the early 2000s. Ramaswami credits Krishnamacharya with the following features of classical vinyasa practice:

- A focus on slowing the breath, preferably to six or fewer breaths per minute.
- Specific instructions for the types of movements to be performed while exhaling and others to be done while inhaling. Krishnamacharya specified that deep forward bending and twisting movements are always done while breathing out, while expansive movements or backbends are typically done while breathing in.
- The notion that vinyasa should be a way of life, not just confined to the practice of asanas. Krishnamacharya exemplified this belief by greeting his students at the gate to his house, guiding them through their practice with him, and then bringing their session to completion by escorting them back to the gate.

Krishnamacharya was noted for tailoring his instruction to the needs and capacities of each individual or small group. As a result, some of his former students find it difficult to summarize his teaching briefly or to explain it in full.

Description

Some practitioners of yoga think of vinyasa as referring primarily to the six series of specific asanas recommended by K. Pattabhi Jois (1915–2009), the founder of ashtanga yoga. In Jois's system, the asanas and the order in which they are to be performed are strictly specified. Most yoga teachers, however, maintain that vinyasa can be correctly used to describe any progressive series of asanas that the instructor arranges. In some cases, yoga instructors may speak of "taking a vinyasa" as a shorthand term for a series of breath-synchronized movements performed in sequence between asanas held for longer periods of time.

Ashtanga vinyasa

Vinyasa as practiced in the ashtanga tradition is highly structured; the student is asked to perform a series of asanas in a standard order. There are six series in ashtanga vinyasa: primary, intermediate, and advanced A, B, C, and D.

Each of the six series has the same overall structure:

- Opening sequence: This phase consists of 10 Sun Salutations and several standing poses.
- Poses specific to the student's series, including a back-bending sequence.
- Finishing sequence: This phase contains several inverted poses.

Vinyasa flow

Vinyasa flow classes are less structured than ashtanga vinyasa practice, and often reflect the personality of the individual instructor. They do, however, follow the overall vinyasa pattern of self-evaluation prior to beginning the practice; using vinyasa krama to build toward a peak within a practice session; and bringing the practice to completion in an integrated and satisfactory way.

Preparation

Preparation is an important part of vinyasa yoga. Since the overall structure of a vinyasa practice should be as structured and smoothly integrated as the flow of asanas into one another, preparation involves determining the goals of a practice before beginning, and then setting up a series of steps to attain those goals. This approach to practice is sometimes called vinyasa krama, *krama* being the Sanskrit word for tool.

Vinyasa krama begins with self-assessment in the moment; that is, the person's present **energy** level, any areas of tension or soreness they may note in their body, and other concerns. The goal of the practice as influenced by the person's present condition may be either short-term—for example, deciding on a restorative set of asanas when one is feeling tired or agitated rather than an active set—or long-term, such as learning to meditate on a deeper level or working on overall conditioning of the body. After setting the goal, the practitioner arranges a series of asanas or other aspects of yoga such as pranayama (breathing exercises) or meditation to be performed in order to move toward the goal.

Risks

The National Center for Complementary and Alternative Medicine (NCCAM) recommends that anyone considering any form of yoga practice should consult their health care provider before starting the program. They should not use yoga as a substitute for conventional medical treatment and they should not postpone seeing a doctor about any health problem they already have. The individual should also ask the instructors at a yoga studio about their training and certification, and about the physical demands associated with the type of yoga taught in the studio.

Vinyasa yoga is less risky for beginners or people with physical limitations because its instructors are trained to tailor the asanas and breathing exercises to individual needs. In addition, the variety of instructors claiming to teach one form or another of vinyasa means that a person can usually find a class that fits their level of experience and overall physical fitness. Most instructors of vinyasa yoga maintain that the students at greatest risk of strains, pulled muscles, or other injuries are those who are impatient with vinyasa krama and attempt more advanced poses before they have integrated the work of earlier stages of practice.

Different vinyasa instructors take their classes at different paces. So-called power vinyasa yoga instructors conduct fast-paced classes that are not suited for pregnant women or seniors. Ashtanga vinyasa yoga is also fast-paced. Unless older adults have had a number of years of yoga practice and are in good physical health, they should look into slow- or moderately paced vinyasa classes.

The remaining consideration is the individual instructor's personality and his or her interpretation of vinyasa. Because there is considerable diversity in vinyasa practice, some instructors' teachings reflect their particular quirks or preferences. It may be necessary for a beginner to try several vinyasa classes with different teachers in order to find a classroom setting and pace in which they feel comfortable.

Results

Most people who practice vinyasa yoga report that it lowers stress as well as improving their flexibility and raising their overall energy level. Some also find that it assists their meditations or other spiritual practices.

QUESTIONS TO ASK YOUR DOCTOR

- In what way do you think yoga will benefit me?
- Do I have any physical limitations that would prohibit my undertaking yoga?
- Is there anything in my present or past medical history that I should tell the instructor?
- What is your opinion of vinyasa practices?
- What pace do you think would be best for me?
- Have any of your other patients practiced vinyasa flow yoga or incorporated vinyasa into their practices? Do they find it helpful?
- Do you recommend any vinyasa instructors?

There is relatively little research done on vinyasa by itself because it is considered an approach to yoga that can be blended into more specific schools or traditions rather than a distinctive school in its own right. As of 2011, there was one clinical trial of vinyasa under way. The study began in 2007 and is sponsored by NCCAM. It is a study (currently in Phase 3) of the effectiveness of vinyasa yoga as an aid to smoking cessation for women.

Resources

BOOKS

Bradbury, Alan. *Starting Yoga: A Practical Foundation Guide for Men and Women.* Wiltshire, UK: Crowood Press, 2011.

Butera, Robert J. *The Pure Heart of Yoga: Ten Essential Steps for Personal Transformation.* Woodbury, MN: Llewellyn Publications, 2009.

Lark, Liz. *Personal Trainer: Yoga for Life.* London: Carlton Publishing Group, 2011.

Philp, John. *Yoga Inc.: A Journey through the Big Business of Yoga.* New York: Penguin Global, 2010.

Rountree, Sage. *The Athlete's Pocket Guide to Yoga: 50 Routines for Flexibility, Balance, and Focus.* Boulder, CO: VeloPress, 2009.

Schiffmann, Erich. *Yoga: The Spirit and Practice of Moving into Stillness.* New York: Pocket Books, 1996.

Singleton, Mark. *Yoga Body: The Origins of Modern Posture Practice.* New York: Oxford University Press, 2010.

PERIODICALS

Brown, R.P., et al. "Yoga Breathing, Meditation, and Longevity." *Annals of the New York Academy of Sciences* 1172 (August 2009): 54–62.

Cowen, V.S. "Functional Fitness Improvements after a Worksite-based Yoga Initiative." *Journal of Bodywork and Movement Therapies* 14 (January 2010): 50–54.

Shelov, D.V., et al. "A Pilot Study Measuring the Impact of Yoga on the Trait of Mindfulness." *Behavioural and Cognitive Psychotherapy* 37 (October 2009): 595–98.

Simard, A.A., and M. Henry. "Impact of a Short Yoga Intervention on Medical Students' Health: A Pilot Study." *Medical Teacher* 31 (October 2009): 950–52.

WEBSITES

Corn, Seane. *Vinyasa Flow DVD Preview.* http://www.youtube.com/watch?v=peBNUkSTvi0 (accessed November 16, 2011).

Dale, Daniel. "Vinyasa: About This Form of Yoga." http://www.omagain.com/?page_id=10 (accessed November 16, 2011).

Gaspar, Lori. "The Many Nuances of Vinyasa." *Yoga Chicago.* (November-December 2003). http://yogachicago.com/nov03/vinyasa.shtml (accessed November 16, 2011).

Rea, Shiva. "Consciousness in Motion." *Yoga Journal.* http://www.yogajournal.com/wisdom/909 (accessed November 16, 2011).

Schiffmann, Erich. "The Wind Through the Instrument." *Moving into Stillness.* (December 1, 1996). http://www.movingintostillness.com/book/yoga_breathing.html (accessed November 16, 2011).

Yoga for Health: An Introduction. National Center for Complementary and Alternative Medicine (NCCAM). Publication No. D412 (May 2008). http://nccam.nih.gov/health/yoga/introduction.htm (accessed November 26, 2011).

ORGANIZATIONS

American Yoga Association, P.O. Box 19986, Sarasota, FL, 34276, info@americanyogaassociation.org, http://www.americanyogaassociation.org.

Erich Schiffmann, Exhale Center for Sacred Movement, 245 S. Main St., Venice, CA, 90291, (310) 450-7676, erichyog@earthlink.net, http://www.movingintostillness.com.

International Association of Yoga Therapists (IAYT), 4150 Tivoli Ave., Los Angeles, CA, 90066

National Center for Complementary and Alternative Medicine (NCCAM), 9000 Rockville Pike, Bethesda, MD, 20892, info@nccam.nih.gov, http://nccam.nih.gov.

Seane Corn, P.O. Box 1425, Topanga, CA, 90290, (310) 285-8129, Seane@seanecorn.com, http://www.seanecorn.com.

Shiva Rea: Yoga as Conscious Evolution, P.O. Box 3319, Frederick, MD, 21705, (301) 560-0934, info@yogadventures.com, http://www.shivarea.com.

Yoga Journal, P.O. Box 51151, Boulder, CO, 80322-1151, (303) 604-7435, http://www.yogajournal.com.

Yoga Research and Education Center (YREC), 2400A County Center Dr., Santa Rosa, CA, 95403, (707) 566-0000, http://www.yrec.org.

Rebecca J. Frey, PhD
Laura Jean Cataldo, RN, EdD

VO2 max *see* **Maximum oxygen uptake**

Volleyball

Definition

Volleyball is a widely popular team sport played on a rectangular court divided evenly by a standing net. Two opposing teams, one on each side of the net, use primarily their hands to hit a spherical ball back and forth over an approximate 8 ft (2.4 m) net. The main types of volleyball are those played indoors on a hard floor, those played outside on grass, dirt, or other material, and those played outside on sand, what is commonly called beach volleyball. Because volleyball is an actively played sport, it helps to provide a healthy workout for all parts of the body.

Purpose

The object of volleyball is to score more points than the opposing team. This is done by sending the ball over the net and grounding it inside the opposing team's court before its players are able to hit it back over the net and ground it inside their opposition's court. However, whether one wins or loses, each player's strenuous and constant activities during the play of volleyball results in a physically fit body and good cardiovascular health.

Demographics

People of all ages play volleyball around the world. The international governing body for volleyball—the International Federation of Volleyball (FIVB), headquartered in Lausanne, Switzerland—estimates that about 800 million people annually play the game.

History

Volleyball was invented in 1895, by William G. Morgan, an American physical education director at the Young Men's Christian Association (YMCA) in Holyoke, Massachusetts. Morgan's new game he called Mintonette was invented based on rules found in **handball** and **tennis**. The first volleyball championship in the United States was held in 1922. Six years later, the U.S. Volleyball Association was formed. Today, it is known as USA Volleyball. In 1947, the FIVB was organized. The Olympic Games include volleyball as one of their competitions. Indoor volleyball was first played at the 1964 Olympic Games in Tokyo, Japan. Beach volleyball made its debut at the 1996 Olympic Games in Atlanta, Georgia. Today, national championships are held in the United States for players of different **age** groups, with each championship play geared to a particular five-year age increment.

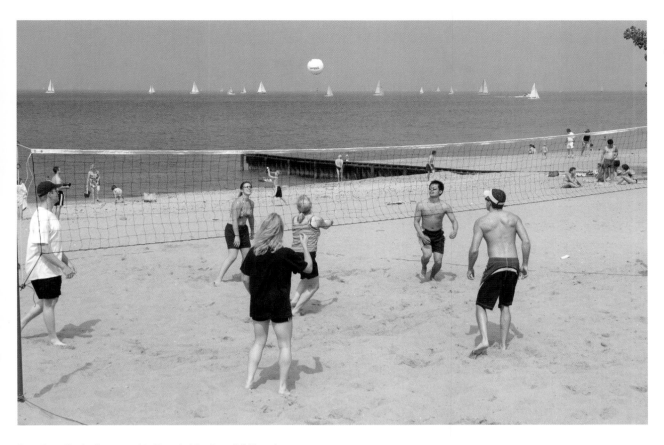

Beach volleyball game. *(© Dennis MacDonald/Alamy)*

Description

In volleyball played indoors and outdoors (except for beach volleyball), six members make up one team. (This article will concentrate on volleyball played with six members.) When played outdoors on sand, only two players form a team. Volleyball players play the game within a area called a court, and they use a ball called a "volleyball."

Playing surface

The rectangular playing surface for volleyball is called a court. For indoor volleyball, this area is 59 ft (18 m) by 29.5 ft (9 m). The ceiling of the building used for indoor volleyball should be at least 23 ft (7 m) in height, and preferably even higher. When played outdoors on sand, the surface area is slightly smaller.

The two sides of the longer dimension of a volleyball court are called the sidelines, one on each side of the court. One center line that is directly below the net divides the longer dimension in half. Thus, each half of the volleyball court consists of a square area 29.5 ft (9 m) by 29.5 ft (9 m). The shorter dimension contains two back lines that are the boundary lines at the furthest points from the center line.

For indoor volleyball, two attack lines are drawn parallel to the center line—with one line 10 ft (3 m) from the centerline on each side of the court. The attack line separates each side into a back row (back court) area and a front row (front court) area. Each of these is further (loosely) divided into three areas (positions). The position of the serving player is called number "1" with the right-side front row person being number "2" and so forth counterclockwise to the number "6" that is positioned next to and to the left of the server.

The service line encompasses the entire back line, however the ball must be contacted within the confines of the sidelines and the serving player must not touch any part of the back line with their foot. When jump serving, the player's feet typically leave the floor behind the back line and may cross over the back line landing inside the court after contact of the ball.

Equipment

A net that is usually made of strong black or brown mesh string divides the court in half lengthwise.

It is positioned directly above the center line. The top of the net has a height of approximately 7 ft 11-5/8 in (2.43 m) above the floor, when played by men, and about 7 ft 4-1/8 in (2.24 m), when played by women. It can be positioned at lower levels for children, seniors, and other groups. The net's width is approximately 40 in (1 m). The poles (also called standards) for the net should be set 36 ft (12 m) apart and 3 ft (1 m) on either side of the sidelines. For competitions, an antenna is placed on top of each pole, about 32 in (81.3 cm) in height. The balls must be hit within the plane of these two antennae (from the floor and upward through the imaginary straight lines going up to the ceiling) when crossing the net.

The ball is an inflated sphere that is about the same size as a **soccer** ball. According to the FIVB, its circumference must be between 25 and 27 in (65 and 67 cm), weigh from 9–10 oz (260–280 g), and have a pressure of 4.267–4.623 lb./sq. in. (0.300–0.325 kg/sq cm). The material used to make the ball's cover is natural leather or a synthetic material made to look like leather.

Game

When a team consists of six players, such as for indoor play, three players play in a row near the front of the net and another three players stand in a row further away from the net. The game begins by deciding who serves first. A server initiates a game by standing behind the end line and serving the ball over the net into the court of the receiving team. The serve may be done by throwing the ball up and hitting it while in the air or holding the ball with one hand while hitting it with the other hand. Only one serve try is allowed. This serve is called the "start of a rally".

The receiving team must hit the ball over the net before it hits the ground. These players can hit the ball up to three times (in addition to the block contact), but an individual player can only hit it once in a row. Typically, the first hit is called a "bump" (or a pass). It is used to position the ball so its flight is directed toward the player called the "setter". The second hit (by the setter) is usually an over-hand pass using the player's wrists to push the fingertips toward the ball so the ball's trajectory is directed in the general area of the attacker. Consequently, the third hit is oftentimes a spike. This consists of the attacker jumping up in the air while raising one arm over the head to hit the ball so it moves in a downward angle toward the opposing team's court while still going above the net. These actions are called the offensive part of the game, while the other players are defending themselves against the return of the ball to their side of the court.

At the same time, the players on defense try to prevent the other team from getting the ball grounded on their side of the court. Players in the front court typically jump up and extend their hands above the top of the net to try to block the ball coming from the offensive team. If the ball is not able to be blocked by them, then the back court players try to prevent the ball from hitting the floor by using a "dig" play that consists of using the forearm to hit the ball upwards. If one of the players is able to successfully dig the ball and the ball goes flying over the net, then this side becomes the defensive team and the other side becomes the offensive team. If the ball remains on their side, the opposite occurs.

Players cannot hold onto the ball while it is in play. Any part of the body may be used to hit the ball, but the hands are used most often. The rally continues as long as each team does not allow the ball to be grounded on their side and they hit the ball only up to three times before it returns to the other side.

A rally is stopped under three circumstances: (1) a team grounds the ball inside the boundary of the opponent's court (they make a "kill"), (2) a team loses the rally (make a "fault"). The ball is in bounds if it touches a sideline or end line, is inside any of these lines, or touches one of the opposing players while going out of bounds., or (3) an illegal play or fault occurs on either side of the court. Some of the more frequently seen faults include the following:

- catching or throwing the ball
- two consecutive contacts (touches) of the ball by one player; what is called a "double hit"
- hitting the ball so it impacts the ground outside the opponent's court (out of bounds) or without first passing it over the net
- touching the net while trying to play the ball
- stepping into the area of the opposing team
- hitting the ball four consecutive times by the members of the same team

Points are awarded to the serving team if the opposing team does not get the ball over the net, such as if the ball hits the ground within the playing area, or if the ball does not go over the net. The server continues to serve as long as points are scored by this person's team. If the point is not awarded to the serving team, then the other team begins to serve. After a team wins back a serve, then a new server is used, with a circular rotation method.

Traditionally, a point was scored by a team only when it serves. When using these rules, if the point is won by the non-serving team, then they get the ball back for serving. In most competitions now, points are scored whether the team is serving or not. This is called "rally scoring."

The first team to score 15 points (in a traditional volleyball game) wins the game. When rally scoring is used, then 25 points are required to win. An indoor volleyball match consists of winning two out of three games or three out of five games—whichever is decided before match play. Beach volleyball usually consists of one game from traditional scoring or two out of three when using rally scoring.

There are many standard plays in volleyball. Some of them are:

- Block: The use of front-row players to jump up high the air near the net with hands and arms held high in the air for the purpose of hitting a spiked ball back to the opposing team or detouring the spiked ball so a teammate can return it over the net
- Dig: An underarm pass made with the forearms
- Set: A well positioned ball placed high in the air and usually near the net for a teammate to hit with a strong overhead shot called spike
- Spike: An aggressively hit ball that goes flying over the net at a high speed; it involves the player jumping very high and hitting the ball while it is high in the air
- Tip: Also called a placement, a slightly hit ball that is deflected or dropped unexpectedly into the court of the opposing team

For serving, players rotate one position clockwise every time their team wins a volley and is allowed to serve again. Only the three players in the front-row are allowed to block, jump, and spike, the ball near the net. The back-row players are only allowed to hit the ball over the net if they jump from behind the attack line.

Officiating

Officials are used during competitive matches in volleyball. They usually include an up-referee, down-referee, scorer, and line judges.

Preparation

Warming up before playing volleyball is critical so muscles can be best prepared for all of the physical activities involved in the game. Five or so minutes of light **exercise** will prepare the body for the physical actions found within volleyball. **Stretching** exercises are also recommended. However, stretching should be done after other exercises so muscles are not injured. After playing volleyball, spend another five minutes to cool-down. Light exercises or **walking** helps to return the body to its resting state. Stretching afterwards is also recommended.

To play volleyball at the utmost level of competition, certain exercises should be performed. When performed on a regular basis, they will provide more agility, endurance, and strength while playing volleyball.

These physical attributes are needed because volleyball players need (1) agility for quick reaction during fast-paced games; (2) endurance to maintain a high level of **energy** throughout games, and (3) strength for spiking, serving, and all of the other moves used in volleyball games. Endurance is especially important because volleyball is a game of near-constant action involving long or short rallies, followed by a very short break, followed by another rally and so forth and so on throughout the game.

Almost all of the muscles of the body are used in volleyball. Some of the more important muscle groups to increase strength for better serving, spiking, blocking, and jumping include abdominal muscles, leg muscles, and arm muscles. For instance, to improve upper body strength, volleyball players will do bench presses, pull-ups, pull-downs, and medicine ball throws. To decrease risk of shoulder injuries, players will do upper **back exercises** such as rows and rotator cuff muscle strengthening exercises.

Risks

Volleyball is a highly competitive sport. Consequently, injuries will happen. Some of the more common injuries are sprains and strains, especially to the ankle. In addition, injuries to the hand and finger, knee, and shoulder also occur. When playing volleyball, the actions of attacking (hitting or spiking) cause the most injuries. Blocking injuries often result in injuries to the finger or ankle, while spiking injuries occur frequently to the shoulder, knee, and ankle.

Results

Volleyball is an all-round good sport to participate in because it helps all parts of the body. The playing of volleyball for at least 45 minutes on a regular basis, along with a balanced and nutritious diet, helps to improve physical strength, mental and physical health, endurance and stamina, and dexterity.

Playing volleyball helps to lose weight when done together with a proper diet. About 45 minutes of volleyball expends (burns) up to 600 **calories**, resulting in **weight loss** over a long period. By losing weight, one has a reduced risk from diabetes, **hypertension** (high **blood pressure**), and heart disease.

Volleyball also helps to improve aerobic endurance, what is often called cardiovascular fitness. It also helps with stamina because one plays volleyball almost continuously for extended periods. Besides improving physical attributes, mental alertness is also improved because players must analyze, evaluate, and react to quick situations and strategies set before them. Players must also have motivation and self-confidence in themselves to play at their best, along with being able to cope with pressure situations.

Strength and power are also important because volleyball players need to exert a large amount of force in a short period, such as when they spike the ball. Speed and quickness is necessary because the ability to move quickly around the volleyball court is essential for scoring points and defending against the other team. Flexibility and dexterity are also improved, as is hand and eye coordination and balance and coordination.

Resources

BOOKS

Crisfield, Deborah W., and John Monteleone. *Winning Volleyball for Girls*. New York: Chelsea House, 2010.

Hanlon, Thomas. *The Sports Rules Book*. Champaign, IL: Human Kinetics, 2009.

Reynaud, Cecile. *Coaching Volleyball Technical and Tactical Skills*. Champaign, IL: Human Kinetics, 2011.

May-Treanor, Misty, with Jill Lieber Steeg. *Misty:Digging Deep in Volleyball and Life.*. New York: Scribner, 2010.

USA Volleyball. *Volleyball Systems & Strategies*. Champaign, IL: Human Kinetics, 2009.

Waite, Pete. *Aggressive Volleyball*. Champaign, IL: Human Kinetics, 2009.

WEBSITES

Selzer, Diane. "Volleyball Conditioning Drills and Exercises to Improve Fitness." Suite101.com. September 1, 2010. http://diane-seltzer.suite101.com/volleyball-conditioning-drills-and-exercises-to-improve-fitness-a281164 (accessed September 26, 2011).

Volleyball Hall of Fame VolleyHall.com. September 1, 2010. http://www.volleyhall.org// (accessed September 26, 2011).

Volleyball Magazine. VolleyballMag.com. September 1, 2010. http://www.volleyballmag.com/ (accessed September 26, 2011).

"What Are the Health Benefits of Volleyball?" LiveStrong.com. June 4, 2011. http://www.athleticscholarships.net/history-of-volleyball.htm (accessed September 26, 2011).

ORGANIZATIONS

International Federation of Volleyball, Chateau Les Tourelles; Edouard-Sandoz 2-4, Lausanne, France, 1006, 4121345-3535, Fax: 4121(345-3545) , info@fivb.org, http://www.fivb.org/.

USA Volleyball, 715 South Circle Drive, Colorado Springs, CO, 80910, (719) 228-6800, Fax: (719) 228-6899, http://usavolleyball.org/.

William A. Atkins, BB, BS, MBA
Emily Darr, MD

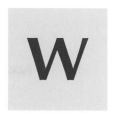

W

Waist circumference and waist-to-hip ratio

Definition

Waist circumference and waist-to-hip ratio are two important measurements that help to determine a person's overall health. Specifically, by measuring the circumference of the waist and the ratio of waist circumference to hip circumference, these two factors provide a good indication of increased risk for getting obesity-related diseases such as diabetes and **cardiovascular disease**.

Obesity is a medical condition in which there is an excess accumulation of fat in the human body. It is associated with increased risk of illness, disability, and premature death. Medical professionals generally consider obesity, or excessively being overweight, to be a chronic illness that is often grouped with other chronic conditions—such as high **blood pressure** and diabetes—that can be controlled but not presently cured.

Good ways to control obesity (and thus to decrease waist circumference and waist-to-hip ratio) is to maintain a healthy body weight by eating modest proportions of balanced and nutritious foods and exercising on a regular basis.

Purpose

The purpose of these two measurements is to help to determine the overall distribution of fat on the human body. Being overweight, especially being obese, places additional stress on the body's organs and puts people at higher risk for many serious and potentially life threatening health problems.

Demographics

Excessive values for waist circumference and waist-to-hip ratio have become much more common in western society as more people become overweight or obese. Being overweight has become a serious public health problem that affects both sexes and all ethnic, racial, **age**, and socioeconomic groups in the United States and around the world. According to the U.S. Centers for Disease Control (CDC), 34% of adults (or about 103 million people) in the United States are obese, as of 2007–2008. As of 2009, approximately 440,000 deaths a year are attributed to obesity.

According to the CDC, childhood obesity has more than tripled from 1980 to 2008. In fact, for children from six to 11 years of age, the rate of obesity has gone from 6.5% in 1980 to 19.6% in 2008. For adolescents from the age of 12 to 19 years, the rate increased from 5.0% to 18.1% in this same year range.

Description

Waist Circumference

The waist is defined as the part of the abdomen between the lowest rib on the rib cage and the upper portion of the hips. Circumference is defined as the distance around an object. For instance, the circumference of a circle is the distance around this geometric figure. In this particular case, circumference refers to the distance around the waist of a person. Waist circumference is determined with the use of a common measuring tape (or sometimes called a tape measure) that is a flexible type of a ruler. Use a measuring tape to determine the circumference of the waist by measuring at or around the navel (medically known as the umbilicus), and commonly called the belly button.

The waist is usually measured at the smallest circumference of the waist. For people of normal weight, the waist is usually just above the navel. This horizontal circle where the waist is the narrowest is generally called the waistline. However, for women who are pregnant or men and women who are overweight or obese, the waist is usually measured one inch vertically above the navel.

KEY TERMS

Cardiovascular—Relating to the heart and blood vessels.

Cholesterol—A steroid alcohol sterol made by the liver, with the formula $C_{27}H_{45}OH$.

Diabetes—Medically called diabetes mellitus, a medical condition that causes the body to produce excessive amounts of urine.

Glucose—A simple sugar with formula $C_6H_{12}O_6$.

HDL cholesterol—High-density lipoprotein cholesterol, commonly called "good" cholesterol.

Hypertension—Another name for high blood pressure.

Kidneys—A pair or organs in the abdomen of vertebrates (such as humans) that filter waste bodily liquids.

LDL cholesterol—Low-density lipoprotein cholesterol, commonly called "bad" cholesterol.

Obesity—Being excessively overweight.

In other words, the National, Heart, Lung and Blood Institute (NHLBI) states: "To correctly measure your waist, stand and place a tape measure around your middle, just above your hipbones. Measure your waist just after you breathe out."

The value found by the waist circumference figure is an important measure for determining obesity-related diseases such as heart disease and diabetes. It has been medically found that people with excessive weight around their waist are at greater risk for such diseases.

Waist-to-hip Ratio

The hip, medically called the coax, is the anatomical region on each side of the human body, being located between the waist and the thigh. Further, the hip is the projection of the pelvis and the upper thighbone on each side of the human body. The waist-to-hip ratio (WHR), or sometimes called the waist-hip ratio, is the ratio of the circumference of the waist to that of the hips. In other words, WHR is equal to the waist circumference (W) divided by the hip circumference (H), where $WHR = W/H$. As such, WHR measures the proportion by which fat is distributed around the central part of the human body (generally called the trunk or torso).

Under most circumstances, the circumference of the waist is measured at the smallest circumference of the waist just above the navel. The circumference of the hip is usually measured at the widest part of the hip. As with the waist circumference measurement, the hip circumference is also determined with a tape measure.

For instance, a woman may state that her measurements are 36-29-38. This group of three dimensions means this particular woman has a circumference around her bust—a measurement of the upper rib cage and the breasts—of 36 in (approximately 91.4 cm), a

circumference around her waist of 29 in (approximately 73.7 cm), and a circumference around her hips of 38 in (approximately 96.5 cm). Therefore, in the case of this women, her waist-to-hip ratio is 29 inches divided by 38 inches, or $WHR = W/H$, equaling approximately 0.76.

Preparation

It is best to use a tape measure that is intended for tailoring or dressmaking. These tapes are made from flexible cloth, plastic, or fiberglass. The tape is marked with numbers representing inches and/or centimeters—beginning at zero and ending at a particular positive number (that is, the length of the tape). For measuring waist circumference and waist-to-hip ratio, the tape should be snuggly wrapped around the portion of the torso that is desired to be measured, in this case, the circumference of the waist or hip. When wrapped around the body in a snug manner, the beginning of the tape (the zero mark) will align with one of the larger markings on the tape. This particular marking is the circumference being measured. For instance, in the case of the woman's waist in the before-mentioned example, the tape will show 29 inches for her waist circumference.

Risks

Waist circumference

The waist circumference measurement is used as an indicator of possible health risks associated with being overweight or obese. As such, it indicates the increased risk of more serious medical problems such as type 2 diabetes, kidney disease, and cardiovascular disease. If more fat is distributed around the waist rather than around the hips, then a person is at higher risk for these obesity-related medical conditions than if less fat was around the waist when compared to the hips.

The National, Heart, Lung and Blood Institute (NHLBI) states that if men have a waist circumference that is greater than 40 in (102 cm) and women have a waist circumference greater than 35 in (88 cm), then they are classified as having increased risk for obesity-related diseases.

Waist-to-hip Ratio

The WHR is used as an indicator of being overweight or obese in people and, as such, is an indication of health risk because being overweight or obese has been shown to lead to more serious health-related problems such as diabetes, kidney disease, and cardiovascular disease.

A waist-to-hip ratio of 0.7 or less for women and a WHR of 0.9 or less for men is generally considered to be healthy. These values may vary depending on the health organization, but for the most part provides a good guide for maintaining a healthy lifestyle. For instance, the National Institute of Diabetes, Digestive and Kidney Diseases (NIDDK) state that women with a WHR of greater than 0.8 and men with a WHR of greater than 1.0 are at increased health risk. On the other hand, the Centers for Disease Control and Prevention (CDC) states that women with a WHR of over 0.8 and men with a WHR of over 0.9 are at increased health risk.

Additional risks

When a person is overweight or obese, then they are at greater risk for heart disease and many other conditions than a person of normal weight. Other factors can increase that risk even more. These factors, according to the NHLBI, include:

• high blood pressure (hypertension)
• high LDL cholesterol ("bad" cholesterol)
• low HDL cholesterol ("good" cholesterol)
• high triglycerides
• high blood glucose (sugar)
• family history of premature heart disease
• physical inactivity
• cigarette smoking

Results

Generally, to maintain a healthy lifestyle keep one's waist-to-hip ratio at a level of 0.7 or less for women and 0.9 or less for men, and one's waist circumference at less than 40 in (102 cm) for men and less than 35 in (88 cm) for women. The primary way for achieving and maintaining a healthy body weight is a lifelong commitment to sensible eating habits and

---

QUESTIONS TO ASK YOUR DOCTOR

• What do my waist circumference and waist-to-hip ratio mean for my general health condition?
• What lifestyle changes should I implement to improve my two measurements?
• Am I not physically fit if these two figures are too high?
• Am I at risk for medical conditions such as heart disease with these measurements?
• What can I do to lower my numbers?
• What types of foods should I avoid? Which ones do you recommend?

---

regular **exercise**. The NHLBI state that even a small weight loss—as small as 5–10% percent of one's current weight—will help lower an individual's risk of developing obesity-related diseases.

Resources

BOOKS

Adolfsson, Birgitta, and Marilynn S. Arnold. *Behavioral Approaches to Treating Obesity*. Alexandria, VA: American Diabetes Association, 2006.

Apovian, Caroline M., and Carine M. Lenders, editors. *Clinical Guide for Management of Overweight and Obese Children and Adults*. Boca Raton, FL: Taylor and Francis, 2006.

Duyff, Roberta Larson. *ADA Complete Food and Nutrition Guide*, 3rd ed. Chicago: American Dietetic Association, 2006.

Finkelstein, Eric A., and Laurie Zuckerman. *The Fattening of America: How the Economy Makes Us Fat, If It Matters, and What To Do About It*. New York: John Wiley & Sons, 2008.

Flamenbaum, Richard K., editor. *Childhood Obesity and Health Research*. New York: Nova Science Publishers, 2006.

Hassink, Sandra Gibson. *Guide to Pediatric Weight Management and Obesity*. Philadelphia: Lippincott Williams and Wilkins, 2007.

WEBSITES

Assessing Your Weight and Health Risk. National Heart, Lung and Blood Institute. http://www.nhlbi.nih.gov/health/public/heart/obesity/lose_wt/risk.htm (accessed September 29, 2011).

Body Measurements. Centers for Disease Control and Prevention. http://www.cdc.gov/nchs/fastats/bodymeas.htm (accessed September 29, 2011).

Childhood Obesity. Centers for Disease Control and Prevention. (September 15, 2011). http://www.cdc.gov/healthyyouth/obesity/ (accessed September 29, 2011).

Choose My Plate. U.S. Department of Agriculture.(September 27, 2011). http://www.choosemyplate.gov/ (accessed September 29, 2011).

Dietary Guidelines for Americans, 2010. Health.gov, U.S. Department of Health & Human Services. (September 29, 2011). http://www.health.gov/dietaryguidelines/ 2010.asp (accessed September 29, 2011).

Excess Fat Around the Waist May Increase Death Risk For Women. National Institute of Diabetes and Digestive and Kidney Diseases, National Institutes of Health. (April 7, 2008). http://www.nih.gov/news/health/ apr2008/niddk-07.htm (accessed September 29, 2011).

Fact Check: The Cost of Obesity. CNN Health. (February 9, 2010). http://www.cnn.com/2010/HEALTH/02/09/fact. check.obesity/index.html (accessed September 29, 2011).

ORGANIZATIONS

American Alliance for Health, Physical Education, Recreation and Dance, 1900 Association Drive, Reston, VA, 20191-1598, (703) 476-3400, (800) 213-7193, http:// www.aahperd.org/.

American Council on Exercise, 4851 Paramount Drive, San Diego, CA, 92123, (888) 825-3636, support@acefitness. org, http://www.fitness.gov/.

Centers for Disease Control and Prevention, 1600 Clifton Road, Atlanta, GA, 30333, (800) 232-4636, odcinfo@ cdc.gov, http://www.cdc.gov.

National Coalition for Promoting Physical Activity, 1100 H Street, N.W., Suite 510, Washington, DC, 20005, (202) 454-7521, Fax: (202) 454-7598, http://www.ncppa.org/ membership/organizations/.

National Heart, Lung, and Blood Institute, NHLBI Health Information Center, P.O. Box 30105, Bethesda, MD, 20824-0105, (301) 592-8573, Fax: (240) 629-3246, nhlbiinfo@nhlbi.nih.gov, http://www.nhlbi.nih.gov.

The Obesity Society, 8758 Georgia Avenue, Suite 1320, Silver Spring, MD, 20910, (301) 563-6526, Fax: (301) 563-6595, http://www.obesity.org.

President's Council on Fitness, Sports and Nutrition, 1101 Wootton Parkway, Suite 560, Rockville, MD, 20852, (240) 276-9567, Fax: (240) 276-9860, http://www.fitness. gov/.

William A. Atkins, BB, BS, MBA

Waist-to-hip ratio *see* **Waist circumference and waist-to-hip ratio**

Walking

Definition

Walking is a low-impact, aerobic activity that can improve heart health, aid in weight-loss, improve mood, and aid in increasing overall health and well-being.

Purpose

The United States Centers for Disease Control and Prevention (CDC) recommends that adults get two hours and 30 minutes of moderate intensity **exercise** every week. This is equivalent to 30 minutes of moderate intensity exercise five days a week. Brisk walking is considered a moderate intensity activity.

Walking is an excellent low-impact, low-cost aerobic activity that can be done by nearly everyone. It is a good way to get the recommended amount of exercise and does not require any special equipment except for a pair of comfortable walking shoes. Walking is recommended as a way to improve health and well-being for all **age** groups and fitness levels.

Description

To start walking, all that is required is a comfortable pair of shoes and 10 minutes. A short walk to the mailbox or around the block during a lunch break can be the first step to better health through walking. Starting to walk for fitness does not require much of a time commitment, and can be fit into even the busiest of schedules.

For individuals who are not at all active, walking should begin slowly and be done for short amounts of time. Walking for 10 minutes at a time just three times a day every day of the workweek can fulfill the CDC recommendations for exercise and have a noticeable impact on health and overall wellness.

For a moderate intensity work-out, walking should be done at a fast enough speed that breathing rate and body temperature are increased but not so fast as to make it difficult to talk or carry on a conversation. As a general rule, if an individual cannot talk easily, the exercise is too vigorous, and if the individual can sing a song the exercise is not vigorous enough.

Wearing a **pedometer** (a device that counts steps) can be a good way to set goals and monitor progress. Wearing one for a few days can provide a good base-line estimate of how active an individual is. Setting a goal of adding a few hundred steps is an easy way to start improving health. Increasing the goal every week or two helps increase health benefits a little bit at a time.

Sometimes staying motivated to exercise can be difficult. Below are some tips for how to stay motivated to keep walking.

• Invite friends or family members to walk. Conversation with loved ones while walking can make the time pass more quickly and add fun to exercise. Also, scheduling a regular time to meet and walk can make staying on track easier because it makes the

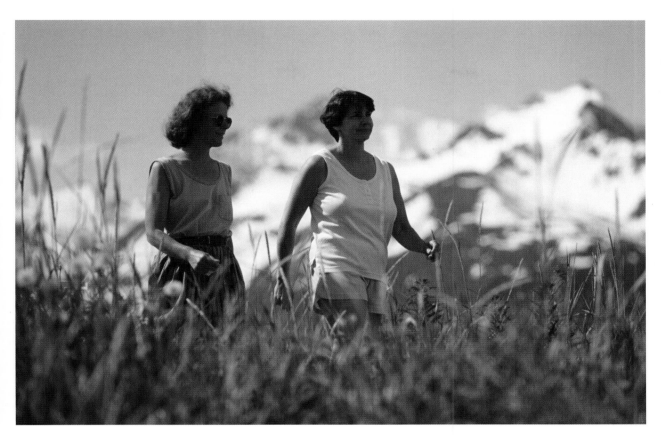

Two women take a walk. (© Bob Rowan/Corbis)

individual is accountable to someone other than him or herself.

- Explore new places. Most towns have a lot of good places to walk. Trying different routes or exploring new parts of town can make walking more interesting and reduce the boredom that can come with repetition.

- Walk to do errands. It often takes only a few more minutes to walk down to the corner store or over to a neighbor's house than it does to drive there. Substituting walking for driving, even once a day, can make a big difference over time.

- Walk as a break. Instead of snacking, or watching television, take a quick walk around the block as a break from work or chores. It is healthier and will help to increase energy levels.

Benefits

Walking has a variety of health and wellness benefits. Regular walking can help strengthen the heart and improve heart health. It also has been found to lower **blood pressure**. Walking also lowers the level of low-density lipoprotein (LDL) **cholesterol**. This is the type of cholesterol that is often called "bad" cholesterol. LDL cholesterol can build up on the artery walls to form plaque and restrict blood flow. Walking not only can decrease LDL cholesterol, it has also been found to increase high-density lipoprotein (HDL) cholesterol, the "good" cholesterol. HDL has been found to prevent heart attack by transporting LDL cholesterol away from the arteries to the liver, where it is processed for removal from the body.

Walking can also help with the management of chronic conditions, such as type 2 diabetes. For individuals who do not have type 2 diabetes, regular walking has been found to decrease the risk of its occurrence.

Regular walking also aids in weight loss and can help with weight maintenance once the desired weight has been achieved. Regular brisk walking also can lead to improved general mobility, and increased muscle tone.

One of the most important benefits of regular walking is improved mood. Having a better mood can lead to a more positive outlook on life and greater enjoyment of many activities.

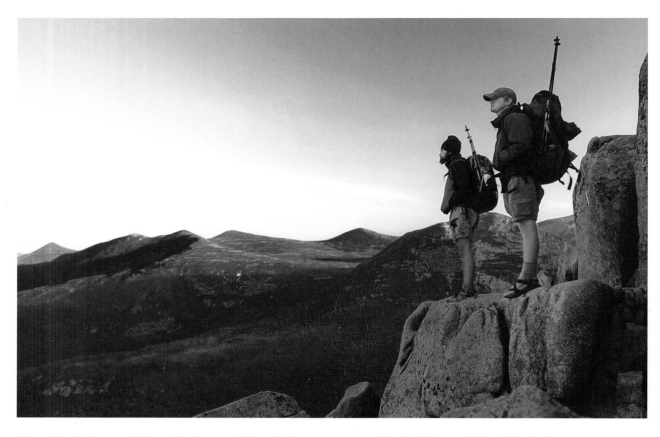

Hikers take in the mountainous landscape while enjoying a strenuous walk. *(© AP Images/Robert F. Bukaty)*

Precautions

Most people can begin walking for health and wellness without concern. However, people with a serious health condition should consult their doctor before beginning any exercise regime. If an individual has a very sedentary lifestyle, walking should be begun slowly and with short walks that gradually lengthen over time.

Preparation

Preparation for a short walk can be very simple. Before taking a 10-minute casual walk to the post office, simply ensuring that comfortable shoes and clothing appropriate for the weather are being worn generally is enough. For longer or more strenuous walks, however, some basic **warm-up** is appropriate.

Before beginning a long or strenuous walk a five-minute warm up walk is a good idea. It does not have to be outside; it can even be as simple as walking in place slowly for five minutes. This helps begin to increase the heart rate and warm and loosen the muscles. After five minutes of slow warm-up walking, about five minutes of gentle **stretching** generally is recommended. Stretching the muscles that will be used during walking such as the hamstrings and calves, helps to ensure that they remain flexible throughout the walk and reduces the risk of damage or strain.

Before beginning a long walk it is important to pick the route. If an individual is going to walk alone it is a good idea to leave a note, or otherwise inform someone else of the planned route. It is also always a good idea to bring along a cell-phone in case of emergencies.

Anyone walking at night should wear reflective clothing to ensure that cars, bikes, and other pedestrians can see them easily. For all walks, it is important to wear weather-appropriate clothing. It often is a good idea to dress in layers so that the amount of clothing can be adjusted as necessary during the walk. For long or strenuous walks it is also important to take a bottle of water to ensure good **hydration**.

Aftercare

After a long or vigorous walk, a cool-down period is recommended. This can consist of walking slowly

KEY TERMS

Low-density lipoprotein (LDL) cholesterol—Cholesterol that is often called "bad" cholesterol, it is the cholesterol that builds up on the artery walls to form plaque which can restrict blood flow and cause heart-attack and stroke.

High-density lipoprotein (HDL) cholesterol—The "good" cholesterol that transports unhealthy cholesterol away from the arteries to the liver that can process it for removal from the body.

Type 2 diabetes—formerly called adult-onset diabetes. In this form of diabetes, the pancreas either does not make enough insulin or cells become insulin resistant and do not use insulin efficiently.

QUESTIONS TO ASK YOUR DOCTOR

- Do I have any diseases or conditions that indicate it may be unsafe for me to walk for long distances or for me to walk briskly?
- What kind of shoes are right to help me walk comfortably?
- Do you have any suggestions for places in the local areas that are good for walking?
- What can I do to make my daily walking more effective?

for about five minutes. The cool-down period reduces strain on the body by allowing it to adjust slowly to a reduced level of exercise. After a five-minute **cool down**, stretching helps to keep the muscles limber and reduces the possibility of **muscle strain** and sprain. Gentle stretching of the muscles involved in walking, such as the hamstrings and calves is generally recommended.

Drinking water both during and after a long or vigorous walk is important to maintaining good hydration. Plain water is generally best for hydration, but flavored waters, low-fat or fat-free milk, or sugar-free juices also can be good choices. Unless the walk has been extremely long or very vigorous, sports drinks are not usually a good choice. They may contain more **calories** than were burned during the walk, and usually only extremely active people will benefit from them.

Risks

Walking is generally considered a low-impact activity that is unlikely to carry any serious risks. However, there are some possible negative outcomes that can occur, which are somewhat more likely with extremely vigorous walking.

Muscle strain or sprain is a possible risk of walking. This risk can be reduced by wearing appropriate walking shoes and warming up and stretching both before and after walking. Walking during daylight hours or in well-lit places can help reduce the risk of stepping incorrectly and injuring oneself on rough or uneven terrain. If an individual is just beginning walking for exercise or is less stable for any reason, finding a place to walk with even terrain is extremely important in reducing the risk of injury. Walking in indoor malls is often a good choice because malls have floors that are flat and even and are not made slippery by rain, wet leaves, snow, or ice.

Anyone who has a serious health condition may be at risk of increased health problems if beginning a new walking program. People with serious health problems should talk to their doctor about possible risks of walking for exercise. The doctor can help to determine what level of exercise is appropriate. Although walking is generally recommended for every individual who is able, even people who are in **cardiac rehabilitation** units of hospitals, this does not mean that it is risk-free. Walking in crowded areas or walking under the supervision of a physical therapist or other health professional can improve the chance of getting help immediately in the case of a heart attack, stroke, or other adverse health event. Starting slowly and walking for only a few minutes at a time, then building up both speed and duration slowly can help reduce the risk of problems, even in those with serious health conditions.

Resources

BOOKS

Kimkio. *Walking your Way to a Better Life*. New York: Vertical, 2009.

Nottingham, Suzanne, and Jurasin, Alexandra. *Nordic Walking for Total Fitness*. Champaign, IL: Human Kinetics, 2010.

Peters, Erika. *The Complete Idiot's Guide to Walking for Health*. Indianapolis, IN: Alpha, 2007.

PERIODICALS

Lee, I-Min, and Buchner, David M. "The Importance of Walking to Public Health." *Medicine and Science in Sports and Exercise,* (July 2008), 40 (7 Supplement): S512–8.

ORGANIZATIONS

American Heart Association, 7272 Greenville Avenue, Dallas, TX, 75231, (800) 242-8721, http://www.americanheart.org.

American Nordic Walking Association, PO Box 491205, Los Angeles, CA, 90049, (323) 244-2519, Fax: (310) 459-8149, info@anwa.us, http://www.anwa.us.

American Volkssport Association, 1001 Pat Booker Road, Suite 101, Universal City, TX, 78148, (210) 659-2112, Fax: (210) 659-1212, avahq@ava.org, http://www.ava.org.

Tish S. Davidson, AM

Warm-up and cool down

Definition

A warm-up and a cool down are slower-paced, reduced-intensity movements that precede and follow exercise, respectively. A warm-up builds gradually toward the pace and intensity of the exercise. A cool down, also called a warm-down, gradually returns the body to its resting state. Both the warm-up and cool down place special emphasis on the muscle groups worked during the exercise session.

Purpose

A warm-up helps prepare the body and mind for more intense exercise. Its primary purpose is to gradually raise the heart and respiratory rates, increasing the activity of the cardiorespiratory system and oxygen and nutrient delivery to the muscles that will be worked during exercise. The warm-up raises core body temperature, as well as muscle temperature. Raising core temperature increases joint mobility, enabling better movement and range of motion, and may reduce the risk of injury. Warmer muscles are more flexible than cool muscles.

Although the purported benefits of a warm-up are based on common sense and experience as well as on scientific evidence, many experts believe that it is very important to warm up before any physical activity. Some athletes advise shortening workout time rather than skipping the warm-up. Some evidence indicates that a warm-up can boost the contractile responses of muscles, through a process called post-activation potentiation (PAP), in which short spurts of strenuous physical activity trigger a biochemical change in muscle. Warming up joints and muscles before any exercise that requires a full range of motion, such as ballet, appears to be especially important. Some running experts believe that warming up, in addition to stretching leg and calf muscles before and after running, can help prevent Achilles tendinitis, a painful inflammation of the Achilles tendon. Some fitness professionals also believe that a warm-up enables one to exercise longer and to burn more calories. Finally, a warm-up can provide a means for gradually building up new skills.

In the past, warm-ups generally involved static or stationary stretching to try to elongate muscles. Some experts still suggest stretching before certain activities—such as shoveling snow—that use muscles not often worked and can be easily strained. These include the muscles between the shoulders and in the upper and lower back, as well as the buttocks and legs. However, it is now generally recognized that stretching should never be performed until muscle temperature has been raised by a warm-up.

A cool down following a workout enables the heart and breathing rates and muscle temperature to gradually return to normal. This is particularly important after intensive exercise. Abruptly halting strenuous cardiorespiratory exercise without a cool down can cause blood that is concentrated in working muscles to pool in the veins, possibly resulting in dizziness or lightheadedness. A cool down also may help the body recover more quickly from intense exercise. Cool downs may be most important for well-conditioned athletes because they help to regulate blood flow. For casual exercisers, a cool down may simply be an enjoyable way to conclude an exercise routine.

Stretching as part of a cool down can relax the mind as well as the muscles. Stretching may help lengthen muscles that have been shortened during exercise such as running, returning the muscles to their resting length. Stretching during a cool down also may increase flexibility and help prevent stiffness.

Demographics

Most exercise regimens include a warm-up and cool down, with or without stretching. Most athletes believe warm-ups and cool downs to be very important and most trainers and coaches insist on them. However workouts, training, and athletic competitions are not the only activities that may require a warm-up and cool down. Any activity, such as yard work or gardening, may benefit, especially activities that involve cramped positions, such as sledding. Automobile and airplane travel can be treated to a warm-up prior to settling in and a cool down, such as a brisk walk to stretch calf and hamstring muscles, after arrival.

Description

Warm-up

There are many different warm-up activities, but the most common is simply performing the primary conditioning activity at a slower pace:

- a slow walk or stroll before a brisk walk or jog
- a brisk walk or light jog before a run, gradually speeding up to one's normal running pace
- swimming slowly for a few laps before gradually picking up speed
- pedaling a bike slowly with no resistance
- moving joints and muscles through appropriate movement patterns before picking up weights for strength training
- slow, sport-specific drills

Warm-ups often focus first on large muscle groups, such as the hamstrings, followed by exercise that is more specific to the activity. Sport-specific warm-up drills often involve extending range of motion and establishing correct rhythm and timing. For example, a running warm-up might include a heel-toe drill to warm up the muscles of the feet, ankles, and calves, while slowly moving the arms. This might be followed by double ankle bounces to continuing warming up the lower legs, adding impact and speed, and raising the arms overhead to warm up the body core. Heel flicks for the front and back of the thighs can improve knee and hip range of motion and begin setting timing and rhythm. Finally, high knees improve hip range of motion, increase stride, begin the use of running arms.

Warm-ups commonly last for five to ten minutes; in general, the more intense and demanding the workout, the longer the warm-up. Strenuous activities may require warm-ups of up to 15–20 minutes. People who are just starting to exercise also may require longer warm-ups. Competitive athletes who, in addition to raising heart rate and body temperature, use warm-ups to condition neuromuscular pathways to increase the speed and efficiency of muscular contraction, may warm up for much longer. For example, sprinters sometimes spend an hour or more warming up. Heavier breathing and very mild sweating usually indicate a sufficient warm-up. However warm-ups should never be tiring.

Warm-ups for **youth sports** generally last 15–30 minutes. They often begin with a brisk walk, running in place, or a slow jog, followed by a sport-specific warm-up and possibly gradual stretching of major muscle groups. It is very important that children receive instruction as to appropriate exercises for their sport.

A warm-up may conclude with gentle dynamic stretching to loosen muscles and joints, increase flexibility and range of motion, and help prevent injury. Proper stretching can also contribute to correct exercise posture and better coordination. The muscle groups to be worked should be gently flexed and extended. Static stretching is not recommended during a warm-up; however dynamic mobility exercises—such as hip circles, lunges, knee lifts, and leg swings—may be beneficial if they are performed in a gentle and controlled manner. Gentle stretching may be particularly beneficial for a tight or previously injured muscle. Movements should never be jerky, bouncy, or painful. Standing stretches are preferable to floor stretches at the end of a warm-up, to keep the heart rate elevated.

Cool down

The cool down from cardiorespiratory exercise is similar to the warm-up. Although it can include a variety of activities, the cool down most often involves continuing the exercise activity while gradually slowing the pace and reducing the intensity:

- walking without moving the arms after a brisk walk or jog
- jogging, then walking briskly following a run
- swimming leisurely laps using various strokes
- pedaling with reduced resistance or spinning bike pedals at about 100 revolutions per minute

As with the warm-up, the duration of a cool down depends on the intensity and duration of the exercise. Strenuous workouts require longer cool downs than more leisurely activity. In general, cool downs should return the body to its resting state over five–ten minutes, with heart and breathing rate gradually returning to normal.

Stretching the worked muscles for a few minutes at the end of a cool down—while they are still warm—may be beneficial. In addition to repeating stretches performed with the warm-up, floor stretches can focus on the muscles that were worked during exercise and those that feel especially tight. Just as there are sport-specific warm-ups, there are sport-specific stretches that focus on the particular muscles used in that sport—for example, the shoulder for throwing a **baseball** or the forearm for batting. Stretches should be performed slowly and gently, just to the point of a slight pull. They should never cause pain. Stretching may include the:

- calf or back of the lower leg and Achilles tendon
- quadriceps (quads) on the front of the thigh
- hamstrings on back of the thigh
- hip flexors or front of the hip

KEY TERMS

Achilles tendinitis—Inflammation of the Achilles tendon—the strong tendon connecting the calf muscles to the heel bone.

Cardiorespiratory—Cardio; aerobic; the delivery of oxygen by the heart, lungs, and blood to large working muscle groups, and the utilization of oxygen by those muscles.

Dynamic stretching—Stretching that involves smooth, gentle movements.

Glutes, glutei—The three muscles of each buttock, especially the outermost gluteus maximus that extends and laterally rotates the thigh.

Hamstrings—The three muscles at the back of the thigh.

Hip flexors—The group of muscles that flex the thigh bone toward the pelvis to pull the knee up.

Post-activation potentiation; PAP—An exercise process that triggers a biochemical change in muscle to maximize muscle performance.

Quads; quadriceps—The large extensor muscle of the front of the thigh that is divided into four parts that join in a single tendon at the knee.

Static stretching—Sustained stretching of muscles without movement.

Triceps—The muscle of the back of the arm.

- glutei (glutes) or buttocks
- lower back
- triceps with an overhead stretch

Preparation

A warm-up prepares the body and mind for exercise. Although various sports and other physical activities have specially designed warm-ups, many people find that they can warm-up and cool down adequately with simple activities, such as **walking** to and from the gym or other exercise facility.

Risks

A warm-up should precede any strenuous activity, not just exercise or sports. Manual labor or lifting significant weight without first warming up can be dangerous. Although there is conflicting evidence about the benefits of a warm-up and cool down, when correctly performed they pose little risk and may help prevent **muscle strain** or injury. However some fitness programs neglect to include a warm-up and cool down before and after strenuous exercise.

Warm-ups that are too taxing can interfere with performance. A 2011 study of highly trained track cyclists found that shorter, lower-intensity warm-ups produced less muscle **fatigue**, increased muscle contractile response as determined by PAP, and improved performance compared with traditional longer warm-ups. However these results were for competitive athletes and they may be sport-specific. Nevertheless, the suggestion is that warm-ups should include just enough activity to promote PAP without causing fatigue.

Stretching as part of a warm-up or cool down entails some risks. Stretching cold muscles can contribute to pulled or torn muscles. Sudden or aggressive stretching can cause injury or worsen an injury. Lengthening tissues by stretching can cause lax muscles, joints, and ligaments that are more susceptible to injury. Although static stretching, if performed correctly, may be beneficial during a cool down, during a warm-up, static stretching relaxes, rather than warms, the central nervous system, and does not significantly raise core body temperature, both of which are required for coordinated muscular contraction. Muscles should be stretched gradually during the cool down. Stretching should never involve force, bobbing, or bouncing that can damage muscle and even lead to scar tissue formation that inhibits flexibility. Static stretches should be held for 10–30 seconds to sufficiently lengthen muscle. Both sides of the body should be stretched equally. Stretches should never be taken to the point of pain. Breathing is as important during stretching as during all other phases of a workout.

Results

When performed correctly, a warm-up and cool down may help reduce the risk of injury, especially strains, sprains, and overuse injuries, and may improve athletic performance. A warm-up also activates the nervous system, possibly improving neuromuscular responses and coordination. A cool down relaxes and loosens muscles that have been tightened during exercise and may help prevent cramping, muscle spasms, or stiff or sore muscles.

Research and general acceptance

The effects of a warm-up and cool down on exercise and athletic performance are active areas of research. However the results often appear to depend on individual fitness and the particular exercise or sport. Research tends to support the premise that athletes can reach metabolic steady state faster and perform better after an active warm-up, compared with a passive warm-up. One study found that there were greater differences in **energy** supply, muscle strength, and performance after an active versus a passive warm-up than between either type of warm-up and no warm-up at all. A British study found that youth **football** players who were in high compliance with a comprehensive injury-preventing warm-up program had a significantly lower risk of injury than players who were in intermediate compliance with the program. Thus, most experts continue to recommend a warm-up and cool down before and after exercise.

Resources

BOOKS

Al-Masri, Lilah, and Simon Bartlett. *100 Questions & Answers About Sports Nutrition and Exercise.* Sudbury, MA: Jones and Bartlett, 2011.

Brandon, Leigh. *Anatomy for Strength and Fitness Training for Speed: An Illustrated Guide to Your Muscles in Action.* New York: McGraw-Hill, 2010.

Colbert, Don, and Kyle Colbert. *Get Fit and Live!* Lake Mary, FL: Siloam, 2010.

Kennedy, Carol A., and Mary M. Yoke. *Methods of Group Exercise Instruction.* 2nd ed. Champaign, IL: Human Kinetics, 2009.

Murphy, Sam, and Sarah Connors. *Running Well.* Champaign, IL: Human Kinetics, 2009.

Page, Portia. *Pilates Illustrated.* Champaign, IL: 2011.

Sandler, David. *Fundamental Weight Training.* Champaign, IL: Human Kinetics, 2010.

Shaw, Beth. *Beth Shaw's Yogafit.* 2nd ed. Champaign, IL: Human Kinetics, 2009.

Ungaro, Alycea. *Pilates Practice Companion.* New York: DK, 2011.

Welsh, Tom. *Conditioning for Dancers.* Gainesville, FL: University of Florida Press, 2009.

PERIODICALS

Ajemian, Robert, et al. "Why Professional Athletes Need a Prolonged Period of Warm-Up and Other Peculiarities of Human Motor Learning." *Motor Behavior* 42, no. 6 (November/December 2010): 381–88.

Brunner-Ziegler, Sophie, Barbara Strasser, and Paul Haber. "Comparison of Metabolic and Biomechanic Responses to Active vs. Passive Warm-Up Procedures Before Physical Exercise." *Journal of Strength and Conditioning Research* 25, no. 4 (April 2011): 909–14.

Fitzgerald, Rob. "Warm Up to a New Idea." *Joe Weider's Muscle & Fitness* 71, no. 11 (2010): 66–73.

"The Lowdown on Warm-Ups and Cool-Down." *University of California, Berkeley, Wellness Letter* 27, no. 4 (January 2011): 6.

WEBSITES

Dallas, Mary Elizabeth. "Athletes May Benefit From Shorter, Less Intense Warm-Ups." *HealthDay.* June 24, 2011. http://www.nlm.nih.gov/medlineplus/news/fullstory_113616.html (accessed July 27, 2011).

Malcolm, Christian, and Steph Twell. "Before You Begin...and After You've Finished." *Guardian.* January 10, 2009. http://www.guardian.co.uk/lifeandstyle/2009/jan/10/running-warm-up-warm-down (accessed July 27, 2011).

Mayo Clinic Staff. "Aerobic Exercise: How to Warm Up and Cool Down." Mayo Clinic. February 26, 2011. http://www.mayoclinic.com/health/exercise/SM00067 (accessed July 27, 2011).

Soligard, Torbjørn, et al. "Compliance with a Comprehensive Warm-Up Programme to Prevent Injuries in Youth Football." *British Journal of Sports Medicine* 44, no. 11 (September 2010): 787–93. http://bjsm.bmj.com/content/44/11/787.full (accessed July 28, 2011).

"Stretching." TeensHealth. April 2009. http://kidshealth.org/teen/food_fitness/exercise/stretching.html# (accessed July 27, 2011).

"Warm Up, Cool Down and Be Flexible." American Academy of Orthopaedic Surgeons. http://orthoinfo.aaos.org/topic.cfm?topic=A00310 (accessed July 27, 2011).

ORGANIZATIONS

American Academy of Orthopaedic Surgeons, 6300 North River Road, Rosemont, IL, 60018-4262, (847) 823-7186, Fax: (847) 823-8125, orthoinfo@aaos.org, http://www.aaos.org.

American Chiropractic Association, 1701 Clarendon Boulevard, Arlington, VA, 22209, (703) 276-8800, Fax: (703) 243-2593, memberinfo@acatoday.org, http://www.acatoday.org.

Margaret Alic, PhD

Water exercise

Definition

Water **exercise** is a type of activity that is done in a body of water, such as a pool, a lake, or the ocean. Sometimes, limited water exercise can be done in a spa or hot tub.

Purpose

The purpose of water exercise is to put the body through activity without adding extra stress and strain on the joints. Though people have been **swimming** and playing water polo for a long time, water exercise grew out of therapeutic exercise for people recovering from injury or conditions such as **bursitis** and sciatica. Water exercise also is used for **arthritis** patients.

Demographics

Anyone can participate in water exercise. Swimming is considered an activity that spans all generations, from infants to octogenarians. Water aerobics, water **walking**, and water **yoga** and **t'ai chi** are most often activities that older adults enjoy. Young people

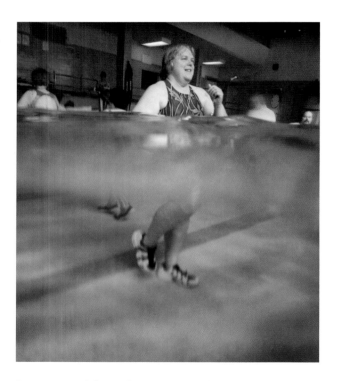

A woman participates in a water aerobics class.
(© AP Images/Scott Anderson)

who have had joint or back injuries may participate for a short time as a rehabilitation activity. Water jogging has become an exercise that even athletes are engaging in because it offers a superior workout with little risk of injury.

History

Water activities have been around since recorded history and the advent of swimming. Water exercise classes began in the 1950s and became very popular with formal water aerobics class offerings in the 1970s and 1980s.

Water aerobics classes have been offered at pools in the United States for more than 50 years. Water exercise has progressed to other varieties such as water ballet and various forms of water yoga. These types of exercise in the water have been popularized and targeted as forms of gentle **stretching** and motion exercise for muscles and joints.

Description

Exercise in the water is a low-impact activity that puts less stress on the joints. When the entire body is underwater, it experiences almost zero gravity since the water carries 90% of the body's weight. This buoyancy helps older adults by improving their balance and strength.

Water also offers resistance. It has 12–14% more resistance than air. This gentle friction aids in strengthening muscles and joints, especially for those recovering from an injury. Resistance can be increased by wearing wrist or ankle weights in shallow water to offer a more challenging workout.

Like land-based exercise, water exercise can increase cardiovascular fitness, lower **blood pressure** and **cholesterol** levels, and increase **energy**. It can also help people lose body fat. Exercising in the water can improve depression, anxiety, and self-esteem. It enhances flexibility, strengthens muscles, and improves circulation. Moreover, the hydrostatic pressure of the water helps increase heart and lung function. It also can encourage better blood flow to the muscles, especially the legs, much like support hosiery does.

Some activities in the water are done by individuals, such as swimming, water jogging, and water walking. Other activities can be done in a group. Those include water polo, water aerobics, water yoga, water t'ai chi, and water **pilates**. All of these individual and group activities, except swimming, do not require skill in the water.

KEY TERMS

Aerobics—Synchronized movements to strengthen muscles while exercising the heart and lungs.

Hydrostatic pressure—The pressure of the water against the body.

Pilates—A form of exercise that combines yoga, dance, and isometric exercises.

T'ai chi—Based on an ancient form of Chinese martial arts, this form of exercise is a series of slow movements that improve balance and strength and also calms the mind.

Water polo—A game played in the water with two teams trying to get a large ball through a hoop on each side of the pool.

Yoga—An ancient form of exercise that strengthens the spine and the muscles of the body while it calms the mind.

Water jogging is a deep-water workout that is done in water over the jogger's head. In order to stay afloat and keep the body upright, joggers wear a buoyancy belt with special floats that keep the person's feet off the bottom of the pool or lake and keep the head above the surface of the water. Water jogging can offer a very intense workout as the jogger does jumping jacks or moves the legs in movements that mimic jogging, cycling, or cross-country skiing on land. These activities place added demand on the heart and lungs, as well as on the jogger's ability to keep his or her balance.

Water exercise is often suggested for people who are obese. It puts less stress on the joints and it fosters more active participation because participants find exercising in water is easier to do. A 2005 study showed that exercising in water to lose weight should be done in warm water, not cold water. The researchers found that participants ate more after exercising in cold water than they did after exercising in warm water.

People who have arthritis often find exercising in warm water easier to do than on land. The warm water soothes stiff joints and muscles and helps people **warm-up** before activity. Warm water raises body temperature, causing the blood vessels to dilate, thus increasing circulation. Water exercises for these patients can help knees, hips, shoulders, elbows, and even ankles and hands. Whatever body part is affected should be submerged in water, and all movements should be done slowly.

People with osteoarthritis often can exercise at higher intensities than they could on a mat on land. A study in 2003 found that not only were osteoarthritis patients who exercised in water able to improve their walking ability on land, but they also increased their independence.

Some people use a spa or hot tub as an adjunct to water exercise. The jet nozzles massage the body and help relax tight muscles. The size of the hot tub will determine what kinds of exercises can be done. If the feet or hands are of concern, then a smaller sized spa can help work these smaller joints and muscles. Obviously, a small spa would not allow for aerobic activities that work the larger muscles and joints. Time in a hot tub should be limited to 10 minutes, and temperatures should not exceed 98–104°F (37–40°C).

Preparation

Before starting any exercise program, older adults should check with their doctors and explain the types of activities they want to do. It is important when starting a new exercise regime to begin slowly and build up gradually. Older adults should go to the pool three times a week and start by doing a few repetitions or a couple of laps, if swimming. Gradually, the person can increase swimming time to 20 or 30 minutes or exercise to 45 minutes.

Equipment

Little is needed in order to participate in water exercise besides swimwear. Some people may want to wear a swimming cap or goggles, but usually those are worn by people who swim laps or engage in water polo. Some swimmers may want to use swim fins or a kickboard.

Training and conditioning

Water exercise is a low-impact activity, however, if done vigorously, it may be a relatively high-intensity activity using multiple muscle groups, and raising the heart and respiratory rate. As such, individuals should begin their exercise regimen slowly and progress toward longer periods of exercise and intensity, while improving cardiovascular fitness. A period of stretching and warm-up activity should be performed and an after-exercise cool down should be conducted at the end of the workout.

Risks

Because exercising in water is easier to do, sometimes beginners can do too much. It is important to

QUESTIONS TO ASK YOUR DOCTOR

- Is water exercise a good form of exercise for me?
- What kinds of water exercise do you recommend?
- How much water exercise should I do to stay fit and healthy?
- Should I combine water exercise with some other exercise? What other type of exercise do you recommend?
- What physical limitations if any, do you foresee?
- Do I need to see a physical therapist?
- Where can I find water exercise programs?

warm up prior to the more vigorous part of the exercise session and to **cool down** afterwards. Warm-ups should include stretches in the areas that will be exercised. Older adults should learn the difference between **muscle pain** and sore muscles. Muscle pain is more intense and lasts longer than a week. If that occurs, older adults should see their healthcare providers.

Most public or therapeutic pools keep water temperatures in the safe range, usually 84–88°F (29–31°C). Home indoor pools and spas should maintain the same temperature range. Spas are usually hotter so older adults should limit their time in hot water to a few minutes. They may be able to stay in a warm pool safely for far longer. In addition, older adults may not realize that the water is too hot.

For water aerobics or other structured activity, a qualified instructor is essential. If older adults have specific problems, such as arthritis, then the instructor should have some knowledge of the disease. The Arthritis Foundation Aquatic Program has qualified instructors who teach at YMCAs and community pools across the United States.

Older adults should never engage in water exercise without someone else near the pool. Most community pools, lakes, and beaches have lifeguards. Therapeutic pools have a therapist available to instruct in the proper exercise techniques. These pools also have pool attendants who keep track of people's time in the pool and are available in case of an emergency.

Results

People who participate in water exercise can expect to have better flexibility, stronger muscles, and improved circulation. Participants can also have lower cholesterol and blood pressure readings. Some people can lose weight using this method of exercise. Most importantly, older people who regularly participate in water exercise have less depression and improved self-esteem, as well as more independence as they gain confidence in a stronger body. Many people report fewer falls after engaging in regular water exercise.

Resources

BOOKS

Harper, Bob. *Are You Ready! Take Charge, Lose Weight, Get in Shape, and Change Your Life Forever*. New York: Broadway Books, 2009.

Hines, Emmett W. *Fitness Swimming*, 2nd ed. Champaign, IL: Human Kinetics, 2008.

Jendrick, Megan Quann, and Nathan Jendrick. *Get Wet, Get Fit: A Complete Guide to a Swimmer's Body*. New York: Fireside, 2008.

Manocchia, Pat. *Anatomy of Exercise: A Trainer's Inside Guide to Your Workout*. Richmond Hill, ONT: Firefly Books, 2009.

Prentice, William. *Get Fit, Stay Fit*, 6th ed. Boston: McGraw–Hill College, 2011.

Ratey, John J., and Eric Hagerman. *Spark: The Revolutionary New Science of Exercise and the Brain*. New York: Little, Brown, 2012.

Salo, Dale, and Scott A. Riewald. *Complete Conditioning for Swimming*. Champaign, IL: Human Kinetics, 2008.

Sheen, Barbara. *Keeping Fit*. Chicago: Heinemann Library, 2008.

Silver, J. K., and Christopher Morin. *Understanding Fitness: How Exercise Fuels Health and Fights Disease*. Westport, CT: Praeger, 2008.

PERIODICALS

Archer, Shirley. "T'ai Chi and Water Exercise Relieve Arthritis Pain." *IDEA Fitness Journal* (October 2007): 95.

"Exercise in Cold Water May Increase Appetite, University of Florida Study Finds." *Ascribe Science News Service* (May 4, 2005).

Mancini, Lee. "Swimming and Water Exercise." *Clinical Reference Systems* (May 31, 2007).

Sato, Daisuke; Kandeda, Koichi; Wakabayashi, Hitoshi; and Nomura, Takeo. "The Water Exercise Improves Health-related Quality of Life of Frail Elderly People at Day Service Facility." *Quality of Life Research*. (December 2007): 1577-1586.

ORGANIZATIONS

American Council on Exercise, 4851 Paramount Dr., San Diego, CA, 92123, (888) 825-3636, http://www.acefitness.org.

American Medical Association, 515 N. State St., Chicago, IL, 60610, (800) 621-8335, http://www.ama-assn.org.

American Physical Therapy Association, 1111 North
Fairfax St., Alexandria, VA, 22314-1488, (703)
684-APTA (2782), (800) 999-APTA (2782),
http://www.apta.org.

National Athletic Trainers' Association, 2952 Stemmons
Freeway, Dallas, TX, 75247-6916, (214) 637-6282,
Fax: (214) 637-2206, http://www.nata.org.

National Institute on Aging (NIA), 31 Center Dr., MSC
2292, Building 31, Room 5C27, Bethesda, MD, 20892,
(301) 496-1752, Fax: (301) 496-1072, http://www.nia.
nih.gov.

President's Council on Fitness, Sports & Nutrition, 1101
Wootton Parkway, Suite 560, Rockville, MD, 20852,
(240) 276-9567, http://fitness.gov.

United States Water Fitness Association, P.O. Box 243279,
Boynton Beach, FL, 33424-3279, (561) 732-9908,
Fax: (561) 732-0950, info@uswfa.org, http://www.
uswfa.com.

Janie F. Franz
Laura Jean Cataldo, RN, EdD

Water intoxication

Definition

It is often recommended that people drink eight
glasses of water each day. However, too much water
suddenly consumed can be dangerous. Excess water—
what is called water intoxication—is a serious and
potentially deadly disorder that occurs when an
abnormally high amount of water is consumed or
when electrolytes are not properly replenished, even
though water is consumed, during intense **exercise**.
Such situations can cause serious disturbances
in brain functions. Water intoxication is also commonly called water poisoning, **overhydration**, or
hyperhydation.

Description

When too much water is consumed, the kidneys
within the body are unable to properly process such
large amounts of water, salts, and other solutes. Consequently, an imbalance of electrolytes occurs. Electrolytes are any substance containing free ions that
makes it electrically conductive—either with an excess
(negative charge) or deficit (positive charge) of
electrons.

The primary electrolytes of the body are sodium
(Na^+), potassium (K^+), calcium (Ca^{2+}), magnesium
(Mg^{2+}), and chloride (Cl^-), along with hydrogen phosphate (HPO_4^{2-}) and hydrogen carbonate (HCO_3^-).

When an imbalance of electrolytes happens, the
kidneys process as much fluids as they can; however,
the excess fluids are forced into the blood, eventually entering the cells of the body. Then, the cells
within the body expand to accommodate the excessive fluids in the body. In essence, the cells become
waterlogged.

When too much water is consumed a lower concentration of electrolytes, especially sodium, are contained on the outside of cells than on the inside. To
correct this imbalance, fluid is moved inside the cells,
causing them to enlarge. At the same time, electrolytes are transferred from inside the cells to the outside, in order to balance their concentration. As this
occurs, more water is transfer inside the cell, again
trying to maintain a balance of electrolytes. Cells
outside of the brain continue this balancing act, swelling larger as more water enters. They are able to
stretch safely because they are contained within flexible tissues. The extra water does not adversely affect
them.

However, the neuron cells in the brain are not
able to swell safely because they are contained within
a rigid skull. Thus, adverse consequences occur
because as the cells swell in the brain, the brain itself
begins to swell, what is called brain edema. This condition leads to increased pressure on the brain, causing the first signs of a problem including headaches,
irritability, and drowsiness. As the problem grows,
further symptoms develop, including difficulties in
breathing, nausea, and vomiting. When a potentially
deadly state occurs, the brain is not receiving an
adequate amount of blood because the enlarged size
of the cells prevents its flow. Pressure to the brain
stem begins to cause the nervous system to fail, eventually leading to brain damage, respiratory arrest,
seizures, brain stem herniation, coma, and even
death.

Water intoxication can occur in athletes, especially when they exercise strenuously. A study published in the August 2004 issue of the *British Journal of
Sports Medicine* is entitled "The Dipsomania of Great
Distance: Water Intoxication in an Ironman Triathlete." The South African authors studied 371 athletes
after finishing the 140-mile (226-kilometer) South
African Ironman Triathlon. The most weight gained
during the competition was approximately 7.9 pounds
(3.6 kilograms). This athlete also developed signs of
hyponatraemia. During his recovery, the athlete
excreted 1.2 gallons (4.6 liters) of urine. The authors
stated, "This case report again confirms that sympto-
matic hyponatraemia is caused by considerable fluid
overload independent of appreciable NaCl [sodium

chloride, also called salt] losses. Hence, prevention of the condition requires that athletes be warned not to drink excessively large volumes of fluid (dipsomania) during very prolonged exercise. This case report also shows that there is a delayed diuresis in this condition and that it is not caused by renal failure."

Demographics

Healthy people normally do not get water intoxication when nutritionally balanced foods and drinks are consumed each day. However, when a situation occurs that involves water intoxication several groups of people are more at risk than are others. Water intoxication is most frequently found in infants six months of age or younger, and sometimes in athletes.

Infants and children with inflammation of the gastrointestinal tract, such as from influenza (flu), are at increased risk from water intoxication because a large electrolyte imbalance can quickly result when vomiting and diarrhea occurs. Infants under the age of one year are also at heightened risk when they have a lower than normal body mass because such a small weight makes it quite easy to take in a relatively large amount of water in a small amount of time.

Athletes that perform strenuous exercises, such as long distance runners, can be at increased risk from water intoxication if they drink too much water, such as while **running** in **marathon** races. Too much water in their systems can cause sodium levels to drop dangerously low. When such a situation occurs, the medical community calls it dilutional **hyponatremia**, or simply hyponatremia. The first symptoms under such cases can be serious, when runners collapse or display obvious signs of confusion.

Any person is at higher risk from water intoxication when conditions cause excess sweating during physical activities or exercising. This is partially because water alone will not replenish needed nutrients into the body. During and after these times, is it extremely important to drink and eat nutritious substances to maintain a balance of electrolytes in the body.

People with the mental condition called psychogenic polydispia are also at heightened risk of water intoxication. The disorder is characterized by a patient unable to stop drinking water due to a compulsion to drinking water or as a result from taking antipsychotic medications used to treat various other mental disorders.

KEY TERMS

Edema—Relating to excess fluids.

Electrolyte—Any ion in cells, blood, or other organic substance, whose purpose is to control fluid levels in the body.

Intoxication—Poisoning by ingestion of a drug, toxic substance, or other such material (such as water).

Intracranial—Within the skull.

Kidney—A pair of organs in the abdomen of vertebrates that filter wastes, which are then excreted as urine from the body.

Mole—A unit within the International System of Units (SI) that measures the amount of a chemical substance, equaling about 6.02214×10^{23} molecules of that substance.

Polydipsia—Extreme thirst.

Solute—A substance dissolved in another substance.

Causes and symptoms

Causes

Water intoxication occurs usually when someone drinks large amounts of water or when intense exercise has been completed and water was been drunk but without proper replenishment of electrolytes.

For athletes, hyponatremia, a type of water intoxication, can often occur. Hyponatremia is a condition in which an electrolyte imbalance occurs with the chemical element of sodium. Sodium concentration in the blood becomes lower than normal when excessive water being consumed. Specifically, it means that a blood sodium concentration becomes lower than 135 millimoles per liter, which is about 0.4 ounces per gallon. A normal concentration in the body is from about 135–145 millimoles per liter. Water intoxication is the result of severe cases of hyponatremia.

Symptoms

Initial symptoms of water intoxication include those that are similar to psychosis, including inappropriate behaviors, confusion, delusions, hallucinations, and disorientation. Associated symptoms include headache, **fatigue**, nausea, vomiting, and frequent urination. These symptoms can progress to acute delirium, seizures, coma, and even death.

Diagnosis

Water intoxication should be diagnosed as early as possible in order to counter its effects in the body. However, in many cases, due to incomplete research and understanding into water intoxication, the problem is not properly diagnosed in its early stages even when clear signs of confusion, disorientation, nausea, and vomiting is present.

Treatment

When mild cases of water intoxication occurs, restriction of water intake is usually the only necessary step. However, in moderate to serious cases, medical professionals are likely to prescribe diuretics in order to increase the rate of urination. Vasopressin receptor antagonists—any substances that interfere with actions at the vasopressin receptors that bind with vasopressin, a hormone that controls the re-absorption of molecules in the kidneys—may also be prescribed.

Prognosis

An early diagnosis and treatment for water intoxication is crucial in order to prevent severe symptoms, including seizures, coma, and possibly death.

Prevention

Restriction of water consumption can prevent water intoxication. Under normal circumstances, people should drink at least 1.0–2.1 quarts (1–2 liters) of water per day or about 34–68 fluid cups (about 4–8 eight-ounce glasses). Water intoxication occurs only when such levels have been far exceeded.

Healthy kidneys can excrete, under normal circumstances, about 27–34 fluid ounces (800–1,000 milliliters, or 0.8–1.0 liters) of fluids per hour without gaining additional water inside the body. However, strenuous exercise can reduce the amount of fluids that can be expelled by the kidneys. The capacity of kidney excretion can reach as low as 100 milliliters per hour. Therefore, for example, drinking 800 milliliters of water per hour (even when sweating profusely) can lead to dangerous conditions within the body.

Medical professionals usually say that a person should only drink water when one is thirsty. In addition, to avoid water intoxication, people should drink small amounts of water throughout the day, rather than taking in a large quantity of water at one time.

Resources

BOOKS

Chernecky, Cynthia C, and Kathleen Murphy-Ende, editors. *Acute Care Oncology Nursing*. St. Louis: Saunders/Elsevier, 2009.

Halperin, Mitchell L, Karmel S. Kamel, and Marc B. Goldstein. *Fluid, Electrolyte, and Acid-base Physiology: A Problem-based Approach*. Philadelphia: Saunders/Elsevier, 2010.

Katch, Victor L., William D. McArdle, and Frank I. Katch. *Essential of Exercise Physiology*. Philadelphia: Wolters Kluwer/Lippincott Williams & Wilkins Health, 2011.

Rennke, Helmut G., and Bradley M. Denker. *Renal Pathophysiology: The Essentials*. Philadelphia: Lippincott Williams & Wilkins Health, 2007.

WEBSITES

Hyponatremia. Mayo Clinic. (July 14, 2009). http://www.mayoclinic.com/health/hyponatremia/DS00974 (accessed June 22, 2011).

Noakes, T. D., K. Sharwood, M. Collins, and D. R. Perkins. *The Dipsomania of Great Distance: Water Intoxication in an Ironman Triathlete*. NCBI. (August 2004). http://www.ncbi.nlm.nih.gov/pubmed/15273209 (accessed June 22, 2011).

Response of the Body to Excess Water. LiveStrong.com. (May 26, 2011). http://www.livestrong.com/article/432756-response-of-the-body-to-excess-water/ (accessed June 22, 2011).

Strange but True: Drinking Too Much Water Can Kill. Scientific American. (June 21, 2007). http://www.scientificamerican.com/article.cfm?id=strange-but-true-drinking-too-much-water-can-kill (accessed June 22, 2011).

Water Works. WebMD. (June 21, 2007). http://www.webmd.com/video/benefits-of-water (accessed June 22, 2011).

ORGANIZATIONS

American College of Sports Medicine, P.O. Box 1440, Indianapolis, IN, 46206-1440, (317) 637-9200, Fax: (317) 637-7817, (888) 463-6332, http://www.acsm.org/.

William A. Atkins, BB, BS, MBA

Weight loss

Definition

Weight loss is defined as any sustained effort to lose excess body mass—most frequently fatty tissue—however, athletes and others may desire to lose fluid or muscle weight for athletic or other purposes.

BMI is described as a measure of body fat that is the ratio of the weight of the body in kilograms to the square of its height in meters. Overweight is defined as having a **body mass index** (BMI) of 25.0–29.9; **obesity** is defined as having a BMI of 30 or greater.

Weight gain, overweight, or obesity is caused by positive energy balance which may occur as a result of a number of intersecting factors. The key reasons have been listed as:

- consistently overeating, or eating foods too high in fats and complex carbohydrates
- getting no physical activity, or not enough physical activity
- genetic predisposition toward overweight or obesity
- medical condition which causes overweight/obesity, such as hypothyroidism

Purpose

Obesity is a leading indicator of chronic disease, and is directly linked to the most prevalent cause of death in men and women—heart disease. In the United States, the occurrence of obesity has doubled in the past twenty years; approximately one third of all adults are now obese. For the same time period, the occurrence of overweight and obesity among children and adolescents has risen markedly. Sixteen percent of children and adolescents are overweight, with the rate doubling for children and tripling for adolescents.

Obesity and excess body fat are significant indicators of the leading causes of chronic disease and premature death including heart disease, type 2 diabetes, stroke, **hypertension**, dyslipidemia (high **cholesterol**), gall bladder disease, respiratory disease, gout, **osteoporosis**, and certain cancers (e.g., colorectal and breast cancer).

Maintaining a healthy weight is important for adults and for young people. Children and adolescents who maintain a healthy weight are more likely to do so throughout adulthood. Those people, young and old, who are obese, see health improvements with even modest weight loss (e.g., ten pounds), and the prevention of even small gains is very important to overall health. However, the most significant impact to overall health is achieved when weight can be brought within the BMI range indicated for ideal weight.

Description

The key to maintaining a healthy weight at any **age** or height is in balancing the total **calories** consumed from food and beverages with those calories expended by physical activity and **exercise**. Most Americans consume more calories well in excess of those they expend by activity and exercise. According to the U.S. Department of Agriculture (USDA), average caloric consumption increased from 2,234 calories per day in 1970 to 2,757 calories per day in 2003. This 500 calorie per day increase accounts in large part for the rise in overweight and obesity rates seen in Americans over the same time period.

The portion size for the average American diet has grown notably larger in recent decades; restaurants are now serving notably larger portions than were customary 20 or even ten years ago. Packets of snack foods in vending machines and in convenience locations are offered frequently in sizes larger than single serving, and economy meals offered in fast food restaurants offer portion increases at inexpensive price points such as the highly popular US$1 menu items found in many fast food franchises. Prepackaging, shipping, and long-term storage of foods for distribution in the global market have driven down the costs of many foods, and therefore the quality, creating a market saturated with cheaply produced foods high in saturated and trans **fats** and low in nutrients. Studies indicate that portion size is directly linked to the amount of food a person will consume in a meal, and that consistently reducing portion size is an effective measure for weight loss.

Access to foods that are nutrient dense and low in saturated and trans fats is more limited in that these foods have grown increasingly more expensive than less healthy choices and are not distributed as widely. Historically, foods higher in fats and sugars were the more expensive choice, but globalization has changed this. Studies reveal the manufacture and global distribution of low cost, high fat and high sugar content foods has made these foods more easily accessible than healthier choices for everyone—all social classes, as well as every age group and gender. In this way, obesity and weight related illnesses are on the rise throughout the world, even in poorer countries.

People seeking to extend health and deter the onset of aging and illness should incorporate healthy nutrition and regular exercise into their lives as much as possible. To that end, incorporating fresh fruits and

RICHARD SIMMONS (1948–)

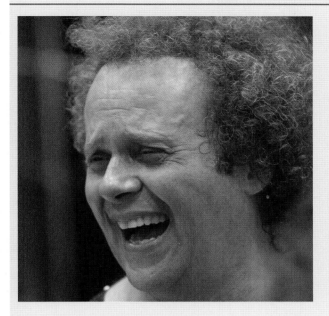

(© Bill Greenblatt/Hulton/Getty Images)

Richard Simmons, born July 12, 1948, weighed almost 200 pounds at age fifteen. Simmons utilized extreme measures to lose his weight rapidly. He lost over 110 pounds in three months, and this extreme weight-loss caused severe side effects, including hair loss and sagging facial skin. Simmons' experience made him realize the importance of a gradual, healthy weight loss program.

In 1975, Simmons established a restaurant and adjoining gym that reflected his nutrition and exercise beliefs. His flamboyant personality, encouraging words, and passion led to a hit television show in 1980.

His first book, *Richard Simmons' Never-Say-Diet Book* is a *New York Times* best seller. Simmons has written three cookbooks and created the "Deal-A-Meal" and the "FoodMover" calorie trackers. He has produced 50 fitness videos that incorporate his zany personality and high-tempo music, including the "Sweatin' to the Oldies" series.

vegetables, whole grains, lean meats, and fat-free, or reduced-fat dairy options are the dietary suggestions for optimum health in adults, children, and adolescents.

Many regimens exist for losing weight, but the most consistently healthy programs, and the most consistently successful over the long term, incorporate the reduction of calories consumed by fat and complex **carbohydrates** along with a program of regular, moderate exercise of 30 or more minutes per day, several days per week. Incorporating a healthy diet with moderate-to-intense exercise on a regular basis is enough to bring the body into balance and allay the risk of chronic disease and many causes of early death. A good, **fat burning** exercise is one that elevates heart rate. A moderate activity such as brisk **walking** can burn approximately 370 calories in a 154 pound individual over a one hour duration. Walking (3.5 mph) can burn 280 calories for the same time period, and jogging/running (5 mph) can burn 590 calories.

Those weight loss programs found to be the most successful over the long term and which bring individuals the healthiest overall benefits are those which:

• help one establish a goal for steady and gradual weight loss (e.g., 1-2 pounds per week)

• offer a wide range of low calorie, delicious, and healthy food choices

• promote consistent physical activity

• teach about the health benefits of good nutrition and regular exercise

• conform to cultural background and personal preferences

• provide tips and support for maintaining a healthy weight as a lifestyle

Precautions

If overweight or obesity are a concern, it is important to have regular health check-ups with one's doctor, particularly if there is a family history of health conditions for which obesity is a risk factor. If one is overweight or obese, and before beginning any exercise program, getting checked for heart disease and type 2 diabetes is important. Children and adolescents with these conditions should also be checked out by a physician, as health related conditions associated with overweight are on the rise in the young.

Weight that is lost gradually is healthier for the body than weight lost suddenly, and is more likely to be kept off over the long term. Research consistently reveals that those weight loss programs that consist in the taking of diuretics or other over-the-counter drugs or supplements by pill, drink, or shake solutions are not the most healthful options and should not be

KEY TERMS

Body mass index—A measure of body fat that is the ratio of the weight of the body in kilograms to the square of its height in meters.

Complex carbohydrates—A polysaccharide built upon hundreds or thousands of monosaccharide units; a food such as rice or pasta made from these poly saccharides.

Dyslipidemia—A condition of high blood cholesterol.

Hypothyroidism—A condition in which the thyroid gland fails to produce enough thyroid hormone; symptoms include sensitivity to cold, depression, constipation, fatigue, weight gain.

considered without the advice of a doctor. Relying solely on such programs for weight loss seldom reveal consistent benefits, and do not reap optimum benefits for health—either for weight loss, healthy weight maintenance, or in the reduction of weight for the purpose of allaying disease.

Aftercare

A "cool down" period is advised after aerobic exercise in order to gradually return the body to its resting heart rate. **Stretching** the muscles after exercise is advised in order to help with the release of lactic acid build-up in the muscles, and to reduce any soreness that may be acquired in the days after exercise. Stretching after the muscles have warmed also helps the body with flexibility and agility, and helps to reduce the possibility of injury during normal movement as well as during future exercise.

Complications

Losing weight too quickly is a often a sign that the body is losing too much weight by fluid loss and is potentially suffering from, or at risk of suffering, **dehydration**. The use of diuretics to lose weight can have the dangerous side effect of dehydration as diuretics cause the body to eliminate fluids more quickly. In a similar fashion, the use of liquid diets may cause dehydration and may also have the side effect of diarrhea that can be dangerous if it persists too long, amplifying dehydration and robbing the body of necessary nutrients and minerals. Some individuals use laxatives in an attempt to lose weight, but this is unsafe, and can come with long term side effects, including bowel irregularities.

Results

The combined effort of regular, near-daily exercise consisting of aerobic activity for 30 or more minutes along with the acquisition of a healthy, well-balanced diet consisting of fresh vegetables, fruits, whole grains, adequate **protein** portions, and vitamins and minerals to include Vitamin C, iron, zinc and vitamins A, E, B_6, and B_{12} have proven to be the best means of achieving healthy weight, and work as a preventative measure in allaying illness and disease—both acute and chronic, current and future. Positive dietary measures combined with consistent moderate exercise are also beneficial in reducing stress hormones, reducing the rate of illness outcomes ever further. Weight loss programs which incorporate these health concepts and teach individuals ways to maintain a healthy weight, as well as offer tips and support for achieving a healthy lifestyle tend to be the most effective over time.

Resources

BOOKS

Karacabey, Kursat, Ozcan Saygin, Recep Ozmerdivenli, Erdal Zorba, Ahmet Godekmerdan, and Vedat Bulut. "The effects of exercise on the immune system and stress exercise in sportswomen." *Neuroendocrinology Letters* 4, 26 (2005): 2-6.

Mahshid Dehghan, Noori Akhtar-Danesh, and Anwar T. Merchant. "Childhood Obesity Prevalence and Prevention," *Nutrition Journal* 4,24 (2005).

National Center for Chronic Disease Prevention and Health Promotion. "Do Increased Portion Sizes Affect How Much We Eat?" *Research to Practice Series* 1,2 (May 2006).

Nieman, David C. "Does Exercise Alter Immune Functions and Respiratory Infections?" *President's Counsil on Physical Fitness and Sports*. 3,13 (June 2001).

World Health Organization. *Diet, Nutrition, and the Prevention of Chronic Diseases*. Geneva, Switzerland: 2003.

WEBSITES

"Assessing Your Weight and Health Risk." NHLBI.nih. gov.com, last modified October 25, 2011, (accessed October 25, 2011).

"Dietary Guidelines for Americans 2005." Nutritionj.com, last modified July 09,2008, (accessed October 25, 2011).

Nutrition Journal. "Childhood Obesity Prevalence and Prevention." Nutritionj.com, last modified September 11, 2011, (accessed September 18, 2011).

"Obesity: Halting the Epidemic by Making Health Easier." CDC.gov, last modified May 26, 2011, (accessed October 26, 2011).

"Overweight and Obesity." CDC.gov, last modified, June 21, 2010. (accessed October 20, 2011).

WHAT TO ASK THE DOCTOR

- May I have my body mass index taken?
- Given the guidelines, am I currently considered overweight or obese?
- Give the medical guidelines, am I currently considered underweight?
- What nutritional or dietary changes do you recommend?
- Given my routine for physical activity, what changes do you recommend?
- Based on my current weight, do I appear to be at risk for disease or early death?
- What recommendations for weight maintenance do you suggest?

"Overweight, obesity, and weight loss fact sheet." Womenshealth.gov, last modified March 06, 2009. (October 17, 2011).

ORGANIZATIONS

American College of Sports Medicine, P.O. Box 1440, Indianapolis, IN, 46206-1440, (317) 637-9200, Fax: (317) 637-7817, (888) 463-6332, http://www.acsm.org/.

American Dietetic Association, 120 South Riverside Plaza, Suite 2000, Chicago, IL, 60606-6995, (800) 877-1600, knowledge@eatright.org

Julie Jordan Avritt

Weightlifting

Definition

Weightlifting is defined as the sport or exercise of lifting barbells. It is often used loosely to refer to several distinctive activities, one of which is a form of exercise—weight training—and three others that are considered competitive sports, namely Olympic weightlifting, powerlifting, and **bodybuilding**.

Purpose

Different forms of weightlifting have somewhat different purposes. The purpose of weight training is to develop the size and strength of skeletal muscles through using the force of gravity (in the form of weighted bars or dumbbells) to oppose the force generated by muscle contraction. Weight training is a form of exercise that can be used by athletes in many sports other than bodybuilding or Olympic weightlifting to prepare for competition; it can also be practiced by amateurs as part of an overall fitness regimen.

The purpose of Olympic weightlifting is to compete in a sport defined by attempting a maximum-weight single lift of a barbell loaded with weight plates. Olympic weightlifting is distinguished from powerlifting by its emphasis on explosive strength—the ability to exert maximal muscular force in minimal time. Powerlifting emphasizes limit strength, defined as the athlete's ability to exert muscular force for a single all-out effort. In contrast to both Olympic weightlifting and powerlifting, bodybuilding is focused on physique, or the external appearance of the body. Bodybuilders use weight training in combination with a dietary regimen to gain muscle and reduce body fat, the goal being an aesthetically pleasing physique with clearly defined muscle groups.

Demographics

Olympic weightlifting and bodybuilding are practiced worldwide in over 160 countries whereas powerlifting is based primarily in the United States, United Kingdom, and Russia. All three types of competitive weightlifting are open to women as well as men. Powerlifting and Olympic weightlifting are open to those 15 and older; however, the minimum age for competition in the Olympic Games themselves is 16.

Weight training is widely used by professional athletes in such other sports as baseball, football, hockey, soccer, and the like as well as by professional bodybuilders and powerlifters. It is also used for muscle building and overall fitness by many people who are not professional or semiprofessional athletes. It is difficult, however, to obtain exact figures for the total number of participants worldwide in weightlifting activities. The Centers for Disease Control and Prevention (CDC) reported in 2006 that 21.9% of men in the United States and 17.5% of women participated in some kind of strength training exercise two or more times per week, with Hispanics being the ethnic group with the lowest rate of participation in this type of exercise. These statistics cover weight training as a form of strength training but do not specify the other forms of exercise included in this category.

Weight training is increasingly used by the U.S. Army as part of physical readiness training (PRT) to prepare soldiers for military operations. Weight training as a part of PRT appears to be effective in reducing the number of injuries among soldiers compared to traditional weightlifting exercises.

JOE WEIDER (1919–)

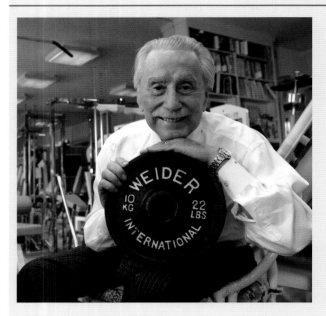

Joe Weider has made a name for himself in the publishing and the bodybuilding worlds. His publishing company, Weider Publications, published several successful fitness magazines, including *Muscle & Fitness*, *Fit Pregnancy*, *Shape*, and *Men's Fitness*. In 1983, he was named "Publisher of the Year" by the Periodical and Book Association, and in 2003, the company was sold to American Media.

Weider also developed a fitness program—The Weider System of Bodybuilding. In 1946, he and his brother Ben created the International Federation of Body-Builders (IFBB)—the highest level of global competitive bodybuilding. Weider also created the Mr. Olympia and Ms. Olympia bodybuilding titles to enable the Mr. Universe champions to continue competing and earning money.

Weider also marketed several weight-loss products (nutritional supplements, vitamins, etc.). Unfortunately, false marketing promises led to several legal claims, resulting in financial settlements to Weider's weight-loss products' customers.

History

The origin of weightlifting can be traced back to origins dating to ancient Chinese and Greek culture, with recordings of physical strength, endurance, and skill found in recorded text. Weightlifting was included as an official sport in the **Olympics**, originating in 1896.

Description

Weight training

Weight training involves a series of exercises intended to strengthen muscles and increase muscle mass. The exercises may involve resistance training—using the body alone with gravity as the opposing force (pushups and pull-ups); using free weights (barbells or **dumbbells**); or using exercise machines with weights or pulleys that force the body to work against their resistance. Free weights generally require more effort to lift, pound for pound, than the weights on weight machines.

Weight training exercises are intended to work specific muscle groups. Each exercise has a specific form that should be maintained by the athlete. The athlete decides how many repetitions (reps) and sets will be included in the exercise. A repetition consists of a single cycle of lifting and lowering a weight in a controlled manner, moving through the form of the exercise, while a set is a number of reps performed without a break. Tempo refers to the speed at which the set is performed. Beginners typically start out with one to five reps per set with one or two sets per exercise, raising the number of reps and sets and increasing the tempo as they gain strength and endurance.

Olympic weightlifting

Olympic weightlifting is a competitive sport and Olympic event in which the goal is a one-time lift of a maximum-weight barbell. It is considered a measure of explosive strength, or the ability to lift a maximum weight in minimal time. The two lifts that must be performed in Olympic weightlifting are the clean-and-jerk and the snatch. In the clean-and-jerk, the athlete begins by squatting down to grasp the bar. In the clean phase of the lift, the lifter uses the hips, knees, and ankles to raise the bar high enough to move underneath it and enter a deep squat position with the bar resting across the muscles of the upper back. The lifter then stands in preparation for the second phase. The overhead jerk phase involves bending the knees from the standing position and then straightening them to push the barbell upward with the help of the arms until the barbell is overhead.

In the snatch, the athlete lifts a barbell from a platform to a locked position overhead in a smooth continuous movement. The barbell is pulled as high as the lifter can manage (in most cases, to mid-chest level) and is then flipped overhead. The snatch requires an excellent sense of balance as well as great muscular strength and explosive speed.

Competitors are classified by body mass in Olympic weightlifting. There are eight divisions for men and seven for women. Athletes in each weight division compete in both the snatch and the clean-and-jerk, and prizes are usually given for the heaviest weights lifted in the snatch, the clean-and-jerk, and the two events combined.

Powerlifting

Powerlifting is a competitive sport that tests limit strength rather than explosive strength. There are three lifts in a powerlifting competition: the squat, the bench press, and the deadlift. In the squat, the lifter begins standing with the loaded bar resting across the shoulders. At a referee's command, the lifter lowers the body into a squatting position and returns to an erect standing position. The bar is then returned to the rack at the referee's command. In the bench press, the lifter lies on his or her back on a flat bench, lowers the weighted bar to the level of the chest, and pushes the bar back upward until the arms are straight and the elbows locked. In the deadlift, the athlete lifts the weighted bar from the floor and assumes an erect standing position with the knees locked and the shoulders back. At the referee's command the athlete returns the bar to the floor while maintaining control of it with both hands.

Competitors in powerlifting are classified by age, sex, and body weight. There are 11 weight categories for men and ten for women. The age categories are sub-junior (15–18); junior (19–23); open (24–39); and masters (40 +).

Bodybuilding

Bodybuilding is a sport involving modification of the body in the form of muscle hypertrophy (overdevelopment). This overdevelopment is achieved through a combination of weight training and a specialized diet. Competitive bodybuilders usually spend most of the year attempting to increase muscle mass (known as bulking) and then reducing body fat about 10 or 12 weeks before a competition by reducing calorie intake. This second process is called cutting. The specialized diet used by bodybuilders contains more calories than the average person of the same weight would require. The bodybuilder's diet is high in carbohydrates and usually includes protein supplements to help build muscle tissue. Current recommendations are that protein should constitute 25–30% of a bodybuilder's diet. Most bodybuilders eat 5 or 7 evenly spaced small meals a day, usually 2–3 hours apart, rather than three larger meals.

A bodybuilding competition is judged on the appearance of the competitor's physique rather than on athletic performance. Competitors are asked by the judges to assume a series of standard poses and are scored on their overall condition, size, and body symmetry. Bodybuilders typically spend a fair amount of time practicing posing before a competition. They also use tanning lotions or oils during a competition to make their muscles stand out under the stage lighting.

Preparation

Preparation for a weight training, weightlifting, or bodybuilding workout includes the following:

- Dressing appropriately. For weight training in a gym or fitness center, a simple tank top or other sleeveless top and exercise shorts are fine. Olympic weightlifting and powerlifting competitions, however, are quite specific about the types of tops and shorts that are acceptable, and competitors should consult the rulebooks for details.

- Adequate **hydration**. Weight training can lead to considerable fluid loss through sweat, so it is important to drink fluids before and during a workout. Some trainers recommend drinking about a cup of water every 15 minutes during weight training.

- Warming up and stretching. Most people in weight training spend between 5 and 20 minutes warming up and stretching before beginning the workout proper. Warming up is thought to lower the risk of **delayed-onset muscle soreness** (DOMS) as well as reduce the risk of damaging muscles, ligaments, or tendons during weight training.

- Using a spotter as a safety precaution for any exercise involving holding a barbell above the head, face, or chest. A spotter is a person who monitors and assists the athlete by making sure that they are maintaining proper form and that they are not in danger of dropping the weight or barbell from sudden muscle **fatigue**. A spotter can prevent such an accident by taking the weight or barbell before it falls on the athlete's head or chest.

People should consult their primary care physician for a general physical examination before undertaking a weight training or weightlifting regimen. Those considering bodybuilding should consult a dietitian about the adequacy of specialized nutrition and **protein** or food supplements, as well as the practice of eating smaller meals frequently. Adolescents who have not yet reached their full growth should consult a specialist in sports medicine or a coach with expertise in this area to reduce the risk of accidental or overuse injuries during weight training or weightlifting competitions.

Risks

Some people may experience some muscular soreness after a workout, particularly if they are new to weight training or were previously deconditioned. While some discomfort or a slight burning sensation in the muscles is normal during weight training or weightlifting, a sudden sharp severe pain or popping sensation in a muscle, tendon, or ligament is not normal. A person who experiences sudden severe pain or popping should stop the exercise at once to prevent further injury.

Physical injuries

Weight training is generally a safe form of exercise when done while maintaining good form with appropriate spotting and other supervision; however, the number of people treated in hospital emergency departments for injuries sustained during workouts is rising. Overly ambitious training, failure to **warm up** properly, or improper execution of the exercises can lead to pulled muscles, joint damage, or overuse injuries. Competitive weightlifting is a fairly high-risk sport; a study of injuries among athletes in the 2008 Olympic Games classified weightlifting as one of the riskiest sports, along with tae kwon do, soccer, hockey, and boxing. Fatal weightlifting accidents are rare, but there have been reports of fatalities from barbells falling on an athlete's head or chest due to muscle fatigue when the person was working out without a spotter.

There are differences between men and women with regard to weightlifting injuries. A study published in 2009 reported that women are more likely to be injured accidentally whereas men are at greater risk of sprains and strains from overexertion. Women are at greater risk of foot injuries whereas men are more likely to be injured in the chest region. With regard to age, children between the ages of 8 and 13 are at greater risk of injuries than older teenagers or young adults. Like adult women, children are at greater risk of accidental injuries than sprains or other injuries caused by overexertion. The authors of this study conclude that "The majority of youth resistance training injuries are the result of accidents that are potentially preventable with increased supervision and stricter safety guidelines."

A specific form of pain common in weightlifters and bodybuilders is delayed-onset muscle soreness, or DOMS. Also called muscle fever, DOMS is a sensation of pain or tenderness in the affected muscles that begins between 24 and 72 hours after a workout and resolves within two or three days. The most recent theory regarding the cause of DOMS is that it results from the breakdown of muscle fibers during the strong contractions involved in weight training. The body's response to this breakdown is inflammation. DOMS typically causes stiffness, swelling, strength loss, and pain in the affected limb or muscle group. Stretching as a warm-up before weight training is thought to lower the risk of DOMS. A common recommendation for treating the condition is contrast showers—alternating between hot and cold showers as a way to increase blood circulation in the affected area.

Failure to drink enough fluid before and during weight training or weightlifting can lead to **dehydration**. Overly shallow breathing during weight training has in a few cases led to blackouts or even brain aneurysms and stroke.

Steroid abuse

Many people interested in competitive weightlifting or bodybuilding are tempted to use **anabolic steroids** to build muscle. These drugs, given by injection or taken by mouth or in patches worn on the skin, are synthetic forms of the male sex hormones testosterone and dihydrotestosterone. They have a legitimate medical use in inducing male puberty and treating such chronic wasting conditions as AIDS and cancer. Anabolic steroids can also be used to increase lean muscle mass in combination with exercise and diet. They began to be abused to gain an advantage in bodybuilding competitions in the 1970s and in other sports a few years later. The International Olympic Committee (IOC) placed steroids on the list of banned substances in 1976. In the United States, these drugs were placed on Schedule III of the Controlled Substances Act in 1990.

There are numerous health risks associated with doping, or the use of anabolic steroids. These risks range from hypertension (high blood pressure), high blood cholesterol levels, and an increased risk of liver damage and cardiovascular disease to baldness and reduced sexual function. Sex-specific adverse effects include gynecomastia and shrinkage of the testicles in men; in women, these effects include deepening of the voice, hair loss, temporary cessation of menstruation, and growth of body hair. Steroid hormones taken during pregnancy can harm the fetus, causing the development of male features in a female fetus and female features in a male fetus. In adolescents, the use of anabolic steroids can lead to premature closure of

KEY TERMS

Anabolic steroids—Synthetic drugs that mimic the effects of male sex hormones in building up body tissue, specifically muscle tissue.

Deadlift—A weight training exercise in which the athlete lifts a loaded barbell from the ground in a stabilized bent-over position and then stands fully upright holding the barbell. It is one of three events in a powerlifting competition.

Doping—The illicit use of steroids or other performance-enhancing drugs in athletic competitions.

Explosive strength—In sports medicine, the ability to exert maximal muscular force in minimal time.

Gynecomastia—Abnormal development of the mammary glands in males, resulting in breast enlargement. It is an occasional side effect of anabolic steroid abuse.

Limit strength—The amount of muscular force that an athlete can generate for a single all-out effort.

Physique—The outward shape, form, or appearance of the body.

Resistance training—A form of strength training in which the athlete performs an effort against an opposing force generated by resistance to being pushed, pulled, stretched, or bent. It is done to strengthen and tone muscles and increase bone mass.

Spotter—A person who monitors and assists an athlete during weight training or powerlifting exercises to prevent injuries and accidents.

Squat—An exercise in which the athlete begins in a standing position with a bar loaded with weights resting on the shoulders. The athlete then bends the knees until he or she is in a squatting position, then stands erect again. The squat is one of three events in powerlifting competitions.

Tanner scale—A series of five stages used to measure the development of primary and secondary sexual characteristics in children and adolescents. It is named for the British pediatrician who developed it in the 1960s.

the growth plates at the end of the long bones, leading to stunted growth. There is also evidence that anabolic steroids can lead to psychiatric disorders, including depression and other mood disorders.

There is growing concern among health care professionals that steroid abuse is no longer limited to professional or semi-professional athletes; it is now widespread in the general population, particularly among males. In Europe as well as North America, most men who take illicit anabolic steroids do so for the sake of improving their appearance rather than athletic performance.

Precautions

In addition to the general precaution of consulting a physician before participating in any form of vigorous exercise, there are several additional precautions needed before beginning weight training, weightlifting, or bodybuilding:

• Adolescents interested in weight training should be evaluated for their present stage of physical maturation (Tanner stage). While there is a growing consensus that properly supervised weight training appropriate to a child or adolescent's stage of physical development is beneficial to health and may even lower the risk of certain musculoskeletal disorders in adult life, it is also

important not to damage the growth plates at the ends of the long bones. In addition, children and adolescents can develop overuse injuries to the lower back from competitive weightlifting or bodybuilding, and are advised against entering these sports until they have reached their full adult height.

• Persons of any age beginning weight training should start with low-key workouts and gradually increase the number, weight load, and speed of repetitions. Too ambitious a workout too early can damage muscles and joints.

• It is also important to learn and practice the proper form during weight training. Form in this context refers to correct body posture and alignment. Maintaining good form during weight training is essential to preventing injury and gaining the maximal benefit from the exercise. An example is the squat, which is intended to exercise the largest muscles in the body—the leg and buttock muscles. People are often tempted to "cheat" by rounding their back during the squat. This deviation from good form draws upon the lower back muscles to perform part of the work in lifting the weights, thus increasing the risk of a lower back injury and reducing the benefit of the exercise for the leg muscles.

• Most trainers recommend alternating weight training with other forms of aerobic exercise like **running**, or with flexibility exercises like **yoga**.

QUESTIONS TO ASK YOUR DOCTOR

- What is your opinion of weight training for the average adolescent or adult who simply wants to improve their overall fitness?
- What precautions would you recommend?
- Have you ever tried weight training yourself?
- What do you consider the most serious risks of weight training or weightlifting?
- What is your opinion of bodybuilding? Are the specialized diets and protein supplements safe to use over long periods of time?
- How can I tell if I am getting the right nutrients?
- What dietary changes, if any, would you recommend for me?
- What tests or evaluation techniques can you perform to see if my fitness and nutritional choices promote a healthy condition?
- What physical or health limitations if any, do you foresee?
- How can I tell whether a friend or family member is abusing steroids?

Results

Weight training and weightlifting regimens offer specific physical benefits: increased muscle mass and strength; stronger tendons and ligaments; increased bone density and metabolic rate; and better postural support. Some people also notice improved endurance and lowered blood pressure as well as greater muscular strength.

The benefits of bodybuilding for many people include a more attractive physique as well as increased muscular strength and better posture.

Resources

BOOKS

Barber, Tiki. *Tiki Barber's Pure Hard Workout: Stop Wasting Time and Start Building Real Strength and Muscle.* New York: Gotham Books, 2008.

Fahey, Thomas D. *Basic Weight Training for Men and Women*, 7th ed. New York: McGraw-Hill Higher Education, 2010.

Manocchia, Pat. *Anatomy of Exercise: A Trainer's Inside Guide to Your Workout.* Richmond Hill, ONT: Firefly Books, 2009.

Marcher, Lisbeth., and Sonja Fich. *Body Encyclopedia: A Guide to the Psychological Functions of the Muscular System.* Berkeley, CA: North Atlantic Books, 2010.

Murray, Thomas H., Karen J. Maschke, and Angela A. Wasunna, eds. *Performance-enhancing Technologies in Sports: Ethical, Conceptual, and Scientific Issues.* Baltimore, MD: Johns Hopkins University Press, 2009.

National Strength and Conditioning Association (NSCA). *Essentials of Strength Training and Conditioning*, 3rd ed. Champaign, IL: Human Kinetics, 2008.

Rizzo, Donald C. *Introduction to Anatomy and Physiology.* Clifton Park, NY: Delmar, 2011.

Shepard, Greg. *Bigger, Faster, Stronger*, 2nd ed. Champaign, IL: Human Kinetics, 2009.

PERIODICALS

Busche, K. "Neurologic Disorders Associated with Weightlifting and Bodybuilding." *Physical Medicine and Rehabilitation Clinics of North America* 20 (February 2009): 273–86.

Centers for Disease Control and Prevention (CDC). "Trends in Strength Training, United States, 1998–2004." *Morbidity and Mortality Weekly Report* 55 (July 21, 2006): 769–772.

Faigenbaum, A.D., et al. "Youth Resistance Training: Updated Position Statement Paper from the National Strength and Conditioning Association." *Journal of Strength and Conditioning Research* 23 (August 2009): Suppl. 5, S60–S79.

Junge, A., et al. "Sports Injuries during the Summer Olympic Games 2008." *American Journal of Sports Medicine* 37 (November 2009): 2165–72.

Knapik, J.J., et al. "United States Army Physical Readiness Training: Rationale and Evaluation of the Physical Training Doctrine." *Journal of Strength and Conditioning Research* 23 (July 2009): 1353–62.

Melnik, B.C. "Androgen Abuse in the Community." *Current Opinion in Endocrinology, Diabetes, and Obesity* 16 (June 2009): 218–23.

Myer, G.D., et al. "Youth Versus Adult 'Weightlifting' Injuries Presenting to United States Emergency Rooms: Accidental Versus Nonaccidental Injury Mechanisms." *Journal of Strength and Conditioning Research* 23 (October 2009): 2054–60.

Quatman, C.E., et al. "Sex Differences in 'Weightlifting' Injuries Presenting to United States Emergency Rooms." *Journal of Strength and Conditioning Research* 23 (October 2009): 2061–67.

WEBSITES

Cassas, Kyle M., and Amelia Cassettari-Wayhs. "Childhood and Adolescent Sports-Related Overuse Injuries." *American Family Physician* 73 (March 15, 2006): 1014–22. http://www.aafp.org/afp/2006/0315/p1014.html (accessed December 28, 2011).

International Weightlifting Federation (IWF). *What Is Weightlifting?* http://www.iwf.net/# (accessed December 28, 2011).

Lift Up. *Olympic Snatch Techniques*. This is a set of online videos of athletes performing the snatch in Olympic weightlifting. http://www.chidlovski.net/liftup/web_external_modules.asp?s_module=mod_snatch_classics (accessed December 28, 2011).

National Strength and Conditioning Association (NSCA). *Combating Anabolic Steroid Abuse*. This is a 17-page document that includes information about the nature, effects, and health risks of steroids as well as advice about policies for deterring the use of steroids among high school and college athletes. http://www.nsca-lift.org/Publications/Combating%20Anabolic%20Steroid%20Abuse.pdf (accessed December 28, 2011).

National Strength and Conditioning Association (NSCA). *Video Library*. This is a collection of 47 videos illustrating different weightlifting and strength training exercises and techniques. http://www.nsca-lift.org/videos/displayvideos.asp (accessed December 28, 2011).

TeensHealth. *Strength Training*. http://kidshealth.org/teen/food_fitness/exercise/strength_training.html (accessed December 28, 2011).

ORGANIZATIONS

American College of Sports Medicine (ACSM), P.O. Box 1440, Indianapolis, IN, 46206, (317) 637-9200, Fax: (317) 634-7817, http://www.acsm.org/.

American Council on Exercise (ACE), 4851 Paramount Drive, San Diego, CA, 92123, (858) 279-8227, (888) 825-3636, Fax: (858) 279-8064, http://www.acefitness.org/default.aspx.

American Sports Medicine Institute (ASMI), 2660 10th Avenue South, Suite 505, Birmingham, AL, 35205, (205) 918-0000, Fax: (205) 918-0800, http://www.asmi.org/.

International Weightlifting Federation (IWF), Maison du Sport International, Av. de Rhodaine 54, Lausanne, Switzerland, 1007, +36 1 353 0530, Fax: +36 1 353 0199, iwf@iwfnet.net, http://www.iwf.net/.

National Athletic Trainers' Association., 2952 Stemmons Freeway, Dallas, TX 75247-6916., Telephone: (214) 637-6282., Fax: Fax: (214) 637-2206., http://www.nata.org.

National Strength and Conditioning Association (NSCA), 1885 Bob Johnson Drive, Colorado Springs, CO, 80906, (719) 632-6722, (800) 815-6826, Fax: (719) 632-6367, nsca@nsca-lift.org, http://www.nsca-lift.org/.

U.S.A. Powerlifting (USAPL), P.O. Box 668, Columbia City, IN, 46725, (260) 248-4889, Fax: (260) 248-4879, http://www.usapowerlifting.com/index.shtml.

World Anti-Doping Agency (WADA), Stock Exchange Tower, 800 Place Victoria, Suite 1700, MontrealQuebec, Canada, H4Z 1B7, +1 514 904 9232, Fax: +1 514 904 8650, info@wada-ama.org, http://www.wada-ama .org/.

Rebecca J. Frey, PhD
Laura Jean Cataldo, RN, EdD

Windsurfing *see* **Ocean sports**

Winter sports

Definition

Winter sports are those that are played on snow or ice. The most common winter sports are skiing, **snowboarding**, **ice hockey**, and sledding.

Purpose

The purposes of winter sports vary. People do some purely for fun and recreation. For example, they may ski or snowboard just to enjoy scenery and a trip to the mountains in the winter. They also may enjoy the **exercise**. Cross-country skiing, in particular, provides an excellent workout in the winter months, when people cannot get outside as often for exercise. Athletes may participate in some individual and team winter sports for competition. There are numerous ski and snowboard events that involve everything from downhill racing to jumping and aerial tricks. Ice hockey is a team sport, usually played indoors, that offers the chance for one team to score more goals with a puck than the opposing team. People compete in winter sports at the amateur and professional level, and many, such as ice skating, snowboarding, skiing, and even curling, are popular Olympic events. Likewise, most people sled for fun, but there also is a highly competitive Olympic event for sledding called luge.

Demographics

Winter sports are enjoyed by people of all ages. For example, sledding and downhill skiing are favorite family activities. According to the National Sporting Goods Association, the following number of people over age seven years old participated in these winter sports in 2010:

- alpine skiing: 7.4 million
- cross-country skiing: 2 million
- snowboarding: 6.1 million
- ice hockey: 3.3 million
- snowboarding: 6.1 million

It is difficult to number how many people sled each year, because it is a mostly informal activity, not an organized sport. There are reports of more than 700,000 injuries a year from sledding. U.S. Figure Skating says it has more than 176,000 members. It also can be difficult to measure skiing and snowboarding participation, because some ski resorts measure visits (and one skier may visit, or ski, several times a year or not at all). The average age of skiers and

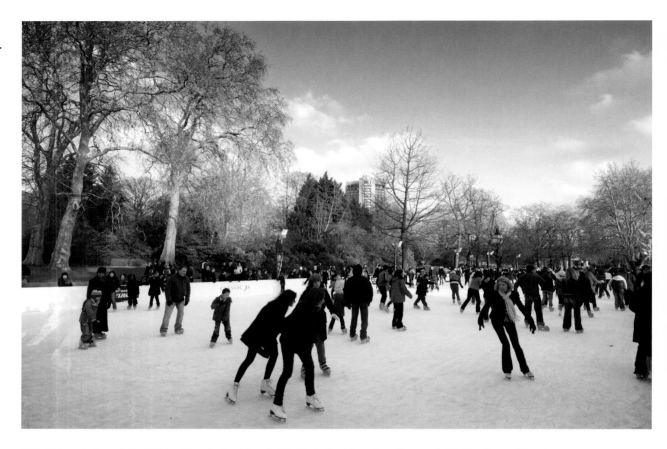

People ice skating at the Winter Wonderland ice rink in Hyde Park London, England. *(© Alex Segre/Alamy)*

snowboarders is rising. It was about 36.6 years in the 2006/2007 season.

History

Skiing may have been around since 5,000 B.C., as shown in cave drawings in Norway, and parts of skis discovered in Switzerland. Swedish soldiers used two pieces of wood to help them reach remote towns in the sixteenth century. It became popular as a sport in the early twentieth century when T-bars, tows, and eventually ski lifts, were added to take skiers back up hills. Skiing competitions probably started in the 1800s in Norway. The first cross-country skiing event in a Winter Olympic games was held in 1924. Legend says that the Vikings raced sleds with two runners in about 800 B.C. This was an early form of luge, an event that today has singles and doubles events and is a crowd favorite at Olympic events, where competitors steer their sleds down icy courses. Snowboarding is a much newer sport; the first mass-produced snowboard, named a "snurfer," appeared in 1965, and the first U.S. snowboarding championships were held in 1982. Ice hockey

probably got its start as a winter version of **field hockey**. The first artificial ice rink was built in England in 1876. The National Hockey League officially began in 1917.

Description

There are many winter sports, and some, such as figure skating and ice hockey, can be enjoyed year-round at indoor ice rinks. Others only can take place outdoors in winter conditions, and often at high altitudes or in rough terrain. For example, snowmobiling and cross-country skiing by nature involve trekking through snowy mountain backcountry. The major winter sports usually take place at special facilities, such as ski resorts, ice rinks, or sledding parks.

Skiing

Alpine, or downhill, skiing is an enjoyable athletic activity that requires balance, coordination, and confidence. Downhill skiing combines the skier's skill with the gravity of steep slopes to produce speeds up to 90 miles per hour. Beginning skiers should not go that fast,

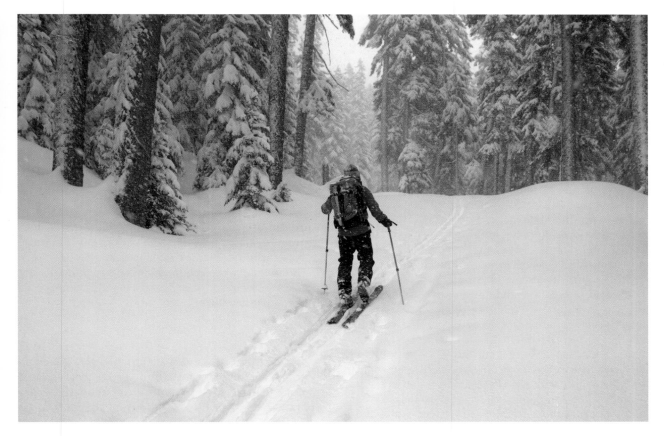

Cross-country skiing. *(© Kurt Werby/First Light/Getty Images)*

however, and the first skill they should learn is how to stop effectively. Ski instructors also teach them how to turn, along with safety and etiquette on the slopes. Professional skiers may compete by racing around gates. The ancient cave drawings are more like cross-country skiing, which takes place on flatter terrain. Skiers must condition themselves to handle tougher and longer terrain. There are classical and free techniques. Competitive skiing also may involve freestyle, aerial, and mogul skiing, along with ski jumping.

Snowboarding

Snowboarding is similar to slalom waterskiing in many ways because both feet can be placed on a wider board that resembles a skateboard, but has no wheels. It takes place on downhill courses, although snowboarding competitions now involve freestyle, racing, and half-pipe events. Competition names are alpine, freestyle, and boardercross. Snowboard competition classes run from age 12 years and younger through age 50 years and older (named "Methusalah"). In downhill skiing, the skier shifts his or her weight from one side to side, but in snowboarding, the weight shift occurs from heels to toes to create edges on the board. The techniques resemble **skateboarding** or surfing more than skiing.

Sledding

It might be called a toboggan or a sledge in another country, but in the United States, people call the sleek seat that rides on snow a sled. Usually made of plastic, a sled fits one or two people and is light enough to easily pull back up a hill. There are different types of sleds, and most cities and mountain areas in snowy climates have parks used just for sledding or tubing. Some runner sleds can be steered. Competitive sledding includes the luge, toboggan, or bobsled.

Ice hockey

Ice hockey is played on an ice rink 200 ft long and 85 ft wide. Each team has 20 players, two of whom are goalkeepers. Only six players from each team are allowed on the rink at a time, and one of these is the goalkeeper. The five players pass the puck around in an attempt to score at their goal and help the goalkeeper defend his or her own team's goal. When players commit penalties that are called by referees, they are sent to a penalty box for a period of time. During this time, the team is short a player for two to five minutes, giving an advantage to the other team. A professional game takes place in three periods, each 20 minutes long.

Preparation

Winter sports require more equipment and preparation than many other sports because of cold temperatures and risk of injury. It is important that people preparing to participate in winter sports, especially skiing and snowboarding, begin conditioning before heading to the slopes. **Running** trails and jogging, mountain biking, and doing exercises that strengthen quadriceps and hamstrings (such as leg curls and leg lifts) can help prevent injury. It also is important to strengthen the body core, the calves, and shins. Anyone who is not used to living and exercising at high altitudes should take particular care to be in good physical condition and health before participating in winter sports at high altitude locations. Many competitive winter sports are high-intensity workouts. People who participate in them should advance with time to the appropriate levels. For example, a person should not head out to the ice rink to play hockey without learning how to ice skate, and a skier should not race before he or she has mastered the sport well enough to do so safely. **Stretching** and warming up before playing winter sports such as ice hockey can help prevent injuries. The following lists some of the specific equipment needs for common winter sports:

- Skiing requires ownership or rental of skis, special boots that fit the skis' bindings, and poles. Cross-country skis and downhill skis are designed differently. Skiers also need ski goggles, a helmet, gloves, a warm and waterproof jacket, and other accessories to keep the head and body warm and dry.
- Snowboarders must have a board and special boots that work with the board's bindings. They also should have a helmet, goggle, warm jacket, gloves, and accessories to keep them warm and dry.
- Sledding requires a sled, and the type depends on the speed, steering, and bounce desired. Sledders need layers of clothing to keep warm and dry, including waterproof boots and gloves. Professionals wear special suits, shoes, helmets and goggles.
- Ice hockey. Like many other winter sports, hockey equipment is used to help play the game and to help protect players from injury. Hockey players need ice skates and special sticks, along with pucks, which are rubber discs that are an inch thick and about three inches around. Players wear helmets, mouth guards, and sometimes face visors. Neck pads or guards,

shoulder pads, elbow pads, and special pants with pads in several places also help. Shin guards help protect against pucks. Hockey players also use pelvic protectors or jock straps. Goalkeepers wear additional arm and chest protection, a special goalie mask, and have a stick with a larger blade. They also wear special gloves that help them catch pucks.

Risks

In 2009, more than 350,000 people were treated in hospitals and physician offices for winter sports-related injuries. Injuries to knee joints are common in winter sports, especially ice hockey, downhill skiing, and ski jumping. Ice hockey players also suffer neck and shoulder injuries and cuts from skate blades. Wrist and elbow injuries are common for people who snowboard because boarders tend to fall on outstretched hands. Emergency physicians say it is foolish to be pulled on sleds behind vehicles along icy streets, as this can lead to serious injuries. Finally, all snowboarders and downhill or freestyle skiers should wear helmets. Of the 600,000 accidents in North America each year from skiing and snowboarding, doctors say 15% to 20% are head injuries. The National Ski Association says that helmet use has gone up in the past few years. Sledders also should consider wearing helmets. Of the 700,000 injuries from sledding in the United States in 2010 (the most of any winter sport), many were head injuries and 30% of them were caused by collisions.

Results

Winter sports can be very gratifying, bring family fun to the colder winter months and vacations, and help people stay in shape. Just 30 minutes of sledding burns 221 **calories**. Skiing downhill for 90 minutes burns 567 calories and cross-country skiing for 60 minutes burns about 500 calories. Snowboarding for 45 minutes can burn about 285 calories; ice skating for recreation or hockey competition can burn at least 173 calories in just 30 minutes. By dressing appropriately for warmth and safety, winter sports can be fun and improve fitness. Experts also recommend that people always participate in winter sports with someone, and never go alone. Backcountry skiing, for example, can be particularly dangerous if a skier gets lost or an avalanche occurs. Skiers, boarders, and sledders should have partners that they stop and wait for if they lose sight of one another.

Resources

PERIODICALS

Joffe, Alain. "Use a Helmet with Skis and Snowboards."- *Journal Watch Pediatrics and Adolescent Medicine* (October 6, 2010).
"Orthopaedic Surgeons Offer Safety Tips for Winter Sports."*Health and Beauty Close-up* (December 23, 2010).
Rushlow, Amy. "Burn Calories Like an Olympian." *Women's Health* 7 (March 2010):25.
"Sledding Source of Most Winter Sports Injuries: Report, more than 700,000 Injuries Linked to the Activity in U.S. Each Year, Surgeon Says."*Consumer Health News* 7 (March 6, 2011):25.
"Winter Activities that Can Land You in ER."*UPI News Track* (February 25, 2011).
"Workouts for Skiers and Snowboarders."*USA Today* 139 (October 2010):10.

WEBSITES

SnowSleds.net. "Snow Sleds for Kids." http://www.snowsleds.net/infosnowsledsforkids.html (accessed September 12, 2011).

ORGANIZATIONS

National Hockey League, St. Paul, MN, http://www.nhl.com.

United States Ski and Snowboard Association, 1 Victory Lane, Park City, UT, 84060, (435) 649-9090, Fax: (435) 649-3613, http://www.ussa.org.

USA Luge, 57 Church Street, Lake Placid, NY, 12946, (518) 523-2071, Fax: (518) 523-4106, (800) 872-5843, info@usaluge.org, http://www.usaluge.org.

Teresa G. Odle, BA ELS

Women's fitness

Definition

Women's fitness refers to the condition of optimum health in the lives of women.

Purpose

According to the Centers for Disease Control and Prevention (CDC), 60% of women do not achieve an adequate amount of physical activity, and of those, 25% receive no physical activity. Sedentary lifestyles, or not enough physical activity, is more common in women than in men, and among women, women of color are more likely to lead sedentary lifestyles.

Beyond controlling weight, the building of lean muscle mass, and the reduction of excess fat, regular physical activity helps women maintain joint health and to fight against **osteoporosis** and the weakening of bones. Regular **exercise** has been shown to greatly reduce the risk of heart disease that is the leading cause of death among women. It is also shown to help fight against other forms of chronic disease such as diabetes, some cancers (e.g., colorectal and breast cancer), and **hypertension**. Regular exercise also helps to reduce stress hormones (i.e., cortisol levels), and has been shown to decrease anxiety, and depression. (About twice as many women suffer depression as men.)

According to the U.S. Department of Health and Human Services (DHHS), being overweight or obese is strongly linked with heart disease, type 2 diabetes, stroke, high **blood pressure**, breathing problems, osteoarthritis, gall bladder disease, and certain cancers. Regular physical activity, reduced calorie consumption, and positive nutrition are the best measures toward the prevention of these diseases or medical conditions. Regular physical activity improves cardiorespiratory (heart, lung, and blood vessel) health, and may help with the prevention of reduced cognitive functioning, such as in the case of dementia and **Alzheimer's disease**.

Women's health and fitness, and the prevention of disease, is also strongly contingent upon nutrition. The "Dietary Guidelines for Americans," published in 2010 by DHHS in partnership with the Office of Disease Prevention and Health Promotion, puts forth three major goals for Americans:

- Balance caloric intake with physical activity.
- Consume greater quantities of certain foods like fruits, vegetables, whole grains, and seafood, and consume fat-free or reduced fat dairy products.

• Reduce the consumption of foods containing sodium, saturated and trans fat, cholesterol, added sugars, and refined grains.

The guidelines further recommend the consumption of nutrient-dense foods. Nutrient-dense foods are those foods in which the naturally occurring vitamins and minerals have not been diluted or supplanted by the addition of solid **fats**, sugars, or starches—or by those solid fats natural to the food. Nutrient-dense foods include all vegetables, fruits, whole grains, seafood, eggs, beans, peas, and unsalted nuts and seeds. Fat-free or reduced-fat dairy and lean meats cooked without the addition of fats and sugars are included in the list.

According to United States Department of Agriculture (USDA), half of one's daily consumption should consist of fruits and vegetables, and these items should be varied. Half of all grains consumed should be whole grain; meats and other proteins should be lean; and dairy should consist of low-fat or reduced-fat options.

Research indicates that most diets are too low in specific nutrients, and that special attention should be paid to the diet in order to ensure appropriate levels are being consumed. These nutrients are potassium, dietary fiber, calcium, and vitamin D. Adequate consumption of iron, folate, and vitamin B_{12} are also important, as these nutrients are found lacking in the diets of many women.

Description

In order to achieve and maintain fitness, regular physical activity or exercise does not need to be strenuous. Mild-to-moderate but regular exercise such as **walking** for about 30 or more minutes several days per week can result in higher levels of fitness, and reduced expectation of chronic disease. This kind of mild-to-moderate physical activity is enough to improve **bone health**, and can reduce stress, depression, and anxiety.

Two types of exercise are necessary in order to achieve best fitness: aerobic exercise and strengthening exercise. Aerobic activity is any activity that increases heart rate; and strengthening activities are those which focus on resistance effort in any of the muscle groups. The President's Counsil on Physical Fitness and Sport's Research Digest "2008 Physical Activity Guidelines for Americans" recommends at least 2.5 hours per week of moderate intensity aerobic activity, such as produced by brisk walking. The guidelines also recommend muscle-strengthening activities 2 or more days per week which will exercise all major muscle groups (e.g., legs, hips, back, stomach, shoulders, and arms).

Greater levels of regular physical activity produce greater health benefits, so moderate intensity aerobic activity (such as brisk walking, cycling on a level surface, water aerobics, or lawn mowing) can be supplemented with vigorous activity (such as produced by jogging or **running**, cycling on a non-level surface, **swimming** laps, or most aerobic sports like singles tennis, **basketball**, etc.). Five hours per week of moderate intensity activity along with muscle strengthening two or more days per week yields better health benefits. This activity doesn't need to take place at once in order to yield results; separating out the activity into ten minute intervals can be just as effective.

Strength training activities can be done with or without equipment such as in the case of **calisthenics** (e.g., sit-ups, pushups, and pull-ups). The use of arm-bands, dumb bells, or even soup cans may be employed in order to add resistance. As with any repetitive exercise, intervals should be gradually increased, different muscle groups should be worked, and periods of rest should be provided so that the muscles have time to recover and strengthen.

Preparation and aftercare

Some research indicates that warming up the muscles before exercise, and a period of muscle "cool down" is appropriate and may reduce the number of injuries sustained during exercise. Slowly warming the muscles before exercise with the implementation of low-impact calisthenics helps to prepare the muscles for a higher impact workout. Rather than stopping aerobic activity suddenly, slowing movement to gradually return the heart to a normal rate, and **stretching** the muscles (to help reduce lactic acid build-up) are recommended.

Stretching the muscles after a workout helps to improve flexibility. This will ensure ease of movement for all tasks such as bending to put on or remove shoes, or turning to check the blind spot when changing lanes or backing out of a parking space. Stretching should be avoided before beginning exercise when the muscles are "cool" as this can increase the possibility of injury.

Ample research indicates the benefits of **yoga**, a 5,000 year practice that incorporates stretching, strengthening, and balance, as well as meditation and breathing exercises to help with fitness of the mind and body and the reduction of stress.

Precautions

Women who are pregnant or those with medical conditions such as diabetes, heart disease, or hypertension should consult their doctors before initiating any exercise routines. Women over the age of 50 should also consult their physicians if they plan to initiate or continue a vigorous exercise routine. Women over 50 should be tested for heart disease or other medical conditions prior to beginning a new exercise program.

If ongoing physical activity is too strenuous, women may run the risk of weakening their bones rather than strengthening them, and menstrual irregularities may result. Women who exercise too strenuously also put themselves at risk of greater opportunity for injury. When activity becomes strenuous over a lengthened period of time, immunological suppression may also result.

Results

Women and girls remain less physically active than men and boys. The World Health Organization and other research institutions explain this differential with the historical disparity between opportunities for females and males. In 1972 when Title IX was implemented, more athletic opportunities were made available for females, however the data does not yet accurately reveal a change in the outcome on life expectancy. The data is clear, however, that regular exercise prevents chronic disease and extends life.

QUESTIONS TO ASK YOUR DOCTOR

- Do my current dietary routines provide adequate nutritional support for my gender, age, and any medical needs I may have?
- What further dietary or nutritional supplementation should I consider?
- Is my current fitness routine adequate for my gender, age, and any medical needs I may have?
- Given my gender, age, and current medical fitness, should I consider adding anything new to my fitness routine?
- Should I be tested for heart disease or any other conditions prior to implementing a moderate exercise routine?
- Should I be tested for heart disease or any other conditions prior to implementing a vigorous exercise routine?

Social support is strongly positively related to physical activity. Women who receive consistent social support by way of encouraging family and/or friends, or who exercise with a partner or group, are more likely to maintain regular exercise programs. Those women who do maintain consistent physical activity are at lower risk for disease, and experience an increased quality of life.

The diets of women, and particularly women of color and those women falling into lower socioeconomic strata, are found to be less nutrient-rich than the diets of other groups. Maintaining a consistent diet of nutrient-rich foods, especially vegetables, fruits, whole grains, low-fat dairy, and lean proteins is proven to help reduce the risk of chronic disease and premature death. If possible, women should be paying particular attention in order to ensure they are receiving enough potassium, dietary fiber, calcium, vitamin D, iron, folate, and vitamin B_{12}. These nutrients are found to be more frequently lacking in the diets of women, however they are necessary for best health and fitness, and the reduction of rates of chronic disease and early or preventable death.

Resources

BOOKS

President's Counsil on Physical Fitness and Sports. "2008 Physical Activity Guidelines for Americans." *Research Digest* 9,4 (2008): 1–8.

Wells, Christine L. "Physical Activity and Women's Health." *Research Digest* 2,5 (2008): 1–12.

William J. Kramer, Scott A. Mazzetti, Bradley C. Nindl, et al. "Effect of resistance training on women's strength/power and occupational performances." *Med. Sci. Sports Exerc.*, 33, 6, (2001) 1011–1025.

WEBSITES

"Choose My Plate." health.gov, last modified October 18, 2011 (accessed October 18, 2011).

"Dietary Guidelines for Americans 2010." http://www.choosemyplate.gov, last modified September 30, 2011 (accessed October 16, 2011).

"Health Benefits of Yoga." http://www.webmd.com, last modified March 06, 2011 (accessed October 16, 2011).

"Physical Activity and Health: Women." http://www.cdc.gov, last modified Novermber 17, 1999 (accessed October 15, 2011).

"Women's Health." http://who.int, last modified 2011 (accessed October 15, 2011).

"Women's Health Publications." http://www.womenshealth.gov, last modified, February 26, 2009 (accessed October 16, 2011).

ORGANIZATIONS

American College of Sports Medicine, P.O. Box 1440, Indianapolis, IN, 46206-1440, (317) 637-9200, Fax: (317) 637-7817, (888) 463-6332, http://www.acsm.org/.

American Dietetic Association, 120 South Riverside Plaza, Suite 2000, Chicago, IL, 60606-6995, (800) 877-1600, knowledge@eatright.org

Centers for Disease Control and Prevention, Div. of Nutrition and Physical Activity, 4770 Buford Highway, NE, Atlanta, GA, 30341-3724, (888) 232-4674, http://www.cdc.gov.

Julie Jordan Avritt

Workplace and fitness

Definition

The modern sedentary workplace appears to be an important contributor to the current epidemics of poor physical fitness, **obesity**, type 2 diabetes, and heart disease. Increasingly, employees and employers are recognizing the benefits of promoting fitness in the workplace, with incentive programs and on-site fitness instructors and facilities.

Purpose

Promoting fitness in the workplace can lower employee medical costs and increase productivity and job satisfaction. A workforce that is overweight or obese and physically unfit has major economic ramifications for business and industry, as well as for the population as a whole. Numerous studies have shown that a significant proportion of escalating employer and employee healthcare costs is due to obesity-related conditions caused, in part, by lack of physical activity. The U.S. National Center for Health Statistics estimates that healthcare expenses for obese employees are 42% higher than for those who are of healthy weight. Healthy, active workers have lower healthcare costs, lower rates of absenteeism, and are more productive.

Research has demonstrated that aerobic **exercise** increases blood flow to the brain, strengthens connections between neurons in the brain, and promotes the formation of new brain cells. This makes for smarter, more productive employees who are less likely to experience cognitive decline as they **age**. Studies also indicate that exercise is important for relieving chronic job stress that contributes to obesity, absenteeism, and reduced productivity. Since most adults spend more than half of their waking hours at work, the workplace is a natural setting for implementing fitness and other wellness programs.

Demographics

Obesity and lack of physical fitness have reached epidemic proportions in the United States and other parts of the developed world. Two-thirds of adult Americans are overweight, including about one-third who are obese. Obesity accounts for 63 million physician visits annually. Furthermore, three-quarters of adult Americans participate in little or no daily physical activity. A study published in 2011 found that, in addition to poor eating habits and lack of leisure-time physical activity, the American workplace is contributing to the obesity epidemic. In 1960, 50% of American jobs required moderate physical activity; today, 80% of jobs are sedentary or require only light activity. This corresponds to a daily decline of about 120–140 **calories** of **energy expenditure**, approximately equivalent to the average weight gain over five decades. The study may have overestimated even light-activity jobs, since it did not take into account technological advances, such as e-mail and the Internet, that have further decreased the need to rise from one's office chair.

Employers are beginning to recognize the importance of fitness in the workplace. According to a 2011 survey by the corporate benefits group, Workplace Options, 36% of employees report that their jobs offer wellness benefits such as fitness programs, and approximately 70% of Fortune 200 companies offer

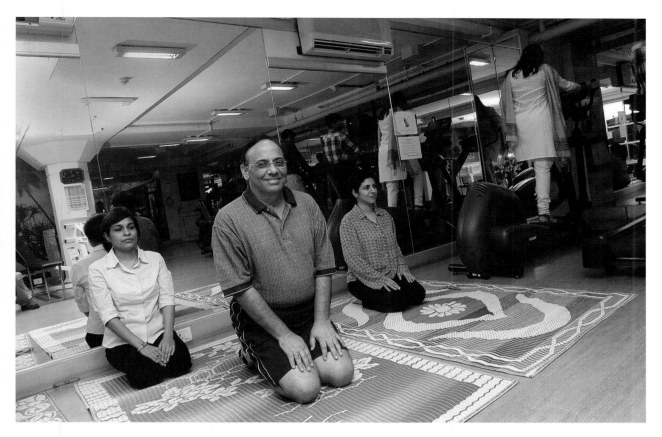

Johnson and Johnson staff doing yoga at the office gym in Mumbai, India. (© The India Today Goup/Getty Images)

physical fitness programs. Among employees of small and mid-sized companies, 47% participate in wellness programs—or would if their companies made them available—and 45% report that they would stay at their jobs longer because of employer-sponsored wellness programs.

Among the *Working Mother* 100 Best Companies to work for, 98% offer health screenings and 97% offer gym discounts. Almost 98% offer on-site fitness facilities and showers that employees are encouraged to use whenever they can, and 62% offer financial incentives for working toward or reaching fitness and wellness goals. Many of the companies also provide "mommy benefits," such as meal or grocery deliveries to afford mothers leisure time for physical activity.

Description

More than fifty years ago, research on the health of sedentary London bus drivers found that they had higher rates of heart disease than bus ticket-takers who were on the move all day. Since then, studies have consistently shown that the rates of obesity, heart disease, and various other chronic diseases, as well as psychological stress, are higher for people who have sedentary jobs. Recent studies indicate that even people who are physically active outside of the workplace are at increased risk of heart disease from sedentary jobs.

It is unlikely that physical activity will once again become an integral component of most occupations; however, there are numerous ways that employers can encourage fitness in the workplace. These include permitting or encouraging individual fitness initiatives, sponsoring onsite or offsite fitness programs, and instituting fitness incentive programs.

Employee initiatives

Employees can take steps to improve their fitness at work: by making an effort to walk as far and as fast as possible during the working day; taking the stairs instead of the elevator; parking at the far end of the lot; and **walking** to confer with coworkers in person, rather than using the phone or e-mail. Many employees work out during lunch breaks or use shorter breaks for **stretching** or a brisk walk. Squeeze balls can tone the arms and hands while **sitting** at a desk. Resistance

KEY TERMS

Calorie—A unit of food energy.

Ergonomic—Furniture or equipment designed to interact effectively and safely with the human body.

Fitness ball—Exercise ball; Swiss ball; a large, well-inflated ball that can be used as a chair, as well as for performing various exercises.

Flextime—A variable work schedule that enables employees to schedule at least some of their own working hours.

Obesity—Excessive weight due to accumulation of fat, usually defined as a body mass index (BMI) of 30 or above or body weight greater than 30% above normal on standard height-weight tables.

Overweight—A body mass index (BMI) between 25 and 30.

Pedometer—Step counter; a device that counts each step taken by detecting hip motion.

Resistance bands—Exercise bands; elastic bands that are extended for exercising muscles and weight training.

Squeeze ball—Stress ball; a small rubber ball that is squeezed by the hand to exercise muscles and relieve stress.

Treadmill desk—A work desk built around a treadmill that enables the user to slowly walk while performing desk work.

bands, hand weights, or other small fitness equipment can be kept in a drawer for use during meetings. Some employees may be able to replace their office chair with a firmly inflated fitness or stability ball to improve balance and tone core muscles while sitting and for exercise during breaks. Others can position their computer screen on a stand and their keyboard on a table above a **treadmill** or use a specially designed treadmill desk.

Social networks and peer-to-peer encouragement can be excellent ways to promote fitness in the workplace. "Walking meetings" can be arranged indoors or out. Lunchtime walks with coworkers or friendly fitness competitions can be organized outside of the workplace hierarchy. The latter might involve wearing pedometers to count daily steps or logging time spent in physical activity.

Employees who travel for work should try to maintain the same fitness routine that they follow when at home. They should pack workout clothes, equipment, and exercise DVDs. Walking briskly through airport terminals between flights, walking up and down train cars, or doing laps around the ferryboat can add **pedometer** steps to travel. Frequent stretching and walking breaks can add exercise and reduce stress when driving for work. Hotels often have onsite or nearby fitness facilities, **swimming** pools, or hiking or **running** trails and guests can use the stairs and walk the hallways.

Workplace programs

Some employers have redesigned the workplace to promote fitness. Office spaces can be designed to encourage walking by employees. Some ergonomic desks function as simple weight machines with attached rubber or resistance bands. Standing workstations, exercise bikes attached to laptop stands, and treadmill desks are also available.

Walking meetings, known as "walk and talk" programs or structured ten-minute exercise breaks, sometimes called "instant recess," two or three times daily are one way employers promote fitness during the day. Some workplaces provide bicycles for lunchtime rides. Flexible scheduling can enable employees to workout whenever it is convenient, not just during lunch breaks. Workplaces without onsite fitness facilities can still hold onsite workshops, seminars, classes, and other programs or bring in fitness, **yoga**, or **t'ai chi** instructors. An increasing number of employers subsidize or reimburse gym memberships for their employees. Some even conduct individual fitness counseling interventions. Such simple initiatives as allowing employees to wear sneakers or running shoes and other casual clothing at work have been shown to significantly increase the number of steps taken during the workday. Finally, there are employer-sponsored sports teams that can be extended to walking and other exercise groups.

Worker incentive programs

Some companies offer employees financial incentives for achieving physical activity goals or sponsor employee participation in charitable runs or walks, such as Race for the Cure. Others reduce employee-paid health insurance premiums in return for participation in fitness programs or health screenings. There are many simple incentives, such as providing scales, **blood pressure** machines, and other measuring tools in the workplace. Some businesses give daily awards for employees who park the farthest from the building. Others institute employee challenges for using the stairs. Still others recognize employees who have reached their fitness goals.

Preparation

Whereas large organizations may be able to afford investments in expensive office equipment, facilities, and programs, there are many low- or no-cost options for small businesses to encourage employee fitness. There are various resources, both public and private, for helping businesses and employers develop practices that encourage employee physical fitness. For example, the American Diabetes Association's Winning at Work program provides employers with resources for helping their employees prevent or manage diabetes, including resources on physical fitness.

The National Prevention Strategy, released in June 2011, promotes workplace programs and policies for increasing employee physical fitness during the working day. These initiatives include:

- flextime
- lunchtime walking groups
- access to fitness facilities
- bicycle racks
- walking paths
- changing facilities with showers
- employer-sponsored community design or redesign to increase active transportation, including sites for physical fitness
- employer-sponsored parks, playgrounds, trails, and recreation programs

Risks

Unfortunately, many workplace fitness initiatives fail or achieve only very modest success. Failures are usually attributed to lack of employee engagement or inadequate employee motivation, since employee participation rates are generally below 10%.

The risk of not achieving higher rates of participation in workplace wellness programs is continued increases in obesity, diabetes, and heart disease. These health conditions in employees lead to further problems with absenteeism, poor productivity, and higher healthcare costs.

Results

Although initiatives to improve fitness in the workplace often fade away or fail outright, successful programs result in healthier, more productive employees, increased employee retention rates, and

QUESTIONS TO ASK YOUR DOCTOR

- Will improving my physical fitness reduce my healthcare costs and/or health insurance premiums?
- What are some ways I can increase my physical activity while at work?
- What steps can I take to encourage physical fitness among my employees?

reduced healthcare costs. Studies have shown that for every dollar spent on promoting health and fitness in the workplace, between US$2 and US$6 are returned to employers in reduced healthcare premiums, lower absenteeism, increased productivity and employee job satisfaction, and overall improvements in workplace morale. The most effective plans achieve net cost savings within three years and sometimes within just one year. The most effective programs for improving overall workforce fitness appear to be less organized approaches that promote more casual and incidental physical activity in and around the workplace.

An employee-sponsored health and fitness challenge in Rochester, New York, eventually grew to involve 125,000 employees from more than 300 businesses and other organizations. The employees walked a total of 49 billion steps and consumed 20 million cups of fruits and vegetables. The key to the program's success appeared to be that it was both collaborative and competitive, as well as fun and social. The latter may be particularly important, since research demonstrates that behaviors—both healthy and unhealthy—spread through social networks at a surprisingly efficient speed. Therefore, behavior modification programs seem to be most successful when they occur within social networks and involve peer support rather than individual interventions.

It remains unclear why some initiatives to improve fitness in the workplace have achieved remarkable successes, whereas others have suffered from low employee participation and, at most, only temporary changes in behavior. Financial incentives, especially those that lower employee-paid healthcare premiums, and social networking strategies may hold the most promise. More research is needed to define the components that make for successful workplace fitness programs with high participation rates.

Resources

BOOKS

Armiger, Phil. *Stretching for Functional Flexibility*. Philadelphia: Wolters Kluwer Health/Lippincott, Williams, & Wilkins, 2010.

Bray, Ilona M. *Healthy Employees, Healthy Business: Easy, Affordable Ways to Promote Workplace Wellness*. Berkeley, CA: Nolo, 2009.

PERIODICALS

Berry, Leonard L., Ann M. Mirabito,ÉandÉWilliam B. Baun. "What's the Hard Return on Employee Wellness Programs?" *Harvard Business Review* (December 2010).

Bill, D.E. "Instant Recess: Building a Fit Nation 10 Minutes at a Time." *Choice* 48, no. 10 (June 2011): 1953.

Bowers, Katherine. "'Me Time.'" *Working Mother* 33, no. 7 (October 2010): 88–92.

Conn, V.S. "Meta-Analysis of Workplace Physical Activity Interventions." *American Journal of Preventive Medicine* 37, no. 4 (2009): 330–39.

Gabel, Jon R., et al. "Obesity and the Workplace: Current Programs and Attitudes Among Employers and Employees." *Health Affairs* 28, no. 1 (January/February 2009): 46–56.

Kaplan, Ben. "Running for a Better Workplace; Science Backs Up What Top Entrepreneurs Have Always Known—Fitness is Good for the Mind." *Vancouver Sun* (April 16, 2011): G12.

Khazan, Olga. "Companies Tell Their Employees to Get a Move On." *Los Angeles Times* (May 15, 2011): A25.

Parker-Pope, Tara. "Sedentary Work Cited as Factor in Rising Obesity." *New York Times* (May 26, 2011): A1.

Tamim, H., et al. "T'ai Chi Workplace Program for Improving Musculoskeletal Fitness Among Female Computer Users." *Work* 34, no. 3 (2009): 331–38.

Wells, Susan J. "Does Work Make You Fat?" *HR Magazine* 55, no. 10 (October 2010): 26–31.

WEBSITES

Church, T.S., et al. "Trends over 5 Decades in U.S. Occupation-Related Physical Activity and Their Associations with Obesity." *PLoS ONE* 6, no. 5 (May 2011): e19657. http://www.plosone.org/article/info%3Adoi%2F10.1371%2Fjournal.pone.0019657 (accessed November 10, 2011).

National Employees Wellness Month. (June 2011). http://www.nationalemployeewellnessmonth.com (accessed November 10, 2011).

National Prevention, Health Promotion, and Public Health Council. HealthCare.gov http://www.healthcare.gov/prevention/nphpphc/index.html (accessed November 10, 2011).

"Office Exercise: How to Burn Calories at Work." Mayo Clinic. (September 24, 2009). http://www.mayoclinic.com/health/office-exercise/SM00115 (accessed November 10, 2011).

"Travel Workout: Fitness Tips for Business Travelers." Mayo Clinic. (July 23, 2010). http://www.mayoclinic.com/health/exercise/HQ01556_D (accessed November 10, 2011).

Winning at Work. American Diabetes Association. http://www.diabetes.org/in-my-community/programs/winning-at-work/ (accessed November 10, 2011).

ORGANIZATIONS

American Diabetes Association, 1701 N. Beauregard St., Alexandria, VA, 22311, (800) DIABETES (342-2383), AskADA@diabetes.org, http://www.diabetes.org.

U.S. Department of Health and Human Services, 200 Independence Ave., SW, Washington, DC, 20201, (877) 696-6775, http://www.hhs.gov.

Margaret Alic, PhD

Wrestling

Definition

Wrestling is a sport or contest in which two unarmed individuals struggle hand to hand with each other attempting to subdue or unbalance the other. Wrestling may consists of professional or amateur wrestlers. Widely recognized as the world's oldest competitive sport, amateur wrestling has featured in every Olympic games since its ancient conception.

Purpose

The principal object of wrestling is to overcome the opponent either by throwing or pinning him to the ground or by causing him to submit. Submission occurs when one opponent put the other in a submission hold, a maneuver that locks the other wrestler into a painful position. Eventually he or she will signal to the referee that the pain is too great, and will simply give up.

Demographics

According to the WWE, formerly World Wrestlng Entertainment, until WWE became its official name in 2011; 61% of wresting fans are male, 39% are women; 15% are ages 12–17, 67% are ages 18–49, 41% are males 18–34, 33% are non-white, 29% have a household income of US$75K or higher, and 15% have a household income of US$100K or higher.

WWE, Inc. is an American publicly traded, privately controlled entertainment company dealing primarily in professional wrestling. As of 2011, it is the

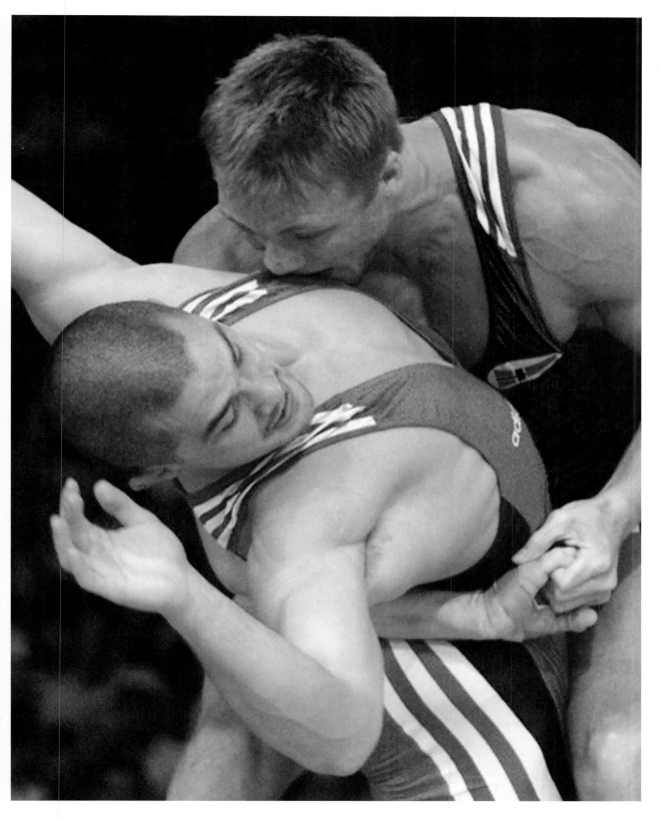

Wrestlers from Hungary and Norway test each other's strength at the Sydney 2000 Olympic Games in Australia. *(© Reuters/Corbis)*

largest professional wrestling company in the world, reaching 13 million viewers in the United States and broadcasting its shows in 30 languages to more than 145 countries. It promotes under two brands, known as Raw and SmackDown. Over the past quarter century, Vince and Linda E. McMahon have built the WWE from a small regional operation into a US$1.2 billion empire operating in 145 countries.

History

The Greeks engaged in a form of wrestling that is known today as freestyle wrestling. The Roman Empire adopted elements of Greek wrestling with an emphasis on brute strength, which is known as Greco-Roman wrestling. It requires wrestlers to perform all moves on the upper body only. Freestyle and Greco-Roman wrestling are the two international amateur forms practiced today in the Olympic Games. They have clear rules and weight classes. Points determine winners, and violations result in disqualifications.

In the United States, wrestling grew out of the traveling carnival strongman, who would challenge anyone to beat him in the ring, or even to last 10 minutes. Challengers almost never won the prize money, since the strongman had helpers who would cheat to ensure his victory. Eventually, carnies realized they could make more money off the crowd than the entry fees of the fighters. They started accepting wagers on the fights that were always fixed. Sometimes, the local fighter was even in on the fix, helping to hype the fight. These wrestlers used fake names and played up the animosity of the crowd to encourage betting. In 1901, the National Wrestling Association (NWA) was formed.

After WWII, the NWA divided wrestling into regional leagues. The leading league was the World Wide Wrestling Federation (WWWF). By the 1980s, there was only one league in existence, World Championship Wrestling. Today, the WWE is the largest wrestling organization in the world.

WrestleMania

WrestleMania is the Super Bowl of wrestling. It was first produced in 1985, and occurs annually in late March or early April as a professional wrestling pay-per-view event. All WrestleMania events are sold out within a short period of time, with recent editions being sold out within minutes of tickets going on sale. WrestleMania has also featured celebrity appearances with varying levels of involvement. In 2012, WrestleMania XXVIII took place in Miami, Florida, featuring The Rock and John Cera.

Description

Wrestling, a sport in which two competitors attempt to throw or immobilize each other by grappling, may consist of professional or amateur bouts. Unlike amateurs, professional (pro) wrestlers are paid. Professional wrestlers also are more skilled. A sporting commission regulates amateur wrestling, but professional wrestling is intentionally unregulated. In its early days, wrestling fell under the state sporting commission authority. League owners soon realized that they could avoid the hassle by classifying their shows as entertainment, not a competitive sport.

Professional wrestling does have rules, however, the rules are loosely defined and loosely enforced. The skills of the wrestlers do not determine the outcome of the match. Instead, writers work on plots and storylines well in advance, and every match is another chapter in the story. Who wins and who loses is all in the script. Professional wrestling matches are scripted, amateur matches are not.

Professional wrestling is in a boxing-like ring and it is scripted show for entertainment, for example WWE, TNA, and ROH. Amateur wrestling usually takes place on a gym mat in a one on one competition only. The outcome of matches are based on the athleticism of the wrestlers. Amateur wrestling matches are seen mostly in high schools, colleges, and the **Olympics**. In amateur wrestling, you cannot use pro wrestling moves. It is mostly about grappling and takedowns. At its highest level, professional wrestling is a combination of athletic display, scripted drama, and media spectacle.

Preparation

To become a wrestler, you must attend wrestling school. There are several schools scattered throughout the United States and Canada. Tuition is usually a few thousand dollars, and the training is extremely difficult. There will be constant endurance and weight training, combined with endless repetition of falls, slams and throws. Once a prospective wrestler has completed wrestling school, his instructor will use his contacts to try to place him in the major promotions. There are no guarantees. However, many graduates have to pay their dues in smaller promotions and work their way to the top.

Equipment

For professional wrestling, each opponent must wear tights for better movement and they can also be used for performance standout to show the wrestler's physique. Boots are worn to prevent angle strains and sprains. Kickpads are a thick leather (or imitation leather) pad worn over the shin to guard against kicks and other potentially damaging blows. Like most other pieces of wrestling gear, kick pads are available in a variety of patterns to complement the wrestler's character. The ring is the most important equipment in professional wrestling. It is a large square that is between 16 and 20 feet wide. The ring is surrounded by three to four ropes which prevent the athletes from falling off the raised platform. The ropes are also used for a variety of acrobatic stunts. To provide the surface needed, a thin foam mat is placed over the stiff platform that is supported by flexible steel beams. The beams flex to absorb the force of the athletes when they fall on it, helping to prevent injury. A canvas sheet is stretched over the platform, providing traction.

In the United States, high school and college wrestlers must wear a wrestling singlet, or a one-piece tight fitting lycra uniform; boots or shoes to prevent ankle injuries and to provide the best traction; kneepads are recommended; and mandatory headgear to protect the ears from cauliflower ear and other injuries. Wrestling is conducted on a padded mat that must have excellent shock absorption, tear resistance, and compression qualities. Most mats are made of PVC rubber nitrile foam. Recent advances in technology have brought about new mats made using closed cell, cross-linked polyethylene foam covered in vinyl backed with non-woven polyester.

Training and conditioning

To become a professional wrestler you will need an overall strong body to be able to take punishment. You must have great cardiovascular strength, as well as just being in good shape you need to be in "ring shape. This means you need to contact a professional wrestling school and sign up for wrestling lessons so your body can get used to taking bump from grappling and bouncing off of the ropes.

In order to increase strength as much as possible, **weightlifting** is a must. To get the best results in the weight room, compound, multi-joint exercises should be emphasized over single-joint, isolation type exercises. For most trainees, the only exercises that should be emphasized are variations of the squat, bench press, deadlift, military press, pullups, rows and dips. In

KEY TERMS

Babyface—The good guy or hero in a wrestling angle. This is the wrestler the fans are supposed to cheer for. A babyface is also known as a face for short.

Blading—The object used by wrestlers to cut themselves. Also, a term used to describe wrestlers cutting themselves to get blood in their matches. This is done to add drama to a match.

Booker—The person who writes (books) the wrestling angles. The booker decides who wins and loses the matches.

Gimmick match—A match with stipulations that differ from the normal rules (ex: steel cage match)

Grappling—Engage in a close fight or struggle without weapons.

Heel—The bad guy or villain in a match.

House show—An event that is not televised.

Push—When league management directs the storylines to make a certain wrestler a big star.

Selling—The art of making your opponents moves look as though they hurt.

Shoot—When something is done not according to the script. This can be either really trying to hurt your opponent or making comments out of character.

Smark—A fan that knows what goes on behind the scenes, but still enjoys watching the events.

Squash—A match in which a big name wrestles a nobody and beats him easily.

Turn—When a face becomes a heel or when a heel becomes a face.

Work—Anything in wrestling that follows the bookers script. The opposite of a shoot.

Worked Shoot—A work that has some real life elements in it. Anything in wrestling that follows the bookers script.

2007, research in the *Journal Sports Medicine* showed that lifting heavy weight for low reps has much more of a neural effect and is better for improving raw strength, while higher volume routines with less weight are better for building muscle. For a wrestler who wants to build strength but does not want to move up to a heavier weight class because of muscle gain, training with heavy weight in the low rep range is the superior option. Other training may include push-ups and other strength and muscle-building exercises.

Risks

Wrestling can be a dangerous sport and there are many risks associated with wrestling. For example:

• Professional wrestling can cause sudden deaths due to over exertion.

• It has been observed that people who have chosen professional wrestling as their career eventually develop health problems.

• Many wrestlers take painkillers to get temporary relief from these injuries but these painkillers give rise to a number of side effects.

• Some wrestlers have died due to extensive steroid use. Drugs and steroids are frequently taken by athletes to enhance the performance. Due to this, majority of wrestlers die in their middle age from steroid related illnesses.

• A lot of physical activity is involved in professional wrestling, making their bodies susceptible to injuries

• Stunts can go wrong causing serious injury, and sometimes death.

Results

Wrestling is one of the few sports that can be traced back to the beginnings of recorded history. There are cave drawings in France that are over 15,000 years old. Babylonians and Egyptians depict wrestling bouts where wrestlers are using most of the holds known to the modern-day sport. Today, people enjoy watching both professional and amateur wrestling. Some consider amateur wrestling more enjoyable because it does not include scripts, and

---

QUESTIONS TO ASK YOUR DOCTOR

• Is there a proper way of grappling to avoid injury?

• How is amateur wrestling different than professional?

• What are the major risks involved with wrestling?

• At what age should you stop wrestling?

• Can you get a closed head injury from wrestling?

---

according to some, is not fake. Nonetheless, wrestling is a sport that can build the strength and fame of the competitors, while providing entertainment for the viewers.

Resources

BOOKS

Albano, Captain Lou, et al. *The Complete Idiot's Guide to Pro Wrestling*. Alpha Books, 2000.

Lentz, Harris M. III. *Biographical Dictionary of Professional Wrestling*. McFarland, 1997.

Strauss, Gerry *Pro Wrestling: The Definitive Reference Guide*. Greenwood Press, 2012.

PERIODICALS

"A Senate Run Brings Wrestling Into Spotlight." *The New York Times*, July 15, 2010.

ORGANIZATIONS

WWE, 1241 East Main Street, Stamford, CT, 06902, (203) 352-8600, http://www.wwe.com.

Karl Finley

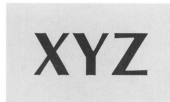

XYZ

Yoga

Definition

The term *yoga* comes from a Sanskrit word that means yoke or union. Traditionally, yoga is a method joining the individual self with the Divine, Universal Spirit, or Cosmic Consciousness. Physical and mental exercises are designed to help achieve this goal, also called self-transcendence or enlightenment. On the physical level, yoga postures, called *asanas*, are designed to tone, strengthen, and align the body. These postures are performed to make the spine supple and healthy and to promote blood flow to all the organs, glands, and tissues, keeping all the bodily systems healthy. On the mental level, yoga uses breathing techniques (*pranayama*) and meditation (*dyana*) to quiet, clarify, and discipline the mind. Yoga is not a religion, but a way of living with health and peace of mind as its aims.

Purpose

The purpose of yoga is to help individuals in all **age** groups improve strength and flexibility, rejuvenate the body, and work toward greater integration of soul and body as well as better physical health. Yoga can also be used as a complementary therapy for such disorders as osteoarthritis, lower back pain, depression, chronic headaches, high **blood pressure**, and **asthma**.

Demographics

Although yoga originated in a culture very different from modern America, it has been accepted and its practice has spread relatively quickly. A 2008 Roper poll, commissioned by *Yoga Journal*, found that 11 million Americans do yoga at least occasionally and six million perform it regularly. Yoga stretches are used by physical therapists and professional sports teams, and the benefits of yoga are being touted by movie stars and Fortune 500 executives. Many prestigious schools of medicine have studied and introduced yoga techniques as proven therapies for illness and stress. Some medical schools even offer yoga classes as part of their physician training program.

History

Yoga originated in ancient India and is one of the longest surviving philosophical systems in the world. Some scholars have estimated that yoga is as old as 5,000 years; artifacts detailing yoga postures have been found in India from over 3000 B.C. Yoga masters (yogis) claim that it is a highly developed science of healthy living that has been tested and perfected for all these years. Yoga was first brought to America in the late 1800s when Swami Vivekananda, an Indian teacher and yogi, presented a lecture on meditation in Chicago. Yoga slowly began gaining followers, and flourished during the 1960s when there was a surge of interest in Eastern philosophy. There has since been a vast exchange of yoga knowledge in America, with many students going to India to study and many Indian experts coming here to teach, resulting in the establishment of a wide variety of schools. Yoga is thriving, and it has become easy to find teachers and practitioners throughout America.

Description

Classical yoga is separated into eight limbs, each a part of the complete system for mental, physical, and spiritual well-being. Four of the limbs deal with mental and physical exercises designed to bring the mind in tune with the body. The other four deal with different stages of meditation. There are six major types of yoga, all with the same goals of health and harmony but with varying techniques: hatha, raja, karma, bhakti, jnana, and tantra yoga. **Hatha yoga** is the most commonly practiced branch of yoga in America. It is a highly developed system of nearly 200 physical postures, movements, and breathing techniques designed to tune the body to its optimal health. The yoga philosophy believes the breath to be the most important facet of health, as the breath is the largest source of *prana*, or

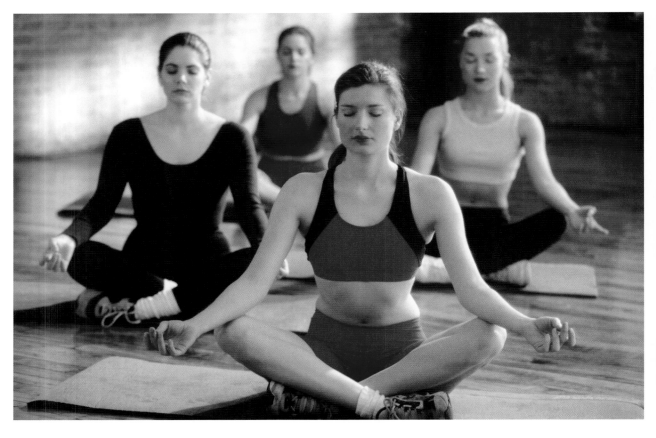

Women sit in sukhasana, or Easy Pose, during yoga. *(© Jose Luis Pelaez, Inc./Corbis)*

life force, and hatha yoga utilizes *pranayama*, which literally means the science or control of breathing. Hatha yoga was originally developed as a system to make the body strong and healthy enough to enable mental awareness and spiritual enlightenment.

There are several different schools of hatha yoga in America; the two most prevalent are Iyengar and ashtanga yoga. **Iyengar yoga** was founded by B.K.S. Iyengar, who is widely considered one of the great living innovators of yoga. Iyengar yoga puts strict emphasis on form and alignment, and uses traditional hatha yoga techniques in new manners and sequences. Iyengar yoga can be good for physical therapy because it allows the use of props like straps and blocks to make it easier for some people to get into the yoga postures. Ashtanga yoga can be a more vigorous routine, using a flowing and dance-like sequence of hatha postures to generate body heat, which purifies the body through sweating and deep breathing.

The other types of yoga show some of the remaining ideas that permeate yoga. Raja yoga strives to bring about mental clarity and discipline through meditation, simplicity, and non-attachment to worldly things and desires. Karma yoga emphasizes charity, service to others, non-aggression and non-harming as means to awareness and peace. Bhakti yoga is the path of devotion and love of God, or Universal Spirit. Jnana yoga is the practice and development of knowledge and wisdom. Finally, tantra yoga is the path of self-awareness through religious rituals, including awareness of sexuality as sacred and vital.

A typical hatha yoga routine consists of a sequence of physical poses, or asanas, and the sequence is designed to work all parts of the body, with particular emphasis on making the spine supple and healthy and increasing circulation. Hatha yoga asanas utilize three basic movements: forward bends, backward bends, and twisting motions. Each asana is named for a common thing it resembles, like the sun salutation, cobra, locust, plough, bow, eagle, and tree, to name a few. Each pose has steps for entering and exiting it, and each posture requires proper form and alignment. A pose is held for some time, depending on its level of difficulty and one's strength and stamina, and the practitioner is aware of when to inhale and exhale at certain points in each posture, as breathing properly is another fundamental

PATANJALI (SECOND CENTURY B.C.)

There is little historical information available on Patanjali, who is credited with developing yoga, one of the six systems of Hindu philosophy. Many scholars suggest several persons may have developed yoga under the pseudonym of Patanjali. In any case, Patanjali existed around 150 B.C. in India. He developed yoga based on a loose set of doctrines and practices from the Upanishads, themselves a set of mystical writings. The Upanishads are part of the Aranyakas, philosophical concepts that are part of the Veda, the most ancient body of literature of Hinduism. Patanjali gave these combined philosophical and esoteric writings a common foundation in his *Yoga Sutra*, a set of 196 concise aphorisms (wise sayings) that form the principles of yoga. He also drew upon Samkhya, the oldest classic system of Hindu philosophy. Patanjali's yoga accepted Samkhya metaphysics and the concept of a supreme soul. He established an eight-stage discipline of self-control and meditation. The individual sutras (verses) lay out the entire tradition of meditation. They also describe the moral and physical disciplines needed for the soul to attain absolute freedom from the body and self.

aspect of yoga. Breathing should be deep and through the nose. Mental concentration in each position is also very important for improving awareness, poise, and posture. During a yoga routine there is often a position in which to perform meditation, if deep relaxation is one of the goals of the sequence.

Yoga routines can take anywhere from 20 minutes to two or more hours, with one hour being a good time investment to perform a sequence of postures and a meditation. Some yoga routines, depending on the teacher and school, can be as strenuous as the most difficult workout, and some routines merely stretch and align the body while the breath and heart rate are kept slow and steady. Yoga achieves its best results when it is practiced as a daily discipline, and yoga can be a life-long **exercise** routine, offering deeper and more challenging positions as a practitioner becomes more adept. The basic positions can increase a person's strength, flexibility, and sense of well-being almost immediately, but it can take years to perfect and deepen them, which is an appealing and stimulating aspect of yoga for many.

Yoga is usually best learned from a yoga teacher or physical therapist, but it is simple enough that one can learn the basics from good books on the subject, which are plentiful. Yoga classes are generally inexpensive, averaging around US$20 per class, and students can learn basic postures in just a few classes. Many YMCAs, colleges, and community health organizations offer beginning yoga classes, often for nominal fees. If yoga is part of a physical therapy program, the cost may be reimbursed by insurance.

Many different schools of yoga have developed in America, and beginners should experiment with them to find the best-suited routine. Hatha yoga schools emphasize classical yoga postures, and raja yoga schools concentrate on mental discipline and meditation techniques. Beginners should search for teachers who show respect and are careful in their teaching, and should beware of instructors who push them into poses before they are ready.

Preparation

Yoga can be performed by individuals of any age and condition, although not all poses should be attempted by everyone. Yoga is a very accessible form of exercise; all that is needed is a flat floor surface large enough to stretch out on, a mat or towel, and enough overhead space to fully raise the arms. It is a good activity for those who can not go to gyms, who do not like other forms of exercise, or have very busy schedules. Yoga should be done on an empty stomach, and teachers recommend waiting three or more hours after meals. Loose and comfortable clothing should be worn.

Risks

People with injuries, medical conditions, or spinal problems should consult a doctor before beginning yoga. Those with medical conditions should find a yoga teacher who is familiar with their type of problem and who is willing to give them individual attention. Pregnant women can benefit from yoga, but should always be guided by an experienced teacher. Certain yoga positions should not be performed with a fever, or during menstruation.

Beginners should use care and concentration when performing yoga postures, and not try to stretch too much too quickly, as injury could result. Some advanced yoga postures, like the headstand and full lotus position, can be difficult and require strength, flexibility, and gradual preparation, so beginners should get the help of a teacher before attempting them.

GALE ENCYCLOPEDIA OF FITNESS

937

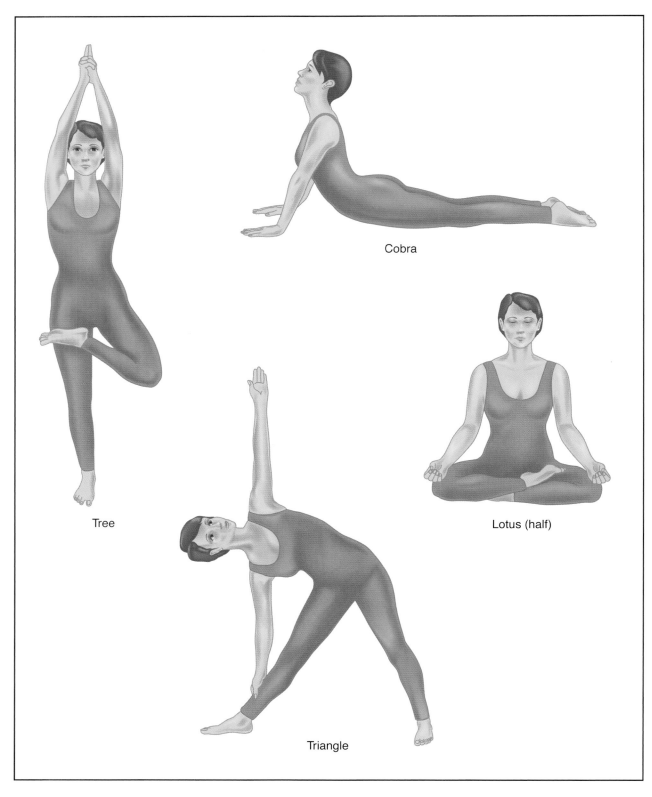

Tree

Cobra

Lotus (half)

Triangle

These poses are an introduction to the variety of ways the body can be used to achieve optimal health through the practice of yoga. *(Illustration by Electronic Illustrators Group. Reproduced by permission of Gale, a part of Cengage Learning.)*

KEY TERMS

Asana—A position or stance in yoga.

Dyana—The yoga term for meditation.

Hatha yoga—Form of yoga using postures, breathing methods and meditation.

Meditation—Technique of concentration for relaxing the mind and body.

Pranayama—Yogic breathing techniques.

Yogi (feminine, yogini)—A trained yoga expert.

In yoga, it does not matter how a person does in comparison with others, but how aware and disciplined one becomes with one's own body and limitations. Proper form and alignment should always be maintained during a stretch or posture, and the stretch or posture should be stopped when there is pain, dizziness, or **fatigue**. The mental component of yoga is just as important as the physical postures. Concentration and awareness of breath should not be neglected. Yoga should be done with an open, gentle, and non-critical mind; when one stretches into a yoga position, it can be thought of as accepting and working on one's limits. Impatience, self-criticism, and comparing oneself to others does not help in this process of self-knowledge. While performing the yoga of breathing (pranayama) and meditation (dyana), it is best to have an experienced teacher, as these powerful techniques can cause dizziness and discomfort when done improperly.

Some people have reported injuries by performing yoga postures without proper form or concentration, or by attempting difficult positions without working up to them gradually or having appropriate supervision. Beginners sometimes report muscle soreness and fatigue after performing yoga, but these side effects diminish with practice. The National Center for Complementary and Alternative Medicine (NCCAM) recommends that anyone considering any form of yoga practice should consult their health care provider before starting the program. They should not use yoga as a substitute for conventional medical treatment and they should not postpone seeing a doctor about any health problem they already have. It is important to ask the instructors at a yoga studio about their training and certification, and about the physical demands associated with the type of yoga taught in the studio.

Results

Yoga has been used to alleviate problems associated with high blood pressure, high **cholesterol**, migraine

QUESTIONS TO ASK YOUR DOCTOR

- In what way do you think yoga will benefit me?
- Do I have any physical limitations that would prohibit my undertaking yoga?
- Is there anything in my present or past medical history that I should tell the instructor?
- What tests or evaluation techniques will you perform to see if yoga has been beneficial for me?
- Will yoga interfere with my current medications?
- What symptoms are important enough that I should seek immediate treatment?

headaches, asthma, shallow breathing, backaches, constipation, diabetes, menopause, multiple sclerosis, varicose veins, and many chronic illnesses. It also has been studied and approved for its ability to promote relaxation and reduce stress. However, some researchers are now questioning claims that yoga is beneficial for such conditions as carpal tunnel syndrome.

The use of yoga is increasingly recommended for dysmenorrhea (pain during menstruation), premenstrual syndrome (physical or emotional symptoms that typically begin about one week before menstruation), and other disorders in premenopausal women in Europe and in the United States.

Yoga can provide the same benefits as any well-designed exercise program—increasing general health and stamina, reducing stress, and improving those conditions brought about by sedentary lifestyles. It has the added advantage of being a low-impact activity that uses only gravity as resistance, which makes it an excellent physical therapy routine; certain yoga postures can be safely used to strengthen and balance all parts of the body.

Meditation has been studied and approved for its benefits in reducing stress-related conditions. The landmark book, *The Relaxation Response*, by Harvard cardiologist Herbert Benson, showed that meditation and breathing techniques for relaxation could have the opposite effect of stress, reducing blood pressure and other indicators. Since then, much research has reiterated the benefits of meditation for stress reduction and general health. The American Medical Association recommends meditation techniques as a first step before medication for borderline **hypertension** cases. Some studies indicate that yogic meditation by itself is effective in lowering serum cholesterol and blood pressure.

Modern psychological studies have shown that even slight facial expressions can cause changes in the involuntary nervous system; yoga utilizes this mind/body connection. That is, yoga practice contains the central ideas that physical posture and alignment can influence a person's mood and self-esteem, and that the mind can be used to shape and heal the body. Yoga practitioners claim that the strengthening of mind/body awareness can bring eventual improvements in all facets of a person's life.

Resources

BOOKS

Bradbury, Alan. *Starting Yoga: A Practical Foundation Guide for Men and Women.* Wiltshire UK: Crowood Press, 2011.

Butera, Robert J. *The Pure Heart of Yoga: Ten Essential Steps for Personal Transformation.* Woodbury, MN: Llewellyn Publications, 2009.

Coulter, David H. *Anatomy of Hatha Yoga: A Manual for Students, Teachers, and Practitioners.* Honesdale, PA: Body and Breath, Inc., 2010.

Lark, Liz. *Personal Trainer: Yoga for Life.* London: Carlton Publishing Group, 2011.

Iyenger, B. K. S. *Yoga Wisdom & Practice.* New York: DK Publishing, 2009.

Philp, John. *Yoga Inc.: A Journey through the Big Business of Yoga.* New York: Penguin Global, 2010.

Rountree, Sage. *The Athlete's Pocket Guide to Yoga: 50 Routines for Flexibility, Balance, and Focus.* Boulder, CO: VeloPress, 2009.

Singleton, Mark. *Yoga Body: The Origins of Modern Posture Practice.* New York: Oxford University Press, 2010.

Williams, Nancy. *Yoga Therapy for Every Special Child: Meeting Needs in a Natural Setting.* Philadelphia: Jessica Kingsley Publishers, 2010.

PERIODICALS

Engebretson, J. "Culture and Complementary Therapies" *Complementary Therapies in Nursing and Midwifery* 8 (November 2002): 177–184.

Gerritsen, A. A., M. C. de Krom, M. A. Struijs, et al. "Conservative Treatment Options for Carpal Tunnel Syndrome: A Systematic Review of Randomized Controlled Trials." *Journal of Neurology* 249 (March 2002): 272–280.

Kronenberg, F., and A. Fugh-Berman. "Complementary and Alternative Medicine for Menopausal Symptoms: A Review of Randomized, Controlled Trials." *Annals of Internal Medicine* 137 (November 19, 2002): 805–813.

Manocha, R., G. B. Marks, P. Kenchington, et al. "Sahaja Yoga in the Management of Moderate to Severe Asthma: A Randomized Controlled Trial." *Thorax* 57 (February 2002): 110–115.

Raub, J. A. "Psychophysiologic Effects of Hatha Yoga on Musculoskeletal and Cardiopulmonary Function: A Literature Review." *Journal of Alternative and Complementary Medicine* 8 (December 2002): 797–812.

Vyas, R., and N. Dikshit. "Effect of Meditation on Respiratory System, Cardiovascular System and Lipid Profile." *Indian Journal of Physiology and Pharmacology* 46 (October 2002): 487–491.

WEBSITES

Pizer, Ann. "Yoga Poses for Menstruation." About.com. (July 29, 2011). http://yoga.about.com/od/yogatherapy/tp/Yoga-Poses-For-Menstruation.htm (accessed November 17, 2011).

Yoga Finder Online. *http://www.yogafinder.com* (accessed November 17, 2011).

ORGANIZATIONS

American Yoga Association, P.O. Box 19986, Sarasota, FL, 34276, info@americanyogaassociation.org, http://www.americanyogaassociation.org.

International Association of Yoga Therapists (IAYT), 4150 Tivoli Ave., Los Angeles, CA, 90066

National Center for Complementary and Alternative Medicine (NCCAM), 9000 Rockville Pike, Bethesda, MD, 20892, info@nccam.nih.gov, http://nccam.nih.gov.

Yoga Journal, P.O. Box 51151, Boulder, CO, 80322-1151, (303) 604-7435, http://www.yogajournal.com.

Yoga Research and Education Center (YREC), 2400A County Center Dr., Santa Rosa, CA, 95403, (707) 566-0000, http://www.yrec.org.

Douglas Dupler, MA
Rebecca J. Frey, PhD
Laura Jean Cataldo, RN, EdD

Youth sports

Definition

The term youth sports refers to sports programs designed specifically for young people. Although no consistent definition is available, the term youth most commonly applies to boys and girls under the age of 18.

Purpose

The major purpose of youth sports programs is to provide young people with an opportunity to participate in a sport of their own choosing, under adequate adult supervision, as a form of recreation. For some small percentage of participants in youth sports programs, such programs also provide an entre into the more competitive field of professional sports at some later time in their lives.

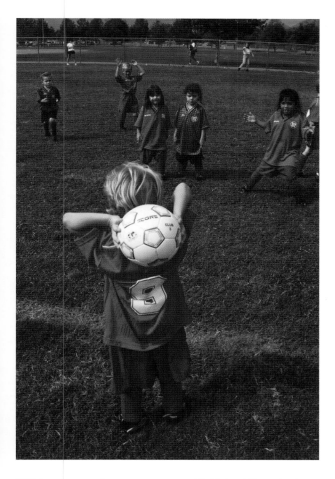

Children engage in a soccer game. *(© Richard Cummins/ Corbis)*

Demographics

In 2008, the National Council of Youth Sports conducted a survey of its members to determine participation in youth sports programs in the United States. That study found that the 112 member organizations that responded reported a total of 44,031,080 participants, of whom two-thirds were boys and one-third, girls. By comparison, a similar survey conducted ten years earlier found a total of 32,822,352 participants, with an almost identical boy/girl breakdown. The age distribution of participants was almost the same for boys and girls, with the largest group being those between the ages of 16 and 18 (35 percent and 39 percent, respectively), followed by the 10-12 age group (23 and 19 percent), and 13-15 age group (17 and 12 percent). The study found that only in the youngest age group, 6 and under, was there a decrease in inequity between boy and girl participation between 1997 and 2008.

A more recent study by the National Sporting Goods Association provides information about the most popular sports among young Americans. In that study, completed in 2010, the most popular sport among boys and girls under the age of 19 was bicycle riding, with 39,789,000 participants, followed by bowling (38,980,000) and freshwater fishing (29,927,000). Better known sports had significantly fewer participants, including **baseball** (12,533,000), **basketball** (26,875,000), **golf** (21,872,000), tackle **football** (9,318,000), **ice hockey** (3,299,000), and **soccer** (13,534,000). Obviously, individual sports, such as bicycling and bowling, are likely to have more participants since they do not require the organization of groups of people to play a sport.

History

Boys and girls have, of course, participated in sports for as long as sports existed. Organized sports, such as Little League Baseball and Pop Warner Football, are, however, more recent phenomena. Local, regional, and national organizations devoted to the supervision and promotion of youth sports are an even more recent development. The National Alliance for Youth Sports, for example, was founded in 1981 to focus on training adult coaches to work in a variety of youth sports. The mission of the organization now is "to make the sports experience safe, fun and healthy for all children." The National Council of Youth Sports was founded in 1979 to provide a unified voice for amateur youth sports. It currently is a membership organization with 185 members. Some individual youth sports organizations are older than they two national organizations. For example, Little League Baseball was founded in June 1939 and now consists of an estimated 2.2 million players worldwide in more than 7,000 leagues.

Description

Youth sports is a very large field that includes opportunities for boys and girls under the age of 19 to participate in virtually every type of sporting activity. Some examples of organizations subsumed under this term are Little League Baseball (which itself has a number of divisions that include Tee Ball, Minor League Baseball, 9–10 Year Old Baseball, Junior League Baseball, Senior League Baseball, Big League Baseball, the Challenger Division, and Girls and Boys **Softball**); Babe Ruth Baseball, Dixie Youth Baseball, Pony Baseball, American Youth Football, Pop Warner Football, the NIKE Elite Youth Basketball League, the American Youth Soccer Organization, and the Junior National Team Squads of the USA **Field Hockey** organization.

In addition to well-known national organizations such as these, there are an almost endless list of local and regional youth sport organizations. As an example, the DMOZ online Open Directory Project lists almost 2,000 individual leagues for youth baseball, basketball, football, hockey, wrestling, and many other sports. As an example, the youth ice hockey page lists 116 leagues ranging from the Alaska Allstar Hockey Association and Alexandria Area Hockey Association to the Wilmette Hockey Association and York Ice Hockey Club. Even that list is probably not inclusive of all such leagues and organizations in the United States.

Each youth sports organizations has its own goals and activities. As an example, the National Alliance of Youth Sports has a Start Smart program for young participants and parents designed to help boys and girls get started in one or another sport, and to help parents guide their children in this endeavor. The organization currently offers two specialized activities in that program. One, called Start Smart Sports Development provides recreation agencies with motor skill development programs that help children get ready for sports such as baseball, basketball, football, soccer, tennis, and golf. The second program is called Start Smart at Home that has suggestion as to how parents can prepare their children for participation in various sporting activities. The National Council for Youth Sports offers resources for the development of adult volunteer participation in youth sports and promotes safety education for participants in youth sports.

Risks

The issue of physical injuries to boys and girls who participate in sports is one of considerable importance. Young people's bodies are still growing and so there is likely to be an increased risk for physical injury not experienced by older competitors. In addition, many young participants are less experienced and less skillful than are older players. An overview of the extent of the risk to young participants in sporting activities was provided at the December 2010 conference of the National Athletic Trainers' Association. A special committee studying youth sport injuries gave the nation a grade of C+ for its efforts in preventing such injuries. The committee pointed out that an average of 8,000 young people are treated in emergency departments each day of the year as a result of sporting injuries. On average 63,000 young people suffer brain injuries during sporting events each year, and in 2010, 48 youths died while participating in sporting events, about half of them as the result of a brain injury. The committee also noted that high school

athletes suffer injuries at a rate twice that of college-level athletes. Gender differences are also not uncommon in youth sport injuries. For example, female basketball players are 240 percent as likely to suffer from a physical injury than are male basketball players (a total of 13,000 such injuries in 2010).

Resources

BOOKS

Ginsburg, Richard D., Stephen Durant, and Amy Baltzell. *Whose Game Is It, Anyway?: A Guide to Helping Your Child Get the Most from Sports, Organized by Age and Stage.* Boston: Houghton Mifflin, 2006.

Harris, Sally S., Steven J. Anderson, and Andrew J. M. Gregory. *Care of the Young Athlete.* Elk Grove Village, IL: American Academy of Pediatrics, 2010.

Herring, Stanley A. *Youth Sports Concussions.* Philadelphia: Saunders, 2012.

Hyman, Mark. *Until It Hurts: America's Obsession with Youth Sports and How It Harms Our Kids.* Boston: Beacon Press, 2009.

Patel, Dilip R., et al., eds. *Adolescence and Sports.* New York: Nova Science Publishers, 2010.

WEBSITES

National Athletic Trainers' Association Issues 2010 Report Card on the Youth Sports Safety Crisis at Washington, D.C., Summit Source. http://www.nata.org/NR120710b (accessed October 17, 2011).

Sports: Youth and High School Source. http://www.dmoz.org/Sports/Youth_and_High_School/ (accessed October 17, 2011).

Troubling Signals from Youth Sports Source. http://sportsforalifetime.com/troublingsignals.pdf (accessed October 17, 2011).

ORGANIZATIONS

National Council of Youth Sports, 7185 S.E. Seagate Lane, Stuart, FL, 34997, 1(772) 781-1452, Fax: 1(772) 781-7298, youthsports@ncys.org, http://www.ncys.org/index.php.

National Alliance For Youth Sports, 2050 Vista Pkwy, West Palm Beach, FL, 33411, 1(561) 684-1141, Fax: 1(561) 684-2546, (800) 729-2057, nays@nays.org, http://www.nays.org/index.cfm.

David E. Newton, A.B., M.A., Ed.D

Zumba

Definition

Zumba is a form of aerobic **dance exercise** similar to Jazzercise; its distinctive characteristic is its use of Latin American music and dance rhythms to create a party-like atmosphere in class sessions. The name comes from a Colombian slang word meaning "to buzz like a bee" or "fast-moving."

Purpose

Zumba appeals to people's wish to have fun while exercising as well as lose weight and improve their overall fitness, flexibility, and endurance. The program's official slogan is "Ditch the Workout, Join the Party!" Some forms of Zumba involve resistance training intended to build strength while the more basic forms are lower-impact and usually slower-paced.

Demographics

According to the Zumba website, as of July 2009 there are 5 million people participating in Zumba classes at 40,000 locations in 75 different countries around the world. It is likely that most of these are young or middle-aged adults, although Zumba has also introduced special programs for children and seniors.

In the United States, Zumba appears to have a special appeal for Hispanics, although there are no precise statistics about ethnic or racial groups represented in most Zumba classes. Although classes are open to men and women, most Zumba instructors in North America are women, as are the majority of class participants.

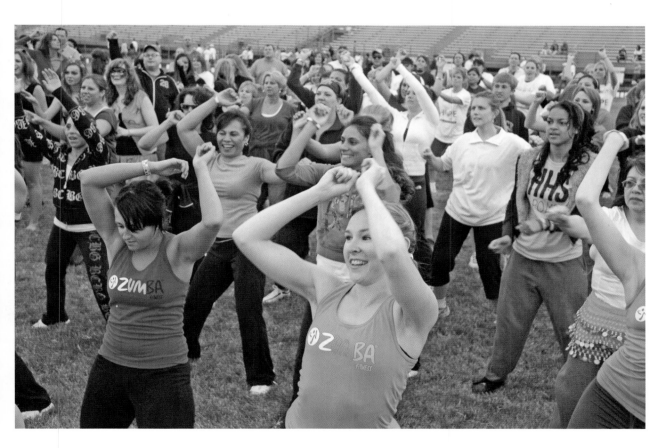

Participants enjoy an outdoor Zumba session. (© Pete Selkowe)

Precautions

People should always check with their primary care physician before beginning any exercise program, including an aerobic program like Zumba. Children and seniors should ask about the special Zumba classes available for their **age** groups. Children should be at least 4 years old to participate in a Zumba children's class.

People who have **arthritis** or other disorders affecting the knee joint should check with their doctor before taking a Zumba class, as the dance routines involve frequent pivoting on the knee joint.

Description

Zumba is a form of aerobic fitness exercise based on Latin American dance rhythms. Participants are taught some basic easy-to-learn movements; they do not have to learn complicated balance techniques or body poses as in **yoga**. The simplicity of the movements is part of the program's appeal, as one instructor explains: "[Zumba] is easy to follow so people don't have to think too much about what they're doing and can just get into it. And the music makes you want to dance." In addition, participants do not need a partner to learn or perform the basic dance steps.

Zumba classes

Zumba classes in North America are offered in a wide variety of locations across the United States and Canada. Most are held in dance studios or fitness centers, although classes are also offered in community centers, senior centers, and college physical education departments. The average fee per class is $10–$15, although a few instructors charge as little as $5 per class.

The average Zumba class session is an hour in length. Participants usually wear standard workout gear (most often T-shirts and loose pants) for vigorous exercise, as the room can get quite warm during a class. Sneakers or fitness shoes are worn to prevent slipping on the dance floor. The company also markets a line of clothing called Zumbawear, which includes caps and headbands as well as crop tops, T-shirts, muscle shirts, capri pants, and cargo pants. An hour-long class alternates between fast and slow dance rhythms and incorporates a variety of musical styles to keep the session interesting. The four basic dance styles are salsa, merengue, cumbia, and reggaeton, with some rumba, mamba, flamenco, and calypso rhythms mixed in.

Practicing at home

People who want to practice Zumba at home can order one or more DVDs (US$10 each). There are four: Original Soundtrack, Vibe Tribe, Cardio Party, and Party Nation.

Zumba instructors

Zumba instructors are trained at Zumba Academy, which is not a brick-and-mortar institution but the company's name for the various workshops offered around North America to train Zumba instructors. Zumba requires prospective instructors to be 18 years of age or older (16- and 17-year-olds can attend a workshop with a letter of permission from their parent(s) and signing a liability form.) The instructors do not need to have taken a Zumba class themselves; they need only complete an eight-hour workshop satisfactorily. Instructors must renew their Zumba certification annually, either by attending another workshop or by preparing to teach one of the more specialized Zumba fitness routines. The average cost to the instructor of attending a Zumba workshop is $225–$260, in addition to transportation costs.

Although Zumba encourages instructors to acquire a general group exercise certification either from the American Council on Exercise (ACE) or the Aerobics and Fitness Association of America (AFAA) on the grounds that many fitness centers and gyms require all personnel to have such certification, ACE or AFAA credentials are not needed to become a Zumba instructor.

Presently, there are six types of workshops that instructors may take:

- Zumba Basic Steps Level 1: Instructors learn how to teach the four basic Zumba rhythms and steps.
- Zumba Basic Steps Level 2: Instructors learn four more rhythms to incorporate into their classes and how to do their own choreography.
- Zumba Gold: Instructors learn how to work with older adults who are still active. This program is also intended for younger adults who are deconditioned and unused to exercise.
- Zumba Toning: Instructors learn how to offer faster-paced and more intense workouts intended for participants interested in body sculpting and toning. This program involves the use of weighted toning sticks to add to the rhythm and build strength.
- Aqua Zumba: Aqua Zumba is a form of Zumba modified for fitness workouts in a swimming pool.
- Zumbatomic: Zumbatomic is the children's version of Zumba, for children from 4 to 12 years of age. Instructors are given tips about class management and discipline as well as dance techniques appropriate for this age group.

KEY TERMS

Aerobic fitness—A measure of the amount of oxygen delivered to muscle tissue to keep it working. Any type of exercise that raises the heart rate and keeps it up for a period of time improves aerobic fitness.

Cumbia—A type of folk dance that developed along the Caribbean coast of Colombia.

Merengue—A style of Latin American music and dance with a two-step beat.

Reggaeton—A form of urban music that developed in Panama and blends reggae from the West Indies with musical influences derived from salsa, cumbia, and merengue.

Resistance training—A form of strength training that uses some form of physical resistance to muscular contraction in order to build up muscular strength.

Salsa—A type of Latin American music and dance that originated in Cuba and became popular in the 1960s among Cuban and Puerto Rican immigrants in New York City.

Origins

Zumba originated in Cali, Colombia, in the late 1990s with a dance and fitness instructor named Alberto (Beto) Pérez. On his way to teaching an aerobics class one day, he realized he had forgotten his usual tapes. He improvised by playing salsa and meringue music recorded by various popular bands. The class enjoyed the dance music so much that they didn't want to go back to the old rigid aerobics tapes.

Pérez moved to Miami, Florida, in 1999 and began teaching his new combination of dance and resistance training there. In 2001, he was approached by two entrepreneurs, Alberto Perlman and Alberto Aghion, to create a worldwide fitness company based on his new approach to exercise. In 2002, the company began to advertise, resulting in wide demand for Zumba classes across the United States. The need for a large number of new instructors led the company to develop its training workshops. Zumba expanded into the Hispanic market in the United States in 2003 and 2004, and went worldwide in 2007. Since 2004, it has offered DVDs for people to use at home.

Preparation

No particular preparation is needed for taking a Zumba class other than a basic health checkup.

QUESTIONS TO ASK YOUR DOCTOR

- What is your opinion of Zumba?
- Is Zumba safe for older adults?
- Have any of your other patients tried Zumba?
- What are the benefits of aerobic exercise?

Aftercare

No particular aftercare is needed other than showering and changing clothes.

Risks

The main risk from a Zumba workout is to the knee joint (assuming the person is otherwise fit and has no chronic cardiovascular or respiratory disorders). Participants are advised to wear shoes without a flat base to minimize stress on the knee joint.

Results

Zumba appears to maintain a long-lasting appeal with most people who try it. Some report losing considerable amounts of weight, while others maintain that the upbeat music and lively rhythm of the movements are a form of emotional as well as physical therapy. One instructor is quoted as saying that "People love it and get addicted to it."

Research and general acceptance

Most media accounts of Zumba have appeared in general-interest newspapers or women's magazines. There are no published studies of Zumba in the mainstream medical literature most likely because this form of exercise became popular worldwide only after 2005. As of November 2009, however, there was one clinical trial in progress sponsored by the Mayo Clinic and the Alzheimer's Association. The trial is intended to determine whether Zumba is superior to an educational program on exercise in improving attention and memory functioning in carriers and noncarriers of a gene associated with **Alzheimer's disease** (APOE e4).

Caregiver concerns

Caregiver concerns regarding seniors or children are to make sure that they are basically healthy enough for aerobic exercise, do not have any major cardiovascular, respiratory, or musculoskeletal disorders, and are enrolled in the appropriate Zumba class for their age group.

Resources

BOOKS

Pérez, Beto. *Zumba: Ditch the Workout, Join the Party: The Zumba Weight Loss Program.* New York: Wellness Central, 2009.

OTHER

Alexander, Jane. "Get Fit Dancing: Dance to a Different Beat with Zumba." *Telegraph (UK)*, March 30, 2009. http://www.telegraph.co.uk/health/dietandfitness/5050441/Get-fit-dancing-Dance-to-a-different-beat-with-Zumba.html

Fortin, Judy. "Zumba Zooms to the Top of the Exercise World." *CNN News*, December 9, 2008. http://edition.cnn.com/2008/HEALTH/diet.fitness/09/22/hm.zumba.dance.exercise/

Navarro, Mireya. "Samba Lines at the Gym." *New York Times*, July 10, 2008. http://www.nytimes.com/2008/07/10/fashion/10fitness.html?_r = 1&pagewanted = all

ORGANIZATIONS

Aerobics and Fitness Association of America (AFAA), 15250 Ventura Blvd., Suite 200, Sherman Oaks, CA, 91403, 877-968-7263, http://www.afaa.com/.

American Council on Exercise (ACE), 4851 Paramount Drive, San Diego, CA, 92123, 858-279-8227, 888-825-3636, Fax: 858-279-8064, http://www.acefitness.org/default.aspx.

Zumba Fitness, LLC., 3801 North 29th Avenue, Hollywood, FL, 33020, 954-925-3755, Fax: 954-925-3505, http://www.zumba.com/us/.

Rebecca J. Frey, PhD

GLOSSARY

The glossary is an alphabetical compilation of terms and definitions listed in the *Key Terms* sections of the main body entries. Although the list is comprehensive, it is by no means exhaustive.

A

ABDOMINAL. Relating to the muscles in the abdomen.

ABDUCT. To pull away.

ABDUCTION. To pull away.

ABNORMAL HEART RHYTHM. Refers to an irregularity in the normal beating pattern of the heart.

ACCELEROMETER. An instrument typically worn on the trunk or limbs that determines physical activity. Measurement is obtained by quantifying the acceleration and deceleration of the body.

ACCLIMATIZE. The process of adapting to a new climate, altitude, or temperature.

ACETYL COA. Acetyl-coenzyme A; a molecule with various functions in metabolism, including transporting carbon (acetyl) groups from the beta-oxidation of fatty acids to the citric acid cycle for further breakdown.

ACETYLCHOLINE. A chemical messenger of the nervous system that is also known as a neurotransmitter.

ACHILLES TENDINITIS. An inflammation of the Achilles tendon—the strong tendon connecting the calf muscles to the heel bone—that occurs with overuse of the affected limb (posterior leg).

ACHILLES TENDON. The tendon that connects the heel bone to the calf muscles, also known as tendo calcaneus.

ACIDOSIS. Excess acidity in muscle due to an accumulation of protons from ATP hydrolysis, causing muscle soreness and fatigue.

ACROSOME. A compartment in the head of the sperm that contains enzymes that allow the sperm to penetrate the protective layers of an egg.

ACTIN. A protein found in muscle tissue involved in the process of muscle function.

ACTINIC KERATOSIS. A condition of premalignant lesions resulting from excessive sun damage and usually occurring after middle age. It lesions are flaky, scaly, or warty in nature and may result in malignancy.

ACTIVE ISOLATED STRETCHING: AIS. A stretching technique that relaxes and lengthens a muscle group by working the opposing group, usually with a rope or strap.

ACTIVITIES OF DAILY LIVING (ADLS). Refers to the daily self-care activities performed by an individual in his/her place of residence and in outdoor environments; people with disabilities and the elderly are often classified as to whether than can or cannot perform ADLs.

ACTIVITY ENERGY EXPENDITURE (AEE). The component of total energy expenditure that refers to the energy expenditure resulting from physical activities.

ACUPRESSURE. A form of acupuncture in which certain points of the body are pressed with the fingers and hands to release energy blocks.

ACUPUNCTURE. An ancient Chinese alternative medicine technique that treats conditions by inserting and manipulating thin needles under the skin.

ADAPTED SPORT. A sport whose equipment, rules, or other characteristics have been changed in some way or another to make it more amenable to play by a disabled person.

ADDUCT. To pull toward the center of the body.

ADDUCTION. The act of pulling toward the center body line.

ADDUCTOR. Any of the three strong triangular muscles of the inside of the thigh.

ADENOSINE TRIPHOSPHATE (ATP). A nucleotide with three high-energy phosphate groups that supplies cellular energy by undergoing enzymatic hydrolysis to adenosine diphosphate (ADP) and adenosine monophosphate (AMP).

ADIPOCYTE. Fat cell.

ADIPOSE. Fat.

ADIPOSE TISSUE. Fat cell tissue.

ADP. Adenosine diphosphate; a nucleotide with two phosphate groups that is converted to and from ATP to store and release cellular energy, respectively.

ADRENAL GLAND. An endocrine gland located above each kidney. The inner part of each gland secretes epinephrine (adrenaline) and the outer part secretes steroid hormones.

ADRENAL GLANDS. The two glands located on top of the kidneys that secrete steroid hormones.

ADRENALINE. Epinephrine.

ADRENERGIC. A substance that acts similarly to epinephrine or that is stimulated by epinephrine.

ADRENOCORTICOTROPIC HORMONE (ACTH). A hormone secreted by the pituitary gland that stimulates the adrenal gland to release epinephrine.

AED. Automatic external defibrillator.

AEROBIC. Strenuous physical exercise that results in a significant increase in respiration and heart rate.

AEROBIC CAPACITY. VO_2max; cardiorespiratory fitness; the maximum amount of oxygen that can be transported by the heart, lungs, and blood to the muscles and utilized by the muscles during exercise.

AEROBIC EXERCISE. Activity that increases the body's requirement for oxygen, thereby increasing respiration and heart rate.

AEROBIC FITNESS. A measure of the amount of oxygen delivered to muscle tissue to keep it working. Any type of exercise that raises the heart rate and keeps it up for a period of time improves aerobic fitness.

AEROBIC RESPIRATION. A form of respiration that uses oxygen to generate energy in the body.

AGGRESSIVE INLINE SKATING. A form of inline skating that involves a variety of challenging maneuvers performed on city streets, in parks, or in a quarter pipe, half pipe, bowl, or other specially built facility.

AGILITY. Moving with quickness.

AGITATION. Excessive restlessness or emotional disturbance that is often associated with anxiety or psychosis; common in middle-stage AD.

AGNOSIA. Inability to recognize familiar people, places, and objects.

AIKIDO. A Japanese martial art of self-defense that uses mainly the arms and hands to immobilize and throw an opponent.

ALBUMIN. A protein in the blood that transports fatty acids to muscle cells.

ALENDRONATE. A non-hormonal drug used to treat osteoporosis in postmenopausal women.

ALKALOSIS. Excessive alkalinity of the blood and body tissue.

ALLERGEN. Any substance that provokes an allergic response.

ALLEVIATE. To make something easier to be endured.

ALPHA-LIPOIC ACID. An antioxidant produced in the body and obtained from the diet that recycles vitamin C in the body.

ALZHEIMER'S DISEASE. A degenerative brain disease of unknown cause that is the most common form of dementia, and that usually starts in late middle to old age, and that results in progressive memory loss, impaired thinking, disorientation, and changes in personality and mood.

AMENORRHEA. Abnormal absence or stopping of menstrual cycles.

AMINO ACIDS. Small organic molecules that are the building blocks of proteins. There are 20 essential amino acids that must be present in the diet.

AMNESIA. Partial or complete loss of memory or gaps in memory.

AMP. Adenosine monophosphate; a nucleotide with one phosphate group that can be converted to and from ADP and ATP.

AMPK. Adenosine monophosphate-activated protein kinase; an enzyme that is activated by AMP and that has a wide variety of physiological effects, including complex roles in the regulation of energy metabolism in muscle during exercise.

AMYGDALA. An almond-shaped brain structure of the limbic system that is activated in stressful situations and triggers fear.

AMYLASE. A digestive enzyme found in saliva and the pancreas that breaks down carbohydrates to simple sugars.

AMYLOIDOSIS. Abnormally high accumulation of protein-based substances in the body.

ANABOLIC. Causing muscle and bone growth and a shift from fat to muscle in the body.

ANABOLIC STEROIDS. Synthetic drugs that mimic the effects of male sex hormones in building up body tissue, specifically muscle tissue.

ANABOLIC-ANDROGENIC STEROIDS (AAS). Anabolic steroids; illegal and prohibited testosterone derivatives that are synthesized as performance-enhancing and muscle-building drugs.

ANABOLISM. The process by which cells use simple molecules, such as simple sugars and amino acids, to build more complex molecules, such as glycogen and proteins.

ANAEROBIC. Pertaining to or caused by the absence of oxygen.

ANAEROBIC EXERCISE. Exercise high enough in intensity that oxygen is required at a greater rate than it can be supplied, for instance heavy weight training and sprinting.

ANAEROBIC RESPIRATION. A form of respiration that occurs in the absence of oxygen.

ANAEROBIC THRESHOLD. An original concept describing increased lactate production during conditions of low blood flow and oxygen.

ANALGESIC NEPHROPATHY. Regular use of analgesics (painkillers) such as acetaminophen (Tylenol) and ibuprofen (Advil) over a long period.

ANAPHYLAXIS. Anaphylactic shock; a severe, potentially fatal hypersensitivity to an allergen that can result in blood vessel dilation and a sharp drop in blood pressure, smooth muscle contraction, and difficulty breathing.

ANDROGEN. A natural or artificial steroid that acts as a male sex hormone. Androgens are responsible for the development of male sex organs and secondary sexual characteristics.

ANDROGENIC. Testosterone-like, masculinizing effects.

ANDROID. An operating system used on mobile devices, which is owned by Google.

ANDROLOGY. The medical specialty area dealing with male health, particularly the male reproductive system.

ANDROSTENEDIONE. Andro; a steroid sex hormone that is secreted by the adrenal glands, testes, and ovaries, as a precursor of testosterone and estrogen, and marketed as a performance-enhancing drug.

ANEMIA. An abnormal condition of the blood in which too few red blood cells are produced or adequate red blood cells are produced but they are lacking in hemoglobin.

ANEROBIC. With respect to living or taking place without the need for oxygen, or in the absence of oxygen.

ANGINA. Chest pain, discomfort, or tightness; stable angina is typically triggered by increased exertion or exercise. The symptoms of angina usually subside with reduced exertion and rest.

ANGINA PECTORIS. A sensation of crushing pain or pressure in the chest, usually near the breastbone, but sometimes radiating to the upper arm or back. Angina pectoris is caused by a deficient supply of oxygenated blood to the heart.

ANGIOPLASTY. A cardiovascular interventional procedure performed by threading a catheter through the arteries around the heart to relieve blockages resulting from cardiovascular disease.

ANKLE DORSIFLEXOR. Muscles responsible for the toe-up motion of the foot at the ankle.

ANKLE PLANTARFLEXOR. Muscles responsible for the toe-down motion of the foot at the ankle.

ANNULUS. The outer portion of a spinal disc.

ANOVULATION. The absence of ovulation in the menstrual cycle.

ANTERIOR. In the front.

ANTHROPOMETRIC. Comparative measurements of the human body.

ANTIBODIES (IMMUNOGLOBULINS). Proteins that bind to their corresponding specific antigen.

ANTIDEPRESSANT. A drug used to prevent or treat depression.

ANTIEMETIC. A type of drug given to stop vomiting.

ANTIGEN. Any substance foreign to the body that evokes an immune response.

ANTIOXIDANT. A substance that prevents the destructive effects of oxidative chemicals in the body.

ANXIETY DISORDER. A group of disorders characterized by anxiety, including panic disorder and post-traumatic stress disorder (PTSD).

APHASIA. Loss of language abilities.

APOLIPOPROTEIN E (APOE). A protein that transports cholesterol throughout the body. One form of this protein, APOE e4, is associated with a 60% risk of late-onset AD.

APP. A small, specialized program designed to be downloaded onto a mobile device, such as a smart phone, that provides information or instruction about some specific topic.

APPETITE SUPPRESSANT. A drug that reduces the desire to eat.

APRAXIA. An inability to perform purposeful movements that is not caused by paralysis or loss of feeling.

AQUA-LUNG. The name of the original type of scuba diving device invented in the 1940s by Jacques-Yves Cousteau and Emile Gagnan.

ARRHYTHMIA. An irregular, abnormal heart rhythm.

ARTERIOLE. A smaller version of an artery.

ARTERIOLES. The small termini of arteries that end in capillaries.

ARTERIOVENOUS OXYGEN DIFFERENCE. The difference in blood oxygen content between arterial and venous blood.

ARTERY. A blood vessel that carries blood away from the heart.

ARTHRITIS. A condition of the joints, which causes stiffness, swelling, or pain.

ARTHROGRAM. A test done by injecting dye into the shoulder joint and then taking x rays. Areas where the dye leaks out indicate a tear in the tendons.

ARTHROSCOPE. A type of endoscope (an instrument used to look inside a hollow cavity or organ of the body) inserted into a joint through a small incision on the surface of the body.

ARTHROSCOPY. A procedure that uses a small fiber optic scope inserted through a small incision in the skin to see inside the shoulder.

ARTICULAR CARTILAGE. Cartilage that covers joint surfaces.

ASANA. A body posture or position used in yoga to promote physical flexibility, improve breathing and well-being, and improve the practitioner's ability to remain in meditation for extended periods of time.

ASCETIC. A type of lifestyle characterized by simplicity and austerity in the use of alcohol or other worldly pleasures in pursuit of religious or spiritual goals.

ASHTANGA YOGA. Astanga, classical, or power yoga; a physically strenuous form of hatha yoga.

ASTHMA. A disease of the respiratory system, which is sometimes caused by allergies; its symptoms include coughing, tightness in chest, and difficulty breathing.

ATHEROSCLEROSIS. A condition in which the buildup of plaque on the inner wall of a blood vessel reduces or interrupts the flow of blood through the vessel.

ATHLETE'S HEART. an enlarged heart due to chronic exercise training that is physiological (normal), not pathological.

ATHLETICS. A term that includes traditional track and field events, as well as a few other sports, such as road running and race walking.

ATOPY. A state that makes people more likely to develop allergic reactions, often including asthma symptoms.

ATP. Adenosine triphosphate; a nucleotide with three phosphate groups that supplies cellular energy by undergoing enzymatic-facilitated hydrolysis to adenosine diphosphate (ADP) and adenosine monophosphate (AMP).

ATRIAL FIBRILLATION. An irregular heart beat.

ATRIAL SEPTAL DEFECT. A condition in which the wall separating the two atria of the heart does not close properly during fetal developments.

ATROPHY. Wasting away of tissues.

ATTACKERS. Lacrosse players primarily responsible for advancing the ball towards the opponent's goal.

AUTOGENIC INHIBITION. Reflex relaxation that occurs when a passive stretch immediately follows an isometric or concentric muscle contraction; used for PNF stretching.

AUTOIMMUNE. A term that refers to a condition in which antibodies or T cells attack the molecules, cells, or tissue of the body organ or system producing them.

AUTOIMMUNE DISEASE. A condition in which the body's immune system produces antibodies to destroy its own tissues or blood components.

AUTONOMIC CONTROL. The combined influence from the sympathetic and parasympathetic nervous system on controlling involuntary functions of the body; for example, heartbeat.

AUTOSOMAL DOMINANT. A gene located on a chromosome other than the X or Y sex chromosomes, whose expression is dominant over that of a second copy of the same gene.

AVALOKITESVARA. The Sanskrit name of Quan yin.

AXIAL. Pertaining to the axis of the body, i.e., the head and trunk.

AXON. Long filament of a neuron that carries outgoing electrical signals from the cell body towards target cells. Each neuron has one axon that can be longer than a foot.

AZOOSPERMIA. The complete absence of sperm in ejaculate.

B

B LYMPHOCYTE. A lymphocyte that contains an immunoglobulin on the surface (the B-cell receptor). B cells mature in the bone marrow.

BABYFACE. The good guy or hero in a wrestling angle. This is the wrestler the fans are supposed to cheer for. A babyface is also known as a face for short.

BAGGATAWAY. A primitive form of lacrosse played by many Native American tribes.

BAIL. One of the two pieces of wood that lie on top of the stumps to form the wicket.

BALANCE. Ability to remain upright and steady.

BALANCE BEAM. A piece of gymnastics equipment consisting of a single piece of wood, 5 meters in length, 10 centimeters wide, and 1.25 meters above the ground, as well as the set of exercises a woman gymnast performs on the apparatus.

BALANCE TRAINING. Exercises designed to improve and maintain balance.

BALLET. A type of dance that features steps, poses, and graceful movements such as spins and leaps; participants are called ballet dancers or ballerinas.

BARIATRIC. Related to or specializing in the treatment of obesity.

BARIATRICS. The branch of medicine that deals with the prevention and treatment of obesity and related disorders.

BASAL METABOLIC RATE (BMR). The component of energy expenditure that refers to the energy expended when an individual is lying down and at complete rest. This measurement is commonly obtained in the morning after a standard night of sleep and in the post-absorptive state.

BAUX SCORE (OR INDEX). A measure used by medical workers to estimate the prognosis for recovery from a burn injury. The Baux is equal to the age of the patient plus the portion of the body damaged by the burn injury.

BELAY. A closeable device to which a climbing rope can be attached.

BETA BLOCKERS. Medications prescribed to patients with heart disease or high blood pressure that lower heart rate at rest and during exercise.

BETA-AMYLOID PLAQUES. Senile plaques; structures in the brain, composed of dead or dying nerve cells and cell debris surrounding deposits of beta-amyloid protein, that are diagnostic of AD.

BETA-2 AGONISTS. Drug that bind to and activate beta-2 receptors, such as bronchodilators used to treat asthma and other lung diseases; sometimes used as performance-enhancing drugs.

BETA-BLOCKER. A drug that slows the heart rate and lowers blood pressure by blocking the beta-receptors for epinephrine and norepinephrine.

BETA-CAROTENE. An antioxidant obtained from dark green and yellow fruits and vegetables.

BETA-OXIDATION. The step-wise breakdown of fatty acids via the removal of two-carbon fragments, with the generation of ATP.

BICEPS BRACHII (OR BICEPS). The two-headed muscle located on the upper arm, both heads flex the arm at the shoulders; and it also flexes and supinates the forearm at the elbow.

BILE. Liquid produced in the liver and stored in the gall bladder that emulsifies fats.

BINGE-EATING DISORDER. A condition characterized by uncontrolled eating.

BIOELECTRICAL IMPEDANCE ANALYSIS (BIA). A method of determining the proportion of body fat by measuring resistance to a weak electrical current in various parts of the body.

BIOENERGETICS. Energy transformations and exchanges in the body.

BIRDIE. A golf score that is one less than par for a hole.

BISPHOSPHONATES. Compounds that slow bone loss and increase bone density.

BLADING. The object used by wrestlers to cut themselves. Also, a term used to describe wrestlers cutting themselves to get blood in their matches. This is done to add drama to a match.

BLOCK. A defensive shot made simply by placing one's racket in front of an opponent's shot, returning at a speed nearly equal to its original speed.

B-LYMPHOCYTES (B-CELLS). A type of white blood cell that originates in the bone marrow and recognizes foreign antigens (or proteins), secreting antibodies in an immune response.

BMX BIKE. A specialized small-framed bike with wide tires used in dirt jumping and other stunt competitions. BMX bikes developed in California in the 1970s from customized alterations of a Schwinn bicycle called the Stingray.

BODHISATTVA. A Buddhist holy person who has attained enlightenment, but postpones nirvana in order to help others become enlightened.

BODY COMPOSITION. The percentage of fat, bone, and muscle tissue in the human body.

BODY DYSMORPHIC DISORDER. A psychiatric disorder marked by preoccupation with an imagined physical defect.

BODY MASS INDEX (BMI). A measure of body fat: the ratio of weight in kilograms to the square of height in meters.

BOGEY. A golf score that is one more than par for a hole.

BONE. Composed primarily of a non-living matrix of calcium salts and a living matrix of collagen fibers, bone is the major component that makes up the human skeleton.

BONE DENSITY. Amount of bone tissue and minerals in a particular area of bone; bone thickness.

BONELESS. A method of taking off and landing on the board while it is in the air.

BOOKER. The person who writes (books) the wrestling angles. The booker decides who wins and loses the matches.

BOULDERING PAD. A padded cushion used to provide protection for climbers who fall during bouldering or other short-distance climbs. Also called a crash pad.

BOX LACROSSE. A form of lacrosse played in an inside facility, often a hockey rink, with somewhat different rules from those used in field lacrosse.

BRACHIAL PLEXUS. A group of lower neck and upper back spinal nerves supplying the arm, forearm and hand.

BRADYKININ. A peptide that causes dilation of blood vessels.

BRAIN STEM. Lowest part of the brain that connects with the spinal cord. It is a complicated neural center with several neuronal pathways between the cerebrum, spinal cord, cerebellum, and motor and sensory functions of the head and neck.

BRAIN-DERIVED NEUROTROPHIC FACTOR (BDNF). A brain protein that helps maintain nerves and promotes the growth of new nerve cells (neurons).

BRANCH-CHAINED AMINO ACIDS (BCAA). The essential amino acids leucine, isoleucine, and valine, which are metabolically important during exercise.

BRONCHI. The trachea branches into two tubes at the base of the trachea called the left and right bronchi, which extend from the trachea to deliver air to the left and right lungs, respectively.

BRONCHIOLES. The bronchioles are no larger than 0.5mm (0.02 inches) in diameter and divide many times in the lungs to form a tree-like structure; they have progressively smaller branches and tiny air sacs called alveoli at the end.

BRONCHOCONSTRICTION. Constriction, or narrowing, of the bronchial air passages that lead to the lungs.

BRONCHODILATOR. Commonly called an inhaler, the small device is filled with medications that can help expand the lungs' capacity for a short time.

BRUGADA'S SYNDROME. inherited heart condition that results in an arrhythmia.

BURPEE. A full body exercise that consists of aerobic exercise and strength training; its basic exercise is beginning in a standing position, dropping into a squat position, kicking feet back while lowering body with a pushup, and returning feet to squat position.

BURSITIS. Inflammation of a bursa, the fluid-filled sacs located between tendons and bones in the joints.

BYPASS SURGERY. A surgical procedure that grafts blood vessels onto arteries to reroute the blood flow around blockages in the arteries.

C

C_AO_2. Arterial blood oxygen content.

C_VO_2. Venous blood oxygen content.

CALCANEUS. The heel bone.

CALCITONIN. A naturally occurring hormone made by the thyroid gland that can be used as a drug to treat osteoporosis and Paget's disease of the bone.

CALCIUM. A naturally occurring element that primarily combines with phosphate to form the nonliving matrix of bones.

CALF MUSCLE. The fleshy part of the back side of the leg, located below the knee.

CALISTHENICS. Physical exercises that improve fitness and muscle tone, such as situps, pushups, and jumping jacks.

CALORIE. A unit used to indicate the potential to produce energy within the human body; although the term "calorie" (small calorie) is used commonly, it actually refers to "kilocalorie" (large calorie).

CAPILLARIES. Tiny blood vessels that lie beneath the mucous membrane, near the surface of the nasal passages.

CAPILLARY DENSITY. The quantity of minute blood vessels connecting the arterioles and venules, where oxygen and carbon dioxide exchange occur at the skeletal muscle tissue level, for a given surface area.

CARABINER. A spring-loaded loop used for attaching various parts of a climbing system to each other.

CARBO LOADING. The process by which a person eats relatively large amonts of complex carbohydrates (such as starches) with the aim of building up a large supply of energy-releasing compounds needed for endurance events, such a marathon races.

CARBOHYDRATE. Any organic compound with the chemical formula $C_x(H_2O)_y$. Most commonly in biochemistry, carbohydrates refer to simple sugars such as glucose or fructose.

CARBON DIOXIDE (CO_2). A gaseous waste product that is dumped into the bloodstream from the cells; a byproduct of respiration, it is released upon exhalation of air from the body.

CARDIAC ARREST. sudden death due to lack of heartbeat.

CARDIAC MUSCLE. The striated muscle tissue of the heart. It is sometimes called myocardium.

CARDIAC OUTPUT. Amount of blood that leaves the heart per heartbeat.

CARDIOMYOPATHY. A disease of the muscles of the heart that leaves them enlarged, weakened, and unable to pump blood effectively.

CARDIORESPIRATORY. Cardiovascular; aerobic; the delivery of oxygen by the heart, lungs, and blood to large working muscle groups and the utilization of oxygen by those muscles.

CARDIORESPIRATORY ENDURANCE. The ability of a person's body to supply nutrients and oxygen for a sustained period of physical activity.

CARDIORESPIRATORY FITNESS. The collective ability of the cardiovascular and pulmonary systems to supply oxygenated blood to the skeletal muscles during exercise and/or physical activity.

CARDIOVASCULAR. Relating to the heart and blood vessels (circulatory system).

CARDIOVASCULAR DISEASE RISK FACTORS. Physiological parameters whereby exceeding threshold values places one at an increased risk for developing cardiovascular disease.

CARDIOVASCULAR DRIFT. Refers to a physiological phenomenon where stroke volume gradually decreases with progressive exercise; this decline is as a result of dehydration and is subsequently accompanied by an increase in heart rate.

CARDIOVASCULAR EXERCISE. Exercise that uses the larger muscles of the body, increases the demand for oxygen, increases the heart rate, and can be sustained for longer than several minutes.

CARDIOVASCULAR SYSTEM. The muscles, tissues, and cells that are involved in the movement of blood and lymph through the body.

CARNITINE. A substance that transports fatty acids into the mitochondria of muscle cells.

CARNOSINE. A dipeptide of the amino acids beta-alanine and histidine; highly concentrated in muscle.

CAROTENOIDS. Various common red and yellow pigments, such as beta-carotene, some of which have antioxidant activity.

CARPAL TUNNEL SYNDROME. A painful progressive condition caused by compression of a key nerve in the wrist, often caused by repetitive motion.

CARTILAGE. Strong, flexible tissue found throughout the body, such as in the nose, throat, ear, and knee.

CATABOLIC. A metabolic process in which energy is released through the breakdown of complex molecules into simpler ones.

CATABOLISM. The process by which cells breakdown molecules, such as glycogen, glucose, proteins, and amino acids into simpler molecules, such as carbon dioxide and water, accompanied by the release of energy.

CATALASE. An enzyme that breaks down hydrogen peroxide into oxygen and water.

CATARACT. A clouding that develops in the lens of the eye or the surrounding transparent membrane that inhibits the passage of light.

CATECHOLAMINES. The so-called "fight or flight" hormones and neurotransmitters epinephrine, norepinephrine, and dopamine that are derived from the amino acid tyrosine.

CELLULITIS. An infection of the tissues under the skin.

CELSIUS. A scale and unit of measurement for temperature, where the freezing point of water is 0°C and the boiling point of water is 100°C.

CENTER LINE. A straight line that bisects a field hockey pitch across its short dimension.

CENTRAL NERVOUS SYSTEM (CNS). One of two major divisions of the nervous system. The CNS consists of the brain, the cranial nerves and the spinal cord.

CEREBRAL EDEMA. Movement of water into brain cells causing the cells to swell, which disrupts normal functioning of the cells.

CERVIX. The narrow, lower end of the uterus forming the opening to the vagina.

CHARLEY HORSE. A common name for a muscle spasm, usually occurring in the leg.

CHECKPOINT. A point on an adventure racing course where participants have to check in and, sometimes, transition to a second event.

CHEMOTHERAPY. A medical treatment for cancer and other disorders using chemical agents (drugs).

CHEST X RAY. A diagnostic procedure in which a very small amount of radiation is used to produce an image of the structures of the chest (heart, lungs, and bones) on film.

CHI. In traditional Chinese culture, the life force or energy flow of all living things.

CHI KUNG. Also known as qigong, a Chinese system of breathing control and exercises to benefit the body and mind.

CHIROPRACTIC MEDICINE. An alternative medicine that focuses on manipulation of the muscles, nervous system, and bones (skeleton).

CHOLELITHIASIS. The formation of gallstones.

CHOLESTEROL. A fat-soluble steroid alcohol found in animal fats and oils and produced in the body from saturated fats. Low-density lipoprotein (LDL) or "bad" cholesterol has a high proportion of cholesterol and increases the risk of coronary heart disease.

CHONDROMALACIA. Abnormal softening or degeneration of cartilage.

CHOP. A defensive shot in which a player strokes downward on the ball, giving it a high degree of topspin.

CHOREOGRAPHY. The planned movements of a dance routine.

CHROMAFFIN CELLS. Cells of the adrenal medulla with epinephrine-containing vesicles.

CHRONIC. A word used to describe a long-lasting condition. Chronic conditions often develop gradually and involve slow changes.

CHYLOMICRON. A lipoprotein that is high in triglycerides and is common in the blood during fat digestion and assimilation.

CILIA. Each epithelial cell is fringed with thousands of these tiny fingerlike extensions of the cells.

CIRCUIT TRAINING. A workout structured around a series of brief exercises or activities that target different muscle groups.

CIRCULATORY SYSTEM. Another name for the cardiovascular system.

CIRCUMDUCTION. Movement of a limb or extremity such that the end closest to the body remains fixed while the other end describes a circle; such as circling the arm from the shoulder.

CLAUDICATION. Cramping discomfort in legs due to poor circulation.

CLAVICLE. The long, curved bone that connects the upper breastbone to the shoulder blade in humans.

CLIMBING HARNESS. A device worn by a climber to which a rope or other safety device can be attached.

CLOSE INFIELD. The area enclosed by a painted circle with a radius of 15 yards measured from the wicket on each end of the pitch.

COGNITIVE IMPAIRMENTS. Dysfunction of the brain that impacts one's ability to concentrate, formulate ideas, reason, and remember; it generally develops later in life as a result of injury or illness.

COLLAGEN. The fibrous, soft protein found in bone, skin, and other connective tissues.

COMBAT SPORT. A competitive contact sport in which the contestants use various striking or grappling techniques that simulate hand-to-hand combat. Kickboxing is considered a combat sport.

COMBINED EVENTS. Track and field events in which a competitor takes part in a number (usually five, seven, or ten) of events, with the winner being the person with the highest total score for those events.

COMMINUTED FRACTURE. A fracture in which the bone shatters rather than breaking cleanly into two places.

COMMOTIO CORDIS. non-penetrating blow to the chest that interrupts a heart beat and causes sudden cardiac death or other serious heart arrhythmia.

CO-MORBIDITIES. The presence of one or more disorders or diseases in addition to the primary disease; for instance an individual with cardiovascular disease and hypertension, obesity, and Parkinson's disease.

COMPLEMENTARY. Something that serves to fill out or complete something else.

COMPLEMENTARY ALTERNATIVE MEDICINE (CAM). A group of medical practices and/or products not considered standard care for a variety of diseases and conditions. Examples include acupuncture, herbal medicine, and chiropractic care.

COMPLEX CARBOHYDRATES. Chemical compounds consisting of carbon, hydrogen, and oxygen of high molecular weight, such as starch and cellulose.

COMPOUND FRACTURE. A fracture in which some part of the broken bone protrudes through the skin. Also known as an open fracture.

COMPRESSION. The state of having been reduced in volume or mass by the application of pressure.

COMPRESSION FRACTURE. A fracture caused by the collapse of a vertebra in the spinal column, usually caused either by trauma or by weakening of the bone in osteoporosis.

COMPUTED TOMOGRAPHY (CT OR CAT). The use of x rays to obtain a three-dimensional image of a part of the body.

CONCENTRIC CONTRACTION. Any activity of a muscle in which it shortens while under tension due to the application of a larger but opposing force.

CONCENTRIC CONTRACTION. Muscle contraction in which the muscles shorten while generating force, as when lifting a weight.

CONCENTRIC EXERCISE. An exercise in which muscles are shortened.

CONCENTRIC PHASE. Muscle contraction in which the muscles shorten while generating force, as when lifting a weight.

CONCURRENT TRAINING. Combining two or more different types of exercise into a single exercise session. For example, including both cardiorespiratory fitness training and resistance training in the same exercise session.

CONCUSSION. The most common injury to the brain caused by a blow to the head, which causes temporary disorientation and other side effects.

CONDYLE. A rounded part at the end of a bone that forms a moving joint with a cup-shaped cavity in another bone.

CONGENITAL. Present at birth.

CONJUGATE PERIODIZATION. A form of periodization training which incorporates a variety of different skills during a single training session.

CONTACT DERMATITIS. An allergic reaction characterized by itchy, blistered skin.

CONTINUOUS GLUCOSE MONITORING (CGM). A system for monitoring blood glucose levels with a tiny sensor inserted under the skin that checks glucose levels in tissue fluid and transmits the information via radio waves to a wireless pager-type device.

CONTRACTION. The shortening and thickening of a functioning muscle or muscle fiber.

CONTRACTURE. A tightening or shortening of muscles that prevents normal movement of the associated limb or other body part.

CONTUSIONS. Bruising.

COOL DOWN. A 5 to 10 minute period of low-intensity activity following the conditioning phase.

CORNEAL ABRASIONS. A scratch on the surface of the cornea. The cornea is the eye's clear outer layer.

CORONARY ANOMALY. congenital anatomical abnormality in coronary artery(s).

CORONARY HEART DISEASE (CHD). A disease involving the blood vessels surrounding the heart; also called coronary artery disease (CAD).

CORTICOSTEROID DRUG. A medication that acts like a type of hormone (cortisol) produced by the adrenal gland of the body. Corticosteroids produced by the body stimulate specific types of functional activity.

CORTISOL. A corticosteroid produced by the adrenal cortex, and which mediates metabolic responses in the body. It has anti-inflammatory and immunosuppressive properties, but may rise in response to physical or psychological stress.

CORTISONE. A hormone produced naturally by the adrenal glands or made synthetically.

COXSWAIN. A non-rowing member of a rowing team who sets the pace for rowers and keeps them informed of their status in a race.

CRANIAL NERVE. In humans, there are 12 cranial nerves. They are connected to the brain stem and basically "run" the head as well as help regulate the organs of the thoracic and abdominal cavities.

CREASE. 1. One of several lines on a cricket pitch near the stumps that delineate the regions in which the bowler and batter must remain. 2. One of two circles at each end of a lacrosse field where the goal is located.

CREATINE. A nitrogen-containing organic acid that supplies muscles with energy.

CREATININE. A waste product of metabolism. Kidney function is measured in part by its ability to filter and remove creatinine from the body. High levels of creatinine often reflect poor kidney function.

CROSS-TRAINING. Cross-conditioning; training in a sport that is complementary to the sport competed in; such as distance running and cross-country skiing or power yoga.

CT SCAN. The abbreviated term for computed or computerized axial tomography. The test may involve injecting a radioactive contrast dye into the body. Computers are used to scan for radiation and create cross-sectional images of internal organs.

CUE. In psychology, a sensory signal that triggers a learned response of some kind. Cues related to eating may involve the smell, taste, or sight of food, or even the sounds of cooking or meal preparation.

CUMBIA. A type of folk dance that developed along the Caribbean coast of Colombia.

CURLING. Curling is a sport played on ice that involves players pushing granite stones across the ice toward a target area.

CURL-UP. A half-sit-up, which does not involve the hip flexors.

CYCLE ERGOMETER. A stationary bicycle with an ergometer to measure work performed; used for cardiorespiratory fitness tests.

CYCLIC ADENOSINE MONOPHOSPHATE (CAMP). A cyclic mononucleotide formed from ATP that carries out hormonal activity within cells; a second messenger.

CYSTITIS. Inflammation of the urinary bladder.

CYTOKINES. A class of proteins, including interleukins, that are released by cells to mediate intercellular communication and regulate immune responses.

CYTOSOL. The aqueous portion of the cell surrounded by the cell membrane.

D

DEADLIFT. A weight training exercise in which the athlete lifts a loaded barbell from the ground in a stabilized bent-over position and then stands fully upright holding the barbell. It is one of three events in a powerlifting competition.

DECOMPENSATED HEART FAILURE. Occurs when the heart cannot adequately pump blood through the body. Signifies worsening heart failure.

DECOMPRESSION ILLNESS. A condition that develops when a diver ascends from a dive at two rapid a rate, resulting in the accumulation of gas bubbles in the bloodstream.

DECONDITIONING. Loss of physical fitness due to illness or inactivity.

DEEP VEIN THROMBOSIS. Abbreviated DVT, a medical condition in which a blood clot forms within a deep vein.

DEFENSEMAN. One of two ice hockey players whose primary responsibility it is to prevent opposing players from successfully advancing the puck into the defending team's zone and, ultimately, its net.

DEFENSEMEN. Lacrosse players whos primary responsibility is to protect against opponent attacks on their goal.

DEFICIENCY. A shortage of something necessary for health.

DEHYDRATION. Excessive loss of water from the body or from an organ or body part, as from illness or fluid deprivation.

DEHYDROEPIANDROSTERONE (DHEA). An androgenic steroid secreted by the adrenal cortex and an intermediate in the synthesis of testosterone; sometimes marketed as a performance-enhancing drug.

DELIRIUM. A disturbance of consciousness marked by confusion, inattention, delusions, hallucinations, and agitation. It is distinguished from dementia by its relatively sudden onset and variation in the severity of symptoms.

DELTOID. Commonly called delt or shoulder muscle, the muscle that forms the rounded contour of the shoulder, the anterior part of the deltoid muscle flexes and medially rotates the arm at the shoulder.

DELUSION. A persistent false belief held in the face of strong contradictory evidence.

DEMENTIA. A group of symptoms (syndrome) associated with a chronic progressive impairment of memory, reasoning ability, and other intellectual functions, personality changes, deterioration in personal grooming, and disorientation.

DENDRITES. Threadlike extensions of the cytoplasm of a neuron.

DENDRITIC CELLS. Any of various antigen-presenting cells with long irregular processes.

DEPARTMENT OF HEALTH (UK). The national agency responsible for public health, adult social care, and the National Health Service.

DEPRESSION. A psychological disorder characterized by feelings of hopelessness, lack of concentration, inability to sleep, and sometimes suicidal thoughts.

DERMATITIS. Inflammation of the skin that causes swelling, redness, itching, or blistering..

DERMATOLOGIST. A medical professional specializing in the care of the skin and skin disorders.

DERMIS. Thicker layer of skin lying below the epidermis.

DEXTERITY. Skills needed to perform physical activity and movements.

DIABETES MELLITUS. The most common form of diabetes, usually developing in obese adults, but becoming increasingly common in young people; characterized by high blood sugar (hyperglycemia) due to impaired insulin utilization.

DIABETIC AUTONOMIC NEUROPATHY. A complication of long-standing diabetes that results in a altered heart rate response; generally characterized by a high resting heart rate and blunted maximal and exercise heart rates.

DIAGNOSTIC. The art or act of identifying a disease from its signs and symptoms.

DIALYSIS. A medical procedure in which waste products are filtered from the bloodstream by a machine.

DIAPHRAGM. The diaphragm is involved in inhalation. It lies just under the lungs and is a muscle shaped like a large dome.

DIAPHRAGMATIC BREATHING. Deep breathing from the diaphragm, utilizing the entire lungs.

DIASTOLIC. The lowest arterial blood pressure of the cardiac cycle.

DIETARY FIBER. also known as roughage or bulk. Insoluble fiber moves through the digestive system almost undigested and gives bulk to stools. Soluble fiber dissolves in water and helps keep stools soft.

DIETARY REFERENCE INTAKE (DRI). The approximate amount of a nutrient that should be ingested daily.

DIETARY SUPPLEMENT. A product, such as a vitamin, mineral, herb, amino acid, or enzyme, that is intended to be consumed in addition to an individual's diet.

DIETARY SUPPLEMENT. Vitamins or minerals taken in the form of pills, powder, or liquid to provide nutrients not produced by the body.

DIHYDROLIPOIC ACID (DHLA). A potent antioxidant that is the reduced (active) form of alpha-lipoic acid obtained from the diet.

DILATED CARDIOMYOPATHY. enlarged, floppy weak heart that does not pump blood effectively and can be due to many different causes.

DIPEPTIDYL PEPTIDASE-4 (DPP-4) INHIBITORS. A class of type 2 diabetes medications that prevent the breakdown of glucagon-like peptide-1 (GLP-1), thereby lowering blood sugar levels.

DIRECT CALORIMETRY. Refers to the direct measurement of heat dissipation from an individual to the calorimeter.

DISC (ALSO INTERVERTEBRAL DISK). Bony structures that lie between adjacent vertebrae in the spine.

DISMISSAL. The act of getting a batsmen out, so that he must discontinue batting.

DISMOUNT. The act of leaving a piece of equipment at the completion of an exercise.

DISTAL. Referring to being away from a point of attachment.

DIURETIC. A substance or drug that removes water from the body by increasing urine production.

DNA. The acronym for deoxyribonucleic acid; the substance that carries a living organism's genetic material.

DOBOK. The uniform worn to practice tae kwon do. Traditionally made of cotton and usually white or black, the dobok has a jacket-like top and wide-legged pants. It is worn with a belt whose color indicates the student's rank.

DOJANG. The Korean word for a tae kwon do school or training hall.

DONEPEZIL HYDROCHLORIDE (ARICEPT). A drug that increases the levels of acetylcholine in the brain.

DOPAMINE. A neurotransmitter in the brain and intermediate in the biosynthesis of epinephrine.

DOPING. The illicit use of steroids or other performance-enhancing drugs in athletic competitions.

DOSE-RESPONSE RELATIONSHIP. The relationship between two variables; where any increase or change in one parameter is associated with a concurrent change in the other parameter.

DOWNHILL SKATEBOARDING. A form of skateboarding in which riders travel down hills.

DRIBBLING. To bounce a ball on a court, such as in basketball.

DRISHTI. "Gazing point;" the focus of the eyes in ashtanga and power yoga.

DUAL ENERGY X-RAY ABSORPTIOMETRY (DXA OR DEXA). A method for measuring the absorption of x rays by body tissues; used primarily to determine bone mineral density for diagnosing osteoporosis and other bone diseases, but also used as a body composition test.

DUMBBELL. A type of exercise weight that is generally composed of bar with a disk or bar at each end.

DYANA. The yoga term for meditation.

DYNAMIC STRETCHING. Stretching with smooth, gentle. continuous movements.

DYNAMOMETER. A device for measuring force, such as the strength of the arms, grip, back, or legs.

DYSLIPIDEMIA. A condition of high blood cholesterol.

DYSMENORRHEA. Painful menstruation.

DYSPESIA. Indigestion.

DYSRHYTHMIA. Irregular heart rhythm.

DYSTROPHY. Any of several disorders characterized by weakening or degeneration of muscle tissue.

E

EAGLE. A golf score that is two less than par for a hole.

EATING DISORDERS. Conditions, such as anorexia nervosa and bulimia nervosa, that are characterized by abnormal attitudes toward food, altered appetite control, unhealthy eating habits, and sometimes compulsive exercise; particularly common in young women.

ECCENTRIC CONTRACTION. Any activity of a muscle in which it lengthens while under tension due to the application of a larger but opposing force.

ECCENTRIC EXERCISE. An exercise in which muscles are lengthened.

ECCENTRIC PHASE. The phase of an exercise in which the muscles elongate under tension because the opposing force is greater than that generated by the muscles.

ECHOCARDIOGRAM. Ultra-sound examination of the heart that provides information about the heart's chambers and valves.

EDEMA. Relating to excess fluids.

EFFECTOR. Any molecule, chemical, organ, structure or agent that regulates a pathway by changing the pathway's reaction rate.

EFFECTOR CELLS. Mature lymphocytes that assist in the removal of pathogens from the system and do not require further differentiation to perform this function.

EJECTION FRACTION. The fraction of blood pumped by the left ventricle each beat; technically, it is stroke volume divided by end-diastolic volume.

EKG. test that examines the electrical conduction of the heart.

ELECTROCARDIOGRAM. A test that records the electrical activity of the heart; commonly term ECG.

ELECTROCARDIOGRAPH. A device that records heart activity.

ELECTROLYTES. Ions in the body that participate in metabolic reactions. The major human electrolytes are sodium (Na^+), potassium (K^+), calcium (Ca^{2+}), magnesium (Mg^{2+}), chloride (Cl^-), phosphate (HPO_4^{2-}), bicarbonate (HCO^{3-}), and sulfate (SO_4^{2-}).

ELITE. In the United States, a rower who has been a member of the U.S. Rowing National Team.

ELITE RUNNER. A runner who runs professionally or who has attained some level of distinction in her or his field of running.

ELLIPSE. A two-dimensional shape similar to a circle (with only one length for its axis) but with a major axis and a minor axis, which makes it longer on its major axis and shorter on its minor axis.

ELLIPTICAL TRAINER. Cross-trainer; a stationary exercise machine that simulates walking, running, or stair-climbing.

EMBOLISM. The blockage of a blood vessel by air, blood clot, or other foreign body.

EMBOLUS. A blood clot, piece of blood clot, air bubble, or other material that travels in the bloodstream forming a blockage at some point beyond its point of origin.

ENDEMIC. Referring to a disease that is prevalent in a particular location.

ENDOCRINE SYSTEM. The glands and their hormones that control metabolic activity, including the adrenal and pituitary glands and the islets of Langerhans of the pancreas.

ENDOCRINOLOGIST. A medical specialist who deals with the endocrine (glands) system and diabetes.

ENDOMETRIUM. The inner lining of the uterus.

ENDORPHINS. A class of peptides in the brain that are produced during exercise and bind to opiate receptors, resulting in pain relief and pleasant feelings.

ENDOTHELIUM. Tissue that is one cell thick that lines many organs in the body, including blood vessels.

ENDOTOXIN. Toxic substances produced by bacteria.

ENDOVER. A skateboard maneuver that involves a 180 degree turn on the board.

ENDURANCE EXERCISE. Exercise, such as running or cycling, that increases stamina.

ENERGY. The ability (capacity) to do work.

ENERGY EXPENDITURE. The collective energy cost for maintaining constant conditions in the human body plus the amount of energy required to support daily physical activities; also called caloric expenditure.

ENZYMES. Protein catalysts that increase the speed of chemical reactions in the cell without themselves being changed.

EPIDEMIC. Affecting many individuals in a community or population and spreading rapidly.

EPIDEMIOLOGY. A branch of medical science that deals with the incidence, distribution, and control of disease in a population.

EPIDERMIS. The outermost of three major layers of the skin.

EPIGLOTTIS. A thin, leaflike flap of tissue that prevents food and fluids from entering the larynx from the pharynx.

EPIMYSIUM. The sheath of connective tissue around a muscle.

EPINEPHRINE. Adrenaline; a hormone that has a variety of effects on metabolism during exercise.

EPITHELIA. A membranous cellular tissue that covers a free surface or lines a tube or cavity of an animal body and serves especially to enclose and protect the other parts of the body, to produce secretions and excretions.

ERECTILE DYSFUNCTION. A medical condition, formerly called impotence, that prevents a male from getting and maintaining an erection.

ERECTOR SPINAE. Also called extensor spinae, a group of muscles and tendons that run primarily vertically within the back, lying in a groove next to the vertebral column and extending throughout the lumbar, thoracic, and cervical regions.

ERGOMETER. A device for measuring work performed.

ERGONOMIC. Furniture or equipment designed to interact effectively and safely with the human body.

ERYTHROPOIETIN (EPO). A hormone made in the kidneys that stimulates red blood cell formation; a synthetic drug sometimes used as a performance enhancer.

ESSENTIAL AMINO ACIDS (EAA). The amino acids histidine, isoleucine, leucine, lysine, methionine, phenylalanine, threonine, tryptophan, and valine, which are required for normal health and growth and must be obtained from dietary protein; arginine is required for growing children, but not for adults.

ESTIMATED AGE-PREDICTED MAXIMAL HEART RATE. Determined using the equation: 206.9 - (age x 0.67).

ESTRADIOL. The most physiologically active form of estrogen.

ESTROGEN. Any of several steroid hormones, produced mainly in the ovaries, that stimulate estrus and the development of female secondary sexual characteristics.

EXCESS POST EXERCISE OXYGEN CONSUMPTION (EPOC). A phenomenon where, after the completion of exercise, oxygen consumption remains elevated for a prolonged period of time.

EXERCISE INTENSITY. The difficulty of the exercise as defined by the increase in oxygen demand and heart rate.

EXERCISE PRESCRIPTION. An individualized exercise and fitness plan drawn up by a specialist in physical therapy or sports medicine.

EXERCISE-INDUCED ANAPHYLAXIS (EIA). A severe, potentially life-threatening, allergic reaction that occurs during exercise.

EXPLOSIVE POWER. The ability to reach maximum strength in a short period of time.

EXPLOSIVE STRENGTH. In sports medicine, the ability to exert maximal muscular force in minimal time.

EXTEND. Straighten.

EXTENSOR. A muscle that serves to extend or straighten a part of the body.

EXTERNAL GENITALS. The greater lips (labia majora), the lesser lips (labia minora), the clitoris, and the opening of the vagina.

F

FACEOFF. An activity in an ice hockey game in which the referee drops the puck between two opposing players, each of whom attempts to deflect the puck to his or her teammates. Also, An action with which a lacrosse game begins, when two players face each other in an attempt to gain control of the ball; also the box at the center of the field at which the action takes place.

FAIRWAY. An extensive manicured plot of grass connecting the tee and the green on a golf course.

FALL PREVENTION. A variety of measures that can be taken to reduce the risk of falling; usually for individuals in the older segment of the population.

FARTLEK. A form of interval training designed to improve one's aerobic functioning.

FASCICULATION. Involuntary contractions or twitchings of groups of muscle fibers. Fasciculations can occur in normal individuals without an associated disease or condition and can also occur as a result of illness, such as muscle cramps, nerve diseases, and metabolism imbalances.

FASCICULUS (PLURAL, FASCICULI). A small bundle of muscle fibers.

FASCIITS. Inflammation of the connective tissue in a muscle.

FASTING PLASMA GLUCOSE (FPG). A measure of blood glucose after fasting for at least eight hours; usually tested in the morning.

FAT. Molecules composed of fatty acids and glycerol; the slowest utilized source of energy, but the most energy-efficient form of food. Each gram of fat supplies about nine calories, more than twice that supplied by the same amount of protein or carbohydrate.

FATTY ACIDS. Fatty acids are a group of carbon chains that make up fat. The body requires some, called essential fatty acids, to form membranes and synthesize important compounds.

FEMUR. Thigh bone.

FERRITIN. A protein complex consisting of iron and phosphate in which iron is stored in the liver, spleen, and bone marrow.

FEUDALISM. A system of legal, economic, and social repression in medieval Europe and Asia from the ninth century to the fifteenth century.

FIBER. Roughage; bulk; indigestible material in food; insoluble fiber moves through the digestive system, giving bulk to stool; soluble fiber dissolves in water and helps keep stool soft.

FIBROMYALGIA. A medical condition characterized by widespread musculoskeletal aches, pain and stiffness, soft tissue tenderness, general fatigue and sleep disturbances.

FICK EQUATION. A mathematical equation used to define maximal oxygen uptake: $VO_2max = Q(C_aO_2-C_vO_2)$. It reflects both the central component (i.e., Q or cardiac output) and peripheral component (i.e., difference between C_aO_2 or arterial blood oxygen content and C_vO_2 or venous blood oxygen content).

FILTRATE. The fluid that results when blood is filtered through the glomerulus; a precursor to urine.

FINE-MOTOR SKILLS. Control of the smaller muscles of the body, especially in the hands, feet, and head, for activities such as writing and crafts.

FINGERBOARD. A strip of wood or plastic with depressions into which the fingers can be placed to provide a training tool for finger strength and placement.

FIRST-CLASS CRICKET. A form of cricket that is usually played at the county, state or international level, consisting of two innings of play per side over three or more days.

FITNESS BALL. Exercise ball; Swiss ball; a large, well-inflated ball that can be used as a chair, as well as for performing various exercises.

F.I.T.T. PRINCIPLE. An acronym that represents exercise frequency, exercise intensity, exercise time, and exercise type.

FLACCID. Flabby, limp, weak.

FLATLAND SKATEBOARDING. A form of skateboarding that is done on a flat, hard-surface area.

FLAVONOIDS. A large group of common plant pigments, some of which are antioxidants.

FLEX. Bend.

FLEXIBILITY. The ability of joints to move through the full range of motion.

FLEXOMETER. An instrument for measuring the flexibility of a joint.

FLEXOR. A muscle that bends a joint or limb when it is contracted.

FLEXTIME. A variable work schedule that enables employees to schedule at least some of their own working hours.

FLIP. A shot made with a short flick of the wrist, rather than a full arm's swing at the ball.

FLOOR EXERCISE. A series of gymnastic activities performed by both men and women on a mat 12 meters square.

FOLATE. Also called folic acid; a B complex vitamin required in the production of red blood cells.

FOLLICLE. A small spherical sac located in an ovary in which an oocyte develops and matures; when the follicle bursts, the mature egg (ovum) is released into the fallopian tube. Only about 300 follicles burst during a woman's lifetime.

FOOT IMPACT. Damage caused to red blood cells in the foot as a result of a repeated running, walking, or jumping exercise.

FORWARD. One of three players on an ice hockey team whose primary responsibility it is to advance the puck into the opposing team's end of the rink and, eventually, into its net. The three forwards are the center, right wing, and left wing.

FOUL LINES. Two lines drawn on the baseball playing field at a 90? angle to each other with home plate at their apex.

14 PADDLEBOARD. A paddleboard of 14 ft (3.6 m) in length.

FRAGILITY FRACTURE. A fracture that occurs because of a fall from standing height or less. A person with healthy bones would not break a bone falling from a standing position.

FREE FATTY ACIDS (FFA). A large family of lipids that are oxidized as fuel and consist of chains of carbon atoms of various lengths attached to an acid.

FREE RADICAL. An especially reactive atom or group of atoms that has one or more unpaired electrons; especially one that is produced in the body by natural biological processes or introduced from an outside source (as tobacco smoke, toxins, or pollutants) and that can damage cells, proteins, and DNA by altering their chemical structure.

FREESTYLE SKATEBOARDING. A form of skateboarding in which riders perform a variety of artistic and demanding maneuvers, often in accompaniment to music.

FRICTION BLISTER. A blister caused when skin rubs against some other material.

FULL-CONTACT SPORT. A sport that allows players to make contact with parts of the body other than the hands.

FUNCTIONAL CAPACITY. The ability to carry out activities of daily living; for example, getting dressed, household chores, and running errands.

FUNCTIONAL FITNESS. The physical ability to safely and effectively carry out tasks of daily life.

FUNCTIONAL LIMITATIONS. Compromised ability to carry out activities of daily living; for instance, requiring assistance with personal hygiene or needing to take an elevator rather than being able to walk up stairs.

FUNCTIONAL STRENGTH. The force exerted by a muscle when it is performing some specific task, such as running or jumping.

FUNGUS. Any type of single- or multi-celled organisms that reproduce with spores and live by absorbing nutrients from organic matter; examples are mildews, molds, mushrooms, and yeasts.

G

GAIT. The manner by which one moves such as walking, jogging, or running.

GALANIN. A neurotransmitter with roles in various physiological processes, including regulation of the stress response.

GAMETE. A one-fold (haploid, that is, having 23 instead of 46 chromosomes) cell involved in sexual reproduction; the male gamete is the sperm; the female gamete is the egg.

GANGLIA. A mass of nerve tissue or a group of neurons.

GASTRIC JUICE. Digestive juice produced by the stomach wall that contains hydrochloric acid and the enzyme pepsin.

GASTRIN. A hormone produced by the stomach lining in response to protein in the stomach that produces increased gastric juice.

GASTROENTERITIS. A condition characterized by severe inflammation of the gastrointestinal tract, usually involving both the small intestines and the stomach; with main symptoms of diarrhea and vomiting.

GASTROESOPHAGEAL REFLUX DISORDER (GERD). A condition in which vapors from the stomach pass upwards through the esophagus into the mouth, causing pain and discomfort.

GASTROINTESTINAL TRACT. The body system that consists of all those organs involved in the digestion of food, as well as its transport into the bloodstream and the elimination of waste products from the body, which includes the esophagus, stomach, small intestine, large intestine, rectum, and anus, along with organs associated with this system, such as the liver, gallbladder, and pancreas.

GASTROPLASTY. A surgical procedure used to reduce digestive capacity by shortening the small intestine or shrinking the side of the stomach.

GHRELIN. A peptide hormone secreted primarily by the stomach that has been implicated in the control of food intake and fat storage.

GIARDIA. A diarrheal disease caused by a protozoa and contracted by swallowing water contaminated with sewage or human or animal feces.

GIMMICK MATCH. A match with stipulations that differ from the normal rules (ex: steel cage match).

GLOMERULONEPHRITIS. Inflammation and damage of the kidney's filtration system.

GLUCAGON. A protein hormone produced by the pancreas that increases the rate of glycogen breakdown in the liver to increase blood sugar.

GLUCAGON-LIKE PEPTIDE-1 (GLP-1). A hormone that controls blood glucose levels by increasing insulin, decreasing glucagon, promoting a feeling of fullness, and slowing the emptying of the stomach contents.

GLUCOCORTICOIDS. A general class of adrenal cortical hormones that are mainly active in protecting against stress and in protein and carbohydrate metabolism. They are widely used in medicine as anti-inflammatories and immunosuppresives.

GLUCOMETER. A device that accurately measures blood sugar levels.

GLUCONEOGENESIS. The formation of glucose in the liver, kidney, or muscle, from amino acids, glycerol, or lactate.

GLUCOSE. A monosaccharide (simple sugar) used for the metabolism of carbohydrates (energy source) in animals. The chemical symbol is $C_6H_{12}O_6$.

GLUCOSE INTOLERANCE. A state where blood sugar levels are elevated beyond normal, though the levels are below those considered to be diabetic; frequently the condition is referred to as pre-diabetes.

GLUTATHIONE. A peptide made of three amino acids that is an important antioxidant, both alone and as part of the enzyme glutathione peroxidase.

GLUTEALS. Any of three muscles that form the buttocks in humans.

GLUTES, GLUTEI. The three muscles of each buttock, especially the outermost gluteus maximus that extends and laterally rotates the thigh.

GLUTEUS MAXIMUS. Also called the glutes, the largest of the three gluteal muscles; it makes up the large portion of the appearance and shape of the buttocks.

GLYCOGEN. A carbohydrate molecule essential to the way glucose is stored in muscle and liver tissues.

GLYCOLYSIS. The series of reactions by which glucose is broken down to produce carbon dioxide, water, and energy.

GLYCOLYTIC FLUX. An increased rate in the transfer of glucose to pyruvate through the reactions of glycolysis.

GOALIE. The member of an ice hockey team whose primary responsibility it is to prevent the puck from entering the net.

GONIOMETER. An instrument that measures the axis and range of motion of a joint.

GOUT. A hereditary metabolic disease that is a form of arthritis and causes inflammation of the joints. It is more common in men.

GRAM. A metric unit of mass.

GRANULOCYTES. A white blood cell with granule-containing cytoplasm.

GRAPPLING. Engage in a close fight or struggle without weapons.

GRAVITY. The attraction due to the gravitational pull of the Earth to another body with mass.

GREENSTICK FRACTURE. A partial break in a bone.

GRIND. A maneuver in which an inline skater slides down an object without using the skate wheels.

GROIN MUSCLES. The muscles located between the top of the thighs and the abdomen.

GROSS-MOTOR SKILLS. Control of the large muscles of the body, including the arms, legs, back, abdomen, and torso, for activities such as sitting and walking.

GROWTH HORMONE (GH). A polypeptide hormone, secreted by the pituitary gland, that regulates growth and fat burning, among other functions.

GURU. In classical Hinduism, a person who has attained great spiritual wisdom and authority and uses it to guide others. Many schools of yoga use the term to refer to their founding teacher.

GYNECOMASTIA. Abnormal development of the mammary glands in males, resulting in breast enlargement. It is an occasional side effect of anabolic steroid abuse.

H

HALF MARATHON. A long distance race that covers half the distance covered in a traditional full marathon.

HALLUCINATION. False sensory perceptions; hearing sounds or seeing people or objects that are not there. Hallucinations can also affect the senses of smell, touch, and taste.

HAMSTRINGS. The three muscles at the back of the thigh that flex and rotate the leg and extend the thigh.

HATHA YOGA. The form of yoga most familiar in the West as a type of physical exercise. It originated in fifteenth-century India as a form of physical preparation for mental purification.

HAVERSIAN SYSTEM. Tubular systems in compact bone with a central Haversian canal that houses blood and lymph vessels surrounded by circular layers of calcium salts and collagen, called lamellae, in which reside osteocytes.

HDL CHOLESTEROL. High-density lipoprotein; "good" cholesterol; a carrier molecule in the blood that is primarily protein with small amounts of triglycerides and cholesterol and that helps protect against heart disease. A healthy adult level should be at least 60 mg/dL.

HEALTH DISPARITIES. Differences in health, health care, and/or health outcomes between different racial and ethnic groups, genders, and geographical locations within a single population.

HEALTH DISPARITIES. Differences in health, health care, and/or health outcomes between different racial and ethnic groups, genders, and geographical locations within a single population.

HEART ATTACK. A serious medical condition caused by a deficient flow of blood to the heart.

HEART MURMUR. A medical condition characterized by an abnormal heartbeat sound caused by any number of anatomical abnormalities in the heart structure, such as a hole in the wall between two parts of the heart.

HEART RATE MAXIMUM (HRMAX). Maximum cardiac activity in beats per minute (bpm); estimated by subtracting one' age from 220.

HEART RATE RESERVE. Refers to the difference between maximal heart rate and resting heart rate.

HEART RATE (HR). Pulse; the number of heartbeats per minute (bpm), determined with an HR monitor or by counting the pulse on the wrist or neck.

HEART-RATE CHECK. Counting the pulse on the wrist or neck during aerobic exercise, to ensure that one is working at aerobic intensity, but not above the maximum intensity for one's age. Generally, the pulse is counted for ten or 15 seconds and multiplied by six or four, respectively, to obtain beats per minute.

HEART TRANSPLANT. Removal of patient's heart and replacement with a donor heart.

HEAT BLISTER. A blister caused by exposure to sunlight or to intense heat.

HEAT CRAMPS. The least serious of the heat-related illnesses, that can quickly develop into heat exhaustion.

HEAT EXHAUSTION. A condition more serious than heat cramp caused by overexercise in hot conditions, characterized by dizziness, nausea, and general bodily weakness.

HEATSTROKE. The most serious stage of overexercise, heat-related medical conditions in which the body is no longer able to disperse heat faster than it is being produced; a potentially life-threatening condition.

HEEL. The back part of the foot just below the ankle.

HEEL. In wrestling, the bad guy or villain in a match.

HELICOBACTER PYLORI. Recently discovered bacteria that live in gastric acids and are believed to be a major cause of most stomach ulcers.

HEMOGLOBIN. An iron-containing protein that transports oxygen molecules throughout the body.

HEMOGLOBIN A1C (HG A1C). Glycated hemoglobin; a stable binding of glucose to hemoglobin A in the blood, which can be used to determine the average blood glucose level for the previous two to three months.

HEMORRHAGIC. Copious discharge of blood from the blood vessels.

HERNIATION. The process of rupturing within the wall of a body cavity, such as the spinal column.

HIGH BAR (ALSO "HORIZONTAL BAR"). A piece of gymnastic equipment 2.4 meters in length, about 2.5 meters above the floor, as well as the exercise performed by men on the apparatus.

HIGH-DENSITY LIPOPROTEIN (HDL) CHOLESTEROL. The "good" cholesterol that transports unhealthy cholesterol away from the arteries to the liver, which can process it for removal from the body.

HILUS. The indentation found along the medial side of the kidney; the point at which blood vessels (the renal artery and renal vein), nerves, and the ureter enter and exit the organ.

HIP FLEXORS. The group of muscles that flex the thigh bone toward the pelvis to pull the knee up.

HIPPOCAMPUS. A part of the brain that is involved in forming, storing, and processing memory, and in regulating mood.

HISTAMINE. A chemical released by mast cells during an allergic reaction that has a variety of effects on cells and tissues throughout the body.

HOGU. The Korean word for the chest protector worn in sport tae kwon do.

HOME RUN. An event in which a batter hits the ball outside the physical limits of the playing field, allowing him or her to pass through all four bases and score a run.

HOMEOSTASIS (WATER). A condition of adequate fluid level in the body in which fluid loss and fluid intake are equally matched and sodium levels are within normal range.

HORMONE. A substance, such as a protein, that is produced in one part of the body and travels through the bloodstream to affect another part of the body.

HORMONE SENSITIVE LIPASE (HSL). An enzyme that releases free fatty acids from triglycerides in response to the hormone epinephrine.

HOUSE SHOW. An event that is not televised.

HPV INFECTION. Infection of the human papillomavirus through sexual transmission.

HUMAN GROWTH HORMONE. A hormone secreted by the pituitary of healthy individuals during childhood and throughout life. It is necessary for normal growth and healthy organs.

HUMERUS. The long bone in the upper arm of humans.

HYDRATION. The act of supplying the body with adequate water.

HYDROGEN PEROXIDE; H_2O_2. An unstable metabolite produced in the body that can cause oxidative damage to cell components.

HYDROSTATIC PRESSURE. The pressure of the water against the body.

HYDROSTATIC WEIGHING. Underwater weighing or hydrodensitometry; an accurate body composition test that determines the proportion of body fat via water displacement.

HYDROXYL RADICAL. OH^-; a highly reactive metabolite produced by the body that can cause oxidative damage to cell components.

HYEONG. The Korean word for the patterns or forms of movement sequences that are a major component of tae kwon do practice. It is also spelled hyung.

HYMEN. Membrane that stretches across the opening of the vagina.

HYPERCHOLESTEROLEMIA. Excess cholesterol in the blood.

HYPERGLYCEMIA. An abnormally high blood glucose level.

HYPERHYDRATION. Accelerated hydration.

HYPERLIPIDEMIA. Abnormally high levels of lipids in the blood.

HYPERPLASTIC OBESITY. Excessive weight gain in childhood, characterized by an increase in the number of fat cells.

HYPERPROLACTINEMIA. The production of too much prolactin, a hormone that normally stimulates the production of breast milk.

HYPERSENSITIVITY. An immune reaction that results from an immune mediated inflammatory response to an antigen that would normally be innocuous.

HYPERTENSION. High blood pressure; systolic blood pressure greater than or equal to 140, and diastolic blood pressure greater than or equal to 90.

HYPERTHERMIA. Refers to an elevated body core temperature due to failed thermoregulation.

HYPERTONIC. Having a greater concentration than some other reference solution, such as body fluids.

HYPERTROPHIC CARDIOMYOPATHY (HCM). pathological, excessive thickening of the heart muscle and the most common cause of sudden death in American athletes.

HYPERTROPHIC OBESITY. Excessive weight gain in adulthood, characterized by expansion of pre-existing fat cells.

HYPERTROPHY. Thickening of muscle fiber, resulting in increased muscle bulk or mass.

HYPERVENTILATION. Rapid, shallow breathing.

HYPOGLYCEMIA. An abnormally low blood glucose level.

HYPOGONADISM. A condition in which there is decreased sexual development and growth of the testes.

HYPOKINETIC DISEASES. Conditions that occur as a consequence of a lifestyle with too little movement; e.g., obesity and Type 2 diabetes.

HYPONATREMIA. An abnormally low level of sodium in blood plasma. It can result from water intoxication.

HYPOPLASTIC ANEMIA. Anemia that is characterized by defective function of the blood-forming organs (such as bone marrow) and is caused by toxic agents such as chemicals or x rays. Anemia is a blood condition in which there are too few red blood cells or the red blood cells are deficient in hemoglobin.

HYPOTENSION. Abnormally low blood pressure.

HYPOTHALAMUS. The hypothalamus is a portion of the diencephalon in the brain. It regulates many functions of the autonomic nervous system as well as communicates with the endocrine system via the pituitary gland.

HYPOTHYROIDISM. A condition in which the thyroid gland fails to produce enough thyroid hormone; symptoms include sensitivity to cold, depression, constipation, fatigue, weight gain.

HYPOTONIC. Having a lesser concentration than some other reference solution, such as body fluids.

HYPOXIA. Low levels of blood oxygen.

HYSTERECTOMY. Surgical removal of the uterus.

I

IDEAL WEIGHT. Weight corresponding to the lowest death rate for individuals of a specific height, gender, and age.

ILIOTIBIAL BAND (ITB). The fibrous tissue along the outside of the hip, thigh, and knee that stabilizes the knee and helps to flex and extend the knee, and is a common problem for runners and other athletes.

ILIOTIBIAL BAND SYNDROME (ITB). A type of hip injury.

ILIUM. The largest and uppermost bone of the pelvis.

IMPACTED FRACTURE. A fracture in which opposite bone ends are driven into each other. Also known as buckle fractures.

IMPAIRED FASTING GLUCOSE (IFG). An abnormally high level of blood glucose after an eight-hour fast.

IMPAIRED GLUCOSE TOLERANCE (IGT). An abnormally high blood glucose level with an oral glucose tolerance test.

IMPERFORATE HYMEN. The lack of an opening in the membranous fold partly or completely closing the opening to the vagina.

INBORN ERRORS OF METABOLISM. Metabolic disorders caused by a genetic error.

INCOMPLETE FRACTURE. A fracture in which a bone breaks, but does not completely separate.

INCONTINENCE. Loss of ability to control urination or to control bowel movements (fecal incontinence).

INCRETIN MIMETICS. GLP-1 receptor agonists; a class of type 2 diabetes medications that mimic the effects of the incretin hormone GLP-1, by binding to GLP-1 receptors, thereby lowering blood sugar levels.

INDIRECT CALORIMETRY. The measurement of oxygen consumption and carbon dioxide production; heat measurement is calculated mathematically using a formula and energy can subsequently be calculated.

INDUSTRIAL REVOLUTION. A time period in the United States during the mid-1800s where there was rapid development of machinery, resulting in a modern urban-industrial state where less physical labor and activity were required.

INFIELD. In cricket, the region of the field that lies inside a 30 yard circle in the center of the playing field.

INFLAMMATION. The reaction of tissue to injury.

INFLUENZA. A contagious viral infection of the respiratory passages; various strains of influenza (e.g., the Spanish flu) have been responsible for the death of millions.

INFRASPINATUS. A muscle at the middle of the shoulder blade.

INNING. The unit of play time in baseball during which the team at bat continues to do so until it has accumulated three outs.

INNINGS. One team's time at bat or at bowling.

INSIDIOUS. Progressing gradually and inconspicuously, but with serious effects.

INSULIN. A protein hormone synthesized in the pancreas and secreted by beta cells of the islets of Langerhans. Insulin is required for the metabolism of carbohydrates, lipids, and proteins, and regulates blood sugar levels by facilitating the uptake of glucose into tissues, converting sugars to glycogen, fatty acids, and triglycerides, and preventing the release of glucose from the liver.

INSULIN RESISTANCE. Reduced sensitivity to insulin, resulting in lower activity of insulin-responsive processes and/or increased insulin production; typically occurring with diabetes.

INSULIN SENSITIVITY. The responsiveness of various physiological processes to the hormone insulin.

INTENSITY VIOLATOR. An individual who consistently exercises at an intensity above their prescribed training intensity range.

INTENSIVE CARDIAC REHABILITATION. New designation for research-proven cardiac rehabilitation, such as the Ornish or Pritikin program.

INTERCALATED GAMES. A proposed series of Olympic Games schedule in the even off years between regularly scheduled Olympic Games, always to be held in Athens. In fact, the intercalated games were held only once, in 1906.

INTERLEUKIN-6 (IL-6). A small molecule produced by various cell types that has a variety of functions, including metabolic regulation during exercise.

INTERMEDIATE. In the United States, a rower who has not yet advanced to the role of Senior or Elite rower.

INTERNAL GENITALS. The vagina, uterus, fallopian tubes, and ovaries.

INTERSTITIAL SPACE. The spaces found within organs and tissues.

INTERVAL TRAINING. A type of endurance training involving very short intervals of very high intensity exercise, followed by equal intervals of active recovery.

INTOXICATION. Poisoning by ingestion of a drug, toxic substance, or other such material (such as water).

INTRACRANIAL. Within the skull.

INTRAMUSCULAR TRIGLYCERIDES; IMTG. The form in which fatty acids are stored in muscle cells.

INTRAVENOUS (IV). The process of giving a liquid through a vein.

IPHONE. A line of Web-based, multimedia-enabled smartphones, which is owned by Apple Inc.

IRON. A type of golf club used to hit for accuracy, generally at distances shorter than those for which woods are used.

ISCHEMIA. An inadequate flow of oxygenated blood to a part of the body.

ISCHEMIC NEPHROPATHY. Another name for atherosclerosis, or the clogging and hardening of the arteries.

ISCHIUM. The bone that forms the lower and back part of the hip bone.

ISOMETRIC. Muscular contraction against resistance without significant change in muscle fiber length.

ISOMETRIC CONTRACTION. Any activity of a muscle in which it neither shortens nor lengthens while under tension due to the application of a larger but opposing force.

ISOTONIC. Having the same concentration as some other reference solution, such as body fluids.

ISOTONIC. Relating to the contraction of a muscle under constant tension.

J

JET LAG. A physiological condition that results when the body's circadian rhythm becomes disoriented by air travel from east to west or west to east across the Earth.

JOGGING. A moderate form of running in which the primary goal is recreational rather than winning a competition.

JOULE. The International System of Units (SI) unit of energy.

JUNIOR. A rower who has not attained the age of 19.

K

KARVONEN FORMULA. Heart rate reserve; maximum heart rate (220 − age) minus resting heart rate.

KATANA. A long, heavy sword originally developed for use by the Japanese samurai.

KERATIN. Insoluble protein found in hair, nails, and skin.

KETONES. Poisonous acidic compounds produced by the body when fat, instead of glucose, is burned for energy. Breakdown of fat occurs when not enough insulin is present to channel glucose into body cells.

KIDNEYS. A pair or organs in the abdomen of vertebrates (such as humans) that filter waste bodily liquids.

KILOCALORIE (KCAL). The actual term used in the United States for a unit of food energy, which is normally called a calorie; the amount of energy needed to increase the temperature of one kilogram of water by one degree of Celsius; one kilocalorie equals 1,000 calories; also defined as the amount of energy that food has the potential to produce when consumed and digested in the body.

KILOGRAM. The International System of Units (SI) unit of mass, where one such unit is equal to one thousand grams.

KINESIOLOGY. The science or study of movement.

KINETIC CHAIN. The connection or relationship between the nerves, muscles, and bones during movement.

KNEELING PADDLEBOARDING. Paddleboarding while one is kneeling on the board.

KUNDALINI. Dormant energy in the body.

KYPHOSIS. The medical term for curvature of the upper spine. Osteoporosis is a common cause of kyphosis in older adults.

L

L/MIN. Liters of oxygen consumed per minute; the absolute expression of maximal oxygen uptake.

LACERATION. Irregular tear-like wound.

LACTATE. This compound is manufactured from pyruvate during higher intensity exercise.

LACTATE THRESHOLD. The point in aerobic metabolism at which lactic acid is being produced more rapidly by muscle cells than it can be removed by the blood.

LACTATION. The secretion of milk by the mammary gland in the breasts.

LACTIC ACID. An organic acid produced by the muscles with chemical symbol $C_3H_6O_3$.

LACTOSE. A sugar found in milk that provides energy.

LACTOVEGETARIAN DIET. A vegetarian diet that includes dairy products, but not eggs.

LAME JACKET. A jacket that contains metallic fibers that allow electronic detection of a touch.

LANUGOS. A soft, downy body hair that develops on the chest and arms of people with anorexia.

LATERALLY. Outwardly.

LATISSIMUS DORSI. Abbreviated lats, the broadest muscle within the back, it adducts, medially rotates, and extends the arm at the shoulder.

LAXATIVE. A substance that stimulates movement of food through the bowels. Laxatives are used to treat constipation.

LDL CHOLESTEROL. Low-density lipoprotein; "bad" cholesterol; a lipoprotein in the blood with a high proportion of cholesterol, which increases the risk of heart disease; less than 100 mg/dL is considered a healthy level in adults.

LEPTIN. A peptide hormone produced by fat cells that acts on the hypothalamus to suppress appetite and burn stored fat.

LEPTOSPIROSIS. A rare bacterial infection that can lead to serious complications, including meningitis, renal failure, and liver failure.

LET'S MOVE. First Lady Michelle Obama's initiative for combating childhood obesity, which incorporates aspects of the President's Challenge.

LEUCINE. A white chrystalline essential amino acid.

LEYDIG CELLS. Found in the interstitial compartment of a testis; responsible for the production and secretion of testosterone.

LIGAMENT. Tissue that connects bones or cartilage at a joint, whose purpose is to support a muscle or other body part.

LIMIT STRENGTH. The amount of muscular force that an athlete can generate for a single all-out effort.

LIPID PEROXIDATION. The oxidative degradation of lipids in cell membranes by free radicals.

LIPIDS. Fats; organic compounds that are stored in the body as energy reserves and that are important components of cell membranes.

LIPOLYSIS. The hydrolysis—breakdown involving water—of fats.

LIPOPROTEIN. A large class of protein-lipid complexes.

LIPOPROTEIN LIPASE (LPL). An enzyme that breaks down triglycerides in lipoproteins to monoglycerides and free fatty acids.

LOB. A defensive shot made by hitting the ball high into the air, allowing the defending player to recover position.

LOCAL AUTHORITY. In the United Kingdom, administrative bodies responsible for policy and programs at the town, city, county, or other local area. The term has somewhat different meanings in England, Wales, Scotland, and Northern Ireland.

LONG. In handball, a served ball that hits the back wall before it hits the floor.

LOOP. A stroke in which the ping pong ball has a great deal of topspin, causing it to jump upward after hitting the table.

LOTUS SUTRA. One of the most sacred texts of Buddhism, regarded as a summary of the supreme Buddhist teaching that leads one directly to enlightenment.

LOW SERUM POTASSIUM LEVELS. Potassium is a normal electrolyte found in the body; lower than normal concentrations in the blood can cause numerous problems including abnormal heart beats and fatigue.

LOW-DENSITY LIPOPROTEIN (LDL) CHOLESTEROL. Cholesterol that is often called "bad" cholesterol, it is the cholesterol that builds up on the artery walls to form plaque which can restrict blood flow and cause heart-attack and stroke.

LOWER ESOPHAGEAL SPHINCTER. A strong muscle ring between the esophagus and the stomach that keeps gastric juice, and even duodenal bile from flowing upwards out of the stomach.

LUMBAGO. Another name for low back pain.

LUMBAR. Relating to the lower back.

LUNGE. A movement in which a fencer thrusts the weapon forward.

LUPUS. Lupus erythematosus, a disease of the connective tissue.

LUPUS VASCULITIS. An inflammation of the blood vessels that sometimes occurs in conjunction with the autoimmune disease known as lupus.

LUTEINIZING HORMONE. A hormone which acts with follicle-stimulating hormone to cause ovulation of mature follicles and secretion of estrogen from the ovary.

LYMPH. The slightly opalescent fluid found within the lymphatic system.

LYMPH NODES. Bean-shaped swellings along the lymphatic vessels that contain macrophages and lymphocytes.

LYMPHATIC SYSTEM. The transport system linked to the cardiovascular system that contains the immune system and also carries metabolized fat and fat soluble vitamins throughout the body.

LYMPHATICS. The system of lymphatic vessels.

LYSOZYMES. A basic bacteriolytic protein that hydrolyzes peptidoglycan and is present in egg white and in human tears and saliva.

M

MACROCYCLE. The major and longest segment of a periodization program that consists of three parts: preparation, competition, and recovery.

MACRONUTRIENT. A substance (protein or carbohydrate) essential in large amounts to the growth and health of an animal.

MACROPHAGES. Cells that are capable of ingesting microorganisms by phagocytosis and have a critical role in the host defense to pathogens.

MAGNETIC RESONANCE IMAGING (MRI) SCAN. A special radiological diagnostic test that uses magnetic waves to create pictures of an area, including bones, muscles, and tendons.

MARFAN'S SYNDROME. genetic connective tissue disorder that increases risk of sudden death by dissection of the aorta.

MARROW. A type of connective tissue that fills the spaces of most cancellous bone. It produces blood cells and stores fat.

MARTIAL ARTS. Various methods of armed and unarmed combat, using the arms, hands, feet, and legs as weapons, that originated centuries ago in Asia, primarily China, Japan, Korea, and the Philippines. The most popular styles include karate, kung fu, jujitsu, judo, aikido.

MASKING AGENT. A drug or other substance that renders another drug undetectable in the urine.

MASTER. A rower who is 21 years of age or older.

MAXIMAL CARDIAC OUTPUT. Total volume of blood capable of being pumped by the left ventricle per minute during intense exercise.

MAXIMAL HEART RATE (HRMAX). The maximal heart rate that can be elicited in an individual during intense exercise or exertion; this value can either be estimated (most commonly using 220-age) or directly measured from a maximal exercise test.

MAXIMAL OXYGEN UPTAKE. The highest rate at which oxygen can be taken up and consumed by the body during intense exercise.

MAXIMAL OXYGEN UPTAKE RESERVE (VO_2R). The difference between maximal oxygen uptake and resting oxygen uptake.

MAXIMAL STROKE VOLUME. Maximal difference between end-diastolic volume and end-systolic volume during intense exercise.

MAXIMAL VOLUNTARY VENTILATION. The highest volume of air that can be breathed per minute.

MECHANORECEPTORS. Receptors specialized to detect mechanical signals and relay that information centrally in the nervous system. Mechanoreceptors include hair cells involved in hearing and balance.

MEDIAL. Inward.

MEDIAL TIBIAL STRESS SYNDROME (MTSS). The technical name for shin splits.

MEDIALLY. Inwardly.

MEDICINE BALL. A weighted exercise ball about 14 in. (36 cm) in diameter that is used for strength training.

MEDITATION. Technique of concentration for relaxing the mind and body.

MELANIN. Brown-black pigment found in skin and hair.

MELANOCYTES. A cell of the epidermis that produces melanin.

MELANOMA. A usually malignant tumor of the melanin-forming cells which is known to metastasize rapidly.

MENARCHE. The first menstrual cycle in a girl's life.

MENOPAUSE. The stage of life during which a woman passes from the reproductive to the non-reproductive stage and she experiences the cessation of menstruation.

MENSTRUATION. The discharge of the lining of the uterus (endometrium) as it sheds during the menstrual cycle when pregnancy does not take place.

MERENGUE. A style of Latin American music and dance with a two-step beat.

MERIDIANS. In traditional Chinese medicine, the channels that run beneath the skin through which the body's energy flows.

MESOCYCLE. A sub-division of a macrocycle in a periodization program, usually lasting a few weeks and consisting of a number of microcycles.

METABOLIC. Referring to the processes involved in which nutrients are converted into energy for a living organism to sustain life.

METABOLIC ACTIVITY. The sum of the chemical processes in the body that are necessary to maintain life.

METABOLIC BONE DISEASE. Weakening of bones due to a deficiency of certain minerals, especially calcium.

METABOLIC EQUIVALENT OF TASK (MET). The energy cost of a physical activity, measured as a multiple of the resting metabolic rate, which is defined as 3.5 milliliters of oxygen consumed per kilogram (kg) of body weight per minute, equivalent to 1 kilocalorie per kg per hour.

METABOLIC PATHWAY. Chemical reactions causing the formation of ATP and waste products.

METABOLIC RATE. The rate (speed) at which biochemical reactions of metabolism take place in living cells, such as those in the human body.

METABOLIC SYNDROME. The name for a group of signs and disorders that put a person at high risk for diabetes and cardiovascular disease.

METABOLISM. The series of chemical processes within a living organism that converts food into energy and products to sustain life.

METANEPHRINE. A breakdown product of catecholamines, including epinephrine, that is found in the urine and some tissues.

MICROCYCLE. The smallest unit of a macrocycle in a periodization training program, typically lasting about a week.

MICRONUTRIENT. An organic compound (vitamin) essential in minute amounts to the growth and health of an animal.

MICROORGANISM. Any tiny organism such as a bacterium or virus, which is only able to be seen under a high-powered microscope.

MICROPHAGES. A small phagocyte.

MIDDLE AGES. The era in European history between the years 476 and 1450.

MIDFIELDERS. Lacrosse players whose primary responsibility is covering the middle part of the playing field.

MILD COGNITIVE IMPAIRMENT (MCI). A transitional phase of memory loss in older people that precedes dementia or AD.

MINDFULNESS. A nonjudgmental conscious awareness of one's present thoughts, feelings, surroundings, and physical sensations.

MITOCHONDRIA. The organelles in cells that produce energy through respiration.

MITOCHONDRIAL ENZYME LEVELS. The concentrations of those enzymes (i.e., biological catalysts) involved with aerobic respiration.

MITOCHONDRIAL RESPIRATORY. Reactions within the mitochondrion that ultimately lead ot the production of ATP and consumption of oxygen.

MIXED MARTIAL ARTS (MMA). A term that is used to describe a recent form of full-contact sport that combines elements of boxing, wrestling, judo, karate, and kickboxing. It is also called ultimate fighting or no-holds-barred fighting.

MOGUL. A mogul is a term for the bumps on certain ski runs (paths) and for the type of freestyle skiing that skis over the bumps and often involves aerial or acrobatic tricks.

MOLE. A unit within the International System of Units (SI) that measures the amount of a chemical substance, which is equal to about 6.02214×10^{23} molecules of that substance.

MONOUNSATURATED FATTY ACID (MUFA). A fatty acid containing one double bond, which lowers plasma cholesterol when replacing SFAs and is believed to be safer than polyunsaturated fats.

MORBIDLY OBESE. defines person who is 100 lb (45 kg) or more than 50% overweight and has a body mass index above 40.

MOTOR NEURON. A nerve cell that specifically controls and stimulates voluntary muscles.

MOUNTAIN BIKE. A lightweight bike with frames designed for off-road use, knobby or studded tires, and disk brakes on the newer models. Mountain bikes are designed to withstand rough trails and such obstacles as logs or rocks.

MRI. The abbreviated term for magnetic resonance imaging. MRI uses a large circular magnet and radio waves to generate signals from atoms in the body. These signals are used to construct images of internal structures.

MUCOSA. The digestive lining of the intestines.

MUCOSAL. Mucus membrane.

MUCUS. A thick, moist fluid that coats epithelial cells and cilia.

MULTI-COMPONENT TRAINING. A specialized type of balance training that requires an individual to perform a balance exercise while simultaneously performing another task; for example, playing catch with a ball while balancing on one leg.

MULTIFIDUS. A muscle of the fifth, deepest layer of the back, extending from the sacrum to the skull, that helps erect and rotate the spine.

MULTINUCLEATED. Having more than one nucleus in each cell. Muscle cells are multinucleated.

MULTIPLE SCLEROSIS (MS). An autoimmune disorder of the central nervous system that is often managed, in part, with endurance training.

MULTIVITAMIN. A nutritional supplement that, usually, contains all of the vitamins and minerals that experts suggest as necessary for a healthy diet.

MUSCLE DIFFUSION CAPACITY. Measure of the capability to exchange carbon dioxide and oxygen between skeletal muscle and the capillary bed.

MUSCLE SPASM. Localized muscle contraction that occurs when the brain signals the muscle to contract.

MUSCULAR FITNESS. An overarching term characterizing the health of an individual's skeletal muscle; can be reflected in the capacity to generate sufficient muscle strength and endurance for various tasks.

MYALGIA. The technical name for muscle pain.

MYASTHENIA GRAVIS. A disease characterized by the impaired transmission of motor nerve impulses, caused by the autoimmune destruction of acetylcholine receptors.

MYELIN. The substance making up the protective sheath of nerve axons.

MYOCARDIAL. Relating to the thick muscular wall of the heart.

MYOCARDIAL INFARCTION. A heart attack. Refers to changes to the heart tissue, with tissue death the principal one, due to sudden disruptions in oxygenated blood flow.

MYOCARDITIS. inflammation of the heart muscle usually due to viral or bacteria infection.

MYOFIBRIL. A long, thin, spaghetti-like strand of actin and myosin that constitutes the basic structure of muscle tissue.

MYOFIBRILLAR HYPERTROPHY. An increase in muscle size because of the addition of actin and myosin proteins to myofibrils.

MYOFIBRILS. Long cylindrical structures that are bundled together within a muscle fiber.

MYOSIN. A protein found in muscle tissue involved in the process of muscle function.

MYOSITIS. Inflammation of muscle tissue.

MYOTONIA. The inability to normally relax a muscle after contracting or tightening it.

I N

NANOPARTICLE. A particle, such as a metal or polymer, that has physical dimensions in the nanometer range, where one nanometer is equal to one billionth of a meter.

NATIONAL CENTER FOR HEALTH STATISTICS; NCHS. The division within the U.S. Centers for Disease Control and Prevention (CDC) that compiles, analyzes, and disseminates health statistics for the nation.

NEOLITHIC AGRICULTURAL REVOLUTION. A time period between 10,000 to 8,000 BC whereby humans gradually transitioned from a society of hunters and gathers to that of agriculture and settlement.

NEOPRENE. Also called polychloroprene, a group of synthetic rubbers produced by the polymerization of chloroprene.

NEPHRITIS. Inflammation of the kidney.

NEPHRON. The individual filtering unit of the kidney; consists of Bowman's capsule, the glomerulus, and the renal tubule.

NEPHROPATHY. A disease or disorder of the kidneys.

NERVOUS SYSTEM. The entire system of nerve tissue in the body. It includes the brain, the brain stem, the spinal cord, the nerves, and the ganglia, and is divided into the peripheral nervous system (PNS) and the central nervous system (CNS).

NEUROFIBRILLARY TANGLES. Accumulations of twisted protein fragments inside nerve cells in the brain that are diagnostic of AD.

NEUROMOTOR FITNESS. Healthy skills in terms of balance, agility, coordination, and gait.

NEURONS. Cells of the nervous system. Usually consist of a cell body, the soma, that contains the nucleus and the surrounding cytoplasm; several short thread-like projections (dendrites); and one long filament (the axon).

NEUROPATHY. A general term describing functional disorders and/or abnormal changes in the peripheral nervous system. If the involvement is in one nerve it is called mononeuropathy, and if in several nerves, mononeuropathy multiplex.

NEUROTRANSMITTER. A chemical—such as norepinephrine or serotonin—that transmits impulses across synapses between nerves.

NEUTRAL SPINE. Good posture; the three natural curves of the spine.

NIACIN. Nicotinic acid; a B-complex vitamin that may help lower cholesterol.

NIRVANA. In Buddhism, release from the cycle of reincarnation through conquering one's hatreds, passions, and delusions.

NITRIC OXIDE (NO). A regulator of various bodily processes, including blood vessel dilation; produced via the oxidation of the amino acid arginine.

NOCICEPTORS. Receptor sites on nerve cells that respond to pain signals.

NOCTURNAL LEG CRAMPS. Cramps that may be related to exertion and awaken a person during sleep.

NON-CALORIMETRIC TECHNIQUES. Methods of predicting the rate of heat production, and therefore energy expenditure, from various physiological measurements and/or observations.

NONESSENTIAL AMINO ACIDS. The 11 common amino acids—glutamate, glutamine, proline, aspartate, asparagine, alanine, glycine, serine, tyrosine, cysteine, and arginine—that are required for health, but which can be synthesized by the body.

NON-EXERCISE ACTIVITY THERMOGENESIS (NEAT). A recently defined concept term that entails the energy expenditure of normal daily physical activities such as fidgeting, maintaining posture when not reclining, and spontaneous muscle contraction.

NONSTEROIDAL ANTI-INFLAMMATORY DRUGS (NSAIDS). A class of drugs that is used to relieve pain, and symptoms of inflammation, such as ibuprofen and ketoprofen.

NOREPINEPHRINE. Noradrenaline; a neurotransmitter in the sympathetic nervous system and some parts of the central nervous system, as well as a blood-pressure-raising (vasoconstricting) adrenal hormone.

NORMAL WEIGHT. A BMI of less than 25.0.

NORMATIVE. Test performance assessment based on results previously achieved by a selected sample of subjects, rather than by independent or absolute standards.

NUTRIENTS. Vitamins, minerals, proteins, lipids, and carbohydrates needed by the body.

NUTRITIONAL SUPPLEMENT. A substance, such as a vitamin, mineral, amino acid, or herb, taken to compensate for the lack of some essential nutrient in one's daily diet.

O

OBESE. Having a body mass index (BMI) of 30–39.9. A BMI of 40 and higher is considered seriously obese.

OBESITY. Excessive weight due to accumulation of fat, usually defined as a body mass index of 30 or above or body weight greater than 30% above normal on standard height-weight tables.

OBLIQUE FRACTURE. A fracture that occurs diagonally to the axis of the bone.

OBLIQUES. The two flat muscles on each side that form the middle and outer layers of the lateral walls of the abdomen.

OCULOMOTOR NERVE. Cranial nerve responsible for motor enervation of the upper eyelid muscle, the extraocular muscle and the eye pupil muscle.

OLLIE. A maneuver in which a skateboard rider lifts the board and himself or herself into the air without the use of hands.

OLYMPIAD. The four-year period between Olympic Games. Also, a synonym for "Olympic Games.".

OMEGA-3 FATTY ACIDS. Any of several polyunsaturated fatty acids found in leafy green vegetables, vegetable oils, and fish such as salmon and mackerel, capable of reducing cholesterol levels and having anticoagulant properties.

ORAL GLUCOSE TOLERANCE TEST (OGTT). A measure of the blood glucose level after a fast of at least eight hours and two hours after drinking a specific glucose solution.

ORIENTEERING. A competitive sport in which participants attempt to find their way across a course using only a map and a compass.

ORNISH. An intensive lifestyle program founded by Dean Ornish, MD, proven to reverse cardiovascular disease. Received the designation of intensive cardiac rehabilitation.

ORTHOPEDIC. Relating to disorders of the bones, ligaments, joints, and muscles.

ORTHOPEDIC SURGEON. A physician and surgeon that specializes in disorders of the bones and associated muscles, tendons, and joints.

OSSIFICATION. The process of replacing connective tissue such as cartilage and mesenchyme with bone.

OSTEOARTHRITIS. A condition of deterioration of the bone and cartilage of joints; marked by pain, swelling, and stiffness in the joints and effecting predominantly older women.

OSTEOBLAST. A type of bone cell that is responsible for bone formation. The number of osteoblasts in a person's body decreases with age.

OSTEOCYTE. Mature bone cell whose main function is to regulate the levels of calcium and phosphate in the body.

OSTEOPENIA. The medical name for low bone mass, a condition that often precedes osteoporosis.

OSTEOPOROSIS. A disease characterized by low bone mass and structural deterioration of bone tissue, leading to bone fragility.

OVER-THE-COUNTER (OTC). A drug that can be purchased without a doctor's prescription.

OVERTRAINING SYNDROME. A state that occurs in athletes or people who exercise regularly when the exercise routine is very strenuous or lasts for excessive amounts of time and rest between exercise sessions is not sufficient for muscle recovery.

OVERWEIGHT. A body mass index (BMI) between 25.0 and 30.0.

OVULATION. The release of a fully mature ovum from the ovary as part of a normal menstrual cycle.

OXIDANT. A substances that oxides another substance.

OXYGEN. An odorless, colorless gas and an element with the symbol "O" (atomic number 8 and chemical formula O_2), which is essential for respiration within most living beings, such as humans.

OXYGEN DEBT. A cumulative deficiency of oxygen for metabolism that develops during intense exercise and must be replenished during rest.

P

PACE/TEMPO TRAINING. High-intensity endurance training designed to improve both aerobic and anaerobic energy production.

PAIDOTRIBE. Physical trainers in ancient Greece who supervised gymnastics at the Palaestra.

PALAESTRA. A public place in ancient Greece devoted to the practice of gymnastics.

PALM SLIDERS. A type of glove worn by inline skaters similar to cycling gloves, with a hard plastic palm to protect the hand while performing certain types of maneuvers.

PALSY. Paralysis.

PAR. In golf, the number of strokes that an average player is expected to take in placing the ball into the cup on a particular hole.

PARALLEL BARS. A set of two bars 3.5 meters in length and 2 meters above the floor, as well as the exercise performed on the apparatus.

PARALLELETTES. Small parallel bars similar in shape, but smaller in size, than parallel bars used in gymnastics.

PARALYMPICS GAMES. An athletic competition held in connection with the Summer and Winter Olympics Games designed for persons who are blind, deaf, or otherwise physically handicapped.

PARAPLEGIC. An individual who is paralyzed from the waist down.

PARASYMPATHETIC. Pertaining to the part of the autonomic nervous system that generally functions in regulatory opposition to the sympathetic system, as by slowing the heartbeat or contracting the pupil of the eye.

PARASYMPATHETIC NERVOUS SYSTEM. One of the two divisions of the autonomic nervous system. Parasympathetic nerves emerge from the skull as fibres from the oculomotor, facial, glossopharyngeal and vagus nerves and from the sacral region of the spinal cord.

PARKINSONISM. A neurological disorder that includes a fine tremor, muscular weakness and rigidity, and an altered way of walking.

PARRY. A defensive action by a fencer.

PATELLA. The medical term for the kneecap.

PATHOGEN. A microorganism that has the potential to cause a disease.

PECTORALIS MAJOR. Sometimes called pectorals, pecs, or chest muscles, the thick, fan-shaped muscles located at the chest of the body; the clavicular part flexes the arm at the shoulder; the sternal part extends the arm at the shoulder; both parts (heads) medially rotate and adduct the arm at the shoulder.

PECTORALS. Any of four flat muscles, positioned two on each side of the front of the chest, which help to move the upper arm and shoulder.

PEDOMETER. Step counter; a device that counts each step by detecting hip motion.

PENALTY. An infraction that occurs because an ice hockey player has violated a rule of the game, resulting in his or her being sent to the penalty box for two, four, or five minutes, or for a longer period of time.

PEPTIDE BOND. A chemical bond between the carboxyl group of one amino acid and the amino nitrogen atom of another.

PERCENTILE. A rank in a population that has been divided into 100 equal groups; thus, test results in the 50th percentile indicate that half of those who took the test scored higher and half scored lower.

PERFORMANCE ENHANCING DRUGS. Any type of drug used to increase performance, such as within an athletic event.

PERIPHERAL NERVES. The nerves outside of the brain and spinal cord, including the autonomic, cranial, and spinal nerves. These nerves contain cells other than neurons and connective tissue as well as axons.

PERIPHERAL NERVOUS SYSTEM (PNS). One of the two major divisions of the nervous system. The PNS consists of the somatic nervous system (SNS), which controls voluntary activities, and of the autonomic nervous system (ANS), which controls regulatory activities. The

ANS is further divided into sympathetic and parasympathetic systems.

PERIPHERAL VASCULAR DISEASE. Abbreviated PVD and also called peripheral artery disease (PAD), a condition involving the obstruction of large arteries excluding those within the heart, aorta, or brain.

PERISTALSIS. The wavelike motion of the digestive system that moves food through the digestive system.

PERSEVERATION. Continuous involuntary repetition of speech or behavior.

PERSONAL FLOTATION DEVICE (PFD). A device such as lifejacket or belt that is designed to keep people afloat with their nose and mouth above the water.

PERTURBATION. A disturbance in the body's equilibrium; within the context of balance it refers to an incident that challenges one's capacity to remain balanced.

PH. the negative logarithm of H^+ (hydrogen) concentration. Acid-base balance can be defined as homeostatis (equilibrium) of the body fluids at a normal arterial blood pH ranging between 7.37 and 7.43.

PHAGOCYTE. A white blood cell that engulfs and consumes foreign material (microorganisms) and debris.

PHALANGES. Bones forming the toes and fingers.

PHOSPHAGEN. Compounds such as phosphocreatine that supply muscles with energy during the initial stages of exercise and high-intensity exercise.

PHOSPHAGEN SYSTEM. Production of energy from coupled reactions of ATP and creatine phosphate.

PHOTOAGING. The effects of long-term exposure to ultraviolet light, either by sunlight or artificial UV light, resulting in wrinkling and spotting of the skin.

PHOTOCONJUNCTIVITIS. Swelling of the conjunctiva of the eye as a result of exposure to ultraviolet light.

PHOTOKERATITIS. Swelling of the cornea of the eye as a result of exposure to ultraviolet light.

PHYSICAL ACTIVITY. Any activity that involves moving the body and burning calories.

PHYSICAL FITNESS. A combination of muscle strength, cardiovascular health, and flexibility that is usually attributed to regular exercise and good nutrition.

PHYSIQUE. The outward shape, form, or appearance of the body.

PHYTOESTROGEN. Phytoestrogens are compounds found in many plants and have mild estrogenic and anti-estrogenic activity. They are known as hormone modulators for their ability to regulate either excess or deficient estrogen states.

PILATES. An exercise regimen specifically designed to improve overall physiological and mental functioning, with special emphasis on core training.

PISTE. A horizontal area 22 meters in length and 1.5 to 2 meters in width within which a fencing competition occurs.

PITCH. In cricket, the rectangular surface, 22 yards long and 10 yards wide, within which bowling and batting take place. Also, the playing field on which field hockey games are conducted.

PITUITARY GLAND. Often referred to as the "master gland," the pituitary is an endocrine gland that secretes several hormones that regulate growth, reproduction and metabolic processes.

PLANTAR FASCIA. Connective tissue that supports the arch in the foot.

PLANTAR FASCIITIS. A painful inflammation of the plantar fascia, or the connective tissue that supports the arch of the foot.

PLAQUE. Deposits of fat, cholesterol, and other substances that accumulate in the lining of the artery wall that can interfere with bloodflow through the vessel.

PLASMA. Clear, yellow- or straw-colored fluid that is the liquid component of blood and lymphatic fluid.

PLASTRON. A half jacket worn underneath the fencing jacket to provide extra protection.

PLATELET. A clotting factor in the blood.

PLATELET ACTIVATION. blood clotting.

PLAY THERAPY. A type of therapy in which a child engages in unstructured play that provides the therapist insight into the child's mind and allows the child to work through problems.

PLEXUS. A network or group of nerves.

PLYOMETRICS. A system of exercise that involves no weights or machines, but emphasizes calisthenics and exercises that use the weight of the body as resistance.

PNEUMONIA. A lung disease usually caused by infection that leads to inflammation. Patients often have fever, chills, cough, and difficulty breathing.

PODIATRIST. A medical professional specializing in the care of the feet and foot disorders.

POLIO. An acute viral disease characterized by inflammation of nerve cells in the brain and spinal cord.

POLYCYSTIC KIDNEY DISEASE. A disorder of the kidneys occurring when cysts are present on the kidneys.

POLYDIPSIA. Extreme thirst.

POLYGENIC. A trait or disorder that is determined by several different genes. Most human characteristics, including height, weight, and general body build, are polygenic. Schizophrenia and late-onset AD are considered polygenic disorders.

POLYMORPHISM. A change in the base pair sequence of DNA that may or may not be associated with a disease.

POLYPEPTIDE. A group of amino acids joined by peptide bonds; proteins are large polypeptides, but no agreement exists regarding how large they must be to justify the name.

POLYUNSATURATED FAT. A fat that contains two or more double per molecule, such as fats from fish and vegetable oils.

POMMEL HORSE. A piece of gymnastics equipment with a shape roughly similar to that of a horse, with a padded body 1.6 meters in length at the top, 35 centimeters wide at the top, and height from surface to floor of 1.15 meters, as well as the exercise performed on the apparatus.

POSITRON EMISSION TOMOGRAPHY (PET) SCAN. A non–invasive scanning technique that utilizes small amounts of radioactive positrons (positively charged particles) to visualize body function and metabolism.

POST-ACTIVATION POTENTIATION (PAP). An exercise process that triggers a biochemical change in muscle to maximize muscle performance.

POSTERIOR. In the rear.

POSTURAL HYPOTENSION (ORTHOSTATIC HYPOTENSION). A sudden drop in blood pressure when rising from a sitting or lying down position.

POTASSIUM HYDROXIDE. An inorganic compound consisting of potassium (K) and hydroxide (oxygen and hydrogen, OH); commonly called caustic potash.

POWER YOGA. A vigorous workout type of yoga that incorporates vinyasa flow at a fast pace. Power yoga emphasizes development of physical strength and flexibility.

PRANAYAMA. The Sanskrit word for the breathing exercises used in hatha yoga.

PREDIABETES. A condition characterized by blood glucose levels above normal, but lower than diabetic levels, that can progress to type 2 diabetes.

PREHYDRATION. Drinking fluid prior to exercise or heavy work in order to maintain proper hydration during the activity.

PREHYPERTENSION. Slightly to moderately elevated arterial blood pressure; usually defined as systolic pressure of 120–139 mm Hg or diastolic pressure of 80–89 mm Hg; a risk factor for hypertension.

PREPARTICIPATION EXAMINATION. A series of tests, inventories, and examinations recommended for a disabled person before she or he participates in a sporting or athletic event.

PRESIDENT'S CHALLENGE. America's primary physical activity and fitness initiative, which includes muscular strength and endurance tests.

PRESIDENTIAL ACTIVITY LIFESTYLE AWARD (PALA). A component of the President's Challenge, the PALA is a six-week commitment to daily physical activity, designed for everyone from young children to seniors.

PRITIKIN. An intensive lifestyle program proven to reverse or reduce several chronic diseases, including cardiovascular disease. Received a designation of intensive cardiac rehabilitation.

PROGESTIN. Female steroid sex hormones.

PROHORMONES. A physiologically inactive precursor of a hormone.

PRONATION. Rotational movement of the foot at the subtalar and talocalcaneonavicular joints.

PRONE PADDLEBOARDING. Paddleboarding while one is lying in the prone position, face down on the board.

PROPRIOCEPTION. The ability to sense the location, orientation, position, and movement of the body and its various parts.

PROPRIOCEPTORS. Sensory receptors located deep within tissues, such as skeletal muscle, that respond to physical or chemical changes in the body.

PROPRIOCEPTIVE MUSCULAR FACILITATION (PNF). A type of stretching with a partner designed to increase range of motion; used by occupational and physical therapists, chiropractors, and sports therapists and trainers.

PROSTAGLANDIN. One of a family of lipid compounds that have a variety of functions in the body.

PROSTATE. A gland found only in men that surrounds the neck of the bladder and secretes fluid that when mixed with sperm becomes semen.

PROSTHESES. Artificial body parts made for individuals who are missing or have a significantly impaired body part, most commonly a limb.

PROTEIN. A complex organic compound that can be used as a source of energy for the body, but that is primarily used for the construction of cells and tissues, for the production of enzymes in the body, and for other functions.

PROTEIN TURNOVER. The balance between protein degradation and synthesis.

PROTON. An elementary particle identical to the nucleus of a hydrogen atom (H^+).

PSEUDOANEMIA. A sport-related condition in which the concentration of red blood cells is less than normal because of an increase in blood plasma volume during exercise; also known as dilutional pseudoanemia and sport anemia.

PSYCHOGENIC POLYDIPSIA. A psychiatric disorder in which patients consume excessive amounts of water, sometimes going to great lengths to obtain it from any source possible.

PTERYGIUM. Thickened growth of the conjunctiva, fleshy and creamy in nature, growing from the inner side of the eyeball and usually covering part of the cornea. Pterygium results in inhibited vision.

PUBIS. Also called the pubic bone, the ventral and anterior of the three main bones on either side of the pelvis.

PUBLIC HEALTH ENGLAND. A new agency in the United Kingdom created to carry out the provisions of the white paper, "Healthy Lives, Healthy People." It is currently within the bureaucratic structure of the Department of Health.

PUCK. The object that hockey players project across the ice in an attempt to score, with a thickness of one inch, a diameter of three inches, and a weight of about six ounces.

PULL-UP. An exercise or test of upper-body strength in which the suspended body is pulled up by the arms.

PULMONARY. Related to or carried by the lungs.

PULMONARY ARTERIES AND VEINS. Blood vessels that carry blood from the heart to the lungs and from the lungs to the hearts, respectively.

PULMONARY DIFFUSION. The volume of gases, principally carbon dioxide and oxygen, that diffuses across the membranes between the alveoli and lung capillaries per minute.

PULMONARY REHABILITATION. Intervention program for people with chronic lung diseases that involves many health disciplines and is tailored for individual patients to help improve their functioning and well-being.

PULSE. Heart rate.

PURGING. The use of vomiting, diuretics, or laxatives to clear the stomach and intestines after a binge.

PUSH. When league management directs the storylines to make a certain wrestler a big star.

PUSH-UP. Press-up; a test or exercise in which the body is lowered and pushed up with the arms.

PUTTER. A golf club with a flat face designed for directing a ball into the hole on a green.

PUTTING GREEN. The destination for a series of golf shots that contains the hole in which one attempts to sink the ball.

PYLOMETRIC EXERCISES. Exercises designed to improve an athlete's neuromuscular control, so as to improve his or her ability to respond quickly and with powerful movements.

PYLOMETRICS. A type of exercise designed to produce fast, powerful movements by strengthening the ability of muscles to expand and contract more quickly and efficiently.

PYRUVATE. Compound derived from metabolism of carbohydrates.

Q

QI. The traditional Chinese term for vital energy or the life force. Also spelled "ki" or "chi" in English translations of Japanese and Chinese medical books.

QUADRICEPS FEMORIS. Also called the quads, the large muscle group consisting of four muscles located on the front of the thigh.

QUADRIPLEGIC. A person who has lost complete or partial use of all four limbs.

QUICKDRAW. A short piece of rope or strap with loops at each end used to attach a rope to a carabiner.

R

RACKET. The paddle with which one hits the ball in table tennis.

RADIATION THERAPY. Also called radiotherapy, the medical treatment of cancer using radiation such as X rays directed from an external source or emitted by radioactive materials within the body.

RADIUS. Shorter bone in the forearm.

RAPIER. A katana-like weapon developed in Western Europe, eventually used widely for dueling.

RAPPEL. A closed device to which a climbing rope can be attached.

RATING OF PERCEIVED EXERTION (RPE). A subjective rating by an individual of their perception of exercise intensity.

REACTION TIME. The time that expires between a stimulus and response to the stimulus.

REACTIVE OXYGEN SPECIES (ROS). Highly reactive molecules containing oxygen that are normal byproducts of metabolism and that have important roles in cells, but can cause cellular damage under conditions of oxidative stress.

RECEPTOR. A molecule, such as a protein, inside or on the surface of a cell, that binds a specific messenger molecule such as epinephrine.

RECIPROCAL INHIBITION. Reflex relaxation or stretching in the muscle opposing the tensed muscle.

RECREATIONAL WATER ILLNESS; RWI. Illnesses that are spread by swallowing, breathing, or contacting contaminated water from pools, lakes, rivers, or oceans; diarrhea is the most common RWI.

REGGAETON. A form of urban music that developed in Panama and blends reggae from the West Indies with musical influences derived from salsa, cumbia, and merengue.

REGULATOR. A device on scuba diving apparatus that controls air pressure within the apparatus.

RELATIVE RISK. The risk of disease in one group compared to another group; where the two groups generally differ in terms of one or multiple key variables (i.e., weekly levels of physical activity).

RELAY. A track and field event in which two or more teams consisting of four members each race against each other.

RENAISSANCE. The era from the 14th through the 17th century when the arts such as dance flourished in Europe.

RENAL. Relating to the kidneys.

RENAL CORTEX. The outer layer of the kidney.

RENAL MEDULLA. The inner region of the kidney.

RENAL PELVIS. The funnel-like reservoir of a kidney that empties to the ureter.

REPETITION TRAINING. The most intense form of aerobic endurance training, with high-intensity intervals usually lasting 60–90 seconds, separated by rest intervals of at least five minutes.

REPETITIVE STRESS OR STRAIN INJURY (RSI). A musculoskeletal injury, such as tendonitis, caused by cumulative damage to muscles, tendons, ligaments, nerves, or joints from highly repetitive movements and characterized by pain, weakness, and/or numbness.

RESIDUAL LUNG VOLUME. The amount of air remaining in the lungs following a maximal exhalation.

RESISTANCE BANDS. Exercise bands; elastic bands that are extended for exercising muscles and weight training.

RESISTANCE EXERCISE. Weight-bearing exercises that primarily use machines, barbells, and dumbbells to increase muscle mass.

RESISTANCE TRAINING. A form of strength training in which the athlete performs an effort against an opposing force generated by resistance to being pushed, pulled, stretched, or bent. It is done to strengthen and tone muscles and increase bone mass.

RESORPTION. The removal of old bone from the body.

RESPIRATORY EXCHANGE RATIO (RER). The ratio of carbon dioxide production to oxygen consumption as measured from expired gas analysis during indirect calorimetry.

RESTING METABOLIC RATE (RMR). A measurement frequently performed in place of basal metabolic rate. Obtained at complete rest in the post-absorptive state.

RETINAL DETACHMENT. Retinal detachment is when the retina separates from the tissues under it. The retina is the transparent tissue on the back wall of the eye.

RHABDOMYOLYSIS. A medical condition resulting from the rapid breakdown of muscle tissue associated with vigorous exercise.

RHEUMATOID ARTHRITIS. A disease characterized by inflammation and degeneration of connective tissue in multiple joints at a young age.

RHOMBOIDS. Rhombus-shaped muscles that are used for retraction; two main ones are called the rhomboid major muscle and the rhomboid minor muscle.

RING-FENCED FINANCING. Financing for a particular project that is protected from use for any purpose than that for which it was specifically designated.

RINK. The arena in which a hockey game is played, usually with dimensions of 61 meters by 26 or 30 meters.

RIPOSTE. In fencing, a riposte is an offensive action mounted by a defender after an attack by an opponent.

RISK STRATIFICATION. A pre-exercise screening process by which individuals at increased risk for an acute cardiac event are identified and subsequently referred for additional medical screening prior to starting an exercise program.

ROAD RASH. An informal term for scrapes and abrasions to the skin resulting from a bicycle accident. Some road rash injuries are severe enough to require surgical repair.

ROTATOR CUFF. The muscles of the shoulder, along with their tendons, that connect the arm to the shoulder joint.

RUBELLA. A contagious viral infection capable of causing birth defects if the mother is infected during pregnancy; symptoms include cough, sore throat, skin rash, and vomiting.

RUPTURE. A tear or break in body tissue of an organ.

S

SALINITY. Consisting of salt.

SALSA. A type of Latin American music and dance that originated in Cuba and became popular in the 1960s among Cuban and Puerto Rican immigrants in New York City.

SARCOMERE. A segment of myofibril in a striated muscle fiber.

SARCOPENIA. The degenerative loss of skeletal muscle mass and strength that occurs with age.

SARCOPLASMIC HYPERTROPHY. An increase in muscle size resulting from an accumulation of fluid in the interior of muscle cells.

SATURATED FATS. A dietary fat usually found in animal products, including meat and dairy, that is considered a "bad" fat.

SATURATED FATTY ACID (SFA). A fatty acid that has no double bonds, is solid at room temperature, and raises blood cholesterol levels.

SAVASANA. Relaxation in the corpse pose at the end of yoga practice.

SCAPULA. Either of two large flat bones that form the back of the shoulder in humans.

SCHIZOPHRENIA. A psychotic disorder characterized by loss of contact with one's environment, deterioration of everyday functioning, and personality disintegration.

SCOLIOSIS. A condition in which there is an abnormal curvature to the spine.

SCULL. A term that refers to a rowing situation in which each rower uses two oars.

SEDENTARY. Inactivity and lack of exercise; a lifestyle that is a major risk factor for becoming overweight or obese and developing chronic diseases.

SEIZURE. A sudden attack, spasm, or convulsion.

SELLING. The art of making your opponents moves look as though they hurt.

SENIOR. In the United States, a rower who has won a certified race over 2,000 meters in the United States or Canada.

SENSORY CELLS. Cells that contain receptors on their surface.

SENSORY CUES. A signal from sensory (e.g., visual or auditory) input that is intended to trigger a specific action within a given time period.

SENSORY NERVE. A nerve that receives input from sensory cells, such as the skin mechanoreceptors or the muscle receptors.

SEQUENCING. The order of different forms of exercise; for instance, sequencing balance training prior to resistance training.

SEROTONIN. A neurotransmitter located primarily in the brain, blood serum, and stomach membrane.

SERTOLI CELLS. Found in the tubular compartment of a testis; aids in the process of spermatogenesis.

SHAPE UP AMERICA!. A public education initiative about the importance of achieving and maintaining a healthy weight through physical activity and healthy eating.

SHELL. The boat used in a rowing competition.

SHIFT. The period of time during which a group of hockey players remain on the ice. A shift typically lasts no more than about a minute.

SHIN. The front part of the leg from below the knee to just above the ankle; also called the shin bone.

SHIN SPLINTS. An aching, painful condition of the skin bone.

SHOOT. In wrestling, a shot is when something is done not according to the script. This can be either really trying to hurt your opponent or making comments out of character.

SHORT. In handball, a served ball that does not return as far as the serving line.

SHORT CORNER. A shot taken by the attacking team from the corner of the defending team's half of the field as the result of an infraction by the defending team.

SICKLE CELL DISEASE. A condition in which red blood cells are crescent-shaped, which is caused by an inherited mutation of hemoglobin.

SIMPLE CARBOHYDRATES. Chemical compounds consisting of carbon, hydrogen, and oxygen or lower molecular weights, such as disaccharide and monosaccharide sugars.

SIMPLE FRACTURE. A fracture in which a bone breaks into two pieces.

SINGLE-COMPONENT TRAINING. In the context of balance training, performance of a balance exercise exclusive of another accompanying task.

SINUS BRADYCARDIA. A heart rate of less than 60 beats per minute while at rest.

SIT-AND-REACH BOX. Equipment of various designs for performing sit-and-reach flexibility tests.

SIT-UP. A common test or exercise for strength and endurance of the abdominal muscles.

SKELETAL MUSCLE. Muscle tissue composed of bundles of striated muscle cells that operate in conjunction with the skeletal system as a lever system.

SKELETON. Consists of bones and cartilage that are linked together by ligaments. The skeleton protects vital organs of the body and enables body movement.

SLALOM SKATEBOARDING. A form of skateboarding in which racers travel downhill following a course laid out by cones.

SMARK. A fan that knows what goes on behind the scenes, but still enjoys watching the events.

SMASH. A rapid, powerful stroke at a ball which has been returned with a significant arc above the table tennis table.

SMOOTH MUSCLE. Muscle tissue composed of long, unstriated cells that line internal organs and facilitate such involuntary movements as peristalsis.

SOCIAL MEDIA. Internet technology and Web sites where people share information and interact socially, such as Facebook, Twitter, and You Tube.

SOLAR LENTIGINES. Spots appearing on the epidermis due to repeated exposure of the skin to ultraviolet rays, either from the sun or from sunbed tanning. Also called age spots or liver spots.

SOLUTE. A substance dissolved in another substance.

SPASM. An involuntary, sudden, violent contraction of a muscle or a group of muscles.

SPEED DRIVE. A table tennis stroke in which the ball is propelled forward at high speed.

SPERMATOGENESIS. The process of the formation of sperm.

SPHINCTERS. Circular muscles that control the flow of urine in to/out of openings to/from the bladder.

SPHYGMOMANOMETER. An instrument for measuring arterial blood pressure.

SPIDER VEINS. Medically called telangiectasias, small dilated blood vessels near the surface of the skin or mucous membranes.

SPINAL CORD. Elongated part of the central nervous system that lies in the vertebral column and from which the spinal nerves emerge.

SPINAL FUSION. A surgical procedure in which adjacent discs are "welded" to each other.

SPINAL STENOSIS. A narrowing of the openings through which the spinal cord runs in vertebrae and discs.

SPIRAL FRACTURE. A fracture that occurs when a twisting force is applied to a bone, causing it to break in a curving shape.

SPIROMETRY. A test that uses an instrument called a spirometer and shows how difficult it is for a person with asthma to breathe. It is used to determine the severity of asthma and to see how well someone with asthma is responding to treatment.

SPONDYLOLISTHESIS. A condition in which two adjacent vertebrae slide forward or backward in relation to each other, causing low back pain.

SPONDYLOLYSIS. A condition where the vertebra disintegrate.

SPORTS ORTHOTICS. Orthotics designed for use during athletic activities.

SPOTTER. A person who monitors and assists an athlete during weight training or powerlifting exercises to prevent injuries and accidents.

SPRING. An adventure race that is completed in six hours or less.

SQUASH. A match in which a big name wrestles a nobody and beats him easily.

SQUAT. An exercise in which the athlete begins in a standing position with a bar loaded with weights resting on the shoulders. The athlete then bends the knees until he or she is in a squatting position, then stands erect again. The squat is one of three events in powerlifting competitions.

SQUEEZE BALL. Stress ball; a small rubber ball that is squeezed by the hand to exercise muscles and relieve stress.

STABILITY BALL. Balance or Swiss ball; an inflated exercise ball, approximately 14–34 in. (36–86 cm) in diameter, with variable air pressure; used for strength training, yoga, Pilates, and other exercises.

STAND-UP PADDLEBOARDING (SUP). Paddleboarding while standing on the board, using a canoe-like paddle for propulsion.

STANDARD ERROR OF THE ESTIMATE (SEE). The standard deviation of observed values about the regression line. SEE is calculated by dividing the error sum of squares by its degrees of freedom.

STATIC STRENGTH. The force exerted by a muscle when it is neither extending nor contracting.

STATIC STRETCHING. Type of stretching in which muscle is gradually lengthened to the point of mild discomfort and then subsequently held for a short period of time (e.g., 30 seconds).

STATINS. HMG-CoA reductase inhibitors; a class of cholesterol- or lipid-lowering drugs that inhibit cholesterol production and release by the liver and usually lower blood LDL and raise HDL slightly.

STENOSIS. Constriction, such as a narrowing of an artery.

STEP TEST. A cardiorespiratory fitness test that involves stepping on and off a bench or step at a specified pace.

STERNUM. The breastbone; the plate covering the abdomen.

STEROIDS. A class of hormones and drugs that includes sex and stress hormones and growth-promoting substances.

STICKBALL. A popular simple variant of baseball played with a broom handle, hockey stick, or similar implement, and a rubber ball or its equivalent.

STILL RINGS. A set of two parallel ropes suspended from a stationary bar on the ceiling, to which are attached two circular rings. The rings have an inner diameter of 18 centimeters and are separated from each other by a distance of 50 centimeters.

STIMULANT. A drug or other substance that produces a temporary increase in activity or efficiency.

STOCK PADDLEBOARD. A paddleboard of less than 12 ft (4 m) in length.

STRATUM LUCIDUM. A layer of dead skin in the epidermis between the stratum granulosum and stratum corneum.

STREET SKATEBOARDING. A form of skateboarding in which the rider performs on the street, sidewalk, parking lot, shopping center, or other flat paved area.

STRENGTH TRAINING. The use of resistance to muscular contraction to improve anaerobic endurance, muscle size, and overall body strength.

STRESS FRACTURE. A fracture in which there is only a hairline break, so small that it may not even be noticeable on an x-ray film of the break.

STRESS TEST. An electrocardiogram recorded before, during, and after a period of increasingly strenuous cardiovascular exercise, usually on a treadmill or stationary bicycle.

STRIKER. In cricket, a striker is another name for the batter, who must hit the ball delivered by the bowler.

STRIKING CIRCLE. The semi-circular area on front of each field hockey goal on the pitch from which shots on the goal may be taken; also known as the "D.".

STROKE. Irreversible damage to the brain caused by insufficient blood flow to the brain as the result of a blocked artery. Damage can include loss of speech or vision, paralysis, cognitive impairment, and death.

STROKE VOLUME. The volume of blood pumped from a heart ventricle in one beat.

SUBAK. The style of unarmed self-defense techniques taught in ancient and medieval Korea.

SUBCHONDRAL. Located beneath cartilage.

SUBCHONDRAL CYSTS. Fluid-filled sacs that form inside the joints in people who have osteoarthritis.

SUBCUTANEOUS LAYER. The innermost of three major layers of the skin.

SUBLUXATION. Partial dislocation.

SUBSTANCE P. A neuropeptide that functions as a neurotransmitter in the transmission of pain signals in the body.

SUBSTRATE. Substance acted upon and changed by an enzyme, such as a foodstuff.

SUDDEN CARDIAC DEATH. Abrupt and unexpected death due to cardiac causes; usually death occurs within one hour of the onset of symptoms.

SUDDEN DEATH. A type of playoff used when a regular game ends in a tie; the first team to score is the winner.

SUN SALUTATION. A flowing series of 12 yoga poses intended to tone the abdominal muscles and increase the flexibility of the spine. It is often used as an introductory or warm-up pose in yoga.

SUPEROXIDE. Oxygen-containing free radicals, especially superoxide anion, O_2^-.

SUPEROXIDE DISMUTASE (SOD). An antioxidant enzyme, containing copper (Cu) and zinc (Zn) or manganese (Mn), that reduces free oxygen radicals to oxygen and hydrogen peroxide.

SUPINATE. To turn palm upward.

SUPRASPINATUS. A muscle at the top of the shoulder blade.

SWEEP. A term that refers to a rowing situation in which each rower uses a single oar.

SWISS BALL. An inflated exercise or fitness ball, also called a balance or stability ball, 14–34 in. (36–86 cm) in diameter, that is used for exercise, athletic training, and physical therapy.

SYMPATHETIC. Pertaining to the part of the autonomic nervous system that regulates such involuntary reactions to stress as heartbeat, sweating, and breathing rate.

SYMPATHETIC DRIVE. The influence of increased impulses from the sympathetic nervous system.

SYMPATHETIC NERVOUS SYSTEM. The portion of the autonomic nervous system that prepares the body to react to stress or emergency; primarily consisting of adrenergic nerve fibers; usually inhibits secretion and increases heart rate.

SYMPATHOMIMETIC AGENTS. Drugs that stimulate the sympathetic nervous system; similar in action to epinephrine.

SYNAPSE. A region in which nerve impulses are transmitted across a gap from an axon terminal to another axon or the end plate of a muscle.

SYNCOPE. partial or complete loss of consciousness.

SYNOVIAL FLUID. Fluid that surrounds a joint.

SYNOVIAL JOINT. One of three types of joints in the skeleton and by far the most common. Synovial joints are lined with a membrane that secretes a lubricating fluid. Includes ball and socket, pivot, plane, hinge, saddle, condylar, and ellipsoid joints.

SYSTOLIC. The maximum pressure of the left ventricle measured during a contraction of the heart.

T

T CYTOTOXIC CELLS (TC). T lymphocytes that kill abnormal cells.

T HELPER CELLS (TH). T lymphocytes that enhance an immune response.

T LYMPHOCYTE. A lymphocyte that matures in the thymus and has receptors related to CD3 complex proteins.

T SUPPRESSOR CELLS (TS). T lymphocytes that diminish the immune response.

T'AI CHI. An ancient Chinese discipline involving controlled movements specifically designed to improve physical and mental well-being.

TALK TEST. Judging exercise intensity by the ability to carry on a conversation.

TANNER SCALE. A series of five stages used to measure the development of primary and secondary sexual characteristics in children and adolescents. It is named

for the British pediatrician who developed it in the 1960s.

TANNER'S STAGES. Stages of physical development in childhood, adolescence and adulthood. They were first described by Drs. Marshall and Tanner in 1969, and are also referred to as pubertal stages 1 through 5.

TAOISM. An ancient Chinese philosophy that advocates simple living and accepting the natural course of life.

TARGET HEART RATE. The heart rate, in beats per minute (bpm), that should be maintained during cardiovascular exercise by an individual of a given age.

TARGET HEART RATE RANGE. A high and low heart rate range based on a percentage of maximal heart rate.

TEEING GROUND. The area from which a golf ball is initially hit.

TENDINITIS. Inflammation of a tendon.

TENDON. A cord or band of dense, tough, fibrous tissue that connects muscles and bones.

TENDONITIS. Inflammation of a tendon.

TENNIS ELBOW. Inflammation and pain over the outside of the elbow, usually resulting from excessive strain on and twisting of the forearm; also called lateral epicondylitis or tendonitis of the elbow.

TESTOSTERONE. A male steroid hormone produced in the testes and responsible for the development of secondary sex characteristics.

TEWARAATHON. A primitive form of lacrosse played by many Native American tribes.

THERAPEUTIC EXERCISE. Physical exercise undertaken to treat an illness or as part of rehabilitation, as distinct from exercise done for general physical fitness in a healthy person.

THERMIC EFFECT OF FOOD (TEF). The component of total energy expenditure referring to the increase in energy expenditure associated with absorption, digestion, metabolism, storage, and transport of food.

THORACIC CAVITY. Also called the chest cavity, it is the portion of the ventral body cavity located between the neck and the diaphragm. It is enclosed by the ribs, the vertebral column, and the sternum. It is separated from the abdominal cavity by the diaphragm.

THROMBOSIS. The formation or presence of a blood clot in the vasculature.

THROMBUS. A blood clot that forms on the inner wall of a blood vessel.

TINEA. Any type of skin infection caused by parasitic fungi living on the outer layer of hair, skin, or nails.

TINEA PEDIS. The medical term for athlete's foot; in Latin it means tinea of the foot.

T-LYMPHOCYTES (T-CELLS). A type of white blood cell that originates in the thymus and attaches to foreign organisms, secreting lymphokines that kill the foreign organisms.

TOLERANCE. The requirement for higher doses of a substance to continue achieving the same effect.

TONSIL. A collection of lymphocytes that form a mass in the back of the pharynx.

TOPICAL. Pertaining to a particular area of the skin.

TOTAL ENERGY EXPENDITURE (TEE). The total energy expenditure is comprised of three major components, including activity energy expenditure, basal metabolic rate, and thermic effect.

TOUCH. An event in fencing in which one competitor's weapon comes into contact with a specified part of an opponent's body, resulting in an award of one point.

TRANS FAT. Any fat containing large amounts of unsaturated trans fatty acids and linked with high cholesterol.

TRANSVERSE ABDOMINIS. The flat muscle that forms the innermost layer of the abdominal wall and that constricts the abdominal organs.

TRANSVERSE FRACTURE. A fracture that occurs at right angles to the direction of a bone.

TRAPEZIUS. Two large flat triangular muscles that are located from the back of the neck to each shoulder blade; which help to move the shoulder blades, support the arms, and move the head backwards.

TREADMILL. An exercise machine that contains a wide moving belt on which a user walks, jogs, or runs.

TREADMILL DESK. A work desk built around a treadmill that enables the user to slowly walk while performing desk work.

TREKKING. A long, often multi-day, hike over difficult terrain.

TRIATHLON. An athletic contest, usually involving swimming, cycling, and running, consisting of three separate events in which points are awarded for each, but an overall best athlete is awarded at the end of the competition.

TRICEPS. The large muscle located along the back of the upper arm.

TRICEPS BRACHII. The muscle group positioned at the upper portion of the inside of the arm and consisting of the long head, lateral head, and medial head, it extends the arm at the shoulder; it also extends the forearm at the elbow.

TRIGLYCERIDES. Neutral fats; lipids formed from glycerol and fatty acids that circulate in the blood as lipoprotein. Elevated triglyceride levels contribute to the development of cardiovascular disease.

TRISTHANA. The three foci of attention in ashanga or power yoga—posture, breathing, and drishti.

TROCHANTER. Either of two knobs on the upper femur, to which the muscles between the thigh and the pelvis are attached.

TRUNK STRENGTH. The strength of muscles in the front and back of the torso, the portion of the body between the neck and the hips.

T-SCORE. The score on a bone densitometry test, calculated by comparing the patient's bone mineral density to that of a healthy 30-year-old of the same sex and race.

TURF TOE. A painful, red, swollen big toe that is caused by inflammation of the tendons within the toe's dorsal and plantar surfaces.

TURN. When a face becomes a heel or when a heel becomes a face.

TYPE 1 DIABETES. A chronic immune system disorder in which the pancreas does not produce sufficient amounts of insulin, a hormone that enables cells to use glucose for energy. Also called juvenile diabetes, it must be treated with insulin injections.

TYPE 2 DIABETES. Formerly called adult-onset diabetes. In this form of diabetes, the pancreas either does not make enough insulin or cells become insulin resistant and do not use insulin sufficiently.

TYPE I FIBERS. Muscle fibers that contract slowly, have a high resistance to fatigue, and are used to almost exclusively support aerobic exercises or activities.

TYPE II FIBERS. Muscle fibers that contract rather rapidly, have a somewhat low resistance to fatigue, and are used to support anaerobic exercises or activities.

U

UBIQUINONE. Any of a family of fat-soluble molecules that function as coenzymes in cellular respiration; especially coenzyme Q (ubiquinone-10) that can function as an antioxidant.

ULNA. Longer bone in the forearm.

ULTRA MARATHON. A long distance race that typically covers 50 miles, 100 miles, 50 kilometers, or 100 kilometers.

ULTRASOUND. A medical technique that uses high-frequency sound waves to perform diagnosis and treatment.

UNDULATING PERIODIZATION. A form of periodization training in which volume and intensity training occur more frequently than they do in a traditional, or linear, training program.

UNEVEN BARS. A pair of fiberglass-covered wood beams parallel to each other, but at different heights, on which contestants perform a variety of exercises.

UNLIMITED PADDLEBOARD. A paddleboard or more than 12 ft (4 m) in length, usually 16 to 19 ft (5 to 6 m) in length.

UNSTABLE ANGINA. Chest discomfort, pain, or tightness that occurs at rest and unpredictably; the severity and duration of the symptoms varies.

UNTOWARD EVENT. Refers to an adverse medical occurrence, for example a heart attack or bout of low blood sugar.

UREA. An end product of protein degradation that is excreted in the urine.

UREMIA. Blood poisoning.

URIC ACID. A nitrogen-containing waste product in the urine; an end product of metabolism and an antioxidant.

UTILITY CYCLING. The use of a bicycle for commuting to and from work or for delivering goods, as distinct from recreational cycling.

V

VAGAL TONE. The impulses from the vagus nerve that contributes to a reduced heartbeat.

VALIDATION. The extent to which a test measures the trait that it is designed to assess.

VANILLYLMANDELIC ACID (VMA). A breakdown product of catecholamines, including epinephrine, that is excreted in the urine.

VARICOCELE. An abnormal swelling of veins in the scrotum.

VARICOSE VEINS. Veins that have become enlarged.

VASCULAR. A term referring to blood vessels.

VASODILATOR. A process involving the widening of the arteries.

VAULT. A gymnastic exercise in which a competitor sprints down a runway, jumps onto a spring board, projects himself or herself onto an apparatus called the "vault" behind the spring board, and then continues with another vault to a mat beyond the sp

VENTRICULAR ARRHYTHMIA. Abnormal heart rate or heart rhythm.

VENTRICULAR FIBRILLATION. severely abnormal heart arrhythmia that will result in death without prompt treatment.

VENTRICULAR TACHYCARDIA. abnormal, rapid heartbeat.

VERT. An abbreviation for "vertical," a form of aggressive inline skating performed in a specially built facility, such as a quarter pipe, half pipe, or bowl.

VERT SKATEBOARDING. A form of skateboarding performed in a half-pipe.

VERTEBRA (PLURAL, VERTEBRAE). One of the segments of bone that make up the spinal column.

VERTEBRATES. Includes all animals with a vertebral column protecting the spinal cord such as humans, dogs, birds, lizards, and fish.

VESICANT. A chemical that causes blistering.

VILLI. Fingerlike projections found in the small intestine that add to the absorptive area for the passage of digested food to the bloodstream and lymphatic system.

VINYASA. The connecting movement and breath between postures in ashanga and power yoga.

VINYASA KRAMA. A step-by-step approach to vinyasa practice; building to a peak within a given practice session after deciding on a series of asanas suited to an individual's energy level and other concerns at the time of beginning practice.

VISUAL DISTURBANCES. A problem that impairs the sense of vision.

VITAMIN C. Ascorbic acid; an antioxidant obtained from fruits and leafy vegetables.

VITAMIN E. Any of several fat-soluble antioxidants obtained from wheat germ, vegetable oils, egg yolk, and green leafy vegetables.

VO$_2$MAX. Maximal oxygen uptake or consumption; the maximum amount of oxygen that can be used during a specified period of usually intense exercise, which depends on cardiac output, lung strength, and body weight; in milliliters of oxygen per kilogram of body weigh

VO$_2$R. The difference between VO$_2$max and resting oxygen uptake.

W

WAIST-TO-HIP RATIO. A body composition test that measures abdominal fat.

WALKING THE DOG. A series of endovers performed continuously.

WARM UP. A 5 to 10 minute period of low-intensity activity preceding the conditioning phase.

WATER HOMEOSTASIS. A condition of adequate fluid level in the body in which fluid loss and fluid intake are equally matched and sodium levels are within normal range.

WATER INTOXICATION. A condition that results from taking in more fluid than is needed to replace fluid losses from sweating, digestion, and other body processes. It is also called overhydration or hyperhydration.

WATER POLO. A game played in the water with two teams trying to get a large ball through a hoop on each side of the pool.

WHEELCHAIR SPORT. A term often used to describe a sport or athletic event in which participants are confined to a wheelchair.

WHIPLASH. An injury to the neck caused by a motion or force.

WHITE KNUCKLE SYNDROME. A situation in which a person grasps an object so tightly that the knuckles turn white from decreased blood circulation.

WILDCARD TEAM. A term referring to a football team that is awarded a position within the NFL playoffs (based on its ratio of wins and loses) after not having won its division during the regular season.

WITHDRAWAL. Unpleasant physiological and/or psychological changes that occur due to the discontinuation of a drug after prolonged regular use.

WOLFF PARKINSON WHITE. abnormal electrical conduction of heart's signal to beat which can increase the risk of developing an arrhythmia.

WOOD. A type of golf club used for hitting long distance. Woods are also called metals or fairway metals.

WORK. Anything in wrestling that follows the bookers script. The opposite of a shoot.

WORKED SHOOT. A work that has some real life elements in it. Anything in wrestling that follows the bookers script.

WORKOUT OF THE DAY (WOD). A set of exercises recommended by CrossFit for participants to complete each day. The WOD is posted on the company's website daily.

Y

YIN AND YANG. The Chinese philosophy that there are two opposing but complimentary forces in the universe.

YOGA. A system of exercises that originated in India 5,000 years ago involving breathing exercises and postures based on Hindu yoga.

YOGI. A trained male yoga expert.

YOGINI. A trained female yoga expert.

Z

ZEN. A form of meditation that emphasizes direct experience.

ZONE OF COAGULATION. The region on the skin at which a burn actually occurs.

ZONE OF HYPEREMIA. The region on the skin most distant from the actual burn site where cells continue to function normally.

ZONE OF STASIS. The region on the skin adjacent to the zone of coagulation where cells may be affected, but not necessarily destroyed by, the causative agent of the burn.

ZYGOTE. A two-fold (diploid, that is having 46 chromosomes) cell resulting from fertilization of the female egg by a sperm.

INDEX

In the index, references to individual volumes are listed before colons; numbers following a colon refer to specific page numbers within the volume indicated. **Boldface** references indicate main topical essays. Photographs and illustration references are highlighted with an *italicized* page number; and tables are also indicated with the page number followed by a lowercase, italicized *t*.

A

AAHPERD (American Alliance for Health, Physical Education, Recreation, & Dance), 2:770
AAOS (American Academy of Orthopaedic Surgeons), 1:369
AAP (American Academy of Pediatrics), 1:105, 2:837, 874
AARP, 2:579, 677
AAT (Alpha-1) related emphysema, 1:176
AAU (Amateur Athletic Union), 1:384, 396, 2:865, 874
ABA (American Burn Association), 2:860–861, 862
Abbott, B. C., 1:255
ABCDE rule, 1:473
Abdominal bracing, 2:812
Abdominal crunch. *See* Sit-ups
Abdominal exercises. *See* Core training
Abdominal fat, 1:103, 2:593, 620
Abdominal strength tests, 2:698
Abducens nerve, 2:605
Ablation
    radiofrequency, 1:442, 2:685
    thermal, 1:442
ABPI (Ankle brachial pressure index), 2:675
Absolute exercise intensity, 1:309–310
Absorbine Jr. *See* Tolnaftate
Acarbose, 1:232
Acceleration, 1:189
Access to Affordable Healthy Food program, 2:874
Accessory nerve, 2:605
ACE. *See* American Council on Exercise
ACEs (Angiotensin-converting enzyme inhibitors), 1:159, 439, 440
Acetaminophen
    for burns, 2:861
    for low back pain, 1:527

for muscle cramps, 2:572
for muscle pain, 2:577
for muscle soreness, 1:531
for muscle strains, 2:580
for osteoarthritis, 1:44
for patellofemoral syndrome, 2:661
Acetyl-CoA, 1:326, 2:558
Acetylcholine (ACh), 2:591, 594, 602, 603, 751
Acetylsalicylic acid. *See* Aspirin
ACh (Acetylcholine), 2:591, 594, 602, 603, 751
Achilles tendon, 1:359
Achilles tendon injuries, 1:*358*, 360–361
    basketball, 1:75
    calf exercises, 1:134
    football, 1:366
    men, 2:549
    older adults, 1:11
    tennis, 2:858
Acid-base balance, 2:738, 742
Acidosis, 1:92, 520, 2:742
Acne, 1:472, 473
Acquired immunity, 1:454, 457–458, 461
Acquired immunodeficiency syndrome. *See* AIDS
Acrobatic gymnastics, 1:385
Acromegaly, 1:265
ACTH (Adrenocorticotropic hormone), 1:263, 279
Actin
    cellular metabolism, 1:26
    muscle contractions, 1:186, 187, 254
    muscle hypertrophy, 2:573
    skeletal muscles, 2:589, 590
    smooth muscle, 2:591
Actinic keratosis, 2:830–831
Active-isolated stretching (AIS), 2:824
Active stretching, 2:682, 824
Active warm-up, 2:903
Activities of daily living (ADL)
    Alzheimer's disease, 1:17, 18
    balance training, 1:61

functional training, 1:372, 373
leg exercises, 1:521
pedometers, 2:664
senior fitness, 2:765
Activity energy expenditure (AEE), 1:275
Actomyosin filaments, 1:534
Actonel. *See* Risedronate
Actors, 2:681–682
Actos. *See* Pioglitazone
Acupressure, 2:622
Acupuncture, 1:126, 2:622, 709, 710
Acute fractures, 2:548–549
Acute phase proteins, 1:455–456
AD. *See* Alzheimer's disease
ADA (American Diabetes Association), 1:148, 230, 2:929
ADA (American Dietetic Association), 1:230, 2:564–565, 807, 808
Adapted aquatics, 2:833–834
Adaptive immunity. *See* Acquired immunity
Addison's disease, 1:265
Adductor muscles, 1:421
Adenine, 2:703
Adenoids, 2:740
Adenoma, pituitary, 1:23
Adenosine diphosphate (ADP), 1:91, 2:557
Adenosine monophosphate-activated protein kinase (AMPK), 1:92, 93
Adenosine triphosphate (ATP)
    anaerobic exercise, 1:37
    epinephrine, 1:279–280
    exercise biochemistry, 1:91–92
    fat burning, 1:326
    lactate threshold training, 1:520
    metabolism, 1:141, 2:557, 558, 703
    muscle contractions, 2:590
    VO$_2$max, 2:544
Adipex-P. *See* Phentermine
Adipocytes, 1:280, 325
Adipose tissue. *See* Body fat

Adjustable weight dumbbells, 1:244

ADL. *See* Activities of daily living

Adolescent Training and Learning to Avoid Steroids (ATLAS), 1:34

Adolescents
aerobic training, 1:290, 308
amenorrhea, 1:22
anabolic steroids, 1:31, 33, 34, 112, 285, 2:916–917
body mass index, 1:103, 105, 107–108, 2:617
bone health, 2:642
boxing, 1:120
calcium status, 1:129, 130
circuit training, 1:182
concussion, 1:193
dietary recommendations, 1:306
energy drinks, 1:272
entertainment media use, 1:309
exercise recommendations, 1:290, 306, 310
female triad, 1:337–340
field hockey, 1:345
gymnastics, 1:384
hypertension, 1:99, 437
ice hockey, 1:453
kickboxing, 1:502, 504
lacrosse, 1:513, 515, 516
lifestyle, 1:406–407
marathons, 2:537
muscle cramps, 2:570
obesity, 1:308, 2:619, 621, 893, 910
osteoporosis prevention, 2:641
overuse injuries, 2:650
patellofemoral syndrome, 2:660
personal training, 2:678
physical activity, 1:306, 2:547
President's Challenge, 2:698–699, 700
skateboarding, 2:780
softball, 2:802
stationary bicycles, 2:817
step aerobics, 2:819
sudden cardiac death, 2:827
tae kwon do, 2:844
track and field, 2:867
undernutrition, 1:139
weightlifting, 2:916, 917
wrestling, 2:932
youth sports, 2:940–943, *941*

Adopted children, 2:618

ADP (Adenosine diphosphate), 1:91, 2:557

Adrenal gland disorders, 1:265

Adrenal gland tumors, 1:438

Adrenal glands, 1:261, 263, 266, 278, 280

Adrenaline. *See* Epinephrine

Adrenergic receptors, 1:279

Adrenergics, 1:279, 282

Adrenocorticotropic hormone (ACTH), 1:263, 279

Adrerenaclick. *See* EpiPen

Adult Fitness Test (President's Challenge), 2:697, 698, 700, 874
cardiorespiratory fitness, 1:154
flexibility, 1:351, 353
muscular strength and endurance, 2:585, 587–588

Adult-onset diabetes. *See* Type 2 diabetes mellitus

Adventure Racer Code of Ethics, 1:2

Adventure racing, 1:**1–5,** *2,* 2:650, 746

Adverse exercise-related events, 2:690–693

Advil. *See* Ibuprofen

Advocate activities, 2:700

AED (Automated external defibrillators), 2:829

AEE (Activity energy expenditure), 1:275

Aerobic capacity, 1:153, 155–156, 310, 475, 2:538

Aerobic fitness. *See* Aerobic capacity; Cardiovascular fitness

Aerobic metabolism, 1:141, 2:557, 558

Aerobic shoes, 1:214, 2:821

Aerobic training, 1:**5–9**
vs. anaerobic exercise, 1:36, 38
children, 1:308
cool down, 2:901
health benefits, 1:5–6, 8, 190, 293–294
cardiac rehabilitation, 1:150
cardiovascular fitness, 1:173
COPD management, 1:177
depression management, 2:551
diabetes management, 1:225
energy expenditure, 1:93
fat burning, 1:326
high cholesterol, 1:170
hypertension, 1:99
immune system, 1:463
lymphatic system, 1:535
men's fitness, 2:547, 736–737
mental health, 2:551
muscular system, 2:592
older adults, 2:765
skin health, 1:473
somatic nervous system, 2:608
weight loss, 2:912
women's health, 2:732, 924
workplace, 2:926
health risks, 1:293
amenorrhea, 1:25
asthma, 1:46, 47
injuries, 1:7–8
intensity of, 1:291, 310–311
maximal heart rate, 1:466
metabolic equivalent of tasks, 2:555
muscle fibers in, 1:187
oxygen consumption, 1:298
prenatal exercise, 2:694, 696
President's Challenge, 2:698

recommendations, 1:139, 267, 306, 2:678
target heart rate, 2:851
techniques, 1:289–290
base-building, 1:518, 519
circuit training, 1:179
concurrent training, 1:190
cricket training, 1:205
CrossFit, 1:207
elliptical trainers, 1:257
endurance, 1:267, 268
field hockey, 1:347
football, 1:365
gymnastics, 1:385
ice hockey, 1:453
indoor cycling classes, 1:466
interval training, 1:475–477
Ironman, 1:483
jumping rope, 1:494
low-impact, 1:57–58
stationary bicycles, 2:814, 815
step aerobics, 2:818–822, *819*
swimming, 2:833
walking, 2:896–900
water exercises, 1:99, 2:904
Wii Fit, 1:321
VO$_2$max, 2:544, 546
weightlifting with, 2:917

Aerobics (Cooper), 1:6, 2:819–820

Aerobics and Fitness Association of America (AFAA), 2:944

AFAA (Aerobics and Fitness Association of America), 2:944

AFC (American Football Conference), 1:363

AFLA (Amateur Fencers League of America), 1:342

Africa, 1:229

African Americans
Alzheimer's disease, 1:16
anorexia nervosa, 1:22
asthma, 1:47
burns, 2:861
cardiovascular disease, 1:158
cardiovascular fitness, 2:546
childhood obesity, 2:873
diabetes, 1:229
eating disorders, 1:247
exercise-related asthma, 1:312
hypertension, 1:98, 437
kidney disease, 1:505
mental illness, 2:550
nerve entrapment, 2:597
obesity, 2:619
osteoporosis, 2:638
physical activity, 2:566
sudden cardiac death, 2:827

Aftate. *See* Tolnaftate

Age and exercise, 1:**9–12,** 2:765
See also Aging; Older adults

Age-predicted maximal heart rate, 2:851, 852

B

CPSC (Consumer Products Safety Commission), 1:471, 526, 2:835, 867, 870–871
Cramps. *See* Muscle cramps
Cranberry extract, 2:883
Cranial bones, 2:785–786
Cranial nerve disorders, 2:607
Cranial nerves, 2:605
C.R.A.S.H.-B Championship, 2:755
Crawl (swim stroke), 2:833
Creatine
  amino acid metabolism, 1:28, 29
  interactions, 2:668
  performance-enhancing effect, 2:666, 667, 668
  side effects, 2:670
Creatine phosphate (CP), 1:28, 2:558, 666, 703
Creatinine, 1:95, 507, 2:881
Creatinine phosphate, 1:141
Creighton, James, 1:449
Cricket, 1:**201–206**, *202, 203*
Cross-country skiing, 2:919, *921, 922*
Cross punch, 1:121
Cross training, 1:267, 470, 2:538, 688
CrossFit, 1:**206–209**
CrossFit Risk Retention Group, 1:209
CRP (C-reactive protein), 1:455–456
Cruciferous vegetables, 1:463
Cruiser bicycles, 1:83
Crunches, 1:136
CSA (Controlled Substances Act), 1:32, 2:916
CT scans
  body composition tests, 1:104
  concussion, 1:194, 195
  COPD, 1:177
  fractures, 1:369
  patellofemoral syndrome, 2:661
  peripheral arterial disease, 2:675
  quantitative, 2:639
Cu/Zn-SOD (Copper/zinc superoxide dismutase), 1:299, 301
Cuba, 1:67
Cubit, William, 2:869
Cumbia, 2:944
Cumulative brain injuries, 1:194
Cumulative trauma injuries. *See* Overuse injuries
Curare, 2:594
Curl-ups, 2:585
Cushing's disease, 1:265
Cushing's syndrome, 1:265, 438, 2:619
CvO$_2$max, 2:544
Cyanocobalamin. *See* Vitamin B$_{12}$
Cycle ergometer tests, 1:154, 155, 156, 2:767
Cyclic adenosine monophosphate (cAMP), 1:279–280

Cycling. *See* Bicycling
Cycling (drug), 1:33, 2:667
Cyclosporine, 2:611
Cypionate, 2:667
Cystic fibrosis, 2:742
Cystitis, 2:883
Cytokines, 1:270, 456, 457
Cytoplasmic fluid, 2:573
Cytotoxic T cells, 1:458
Czech handball, 1:395
Czech Republic, 1:449

D

Daily living activities. *See* Activities of daily living
Dairy products, 1:114, 328
Dalleck, Lance C., 1:308, 2:678
Dance, 1:**211–215**, *212*
  amenorrhea from, 1:25
  ballet, 1:*62,* 62–65, 213, 315
  ballroom, 1:211, 213, 214
  history, 1:211, 424
  metabolic equivalent of tasks, 2:555
  Pilates, 2:681–682
  war, 2:758, *758*
  zumba, 2:*943,* 943–946
Dance Dance Revolution (DDR), 1:320
Dandelion, 2:622
Darby, Newman, 2:628
DASH (Dietary Approaches to Stop Hypertension), 1:101, 439
DDR (Dance Dance Revolution), 1:320
DEA (Drug Enforcement Administration), 1:32
Dead lift
  dumbbells, 1:187, 244
  hamstring exercises, 1:390, *390*
  leg exercises, 1:523
  stiff-legged, 1:244, *529*
  weightlifting, 2:915
Deadlift. *See* Dead lift
"Deal-A-Meal" calorie tracker, 2:911
Deamination, 2:703
Death rate. *See* Mortality
DecaDurabolin. *See* Nandrolone
Decathalon, 2:866
Decline bench press, 1:244
Deconditioning, hospital-related, 2:680
Decongestants, 1:279, 508
Deep breathing, 2:837
Deep tissue hyperthermia, 1:443
Deep vein thrombosis (DVT), 1:157–158, 521
Deep water soloing, 2:747

Defibrillation, 2:829
Dégagé, 1:64
Dehydration, 1:**215–221**, 216*t*
  causes, 1:217–219
    aerobic training, 1:8
    bikram yoga, 1:89, 90
    military fitness tests, 2:561
    soccer, 2:801
    weight loss, 2:912
    weightlifting, 2:916
  diagnosis, 1:218–219
  nutrition timing, 2:613
  prevention, 1:220
  risk factors, 1:217, 433
  sunburn with, 2:830
  symptoms, 1:216*t*, 218, 2:724, 726, 727
    cardiovascular drift, 1:304
    fatigue, 1:331
    kidney function, 2:881
    muscle cramps, 2:571, 572
  treatment, 1:216, 219–220, 433, 2:723–727
Dehydroepiandrosterone (DHEA), 2:667
Delayed hypersensitivity reactions, 1:459
Delayed onset muscle soreness (DOMS), 1:**221–224**, 2:915
Deltoids, 1:40, 41, 166, 244–245
Delts. *See* Deltoids
Delusions, 1:17
Dementia, 1:194
Demi plie, 1:63
Demonstration Centers, 2:700
Dendrites, 2:605
Dendritic cells, 1:457, 459
Denosumab, 1:115, 2:640
Department of Agriculture. *See* U.S. Department of Agriculture
Department of Education, 2:875–876
Department of Health (United Kingdom), 1:403
Department of Health and Human Services (DHHS)
  Dietary Guidelines for Americans, 1:7, 129, 147, 2:875, 923
  exercise recommendations, 1:139, 290
  Healthy People programs, 1:403–408
  men's fitness, 2:547
  Office of Disease Prevention and Health Promotion, 1:404
  "Physical Activity Guidelines for Americans," 1:240, 308, 309, 2:875, 924
  sling training, 2:794, 875
  U.S. President's Council on Fitness, Sports, & Nutrition initiatives, 1:397, 425, 2:697, 875–876, 924
  women's fitness, 2:923

Department of the Interior, 2:874
Depression
    Alzheimer's disease, 1:17
    antidepressants for, 2:550
    demographics, 2:550
    eating disorders, 1:252
    exercise, 1:225, 2:550–553
    fatigue from, 1:330
    osteoporosis risk, 2:638
    prevention, 1:241
    retired football players, 1:193
    t'ai chi for, 2:850
Dermal papillae, 1:472
Dermatitis
    cercarial, 2:835
    contact, 1:96, 473–474
Dermatomyositis, 2:576
Dermis, 1:471, 472
Dervish turn, 1:78
Designer drugs, 1:33
Developmental milestones, 1:392–393
Devi, Indra, 1:400
Dexfenfluramine hydrochloride, 2:622
DHEA (Dehydroepiandrosterone), 2:667
DHLA (Dihydrolipoic acid), 1:299, 300
Di Pasquale, Arnaud, 2:856
Diabeta. *See* Glyburide
Diabetes and exercise, 1:**224–228**
    bodybuilding precautions, 1:112
    cardiac rehabilitation, 1:151–152
    exercise biochemistry, 1:93–95
    target heart rate precautions, 2:852
    upper body exercises, 2:878
Diabetes medications, 1:230–232, 2:668
Diabetes mellitus, 1:**228–233,** 264
    causes, 1:147–148, 225, 228–230, 238, 2:559
    complications, 1:224, 2:674, 675, 923
    demographics, 1:229, 264, 406
    diagnosis, 1:230
    gestational, 1:229, 2:696
    prevention, 1:175, 232, 241
    risk factors, 1:224, 229, 311
    secondary, 1:230
    treatment, 1:148, 230–232, 264
    type 1, 1:147–148, 224, 225, 226, 229, 264
    See also Type 2 diabetes mellitus
Diabetic foot, 1:224, 359
Diabetic nephropathy, 1:505–506
Diabetic neuropathy, 2:607
Diagnostic and Statistical Manual of Mental Disorders (DSM), 1:247, 337
Diagnostic imaging. *See* Imaging studies
Dialectical behavior therapy, 1:252
Dialysis, 1:436–437, 505, 508

Dianabol. *See* Methandrostenolone
Diaphragm, 2:741
Diaphragmatic breathing, 1:200
Diaphysis, 2:785
Diarrhea, 1:217–218, 220, 434, 446, 2:908
Diastolic blood pressure, 1:99, 101, 435, 438
Dichlotride. *See* Hydrochlorothiazide
Diet
    bone health, 2:791
    bursitis from, 1:126
    dehydration, 1:220–221
    demographics, 1:406
    diabetes mellitus, 1:148
    fatigue from, 1:331
    functional food, 2:622
    historical changes in, 2:910
    lymphatic system effects, 1:535
    men's health, 2:737–738
    mindful eating, 2:562–566
    muscular system health, 2:593
    obesity, 2:623
    post-exercise, 2:614
    recommendations, 1:306–307
    recovery period, 2:725–726
    respiratory system health, 2:744
    types
        Bernstein, 1:148
        DASH, 1:101, 439
        fad, 1:328, 2:623
        fat burning, 1:327
        heart healthy, 1:173, 2:732, 737, 744
        high-cholesterol, 1:158, 163
        high-fat, 1:307, 463, 2:604
        high-fiber, 1:171
        high-protein, 1:29, 2:704–705
        high-salt, 1:101
        liquid, 2:621, 911–912
        low-calorie, 2:621
        low-fat, 1:169, 171, 2:619
        low-fiber, 1:307
        low-protein, 2:705
        low-salt, 1:445
        meat-based, 1:28
        vegan, 1:170, 478, 2:704
        vegetarian, 1:170, 478, 2:704
        very-low-calorie, 2:621, 623
        weight loss, 2:912
        yo-yo, 2:621
    urinary system health, 2:882–883
    women's fitness, 2:566, 732, 733, 923–924
Diet pills. *See* Appetite suppressants
Dietary Approaches to Stop Hypertension (DASH), 1:101, 439
Dietary Guidelines for Americans (DHHS), 1:7, 129, 147, 2:875, 923
Dietary reference intake (DRI), 1:28–29
Dietary Supplement Health and Education Act (DSHEA), 2:609, 610

Dietary supplements. *See* Nutritional supplements
Diethylpropion, 2:622
Diflucan. *See* Fluconazole
Digestion, 1:233–237, 238, 375, 376
    autonomic nervous system, 2:603
    carbohydrates, 1:145, *146,* 234–235, 2:557
    fats, 1:235–236, 326, 534, 2:557–558
    lymphatic system, 1:236, 534
    protein, 1:235, 2:702–703
Digestive system, 1:**233–239,** *234,* 2:592
Digoxin, 2:611
Dihydrolipoic acid (DHLA), 1:299, 300
Dilutional hyponatremia, 2:908
Dilutional pseudoanemia, 1:479
Dimick, Keene, 2:816
Dioscorrhea sp. *See* Wild yam
Dipeptides, 2:702
Dipeptidyl peptidase-4 (DPP-4) inhibitors, 1:232
Dips test (muscular strength), 2:586
Dipstick test, 1:507
Direct calorimetry, 1:275
Disabled individuals
    exercise recommendations, 1:310
    Olympics, 2:632
    paraplegic and quadriplegic athletes, 2:*656,* 656–660
    Pilates, 2:680, 681
    swimming, 2:833–834
Disaccharides, 1:142, 145
Disc degeneration, 1:526
Discectomy, 1:527
Discus, 2:863, 866
Disease-modifying antirheumatic drugs (DMARDs), 1:44
Disease prevention, 1:**239–242,** 239*t,* 426
    chronic diseases, 1:7, 172–176
    Healthy Lives, Healthy People program, 1:403–408
Dislocations, 1:11, 2:748, 774–776
Distance running, 1:268, 2:560
Disuse atrophy. *See* Muscle loss
Dityatin, Aleksander, 2:835
Diuretics
    for cardiovascular disease, 1:159
    creatine interactions, 2:668
    dehydration precautions, 1:433, 2:912
    fatigue from, 1:330
    football player abuse, 1:366
    heat exhaustion precautions, 1:412
    heatstroke precautions, 1:418
    for hypertension, 1:439, 440
    hyponatremia precautions, 1:445–446
    for overhydration, 2:645

F

Facial bones, 2:786
Facial injuries, 1:471
Facial nerve, 2:605
Fad diets, 1:328, 2:623
Fair Society, Healthy Lives report, 1:402
Fallopian tubes, 2:728–729, 730
Falls
  concussion from, 1:194
  demographics, 1:59
  exercising at home, 1:318
  prevention
    balance training, 1:59–62, 2:642
    flexibility, 1:190
    tae kwon do, 2:843
    t'ai chi, 2:849–850
  rock climbing, 2:749
  senior fitness, 2:767
  from wheelchairs, 2:658
Familial dysautonomia, 2:603
Familial periodic paralysis, 2:594
Family history, 1:160, 2:618, 829
  See also Genetic factors
Family therapy, 1:252
Famine, 2:615
Famotidine, 1:508
Faremouth, Lisa, 2:819
Fartlek training, 1:268, 347
Fasciculation, 2:570, 571
Fasciculi, 2:590
Fast food, 2:910
Fast-pitch softball, 2:802
Fast-twitch muscle fibers. See Type II muscle fibers
Fasting, 1:328
Fasting plasma glucose test (FPG), 1:230
Fat burning, 1:**325–329**, 2:557–558
  endurance training, 1:267, 268
  interval training, 1:476, 477
  jumping rope, 1:494
  marathons, 2:538–539
  metabolism, 1:92, 325–329, 2:557–558
  target heart rate, 2:852
  weight loss, 2:911
Fat deposits. See Body fat
Fat-free labels, 1:169
Fat metabolism. See Fat burning
Fat oxidation. See Fat burning
Fatal accidents. See Injury-related deaths
Fatigue, 1:**329–332**
  anaerobic exercise, 1:38
  calcium status, 1:130
  carbohydrate replacement, 1:142
  causes, 1:329–331, 2:647, 648
  endurance training, 1:270

lactate, 1:520
Lifestyle changes, 1:331
muscle cramps from, 2:571, 572
muscle toning, 2:584
muscular strength and endurance tests, 2:585
Fats (dietary), 1:**332–337**, *333*
  animal, 1:325, 333
  digestion, 1:235–236, 326, 534, 2:557–558
  food sources, 1:332, *333*
  high-fat diet, 1:307, 463, 2:604
  immunity, 1:463
  intake recommendations, 1:306, 328, 332, 2:624–625
  low-fat diet, 1:169, 171, 2:619
  monounsaturated, 1:325, 334
  muscular system, 2:593
  obesity, 2:619, 624
  periodization, 2:673
  polyunsaturated, 1:325, 334–335
  trans, 1:335–336, 2:733
  unsaturated, 1:*333*
  See also Saturated fats
Fats (lipids), 1:325–326, **332–337**
  exercise biochemistry, 1:91, 92
  kilocalories from, 1:138
  metabolism, 1:26, 92
  role, 1:332–333
Fatty acids, 1:325–326
  catabolism, 1:141
  essential, 1:332–333, 2:615
  free, 1:326
  as fuel, 1:280
  long-chain, 1:92, 334
  metabolism, 2:557–558
  nonessential, 1:332–333
  omega-3, 1:334, 335, 460, 472, 2:737
  omega-6, 1:334–335
  role, 1:332–333
  See also Omega-3 fatty acids; Omega-6 fatty acids
FDA. See Food and Drug Administration
Fedak, Alex, 1:470
Fédération Internationale de Gymnastique (International Gymnastics Federation) (FIG), 1:383
Fédération Internationale de Hockey (FIH), 1:346
Fédération Internationale de Roller Skating (FIRS), 1:469
Federation Internationale des Societes d'Aviron (International Federation of Rowing Associations) (FISA), 2:754, 755
Fédération Internationale d'Escrime (FIE), 1:342, 343
Federation of International Lacrosse (FIL), 1:515
Federer, Roger, 2:*856*, 856–857
Fedorenko, Valery, 1:498, 500

Feldenkrais, Moshe, 1:356
Feldenkrais method, 1:356
Felodipine, 1:440
Female athlete triad. See Female triad
Female athletes
  amenorrhea, 1:21–22
  anabolic steroids, 1:31
  boxing, 1:120
  cricket, 1:201
  gastrointestinal function, 1:375
  gymnastics injuries, 1:386
  ice hockey, 1:451
  iron status, 1:478
  lacrosse, 1:514–515, 516, 517
  performance-enhancing drugs, 1:112
  track and field, 2:867
  See also Women; Women's fitness
Female reproductive system, 2:**727–734**, *728*
Female reproductive system disorders, 2:730–731
Female triad, 1:21–22, 131, **337–340**, 2:638, 642
Fempatch. See Estrogen replacement therapy
Fen/Phen (Fenfluramine-fenfluramine), 2:622
Fencing, 1:**340–345**, *341*
Fenfluramine, 2:622
Fenfluramine-fenfluramine (Fen/Phen), 2:622
Fennel, 1:238
Fenofibrate, 1:171
Feoris. See Ketoconazole
Ferritin, 1:478
Ferritin tests, 1:507
Fertility treatments, 2:730
Fertilization, 2:729, 735
Fetus, 2:729
Fever, 1:456
Fever-range hyperthermia, 1:443
FFA (Free fatty acids), 1:326
FIBA (International Basketball Federation), 1:72–73
Fiber (dietary), 1:146–147
  high cholesterol, 1:171, 336
  high-fiber diet, 1:171
  low-fiber diet, 1:307
  osteoporosis risk, 2:642
  recommendations, 1:306, 2:924
Fibrates. See Fibric acid derivatives
Fibric acid derivatives, 1:171
Fibrin, 1:93
Fibromyalgia, 1:415, 2:575, 849
Fick, Adolf, 1:255
Fick equation, 2:543–544
FIE (Fédération Internationale d'Escrime), 1:342, 343
Field hockey, 1:**345–348**, 449
Field tests, 1:153–154, 156

G

H

M

P

Pathogen-associated molecular patterns (PAMPs), 1:455–456
Pathological fractures, 1:369
Patient education, 1:150
Pattern recognition receptors (PRR), 1:455–456
Patterns (Hyeong), 2:844
PBIC (Pedestrian and Bicycle Information Center), 1:83
PCFSN. *See* U.S. President's Council on Fitness, Sports, & Nutrition
PCFSN Research Digest, 2:875
PCOS (Polycystic ovary syndrome), 1:23, 25–26
Peak bone mass
calcium status, 1:129
development, 1:113, 130–131
osteoporosis risk, 2:637, 638, 639, 641
Peak flow measurement, 1:47
Peak heart rate method, 1:302
Pear-shaped body type, 1:105, 325, 2:620
Pearce, Kevin, 2:797
Pecs. *See* Pectoralis major; Pectoralis minor
Pectineus, 1:421, 422
Pectoralis major, 1:40, 41, 164–167, 244
Pectoralis minor, 1:164–167, 244
Pedestrian and Bicycle Information Center (PBIC), 1:83
Pedestrians, 1:82
Pedometers, 1:276, 2:**663–665,** 896
Pele, 2:800, *800*
Pelliccia, A., 2:829
Pelvic girdle, 2:787
Pelvic muscles, 1:197, 2:881–882
Pelvic tilts, 1:316
Pelvis injuries, 2:539
Penbutolol, 1:440
Penis, 2:735
Pentathalonn, 2:866
Pentoxifylline, 2:675
Pepcid. *See* Famotidine
Pepcid AC. *See* Famotidine
Peppermint, 1:238
Peppers, chili, 1:328, 2:622
Pepsin, 1:235
Pepsinogen, 2:702
Peptic ulcers. *See* Stomach ulcers
Peptides, 1:235, 2:702
Perceived exertion methods, 1:303
Perera, Augurio, 2:856
Pérez, Alberto (Beto), 2:944
Performance-enhancing drinks. *See* Energy drinks; Sports drinks
Performance-enhancing drugs, 1:33, 111–112, 366, 2:*666,* **666–671,** 934
See also Anabolic steroids

Perimysium, 2:590
Perineum, 2:728
Periodization, 2:652, **671–674,** 756
Peripheral acting adrenergic antagonists, 1:440
Peripheral arterial disease (PAD), 2:*674,* **674–676**
Peripheral lymphoid tissue, 1:458
Peripheral nervous system, 2:601, 605, 606
Peripheral nervous system cancer, 2:608
Peripheral neuropathy, 1:232, 2:606–608
Peripheral vascular disease, 1:164
Peristalsis, 1:233, 238
Perlman, Alberto, 2:944
Peroxide, 1:298
Persian Empire, 1:425
Personal training, 1:118, 119, 2:**676–680,** *677,* 694
PET (Positron emission tomography), 1:*16,* 53
Peyer's patches, 1:459
PGA (Professional Golfers Association), 1:378, 379
Phagocytes, 1:462
Phagocytosis, 1:456
Pharynx, 2:740
Pheidippides, 2:537
Phelps, Michael, 2:835, *835*
Phendimetrazine, 2:622
Phentermine, 2:622
Phenylketonuria (PKU), 2:559
Phenylpropanolamine, 2:622
Pheochromocytoma, 1:282
Philippine martial arts, 2:540
Philippoussis, Mark, 2:857
Phillips, Richard, 2:816
Philp, John, 1:88
Phosphagen system, 1:92, 520
Phospholipids, 1:325
Phosphoric acid, 2:641
Phosphorous acid, 1:113, 2:637
Phosphorus, 1:507, 508
Photoaging, 2:830
Photoconjunctivitis, 2:831
Photodynamic therapy, 2:832
Photokeratitis, 2:831
Photoreceptors, 2:606
Physical activity, 1:308–312
definition, 1:308
demographics, 1:308, 424, 2:566
adolescents, 1:306, 2:547
decline, 2:619–620
men, 1:530, 2:547
regional differences, 1:240
women, 1:530, 2:566, 923
female triad, 1:338
green, 2:550, 553

health benefits
disease prevention, 1:240–241, 242
energy expenditure, 1:274–278
gender differences, 1:530, 2:566, 791
immune role, 1:460
mental health, 2:550–554
obesity, 2:621, 624
respiratory rate, 2:742–743
history, 1:424–426, 2:877
leisure time, 1:308, 406, 529–530, 2:566, 873
pre-participation screening, 2:690–693
President's Council on Fitness, Sports, & Nutrition initiatives, 2:874–875
recommendations, 1:240, 310
starting slowly, 2:648–649
workplace, 2:926
Physical Activity (President's Challenge initiative), 2:874
"Physical Activity Guidelines for Americans" (DHHS), 1:240, 308, 309, 2:875, 924
Physical Activity Readiness Questionnaire (PAR-Q), 1:315, 2:691
Physical education, 1:308, 309, 2:677, 873
Physical examination
eating disorders, 1:251
hypertension, 1:438–439
kinesiology, 1:510
low back pain, 1:527
muscle pain, 2:577
obesity, 2:620
osteoporosis, 2:639
patellofemoral syndrome, 2:661
plantar fasciitis, 2:685
pre-exercise, 1:241, 2:690–693
Physical inactivity, 1:**308–312,** *309*
energy expenditure, 1:277
fatigue from, 1:330
muscle loss from, 2:582, 592
osteoporosis risk, 2:638
sitting, 2:777–778
See also Sedentary lifestyle
Physical readiness training (PRT), 2:913
Physical therapy
Alzheimer's disease, 1:20
circuit training, 1:180–181
core training, 1:197
functional training, 1:372–373
hand-eye coordination, 1:394
muscle pain, 2:577
nerve entrapment, 2:599
overuse injuries, 2:651
patellofemoral syndrome, 2:662
vs. Pilates, 2:682
plantar fasciitis, 2:685
shoulder instability, 2:775

S

T

U